Report of the Committee on Infectious Diseases

Twenty-second Edition

1991

Author: Committee on Infectious Diseases
American Academy of Pediatrics

Georges Peter, M.D., Editor
Martha L. Lepow, M.D., Associate Editor
George H. McCracken, Jr., M.D., Associate Editor
Carol F. Phillips, M.D., Associate Editor

American Academy of Pediatrics
141 Northwest Point Blvd.
P.O. Box 927
Elk Grove Village, Illinois 60009-0927

22nd Edition

1st Edition – 1938
2nd Edition – 1939
3rd Edition – 1940
4th Edition – 1942
5th Edition – 1943
6th Edition – 1944
7th Edition – 1945
8th Edition – 1947
9th Edition – 1951
10th Edition – 1952
11th Edition – 1955
12th Edition – 1957
13th Edition – 1961
14th Edition – 1964
15th Edition – 1966
16th Edition – 1970
16th Edition Revised – 1971
17th Edition – 1974
18th Edition – 1977
19th Edition – 1982
20th Edition – 1986
21st Edition – 1988

Library of Congress Catalog Card No. 52-19143

ISBN No. 0-910761-27-2

Quantity prices on request. Address all inquiries to:
American Academy of Pediatrics
141 Northwest Point Boulevard, P.O. Box 927
Elk Grove Village, Illinois 60009-0927

Committee on Infectious Diseases 1988-1991

Chairpersons

Stanley A. Plotkin, M.D. (1987-1990)
Georges Peter, M.D. (Interim Chairman, Nov. 1990 - June 1991)

Committee

Robert S. Daum, M.D.
G. Scott Giebink, M.D.
Caroline Breese Hall, M.D.
Neal A. Halsey, M.D.
Martha L. Lepow, M.D.
Edgar K. Marcuse, M.D.
Melvin I. Marks, M.D.
Georges Peter, M.D., Ex-Officio
George H. McCracken, Jr., M.D.
George A. Nankervis, M.D.
Carol F. Phillips, M.D.
Larry K. Pickering, M.D.
Gwendolyn B. Scott, M.D.
Russell W. Steele, M.D.
Harry T. Wright, Jr., M.D.

Liaison Representatives

Kenneth J. Bart, M.D., National Vaccine Program, Department of Health and Human Services
James G. Easton, M.D., AAP Section on Allergy and Immunology
Elaine C. Esber, M.D., Center for Biologics Evaluation & Research, Food and Drug Administration
Ronald Gold, M.D., Canadian Paediatric Society
M. Carolyn Hardegree, M.D., Office of Biologics Research, Food and Drug Administration
Alan R. Hinman, M.D., Center for Prevention Services, Centers for Disease Control
John R. La Montagne, Ph.D., National Institute of Allergy and Infectious Diseases
Noni E. MacDonald, M.D., Canadian Paediatric Society
Walter A. Orenstein, M.D., Center for Prevention Services, Centers for Disease Control

Consultants to the Editors

Philip A. Brunell, M.D.
James D. Cherry, M.D.
Leigh Grossman Donowitz, M.D.
Walter T. Hughes, M.D.
Sidney Hurwitz, M.D.
Michael Katz, M.D.

Committee on Infectious Diseases

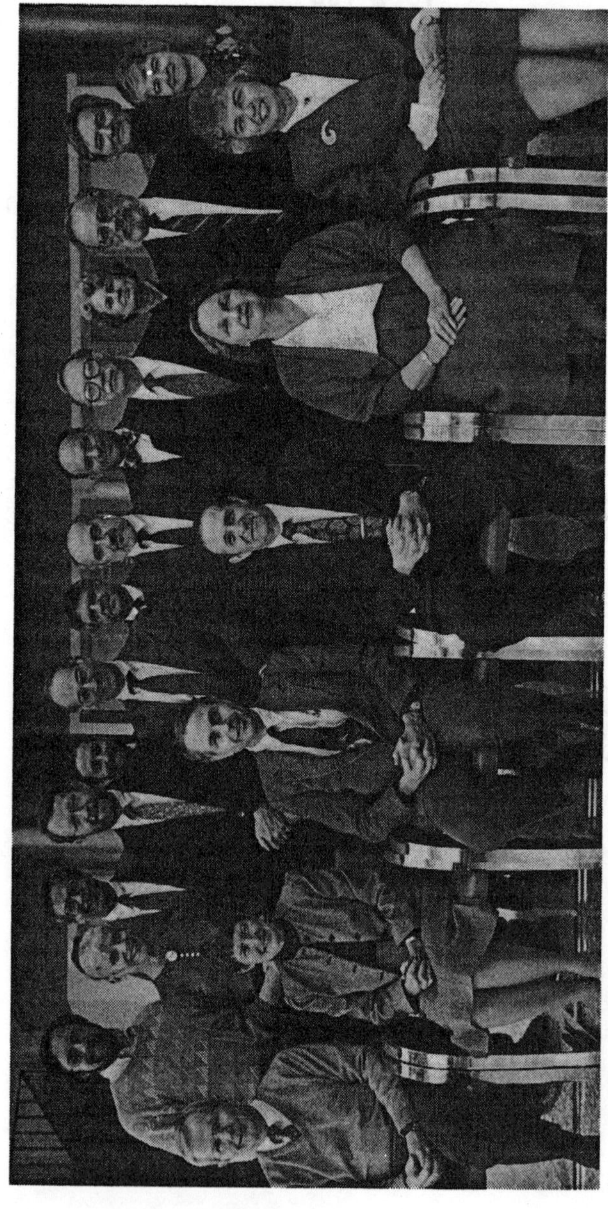

Front row: George H. McCracken, Jr.; Martha L. Lepow; Georges Peter; Stanley A. Plotkin; Carol F. Phillips; Gwendolyn B. Scott *Second row*: Robert S. Daum; Caroline Breese Hall; G. Scott Giebink; Alan R. Hinman; Walter A. Orenstein; John R. La Montagne; George A. Nankervis; Neal A. Halsey; Edgar K. Marcuse; Harry T. Wright, Jr.; M. Carolyn Hardegree; Ronald Gold; Russell W. Steele; Noni E. MacDonald

Preface

There is no reason to alter the sentiments expressed in the Preface to the last edition of the Red Book, reproduced below. Once again, Georges Peter has performed the Herculean task of bringing it all together without adding significantly to the bulk, despite the well-known exponential increase in our knowledge.

I will add only one thought, directed at those who insist on always having simple answers to complicated questions. It has been said that for every complicated problem there is a solution that is simple, straightforward, and wrong. In the *Red Book* you will find answers that are simple when possible, but sometimes complex. However, the Committee prefers complexity to oversimplification.

Stanley A. Plotkin, MD
Chairman, Committee on Infectious Diseases

Preface to the 1988 *Report of the Committee on Infectious Diseases (21st edition)*

The only book written by a committee that is beyond criticism is the King James Version of the Bible. Other books, such as the *Red Book,* though they may be treated as a bible, are written by fallible men and women, attempting to distill the knowledge of the moment. Since the *Red Book* deals with scientific information rather than with eternal verities and received wisdom, it is bound to change from edition to edition, and because of publishing delays it is likely to be partly out of date as soon as it reaches the readers.

The process of creating the *Red Book* is a long and arduous one, which only someone as organized and knowledgeable as Georges Peter could orchestrate. It starts with a review of the previous edition by the Committee members, with laborious correction to introduce new information and to excise yesterday's truths. The articles are reviewed by outside experts who add their points of view, sometimes conflicting. Letters from readers concerning the last edition or omissions in the book receive careful and grateful consideration. Meanwhile, the editors attempt to add new chapters or other helpful material. Particularly controversial areas are then hammered out at Committee meetings. Finally, the Executive Committee of the AAP reviews the final product.

The result is never entirely what one would want. The original author of a section often cannot recognize the final product. Inevitably, extreme points of view, though possibly correct, are overridden for the sake of consensus, and try as we might, many weasel words or phrases remain embedded, such as "may be desirable," or "some experts believe." But, dear reader, why should the *Red Book* not reflect the real world, where facts are often slippery and hard to come by?

Despite all this, the *Red Book* manages to come out as one of the best textbooks of infectious diseases available, and certainly the handiest. Moreover, the creation of this book, difficult and frustrating though it often is, remains a joy and pride for the Committee members, all of whom believe they are contributing to something useful and important. We hope you agree.

Stanley A. Plotkin, M.D.

Introduction

The Committee on Infectious Diseases is responsible for formulating and revising guidelines of the American Academy of Pediatrics for the control of infectious diseases in children. At intervals of approximately 2 to 3 years, the Committee reviews all of its current recommendations and prepares a composite summary, *Report of the Committee on Infectious Diseases (Red Book)*. These recommendations represent consensuses developed by the members of the Committee in conjunction with liaison representatives from the Centers for Disease Control, the Food and Drug Administration, the National Institutes of Health, and the Canadian Paediatric Society; our consultants; and the numerous collaborators whose expert advice the Committee solicits. This edition is based on information available as of October 1990.

Unanswered scientific questions, the complexity of medical practice, new information, and inevitable differences of opinion between experts result in inherent limitations in the *Red Book*, as so aptly expressed by Dr. Plotkin in the Preface to this and the 1988 editions. In the context of these limitations, the Committee endeavors to provide current, relevant, and defensible recommendations for the prevention and management of infectious diseases in children. We hope that most experts agree with these recommendations, but inevitably in some cases other committees and experts may differ in their interpretation of the data and resulting recommendations. In some instances, no single recommendation can be made, as several options for management are equally acceptable. Inevitably in clinical practice, questions arise which cannot be answered on the basis of currently available data, but in such cases the Committee attempts to provide guidelines and information that in conjunction with clinical judgment will facilitate well-reasoned decisions. We welcome questions, different perspectives, and alternative recommendations, as the resulting dialogue helps the Committee in its continuing review and periodic revisions of the *Red Book*. Through this process, the Committee seeks to provide a practical and authoritative (but not authoritarian) guide for physicians in their care of children.

To aid the physician in assimilating changes in the recommendations in the *Red Book*, a summary of major changes has been prepared. However, no list can be complete, and physicians are urged to consult individual chapters for other changes that might have escaped the Editor's scrutiny. New information inevitably outdates some recommendations in the *Red Book* and necessitates that physicians remain informed of new developments and resulting changes in recommendations. Between editions, new recommendations are published in *AAP News* and *Pediatrics*.

Physicians, in using antimicrobials, should review the package inserts prepared by the manufacturers, particularly concerning contraindications and adverse reactions. No attempt has been made in the *Red Book* to provide this information, since it is readily available in the *Physicians' Desk Reference*. As in previous editions, recommended dosage schedules for antimicrobials are given (see Part 5, Antimicrobials). Recommendations in the *Red Book* for drug dosages may differ from those of the manufacturer in the package inserts. Physicians should also be familiar with the information in the package inserts for vaccines and immune globulins as well as the recommendations of this and other committees (see Sources of Vaccine Information, page 8).

This book could not have been prepared without the invaluable and dedicated professional and administrative expertise of Dr. Edgar O. Ledbetter, Director of the Department of Maternal, Child, and Adolescent Health at the American Academy of Pediatrics. I am equally indebted to the Associate Editors, Drs. Martha L. Lepow, George H. McCracken, Jr., and Carol F. Phillips for their competence, tireless efforts, and support. In particular, I am most appreciative of the guidance, wisdom, and infinite knowledge of Dr. Stanley A. Plotkin who served as the Committee Chairman during the preparation of this edition and that of 1988. His leadership, counsel, and support have been invaluable and maintained the exemplary role in pediatric infectious diseases established by previous chairpersons of the Committee. He will be missed but we are fortunate to have worked with him during his four years as Chairman.

Special thanks are also given to Felice Bassuk for editorial assistance, and to Victoria K. Dahl of the American Academy of Pediatrics, and Charlotte A. Gauthier, secretary to the Editor, for their secretarial work, patience, and understanding. These individuals are only a few of the many unrecognized contributors whose long hours of work and sense of responsibility are an integral and essential aspect of the Committee's preparation of the *Red Book*.

Georges Peter, M.D.
Editor

COLLABORATORS

The Committee gratefully acknowledges the invaluable assistance provided by the following individuals who served as contributors, consultants, and/or reviewers in the preparation of this edition of the *Red Book.* Their expertise, critical review, and cooperation are essential to the Committee's continuing review and revisions of its recommendations for the management and control of infectious diseases in children.

David G. Addiss, M.D., M.P.H., Centers for Disease Control, Atlanta, GA
Libero Ajello, Ph.D., Centers for Disease Control, Atlanta, GA
Paul Albrecht, M.D., Food and Drug Administration, Bethesda, MD
Renata Albrecht, M.D., Food and Drug Administration, Bethesda, MD
Mercedes Albuerne, M.D., Food and Drug Administration, Bethesda, MD
E. Russell Alexander, M.D., Centers for Disease Control, Atlanta, GA
James R. Allen, M.D., M.P.H., Dept. of Health and Human Services, Washington, DC
Susan Alpert, M.D., Food and Drug Administration, Bethesda, MD
Miriam J. Alter, Ph.D., Centers for Disease Control, Atlanta, GA
Donna M. Ambrosino, M.D., Harvard University, Boston, MA
Larry J. Anderson, M.D., Centers for Disease Control, Atlanta, GA
William L. Atkinson, M.D., M.P.H., Centers for Disease Control, Atlanta, GA
Col. James W. Bass, M.C., Tripler Army Medical Center, Honolulu, HI
Barbara L. Bavins, A.R.N.P., Children's Hospital and Medical Center, Seattle, WA
Michael G. Beatrice, Food and Drug Administration, Bethesda, MD
Thomas A. Bell, M.D., M.P.H., University of Washington, Seattle, WA
Paul Beninger, M.D., Food and Drug Administration, Bethesda, MD
Renee S. Bergner, M.D., University of Vermont, Burlington, VT
Stuart M. Berman, M.D., Centers for Disease Control, Atlanta, GA
Roger H. Bernier, M.D., Centers for Disease Control, Atlanta, GA
Robin Biswas, M.D., Ph.D., Food and Drug Administration, Bethesda, MD
Paul A. Blake, M.D., M.P.H., Centers for Disease Control, Atlanta, GA
Alan Bloch, M.D., M.P.H., Centers for Disease Control, Atlanta, GA
Michael Blum, M.D., Food and Drug Administration, Bethesda, MD
John C. Bolton, M.D., Presbyterian Medical Center, San Francisco, CA
Debra Bowen, M.D., Food and Drug Administration, Bethesda, MD
Robert F. Breiman, M.D., Centers for Disease Control, Atlanta, GA

Edward W. Brink, M.D., Centers for Disease Control, Atlanta, GA
Claire V. Broome, M.D., Centers for Disease Control, Atlanta, GA
Ralph T. Bryan, M.D., Centers for Disease Control, Atlanta, GA
Sandra K. Burchett, M.D., University of Washington, Seattle, WA
D. Bruce Burlington, M.D., Food and Drug Administration, Bethesda, MD
Willard Cates, Jr., M.D., Centers for Disease Control, Atlanta, GA
Wiley Chambers, M.D., Food and Drug Administration, Bethesda, MD
Sotiros Chaparas, Ph.D., Food and Drug Administration, Bethesda, MD
Robert T. Chen, M.D., Centers for Disease Control, Atlanta, GA
Wallace A. Clyde, M.D., University of North Carolina, Chapel Hill, NC
Stephen L. Cochi, M.D., Centers for Disease Control, Atlanta, GA
Lawrence Corey, M.D., University of Washington, Seattle, WA
Robert B. Craven, M.D., Centers for Disease Control, Atlanta, GA
Adnan G. Dajani, M.D., Wayne State University, Detroit, MI
Jeffrey P. Davis, M.D., State of Wisconsin Dept. of Health and Social Services, Madison, WI
Rebecca Devine, Ph.D., Food and Drug Administration, Bethesda, MD
Raphael Dolin, M.D., University of Rochester, Rochester, NY
Vulus R. Dowell, Jr., Ph.D., Centers for Disease Control, Atlanta, GA
D. Peter Drotman, M.D., M.P.H., Centers for Disease Control, Atlanta, GA
Lee Dupuis, M.Sc.Phm., Hospital for Sick Children, Toronto, Ontario, Canada
Clare A. Dykewicz, M.D., Centers for Disease Control, Atlanta, GA
C. Carnot Evans, M.D., Food and Drug Administration, Bethesda, MD
Laura J. Fehrs, M.D., Centers for Disease Control, Atlanta, GA
Steve Feinstone, M.D., Food and Drug Administration, Bethesda, MD
Patricia E. Ferrieri, M.D., University of Minnesota, Minneapolis, MN
Patricia I. Fields, Ph.D., Centers for Disease Control, Atlanta, GA
Robert Finberg, M.D., Harvard University, Boston, MA
Joyce Fingeroth, M.D., Harvard University, Boston, MA
John S. Finlayson, Ph.D., Food and Drug Administration, Bethesda, MD
Daniel B. Fishbein, M.D., Centers for Disease Control, Atlanta, GA
Edward Fitzgerald, M.D., Food and Drug Administration, Bethesda, MD
Julie Francis, M.D., University of Washington, Seattle, WA
Carl Frasch, Ph.D., Food and Drug Administration, Bethesda, MD
Donna Freeman, M.D., Food and Drug Administration, Bethesda, MD
Julie S. Garner, R.N., M.N., Centers for Disease Control, Atlanta, GA
Lillian Gavrilovich, M.D., Food and Drug Administration, Bethesda, MD
Norma Gibbs, M.D., Centers for Disease Control, Atlanta, GA
Ann E. Giesel, M.D., University of Washington, Seattle, WA
Steve Gitterman, M.D., Food and Drug Administration, Bethesda, MD
Roger I. Glass, M.D., Ph.D., Centers for Disease Control, Atlanta, GA
Mary P. Glode, M.D., University of Colorado, Denver, CO
Mark Goldberger, M.D., Food and Drug Administration, Bethesda, MD
Robert C. Good, Ph.D., Centers for Disease Control, Atlanta, GA

Dwayne J. Gubler, Sc.D., Centers for Disease Control, Atlanta, GA
William Habig, Ph.D., Food and Drug Administration, Bethesda, MD
Stephen C. Hadler, M.D., Centers for Disease Control, Atlanta, GA
John R. Harkess, M.D., Oklahoma Department of Health, Oklahoma City, OK
Lee H. Harrison, M.D., Johns Hopkins University, Baltimore, MD
Kenneth L. Herrmann, M.D., Centers for Disease Control, Atlanta, GA
Barbara L. Herwaldt, M.D., M.P.H., Centers for Disease Control, Atlanta, GA
John C. Hierholzer, Ph.D., Centers for Disease Control, Atlanta, GA
Donald Hill, Food and Drug Administration, Bethesda, MD
Margaret K. Hostetter, M.D., University of Minnesota, Minneapolis, MN
Phyllis Huene, M.D., Food and Drug Administration, Bethesda, MD
David L. Ingram, M.D., Wake Medical Center, Raleigh, NC
Richard F. Jacobs, M.D., University of Arkansas for Medical Science, Little Rock, AR
William R. Jarvis, M.D., Centers for Disease Control, Atlanta GA
Joseph Johnson, Pharm D., Food and Drug Administration, Bethesda, MD
Robert E. Johnson, M.D., Centers for Disease Control, Atlanta, GA
Dennis D. Juranek, D.V.M., Centers for Disease Control, Atlanta, GA
Edward L. Kaplan, M.D., University of Minnesota, Minneapolis, MN
Arnold F. Kaufmann, D.V.M., Centers for Disease Control, Atlanta, GA
Kathi J. Kemper, M.D., University of Washington, Seattle, WA
Keith M. Krasinski, M.D., New York University, New York, NY
Edgar O. Ledbetter, M.D., American Academy of Pediatrics, Elk Grove Village, IL
Bradley Leissa, M.D., Food and Drug Administration, Bethesda, MD
Eileen Leonard, M.D., Food and Drug Administration, Bethesda, MD
Renita Leva-Johnson, Food and Drug Administration, Bethesda, MD
Ralph Lillie, Food and Drug Administration, Bethesda, MD
Sarah S. Long, M.D., Temple University, Philadelphia, PA
Murray M. Lumpkin, M.D., Food and Drug Administration, Bethesda, MD
Charles R. Manclark, Ph.D., Food and Drug Administration, Bethesda, MD
Andrew M. Margileth, M.D., Uniformed SVC-University of Health Sciences, Bethesda, MD
Harold S. Margolis, M.D., Centers for Disease Control, Atlanta, GA
Lauri Markowitz, M.D., Centers for Disease Control, Atlanta, GA
Timothy D. Mastro, M.D., Centers for Disease Control, Atlanta, GA
Cecilia Maxwell, M.D., Food and Drug Administration, Bethesda, MD
Joseph B. McCormick, M.D., Centers for Disease Control, Atlanta, GA
H. Cody Meissner, M.D., Tufts University, Boston, MA
Marion Melish, M.D., University of Hawaii, Honolulu, HI
Paul M. Mendelman, M.D., University of Washington, Seattle, WA
Marco K. Michelson, M.D., Centers for Disease Control, Atlanta, GA

Zachary Miller, M.D., Group Health Cooperative of Puget Sound, Seattle, WA
Nasim Moledina, M.D., Food and Drug Administration, Bethesda, MD
Marguerite A. Neill, M.D., Brown University, Providence, RI
John D. Nelson, M.D., University of Texas Southwestern, Dallas, TX
Jane W. Newburger, Harvard University, Boston, MA
Phillip Noguchi, M.D., Food and Drug Administration, Bethesda, MD
Charles M. Nolan, M.D., Seattle/King County Department of Public Health, Seattle, WA
Richard J. O'Brien, M.D., Centers for Disease Control, Atlanta, GA
G. Richard Olds, M.D., Brown University, Providence, RI
Michael T. Osterholm, M.D., Minnesota Department of Health, Minneapolis, MN
Margaret J. Oxtoby, M.D., Centers for Disease Control, Atlanta, GA
Mark A. Pallansch, Ph.D., Centers for Disease Control, Atlanta, GA
Robertson Parkman, M.D., USC School of Medicine, Los Angeles, CA
Peter A. Patriarca, M.D., Centers for Disease Control, Atlanta, GA
Philip A. Pizzo, M.D., National Institutes of Health, Bethesda, MD
Keith R. Powell, M.D., University of Rochester, Rochester, NY
Paul G. Quie, M.D., University of Minnesota, Minneapolis, MN
Seymour Rand, M.D., Food and Drug Administration, Bethesda, MD
James E. Rasmusen, M.D., University of Michigan Hospital, Ann Arbor, MI
Theresa G. Reed, M.D., Food and Drug Administration, Bethesda, MD
Philip J. Rettig, M.D., Oklahoma University, Oklahoma City, OK
Rosemary Roberts, M.D., Food and Drug Administration, Bethesda, MD
Martha F. Rogers, M.D., Centers for Disease Control, Atlanta, GA
Fred S. Rosen, M.D., Harvard University, Boston, MA
Anne H. Rowley, M.D., Northwestern University, Chicago, IL
Andrea J. Ruff, M.D., Johns Hopkins University, Baltimore, MD
Jean E. Sanders, M.D., University of Washington, Seattle, WA
John Sanders, M.D., Food and Drug Administration, Bethesda, MD
Peter M. Schantz, V.M.D., Ph.D., Centers for Disease Control, Atlanta, GA
David W. Scheifele, M.D., British Columbia's Children's Hospital, Vancouver, Canada
Mark R. Schleiss, M.D., Children's Hospital and Medical Center, Seattle, WA
Lawrence B. Schonberger, M.D., Centers for Disease Control, Atlanta, GA
Anne Schuchat, M.D., Centers for Disease Control, Atlanta, GA
Benjamin Schwartz, M.D., Centers for Disease Control, Atlanta, GA
Ira K. Schwartz, M.D., Centers for Disease Control, Atlanta, GA
Craig Shapiro, M.D., Centers for Disease Control, Atlanta, GA
David D. Sherry, M.D., University of Washington, Seattle, WA
John M. Short, M.D., University of Washington, Seattle, WA
Stanford T. Shulman, M.D., Northwestern University, Chicago, IL

Tor A. Shwayder, M.D., Henry Ford Hospital, Detroit, MI
George Siber, M.D., Harvard University, Boston, MA
Arnold L. Smith, M.D., University of Washington, Seattle, WA
Dixie E. Snider, Jr., M.D., M.P.H., Centers for Disease Control, Atlanta, GA
Anna Standard, M.D., Food and Drug Administration, Bethesda, MD
Jeffrey R. Starke, M.D., Baylor College of Medicine, Houston, TX
Barbara W. Stechenberg, M.D., Tufts University, Boston, MA
Allen C. Steere, M.D., Tufts University, Boston, MA
John A. Stewart, M.D., Centers for Disease Control, Atlanta, GA
Katherine M. Stone, M.D., Centers for Disease Control, Atlanta, GA
Peter Strebel, M.D., Centers for Disease Control, Atlanta, GA
Roland W. Sutter, M.D., M.P.H., T.M., Centers for Disease Control, Atlanta, GA
Ana Szarfman, M.D., Food and Drug Administration, Bethesda, MD
Phillip I. Tarr, M.D., University of Washington, Seattle, WA
Robert V. Tauxe, M.D., M.P.H., Centers for Disease Control, Atlanta, GA
Steven Teutsch, M.D., Centers for Disease Control, Atlanta, GA
Margaret A. Tipple, M.D., Centers for Disease Control, Atlanta, GA
Ella Toombs, M.D., Food and Drug Administration, Bethesda, MD
Thomas J. Torok, M.D., Centers for Disease Control, Atlanta, GA
Carol Trapnell, M.D., Food and Drug Administration, Bethesda, MD
Theodore F. Tsai, M.D., M.P.H., Centers for Disease Control, Atlanta, GA
Paul Turkeltaub, M.D., Food and Drug Administration, Bethesda, MA
Ellen R. Wald, M.D., University of Pittsburgh, Pittsburgh, PA
Mary Jane Walling, Food and Drug Administration, Bethesda, MD
Steven G. Wassilak, M.D., Centers for Disease Control, Atlanta, GA
Paul F. Wehrle, M.D., University of California at Irvine, Orange, CA
Jay D. Wenger, M.D., Centers for Disease Control, Atlanta, GA
Kim R. Wentz, M.D., M.P.H., University of Washington, Seattle, WA
William L. Weston, M.D., University of Colorado, Denver, CO
Richard J. Whitley, M.D., The University of Alabama at Birmingham, Birmingham, AL
William L. Whittington, Centers for Disease Control, Atlanta, GA
Catherine M. Wilfert, M.D., Duke University, Durham, NC
Walter W. Williams, M.D., M.P.H., Centers for Disease Control, Atlanta, GA
Christopher B. Wilson, M.D., University of Washington, Seattle, WA
Joseph Winfield, M.D., Food and Drug Administration, Bethesda, MD
Teresa Wu, M.D., Food and Drug Administration, Bethesda, MD
Paul N. Zenker, M.D., M.P.H., Centers for Disease Control, Atlanta, GA

CONTENTS

Part 2
Recommendations for Care of Children in Special Circumstances

Part 3
Summaries of Infectious Diseases

Part 4
Antimicrobial Prophylaxis

Part 5
Antimicrobials and Related Therapy

Appendices

Tables

SUMMARY OF MAJOR CHANGES IN THE 1991 *RED BOOK*

Major changes in recommendations and related information in the 1991 *Red Book* are summarized as follows:

1. *Immunization recommendations.* The schedules for routine immunization incorporate the changes in recommendations for *Haemophilus* b (as of October 1990)* and measles vaccines (see Tables 2 and 3, pp. 17 and 18). In view of the increased complexity of immunization schedules, particular attention should be given to the footnotes in the immunization schedules. The schedule recommended by the World Health Organization Expanded Programme on Immunization (EPI) is also included (see Table 4, p. 19).

2. *Reporting of adverse events.* The new procedure for reporting adverse events following administration of vaccines (VAERS) is described (see p. 27).

3. *Contraindications to vaccines.* The recommendation concerning a minor illness as a possible contraindication to DTP immunization has been modified (see p. 28). A procedure for desensitization and vaccination with egg-derived vaccines of children with severe egg hypersensitivity and positive skin tests is given (see p. 29).

4. *Indications and use of intravenous immunoglobulin (IGIV).* Relevant recommendations and conclusions of the 1990 National Institutes of Health Consensus Development Panel on use of IGIV are given (see p. 37).

5. *Immunizations in special circumstances.* Recommendations for immunizing preterm infants have been expanded (see p. 46), and guidelines for immunization of transplant recipients have been formulated (see p. 50).

6. *Foreign travel.* Comprehensive and updated recommendations for prevention of infection in travelers are given (see p. 64).

7. *Children in day care.* Recommendations and related information concerning the epidemiology and control of infectious diseases in day care have been extensively revised in accordance with the national standards developed by a joint project of the AAP and the

***After the *Red Book* went to press, a second *Haemophilus* b conjugate vaccine was also approved for use in infants. Since the recommendations for these vaccines differ, subsequent AAP guidelines should also be reviewed.**

American Public Health Association. Exclusion criteria for children in day care are listed (see p. 70). Physicians and providers of day care are urged to review this chapter in detail for further information and recommendations. These recommendations will also be published in the national standards for out-of-home child care.

8. *Infection control in hospitalized children.* Guidelines for sibling visitation (see p. 93) and health care personnel (see p. 92) have been added. Although these guidelines are not new, this information was not previously provided in the *Red Book.* Recommended infection control precautions for hospitalized patients are similar to those in the 1988 *Red Book.* Exceptions include those for patients with amebiasis, newborns whose mothers have active varicella, and persons with parvovirus B19 infection. Physicians should consult the chapters on specific infections *(Part 3 - Summaries of Infectious Diseases),* however, for updated information on patient-specific recommendations.

9. *Sexually transmitted diseases.* New recommendations and information include hepatitis B immunization of persons with sexually transmitted diseases or recent multiple partners (see p. 102); guidelines for use of condoms (see Table 17, p. 106); and advice for the management of sexually abused children (see p. 103).

10. *AIDS and HIV infection.* Current information on HIV infection in pediatrics is provided. Changes in recommendations include indications for zidovudine therapy (see p. 122) and for chemoprophylaxis of *Pneumocystis carinii* pneumonia (see p. 380) in the HIV-infected child. In addition, the Committee's recommendations on informed consent for HIV serologic testing have been revised (see p. 122).

11. *Arbovirus.* Recommendations concerning the Japanese B encephalitis vaccine for those traveling to areas with endemic disease are given (see p. 143).

12. *Cytomegalovirus (CMV).* Updated information on CMV risks and relevant recommendations for day care personnel, children in day care, and their mothers are provided (see p. 189; also see p. 76). In addition, possible indications for the use of CMV immune globulin (see p. 190) and ganciclovir (see p. 189) are given.

13. *Gonococcal infections.* Recommendations for treatment (see p. 213) have been extensively revised in view of the relatively high frequency of penicillin-resistant *Neisseria gonorrhoeae*, and are in accordance with those of the Centers for Disease Control.

For parenteral therapy, ceftriaxone (or cefotaxime in some cases) is the drug of choice unless the *N gonorrhoeae* isolate has been proven to be penicillin susceptible.

14. *Haemophilus influenzae infections.* Vaccine recommendations were revised in October 1990 and now include *Haemophilus* b immunization of infants beginning at 2 months of age. As of October 1990, only one vaccine has been approved for children younger than 15 months (see p. 225). Since one or more additional *Haemophilus* b vaccines is likely to be approved for infants, however, further revision of these recommendations is anticipated, possibly before or shortly after publication of the 1991 *Red Book.*

15. *Hepatitis B.* The recommended indications for hepatitis B vaccination have been increased, and include certain sexually active heterosexual persons; staff and children of nonresidential day care programs exposed to hepatitis B carriers; and children from populations in which hepatitis B virus infection is endemic (see p. 246). Doses and schedules for the several available vaccines are listed (see p. 244). Recommendations concerning children in day care (see p. 242; also see p. 76) and for persons with percutaneous or permucosal exposure to HBsAg-positive blood (see p. 252) are given.

16. *Herpes simplex virus (HSV).* Recommendations for the management of infants whose mother had HSV infection during pregnancy are similar to the recommendations in the 1988 *Red Book.* However, discussion of the management of infants exposed to HSV during delivery has been expanded (see p. 267) in order to provide further guidance in management of this difficult problem. Current recommendations for antiviral therapy of HSV infections in newborns and older children are given (see p. 263).

17. *Kawasaki disease.* Recommendations for treatment with intravenous immune globulin (IGIV), including use of a single-dose IGIV regimen, have been updated (see p. 284).

18. *Lyme disease.* This chapter has been expanded and includes recommendations for antimicrobial therapy (see p. 298) and control measures (see p. 300).

19. *Malaria.* The current recommendations for treatment (see p. 303) and chemoprophylaxis (see p. 305) of malaria, including revised recommendations for prophylaxis of chloroquine-resistant *Plasmodium falciparum* (with mefloquine), are provided.

20. *Measles.* In accordance with the 1989 AAP recommendations for measles reimmunization, usually with MMR, and those for control of measles in areas with outbreaks or recurrent measles transmission, the recommendations for measles immunization have been extensively revised (see p. 312).

21. *Meningococcal infections.* Changes include recommended duration of therapy for invasive infections (see p. 324) and a discussion of alternate chemoprophylaxis regimens to the currently recommended 2-day course of rifampin (see p. 325).

22. *Parvovirus B19.* Previously published information and recommendations for control of infection from the AAP's 1990 statement are included in this chapter (see p. 350).

23. *Pertussis.* Contraindications to pertussis vaccine are no longer considered absolute (see p. 366). A review and assessment of the adverse events related to pertussis vaccine, including the lack of proven relationship between pertussis immunization and brain damage, is given (see p. 363).

24. *Salmonellosis.* Recommendations for the use of the new oral typhoid vaccine are provided (see p. 421).

25. *Shigellosis.* Control measures in day care have been revised (see p. 429).

26. *Syphilis.* The recommendations for treatment of infants with either proven or possible congenital syphilis have been revised and now include indications in some cases for the possible use of benzathine penicillin G (see p. 457).

27. *Tuberculosis.* Recommendations for prophylaxis (see p. 493) and therapy (see p. 496) have been revised and include new recommendations for initial triple drug therapy, duration of therapy, follow-up of isoniazid recipients (see p. 499), and management of the newborn infant whose mother (or other household contact) has tuberculosis (see p. 504). In view of these extensive changes, physicians treating children with tuberculosis should review the recommendations in this chapter in detail.

28. *Prevention of bacterial endocarditis.* The 1990 recommendations of the American Heart Association are reproduced in the 1991 *Red Book* (see p. 536).

29. *Ribavirin therapy.* The earlier Committee statement (see 1988 *Red Book*) has been revised to include a discussion of the risks and adverse events possibly related to ribavirin therapy (see p. 581).

Recommended indications for ribavirin therapy, however, remain unchanged (see p. 581).

30. *New chapters or sections.* The following have been added:
    - Dexamethasone Therapy for Infants and Children With Bacterial Meningitis (as previously published by the AAP, see p. 566)
    - Control Measures for Tick-Borne Infections (see p. 112)
    - Medical Evaluation of Internationally Adopted Children (see p. 109)
    - Sexual Abuse (see p. 103)
    - *Blastocystis hominis* (see p. 152)
    - Ehrlichiosis (see p. 195)
    - *Helicobacter pylori* (see p. 230)
    - Hepatitis C (see p. 256)
    - *Isosporiasis belli* (see p. 281)
    - Pelvic Inflammatory Disease (see p. 354)
    - Directory of Telephone Numbers (see p. 611)

31. *Part 3 - Summary of Infectious Diseases.* Several chapters on specific diseases have been expanded, including Staphylococcal Infections (to include management of coagulase-negative staphylococcal infections; see p. 429) and Disease Due to Nontuberculous Mycobacteria (see p. 508).

32. *Therapeutic recommendations.* Numerous changes have been made in the recommendations for specific diseases (in *Part 3 - Summaries of Infectious Diseases*); examples include a new topical drug of choice for scabies (5% permethrin); possible indications for fluconazole in the treatment of some fungal infections (*Candida* and *Cryptococcus neoformans*); possible indications for acyclovir in otherwise healthy children with varicella; and indications for use of tetracyclines in children younger than 9 years (for example, see Rocky Mountain Spotted Fever, p. 407). Physicians are urged to review specific chapters for current recommendations for therapy of specific diseases.

33. *Antimicrobial tables.* The tables of drug dosages and recommendations have been updated, including those for parasitic infections. A new table on topical drugs for superficial fungal infections is provided (see p. 576).

Every effort in this review has been made to identify major changes in order to aid physicians to rapidly assimilate new recommendations in the care of their patients. However, no list can be complete and physicians are urged to review the *Red Book* in detail.

PART 1

ACTIVE AND PASSIVE IMMUNIZATION

Prologue

The ultimate goal of immunization is eradication of disease; the immediate goal is prevention of disease in individuals or groups. To accomplish these goals, physicians must maintain immunization practices, including both active and passive immunoprophylaxis, as a high priority in the care of children, adolescents, and adults. The eradication of smallpox serves as a model for each disease for which immunization procedures are designed and implemented. Eradication of smallpox was achieved by combining an effective immunization program with intense surveillance and adequate public health control measures on a worldwide basis. No natural instance of smallpox has occurred since October 1977.

Infectious diseases can be prevented by immunoprophylaxis. With active immunization, a person is stimulated to develop immunologic defenses against future natural exposure. With passive immunization, a person already exposed, or about to be exposed, to certain infectious agents is given preformed human or animal antibody.

In the United States, large-scale public health efforts with available vaccines have sharply curtailed, or practically eliminated, diphtheria, measles, mumps, pertussis, poliomyelitis, rubella, and tetanus. Yet because these diseases persist in the United States as well as in other countries, immunizations need to be continued. Research on new vaccines is being actively conducted with the aid of molecular biologic techniques. Some of these experimental vaccines will eventually become used routinely. Physicians must continue to update their knowledge about specific vaccines and their use because information about the safety and efficacy of vaccines and recommendations relative to their administration continue to develop after a vaccine is licensed.

Each edition of the *Report of the Committee on Infectious Diseases (Red Book)* presents recommendations for immunization of children based on current knowledge, experience, and premises tenable at the time of publication. The recommendations represent a consensus with which reasonable physicians may at times disagree. No claim is made for infallibility, and the Committee recognizes that individual circumstances may warrant decisions differing from the recommendations given here.

Sources of Vaccine Information

In addition to the *Red Book,* which is published at approximately 2- to 3-year intervals, physicians can use the scientific literature and other sources for data or answers to specific questions encountered in practice. Among these sources are the following:

- *Pediatrics.* Statements of the Committee on Infectious Diseases and updated recommendations are published in *Pediatrics.* In addition, articles provide new information on infectious diseases and immunizations.
- *AAP News.* Committee statements are often initially published in the Academy's monthly newspaper in order to inform its membership promptly of new recommendations.
- *Morbidity and Mortality Weekly Report (MMWR). MMWR* is published weekly by the Centers for Disease Control (CDC) and contains current vaccine recommendations, reports of specific disease activity, and changes in policy statements. Recommendations of the Immunization Practices Advisory Committee (ACIP) of the United States Public Health Service are published periodically. Subscriptions can be purchased from the following: Superintendent of Documents, U.S. Government Printing Office, Washington, D.C. 20402; Ochsner Clinic, 1514 Jefferson Highway, New Orleans, LA 70121; and
- *New England Journal of Medicine,* MMS Publications, CSPO, Box 9120, Waltham, MA 02254. *MMWR* is now available by computer on DIALCOM.
- *Official package circulars.* Manufacturers provide product-specific information with each package of vaccine; the same information is also usually given in the *Physicians' Desk Reference (PDR).* The package circular must be in full compliance with FDA regulations pertaining to labeling for prescription drugs, including indications and usage, dosages, routes of administration, description, clinical pharmacology, contraindications, and adverse reactions. The circulars list preservatives, stabilizers, antibiotics, adjuvants, and suspending fluids, which may be the cause of allergy or inflammation. Health care providers should be familiar with the circular for each specific product they administer.
- *Health Information for International Travel.* This useful monograph is published annually by the CDC as a guide to requirements of the various countries for specific immunizations. It also provides information concerning vaccines that are not required but are recommended for travel for specific areas, and other helpful information for travelers. It can be purchased from the Superintendent of Documents, U.S. Government Printing Office, Washington, D.C. 20402 (202/738-3238).

- *Control of Communicable Diseases in Man.* The American Public Health Association publishes this manual at approximately 5-year intervals. The most recent edition was published in 1990. It contains valuable information about most infectious diseases, their worldwide occurrence, diagnostic and therapeutic information, immunizations, and recommendations on isolation and other control measures for specific diseases.
- *Guide for Adult Immunization.* This publication by the American College of Physicians (4200 Pine Street, Philadelphia, PA 19104) provides useful information about infectious diseases and vaccine recommendations for patients ranging in age from the late teens to the elderly years. The latest edition was issued in 1990.

In addition, physicians can consult members of the Committee by phone or letter. Specific questions may be addressed directly to the Academy at 141 Northwest Point Boulevard, Elk Grove Village, IL 60009 (708/228-5005). Consultation on immunizations can also be obtained from the Division of Immunization, Centers for Disease Control (404/639-1880). Other resources include infectious disease experts in medical schools, university-affiliated hospitals, and public health departments. Information can be obtained from local and state public health offices about current epidemiology of diseases, immunization recommendations, legal requirements, public health policies, foreign travel, and nursery school, day care, and school health concerns.

Informed Consent

Parents and patients should be informed about the benefits and risks of preventive and therapeutic procedures, including immunizations.

The patient, parent, and/or legal guardian should be educated about the major benefits to be derived from vaccines in preventing disease in individuals and in the community, and about the risks of those vaccines. Benefit and risk statements should be presented in lay terminology. No formal and legally acceptable vaccine information statement has been universally adopted for the private medical sector, but the Centers for Disease Control has developed "Important Information" statements about vaccines, which are revised periodically and made available from state health departments. These statements have been used in public health clinics throughout the United States. Although these statements may include space for the parents' or patients' signatures to indicate that they have read and understood the material, the Committee considers that parents' signatures on a form are not as important as making sure that the information is understood and consent is given. The fact that consent has been given should be recorded on the patient's chart.

The National Childhood Vaccine In jury Act of 1986, which became effective in 1988, includes requirements for detailed notification of patients and parents about vaccine benefits and risks in both the private and public sectors. This legislation requires development and distribution of standardized benefit and risk statements when administering vaccines for which vaccine injury compensation is available (see Federal Vaccine Injury Compensation Table, page 612). These statements are required for fulfillment of the duty to warn. They are in preparation,* and physicians will be notified by the Federal government when their use is mandatory.

Active Immunization

Active immunization involves administration of all or part of a microorganism or a modified product of that microorganism (e.g., a toxoid) to evoke an immunologic response mimicking that of the natural infection but which presents little or no risk to the recipient. The response can result in antitoxic, anti-invasive, or neutralizing activity in the patient. Some immunizing agents provide complete protection for life, some provide partial protection, and some must be readministered at intervals. The effectiveness of a vaccine is assessed by the evidence of protection against the natural disease. Induction of antibodies is frequently an indirect measure of protection, but in some instances the immunologic reaction responsible for protection is poorly understood, and serum antibody concentrations are not always predictive of protection.

Vaccines incorporating an intact infectious agent may be either live and attenuated or killed (inactivated or subunit). Currently licensed vaccines are listed in Table 1. Many viral vaccines contain live attenuated virus. Although active infection (with replication) ensues after administration of these vaccines, little or no adverse host reaction usually occurs. The vaccines for some viruses and most bacteria are inactivated (killed) or subunit preparations. Inactive agents are incapable of replicating in the host; therefore, these vaccines must contain a sufficient antigenic mass to stimulate the desired response. Maintenance of long-lasting immunity with nonliving vaccines often requires periodic administration of booster doses. Inactivated vaccines may not elicit the range of immunologic response provided by live attenuated agents. For example, an injected, inactivated viral vaccine may evoke sufficient serum antibody or cell-mediated immunity but fail to evoke local antibody in the form of secretory immunoglobulin A (IgA). Thus, mucosal protection is not afforded and local infection or colonization with the agent can occur, although systemic infection is prevented or ameliorated

*As of October 1990.

Table 1. Vaccines Licensed in the United States and Their Routes of Administration

Vaccine*	Type	Route†
BCG	Live bacteria	ID (preferred) or SC
Cholera	Inactivated bacteria	SC, IM, or ID‡
DTP	Toxoids and inactivated bacteria	IM
Hepatitis B	Inactivated viral antigen: yeast recombinant-derived, plasma-derived	IM; if risk of hemorrhage, SC
Haemophilus b		
Polysaccharide (HBPV)	Polysaccharide	SC or IM
Conjugate (HbCV)	Polysaccharide-protein conjugate	IM
Influenza	Inactivated virus	IM
	Subvirion (split)	IM
Measles	Live virus	SC
Meningococcal	Polysaccharide	SC or IM
MMR	Live viruses	SC
MR	Live viruses	SC
Mumps	Live virus	SC
Plague	Inactivated bacteria	IM
Pneumococcal	Polysaccharide	IM or SC
Poliovirus (trivalent)		
OPV	Live virus	Oral
IPV	Inactivated virus	SC
Rabies	Inactivated virus	IM or ID‡,§
Rubella	Live virus	SC
Tetanus and Td, DT (adsorbed)	Toxoids	IM
Tetanus (fluid)	Toxoid	SC
Typhoid		
Parenteral	Inactivated bacteria	SC (boosters may be ID‡)
Oral	Live attenuated bacteria	Oral
Yellow fever	Live attenuated virus	SC

*BCG = Bacillus of Calmette and Guérin (tuberculosis); DTP = diphtheria and tetanus toxoids and pertussis vaccine adsorbed; HBPV = Haemophilus b polysaccharide vaccine; HbCV = Haemophilus b conjugate vaccine; MMR = measles, mumps, and rubella vaccines; MR = measles and rubella vaccines; OPV = oral poliovirus vaccine; IPV = inactivated poliovirus vaccine; Td = tetanus and diphtheria toxoid (for children ≥ 7 years old and adults); DT = diphtheria and tetanus toxoids (for children < 7 years old).

†ID = intradermal; SC = subcutaneous; IM = intramuscular.

‡The intradermal dose is different from the subcutaneous and intramuscular doses.

§Used for prophylaxis only.

by the presence of serum and cellular factors. However, killed vaccines cannot adversely affect the immunosuppressed host or be excreted by the vaccinee.

The mechanics of immunization are critical to the success of immunization procedures. Recommendations for dose, route, technique of administration, and schedules must be followed for predictable, effective immunization.

The physician must be certain that vaccines are stored at the appropriate temperature and handled correctly after receipt in the office. When multidose vials are used, scrupulous care must be taken to prevent bacterial contamination.

Immunizing Antigens

Physicians should become familiar with the major constituents of the products they use. These are listed in the package inserts. If a vaccine is produced by different manufacturers, some differences may exist among the various products in the active and inert ingredients. The major constituents of vaccines include the following:

1. *Active Immunizing Antigen.* In some vaccines this antigen is a highly defined, single constituent (e.g., pneumococcal polysaccharide, or tetanus or diphtheria toxoid); in others, it is complex or poorly defined (e.g., live viruses or killed pertussis bacteria).
2. *Suspending Fluid.* The suspending fluid frequently is as simple as sterile water or saline, but it may be a complex tissue-culture fluid. This fluid may contain proteins or other constituents derived from the medium and biologic system in which the vaccine is produced (e.g., egg antigens or tissue-culture-derived antigens).
3. *Preservatives, Stabilizers, and Antibiotics.* Trace amounts of chemicals (e.g., mercurials, glycine, and antibiotics) are frequently necessary to prevent bacterial growth or to stabilize the antigen. Allergic reactions may occur if the recipient is sensitive to one or more of these additives. Whenever feasible, these reactions should be anticipated by identifying known host hypersensitivity to specific vaccine components.
4. *Adjuvants.* An aluminum compound is frequently used to increase antigenicity and to prolong the stimulatory effect, particularly for vaccines containing inactivated microorganisms or their products (e.g., diphtheria and tetanus toxoids).

Because of possible hypersensitivity to vaccine components, vaccines should be administered only when ready access is available to emergency equipment and drugs such as epinephrine (see Hypersensitivity Reactions to Vaccine Constituents, page 29).

Site and Route of Immunization*

Injectable vaccines should be administered in a site as free as possible from the risk of local neural, vascular, or tissue injury. Data in the medical literature do not warrant recommendation of a single preferred site for all injections, and many manufacturers' product recommendations allow some flexibility in site of injection. Preferred sites include the anterolateral aspect of the upper thigh and the deltoid area of the upper arm for vaccines administered either subcutaneously or intramuscularly.

Recommended routes of administration are included in the package inserts of vaccines and are listed in Table 1. The recommended route is based on the results of prior clinical use that demonstrated maximum safety and efficacy. To minimize untoward local or systemic effects and ensure optimal efficacy of the immunizing procedure, vaccines should be given according to the recommended route.

For intramuscular (IM) injections, the choice of site is based on the volume of the injected material and the size of the muscle. In children younger than 1 year (i.e., infants), the anterolateral aspect of the thigh provides the largest muscle and is the preferred site. In older children, the deltoid muscle is usually large enough for IM injection. Some physicians prefer to use the anterolateral thigh muscles for toddlers. Parents and children, however, often prefer the deltoid muscle for children 18 months and older because of less discomfort in the affected extremity and in ambulating.

Ordinarily, the upper, outer aspect of the buttocks should not be used for immunizations in infants because the gluteal region consists mostly of fat until the child has been walking for some time and because of the possibility of damaging the sciatic nerve. When the upper, outer quadrant of the buttocks is used, considerable care must be exercised to avoid injury to the nerve. The site selected should be well into the upper, outer mass of the gluteus maximus and distal from the central region of the buttocks, and the needle should be directed anteriorly—*not* perpendicular to the skin plane. The ventrogluteal site may be less hazardous for IM injection because it is free of major nerves and vessels. This site is the center of a triangle whose boundaries are the anterior superior iliac spine, the tubercle of the iliac crest, and the upper border of the greater trochanter. However, clinical information on the use of this area is limited. Because of diminished immunogenicity, hepatitis B vaccine should not be given in the buttock at any age.

Vaccines containing adjuvants (e.g., aluminum-adsorbed DTP, DT, and Td) must be injected deep in the muscle mass; they should not be administered subcutaneously or intracutaneously because they can cause

---

*An informative review on intramuscular injections is the following: Bergeson PS, Singer SA, Kaplan AM. Intramuscular injections in children. *Pediatrics.* 1982;70:944-948.

local irritation, inflammation, granuloma formation, and necrosis. The needles used for IM injections should be long enough to reach the substance of the muscle. Ordinarily a needle 7/8 inches or longer is required to assure penetration of the muscle in a normal four-month-old infant. A 22- or 23-gauge needle is appropriate for most IM vaccines.

Immunizing agents requiring IM injection include DTP (diphtheria and tetanus toxoids and pertussis vaccine adsorbed); DT and Td (diphtheria and tetanus toxoids products), hepatitis B (in most cases), and rabies (human diploid cell) vaccine for postexposure prophylaxis. Immune Globulin (IG), Rabies Immune Globulin (Human), and other similar products for passive immunoprophylaxis are also injected intramuscularly. Serious complications of IM injections are rare. Reported events include muscle contracture, nerve injury, bacterial abscesses (staphylococcal, streptococcal, and clostridial), sterile abscesses, skin pigmentation, hemorrhage, cellulitis, tissue necrosis, gangrene, local atrophy, periostitis, cyst or scar formation, broken needles, and inadvertent injection into a joint space. Sterile or bacterial abscesses at the injection site are estimated to occur approximately once per 100,000 to 166,000 doses of DTP. The incidence of other complications is unknown.

Subcutaneous (SC) injections can be given in the anterolateral aspect of the thigh or the upper arm by inserting the needle in a pinched-up fold of skin and subcutaneous tissue. Certain vaccines (e.g., pneumococcal polyvalent polysaccharide, meningococcal quadrivalent polysaccharide, and hepatitis B) recommended for IM injection may be given subcutaneously to persons at risk of hemorrhage after IM injection (e.g., persons with hemophilia). For these vaccines, immune responses and clinical reactions have generally been reported to be similar after either IM or SC injection. However, because of suboptimal responses, persons who were given hepatitis B vaccine in the buttock should be tested for immunity. Immune responses after SC administration of recombinant rabies vaccine have been reduced compared to the IM route.

Intradermal (ID) injections generally are given on the volar surface of the forearm. Because of the decreased antigenic mass administered with ID injections, attention to technique is essential to ensure that the material is not injected subcutaneously.

For SC or ID injections, a 25-gauge needle 5/8 to 3/4 inches long is recommended.

Syringes and needles for vaccine injections must be sterile and preferably disposable to minimize the chances of contamination. Changing needles between drawing the vaccine into the syringe and injecting it into the child is not necessary. After use, needles and syringes should not be recapped and should be discarded in specially labeled impermeable containers to prevent accidental inoculation or theft.

The patient should be adequately restrained before any injection. If multiple vaccines are used, each injection should be given at a different site and not mixed in the syringe. A different needle and syringe should be used for each injection. Before the injection is given, the needle should be inserted in the site and the syringe plunger pulled back to see if blood appears; if so, the needle should be withdrawn and a new site selected. The procedure is repeated until no blood appears.

Scheduling Immunizations

A vaccine is intended to be administered to an individual who is capable of an appropriate immunologic response and who will likely benefit from the protection afforded. However, optimal immunologic response for the individual must be balanced against the need to achieve effective protection against disease. For example, DTP and poliovirus vaccines in early infancy are less immunogenic than later in infancy, but the benefit of early protection in infants at high risk from these diseases dictates that immunization should proceed despite a lessened immunologic response. In some situations in the developing world, poliovirus vaccine is given at birth.

With parenterally administered live virus vaccines, the inhibitory effect of residual specific maternal antibody determines the optimal age of administration. For example, live measles virus vaccine in use in the United States has suboptimal rates of successful immunization during the first year of life because of maternal antibody.

An additional factor in selection of an immunization schedule is the need to achieve a uniform and regular response. With some products, a response is achieved after one dose; for others, it is achieved only after multiple doses. Live rubella vaccine is an example of a vaccine that evokes a regular, predictable response at highly acceptable rates after a single dose. In contrast, some individuals respond to only one or two types of poliovirus(es) after a single dose of OPV. Hence, multiple doses are given to produce antibody against all three types, thereby ensuring complete protection for the individual and maximum response rates for the population. A single dose of some vaccines (mostly inactivated or killed antigens) confers less than optimal response in the individual. As a result, several doses are used to complete the primary immunization, and periodic booster doses (e.g., with tetanus and diphtheria toxoids) are administered to maintain immunologic protection.

Most of the widely used vaccines can be safely and effectively administered simultaneously. This information is particularly important in scheduling immunization for children with lapsed or missed immunizations and for persons preparing for foreign travel (see Simultaneous Administration of Multiple Vaccines, page 16). Theoretical concerns exist about impaired immune responses to two live virus vaccines given within 30 days of each other, but no evidence substantiates this possibility. Hence, when feasible, live virus vaccines not administered on the same day should be given at least 30 days apart. Recent receipt of OPV is **not** a contraindication to MMR, which should be given at the first available opportunity (according to age-specific recommendations).

Tables 2 and 3 give the recommended immunization schedules in the United States for infants and children, including those who were not appropriately immunized in the first year of life. Special attention should be given to the "Comments" and boldfaced footnotes in these tables as they indicate the flexibility the physician has in scheduling immunizations, especially during the second year of life. MMR should ordinarily be given at 15 months of age. However, DTP can be given between 12 and 18 months of age and OPV can be administered between 12 and 24 months; DTP and OPV can be given concurrently with either MMR or *Haemophilus* b conjugate vaccine. Although administration of DTP and OPV at 18 months of age is still appropriate, administration of these vaccines at 15 months is equally acceptable and is often the practice in public health clinics in order to enhance immunization rates at the recommended ages. Physicians and families who wish to avoid multiple simultaneous injections can use a multiple visit schedule.

The immunization schedule used in the United States may not be appropriate for developing countries because of different disease risks, age-specific immune responses, and vaccine availability. The schedule recommended by the Expanded Programme on Immunization (EPI) of the World Health Organization should be consulted (see Table 4). Modifications may be made by the ministries of health in individual countries, based on local considerations.

Simultaneous Administration of Multiple Vaccines

No contraindications to the simultaneous administration of multiple vaccines routinely recommended for infants and children are known, and most vaccines can be safely and effectively administered simultaneously. Immune responses to one vaccine do not interfere with those to other vaccines; exceptions include oral poliovirus strains (see Scheduling Immunizations, page 15) and concurrent administration of cholera and yellow fever vaccines. Antibody responses to both cholera and yellow fever vaccines are decreased if given simultaneously or within a short time of each other. If possible, these vaccines should be separated by at least three weeks. Simultaneous administration of MMR, DTP, and OPV has resulted in seroconversion rates and rates of side effects similar to those observed when the vaccines are administered at separate times. Simultaneous administration of *Haemophilus* vaccines and other common vaccines would not be expected to affect the efficacy or safety of

Table 2. Recommended Schedule for Immunization of Healthy Infants and Children*

Recommended Age†	Immunizations‡	Comments
2 mo	DTP, HbCV,§ OPV	DTP and OPV can be initiated as early as 4 wk after birth in areas of high endemicity or during epidemics
4 mo	DTP, HbCV,§ OPV	2-mo interval (minimum of 6 wk) desired for OPV to avoid interference from previous dose
6 mo	DTP, HbCV§	Third dose of OPV is not indicated in the U.S. but is desirable in other geographic areas where polio is endemic
15 mo	MMR,‖ HbCV¶	Tuberculin testing may be done at the same visit
15-18 mo	DTP,**,†† OPV#	(See footnotes)
4-6 y	DTP,§§ OPV	At or before school entry
11-12 y	MMR	At entry to middle school or junior high school unless second dose previously given
14-16 y	Td	Repeat every 10 y throughout life

***For all products used, consult manufacturer's package insert for instructions for storage, handling, dosage, and administration. Biologics prepared by different manufacturers may vary, and package inserts of the same manufacturer may change from time to time. Therefore, the physician should be aware of the contents of the current package insert.**

†These recommended ages should not be construed as absolute. For example, 2 months can be 6 to 10 weeks. However, MMR usually should not be given to children younger than 12 months. (If measles vaccination is indicated, monovalent measles vaccine is recommended, and MMR should be given subsequently, at 15 months.)

‡DTP = diphtheria and tetanus toxoids with pertussis vaccine; HbCV = *Haemophilus* b conjugate vaccine; OPV = oral poliovirus vaccine containing attenuated poliovirus types 1, 2, and 3; MMR = live measles, mumps, and rubella viruses in a combined vaccine; Td = adult tetanus toxoid (full dose) and diphtheria toxoid (reduced dose) for adult use.

§As of October 1990, only one HbCV (HbOC - see page 226) is approved for use in children younger than 15 months (see *Haemophilus influenzae* Infections, page 227).

‖May be given at 12 months of age in areas with recurrent measles transmission.

¶Any licensed *Haemophilus* b conjugate vaccine may be given.

****Should be given 6 to 12 months after the third dose.**

††May be given simultaneously with MMR at 15 months.

#May be given simultaneously with MMR and HbCV at 15 months or at any time between 12 and 24 months; priority should be given to administering MMR at the recommended age.

§§ Can be given up to the seventh birthday.

Table 3. Recommended Immunization Schedules for Children Not Immunized in First Year of Life

Recommended Time/Age	Immunizations*	Comments
	Younger Than 7 Years	
First visit	DTP, OPV, MMR	MMR if child ≥ 15 mo old; tuberculin testing may be done at same visit
	HbCV†	For children aged 15-59 mo, can be given simultaneously with DTP and other vaccines (at separate sites)‡
Interval after first visit		
2 mo	DTP, OPV (HbCV)	Second dose of HbCV is indicated only in children whose first dose was received when younger than 15 mo
4 mo	DTP	Third dose of OPV is not indicated in the U.S. but is desirable in other geographic areas where polio is endemic
10-16 mo	DTP, OPV	OPV is not given if third dose was given earlier
4-6 y (at or before school entry)	DTP, OPV	DTP is not necessary if the fourth dose was given after the fourth birthday; OPV is not necessary if third dose was given after the fourth birthday
11-12 y	MMR	At entry to middle school or junior high
10 y later	Td	Repeat every 10 y throughout life
	7 Years and Older§,‖	
First visit	Td, OPV, MMR	
Interval after first visit		
2 mo	Td, OPV	
8-14 mo	Td, OPV	
11-12 y	MMR	At entry to middle school or junior high
10 y later	Td	Repeat every 10 y throughout life

*Abbreviations are explained in the footnote‡ to Table 2.

†If child is younger than 15 mo, only one HbCV (HbOC), as of October 1990, is approved for use (see *Haemophilus influenzae* Infections, page 227).

‡The initial three doses of DTP can be given at 1- to 2-month intervals; hence, for the child in whom immunization is initiated at age 15 months or older, one visit could be eliminated by giving DTP, OPV, and MMR at the first visit; DTP and HbCV at the second visit (1 month later); and DTP and OPV at the third visit (2 months after the first visit). Subsequent doses of DTP and OPV 10 to 16 months after the first visit are still indicated. HbCV, MMR, DTP, and OPV can be given simultaneously at separate sites if failure of the patient to return for future immunizations is a concern.

§If person is ≥ 18 years old, routine poliovirus vaccination is not indicated in the U.S.

‖Minimal interval between doses of MMR is 1 month.

Table 4. Immunization Schedule Recommended by the Expanded Programme on Immunization (EPI) of the World Health Organization

Age*	Immunization†
Birth	BCG and OPV
6 wk	DTP and OPV
10 wk	DTP and OPV
14 wk	DTP and OPV
9 mo‡	Measles
Women of childbearing age	Tetanus toxoid

*In many countries, OPV is administered to all children on the same day through national immunization campaigns. This strategy has been very effective in eliminating transmission of wild-type poliomyelitis virus.

†BCG = Bacillus of Calmette and Guérin; OPV = oral poliovirus vaccine; DTP = diphtheria and tetanus toxoids with pertussis vaccine.

‡High-titer Edmonston-Zagreb strain measles vaccine is recommended at 6 months of age in countries where measles is an important cause of death in infants younger than 9 months.

any individual vaccine. Therefore, if return of a vaccine recipient for further immunization is doubtful, simultaneous administration of all vaccines (including DTP, OPV, MMR, and *Haemophilus* vaccines) appropriate to the age and previous vaccination status of the recipient is recommended.

For persons preparing for foreign travel, multiple vaccines can generally be given concurrently. An exception is the simultaneous administration of yellow fever and cholera vaccines, but if both vaccines are necessary and time constraints exist, both vaccines can be given with the understanding that antibody responses may not be optimal.

When vaccines commonly associated with local or systemic reactions (e.g., cholera and parenteral typhoid vaccines or influenza and DTP in young children) are given simultaneously, the reactions can be accentuated. Thus, in most circumstances, these vaccines should be given on separate occasions.

Lapsed Immunizations

A lapse in the immunization schedule does not require reinstitution of the entire series. If a dose of DTP or OPV is missed, immunization should occur on the next visit as if the usual interval had elapsed. **The charts of children in whom immunizations have been missed or postponed should be flagged to remind health care providers to complete immunization schedules at the next available opportunity.**

Reimmunization

Epidemics of measles involving large numbers of high school and college-aged students have led to a decision to recommend universal measles reimmunization. Some data also suggest that adequate control of mumps may require reimmunization. A second dose of MMR, therefore, should be given to all children entering middle school, enrolling in college, or traveling abroad. Some states follow the recommendations of the Immunization Practices Advisory Committee (ACIP) of the U.S. Public Health Service and require MMR reimmunization at entry to primary school. In states and localities where the law mandates revaccination at or before school entry, the pediatrician should revaccinate at a younger age, but where the law is mute the pediatrician should explain to the parents why revaccination at a later age (11 or 12 years) is preferred by the Academy. In any case, a child who has received two doses of MMR at least one month apart beginning at age 12 months or older should be considered to be adequately immunized. Reactions to reimmunization are no greater than those seen following primary immunization and are likely to be less common, since many recipients are already immune.

Unknown Immunization Status

The physician may encounter some children with an uncertain immunization status. Many young adults and some children have no adequate documentation of immunizations, and recollection by the parent or guardian may be of questionable validity. In general, these individuals should be considered susceptible and appropriate immunizations should be administered. No evidence indicates that administration of MMR or poliovirus vaccine to already immune recipients is harmful. Td, rather than DTP, should be given to those 7 years or older.

Vaccine Dose

The recommended doses of vaccines are derived from theoretical considerations, experimental trials, and experience. Reduction in the recommended doses can result in an inadequate response and leave the recipient susceptible. Exceeding the recommended dose may also be hazardous because excessive local concentrations of injectable, inactivated vaccines might result or because an excessive dose of a live vaccine might be given (a theoretical, but unproven, risk).

The Committee does not recommend reducing or dividing doses of DTP or any vaccine, including those given to premature or low-birth-weight infants. The efficacy of this practice with DTP in reducing the frequency of associated adverse events and in inducing protection against disease similar to that which is achieved with the recommended DTP dose has not been demonstrated (see Pertussis, Immunization, page 361). A diminished antibody response in both term and premature infants to reduced doses of DTP has been reported (see Preterm Infants, page 46).

Active Immunization of Persons Who Recently Received Immune Globulin

In general, measles, mumps, and rubella vaccines should not be given to individuals who have received immune globulin within the previous 3 months because the desired immune response may be inhibited. If an immune globulin must be administered within 14 days of the parenteral administration of these live virus vaccines, the vaccine should be administered again after 3 months unless serologic testing indicates that antibodies were produced. The immunologic response to OPV vaccine is not inhibited by administration of immune globulins.

In contrast, concurrent administration of recommended doses of Hepatitis B Immune Globulin (HBIG), Tetanus Immune Globulin (TIG) or Rabies Immune Globulin (RIG) and the corresponding inactivated vaccine or toxoid in postexposure prophylaxis does not impair the immune response and provides immediate protection and active/passive immunity. Standard doses of the corresponding vaccines should be used, and increases in the vaccine dose volume or number of immunizations are not indicated. Vaccines should be administered at sites different from that of the immune globulin. (See chapters on specific diseases in Part 3 for further discussion.)

Immune globulins have been reported not to interfere with the immune response to OPV and yellow fever vaccine. Hence, if necessary, these live vaccines can be administered simultaneously with immune globulin to individuals such as travelers whose departure is imminent. Similarly, preliminary data indicate that immune globulins do not significantly affect the responses of infants to DTP. However, maternally acquired passive antibodies may complicate the evaluation of responses in young infants.

Tuberculin Testing

Tuberculin testing at any age is not a prerequisite before administration of live virus vaccines, such as MMR. Recommendations for tuberculin testing (see Tuberculosis, page 489) are independent of those for immunization, and tuberculin testing may be done at the same visit at which the MMR vaccine is given (see Table 2, page 17).

Record Keeping

Each state health department has developed an official immunization record. A form should be given to the parents of every newborn infant; this record should be accorded the status of a birth certificate or passport and should be retained with vital documents for subsequent referral. The Committee urges physicians to cooperate with this endeavor by encouraging patients to preserve the record and to present it at each visit to a health care provider. Physicians and other health care providers should also cooperate by recording immunization data in the record.

The immunization record is especially important for patients who move frequently. It will facilitate accurate record keeping for the patient and assist the physician in evaluating immunizations. It will also fulfill the need for documentation of immunizations for school attendance and admission to other institutions and organizations.

Every physician should maintain a permanent office record of the immunization history for each patient which can be reviewed easily and updated when subsequent immunizations are administered; the format of the record should facilitate identification and recall of patients in need of immunization. **Records of children whose immunizations have been postponed should be flagged to indicate the need to complete immunizations.**

For all immunizations, the following data should be entered into the patient's medical record and the patient-retained record: month, day, and year of administration; vaccine or other biologic administered; manufacturer; lot number and its expiration date; site and route of administration; and health care provider administering the vaccine.

For childhood mandated vaccines (diphtheria, tetanus, pertussis, poliovirus, measles, mumps, and rubella vaccines) the National Childhood Vaccine Injury Act, which became effective in 1988, requires that health care providers record in the patient's permanent medical record the date of administration of the vaccine; manufacturer and lot number; and the name, address, and title of the person administering the vaccine. In addition, reporting of selected events that occur after vaccination is required (see Reporting of Adverse Reactions, page 27).

Vaccine Safety and Contraindications

Risks and Adverse Events

Although modern immunizing agents are generally considered safe and effective, they are neither completely safe nor completely effective. Some vaccinees may have an untoward reaction, and some will not be protected. The goal in vaccine development is to achieve the highest degree of protection with the lowest rate of untoward effects.

Risks associated with the use of vaccines vary from trivial and inconvenient to severe and life threatening. In developing recommendations for the use of a vaccine, vaccine safety is weighed against the benefits of the vaccine and the risks of the natural disease. The resulting recommendations attempt to minimize the risk by providing specific advice on dose, route, and timing of the vaccine and by delineating circumstances that warrant precaution in, or abstention from, administering the vaccine.

Vaccine reactions usually are mild to moderate in severity, with few or no permanent sequelae. Because these reactions are intrinsic to the immunizing antigen or some component of the vaccine, they may occur frequently and are unavoidable. Examples of these side effects include fever or local irritation after administration of DTP vaccine, fever and rash after administration of live measles virus vaccine, and tenderness and induration after administration of cholera or typhoid vaccines.

Sterile abscesses have occurred after immunization with a number of killed vaccines. The abscesses presumably result from the irritating nature of the vaccine or its adjuvant vehicle; in some instances they may be caused by inadvertent subcutaneous inoculation of a vaccine intended for intramuscular use.

Rare, serious consequences of vaccine use that can result in sequelae or may even be life threatening can also occur. These events are not necessarily predictable (e.g., paralytic poliomyelitis after administration of live oral poliovirus vaccine to an otherwise healthy child).

The occurrence of a clinical event after the administration of vaccine does not prove that the vaccine caused the symptoms or signs. Vaccines are administered to infants and children during a period in their lives when certain clinical conditions are common (e.g., convulsions). For most live virus vaccines, definitive etiologic association between the vaccine and a subsequent clinical illness requires isolating the vaccine strain from the patient. However, even this generalization has exceptions. For example, vaccine-type poliovirus is commonly found in the stool of vaccinees for several weeks or more after immunization. The occurrence of a neurologic syndrome during this period (e.g., encephalitis) does not prove that the poliovirus vaccine caused the illness. Firmer evidence may be obtained by isolating the agent from normally sterile body fluids or tissues, such as the brain or the cerebrospinal fluid. Association of an adverse clinical event with a specific vaccine is suggested if vaccinees experience the event at a rate significantly higher than that in nonvaccinated groups of similar age or residence. Unusual clustering of a condition in vaccinees in a limited interval after vaccination may also suggest a causal association.

Although a specific condition occurring in a single individual after immunization does not provide sufficient evidence to link that condition to

Table 5. Reportable Events Following Immunization*

Vaccine/ Toxoid	Event	Interval from Vaccination
DTP, P, DTP/polio-virus combined	A. Anaphylaxis or anaphylactic shock	24 hours
	B. Encephalopathy (or encephalitis)†	7 days
	C. Shock-collapse or hypotonic-hyporesponsive collapse†	7 days
	D. Residual seizure disorder†	†
	E. Any acute complication or sequela (including death) of above events	No limit
	F. (See package insert)§	(See package insert)
Measles, mumps, and rubella; DT, Td, T toxoid	A. Anaphylaxis or anaphylactic shock	24 hours
	B. Encephalopathy (or encephalitis)†	15 days for measles, mumps, and rubella vaccines; 7 days for DT, Td, and T toxoids
	C. Residual seizure disorder†	†
	D. Any acute complication or sequela (including death) of above events	No limit
	E. (See package insert)§	(See package insert)
Oral poliovirus vaccine	A. Paralytic poliomyelitis	
	- in a nonimmunodeficient recipient	30 days
	- in an immunodeficient recipient	6 months
	- in a vaccine-associated community case	No limit
	B. Any acute complication or sequela (including death) of above events	No limit
	C (See package insert)§	(See package insert)
Inactivated poliovirus vaccine	A. Anaphylaxis or anaphylactic shock	24 hours
	B. Any acute complication or sequela (including death) of above event	No limit
	C. (See package insert)§	(See package insert)

From Centers for Disease Control. Vaccine Adverse Event Reporting System–United States: Requirements. *MMWR.* 1990;39:730-732.

continued on next page

*Events listed are required by law to be reported to the U.S. Department of Health and Human Services; however, VAERS will accept *all* reports of suspected adverse events after the administration of *any* vaccine.

†Aids to Interpretation:

- Shock-collapse or hypotonic-hyporesponsive collapse may be evidenced by signs or symptoms such as decrease in or loss of muscle tone, paralysis (partial or complete), hemiplegia, hemiparesis, loss of color or change of color to pale white or blue, unresponsiveness to environmental stimuli, depression of or loss of consciousness, prolonged sleeping with difficulty arousing, or cardiovascular or respiratory arrest.
- Residual seizure disorder may be considered to have occurred if no other seizure or convulsion unaccompanied by fever or accompanied by a fever of < 102°F occurred before the first seizure or convulsion after the administration of the vaccine involved,

  AND, if in the case of measles-, mumps-, or rubella-containing vaccines, the first seizure or convulsion occurred within 15 days after vaccination OR in the case of any other vaccine, the first seizure or convulsion occurred within 3 days after vaccination,

  AND, if two or more seizures or convulsions unaccompanied by fever or accompanied by a fever of < 102°F occurred within 1 year after vaccination.
- The terms seizure and convulsion include grand mal, petit mal, absence, myoclonic, tonic-clonic, and focal motor seizures and signs.
- Encephalopathy means any substantial acquired abnormality of, injury to, or impairment of brain function. Among the frequent manifestations of encephalopathy are focal and diffuse neurologic signs, increased intracranial pressure, or changes lasting ≥ 6 hours in level of consciousness, with or without convulsions. The neurologic signs and symptoms of encephalopathy may be temporary with complete recovery, or they may result in various degrees of permanent impairment. Signs and symptoms such as high-pitched and unusual screaming, persistent unconsolable crying, and bulging fontanel are compatible with an encephalopathy, but in and of themselves are not conclusive evidence of encephalopathy. Encephalopathy usually can be documented by slow wave activity on an electroencephalogram.

§Refer to the CONTRAINDICATION section of the manufacturer's package insert for each vaccine.

VAERS

VACCINE ADVERSE EVENT REPORTING SYSTEM

24 Hour Toll-free information line 1-800-822-7967

Patient identity kept confidential

For CDC/FDA Use Only — VAERS Number — Date Received

Patient Name:	Vaccine administered by (Name):	Form completed by (Name):
Last First M.I.	Responsible Physician ______	Relation to Patient ☐ Vaccine Provider ☐ Manufacturer ☐ Patient/Parent ☐ Other
Address	Facility Name/Address	Address (if different from patient or provider)
City State Zip	City State Zip	City State Zip
Telephone no. (____)______	Telephone no. (____)______	Telephone no. (____)______

1. State
2. County where administered
3. Date of birth __/__/__ (mm dd yy)
4. Patient age
5. Sex ☐M ☐F
6. Date form completed __/__/__ (mm dd yy)

7. Describe adverse event(s) (symptoms, signs, time course) and treatment, if any

8. Check all appropriate:
- ☐ Patient died (date __/__/__ mm dd yy)
- ☐ Life threatening illness
- ☐ Required emergency room/doctor visit
- ☐ Required hospitalization (______days)
- ☐ Resulted in prolongation of hospitalization
- ☐ Resulted in permanent disability
- ☐ None of the above

9. Patient recovered ☐ YES ☐ NO ☐ UNKNOWN

10. Date of vaccination __/__/__ (mm dd yy) Time______ AM PM

11. Adverse event onset __/__/__ (mm dd yy) Time______ AM PM

12. Relevant diagnostic tests/laboratory data

13. Enter all vaccines given on date listed in no. 10

	Vaccine (type)	Manufacturer	Lot number	Route/Site	No. Previous doses
a.					
b.					
c.					
d.					

14. Any other vaccinations within 4 weeks of date listed in no. 10

	Vaccine (type)	Manufacturer	Lot number	Route/Site	No. Previous doses	Date given
a.						
b.						

15. Vaccinated at:
☐ Private doctor's office/hospital ☐ Military clinic/hospital
☐ Public health clinic/hospital ☐ Other/unknown

16. Vaccine purchased with:
☐ Private funds ☐ Military funds
☐ Public funds ☐ Other /unknown

17. Other medications

18. Illness at time of vaccination (specify)

19. Pre-existing physician-diagnosed allergies, birth defects, medical conditions (specify)

20. Have you reported this adverse event previously? ☐ No ☐ To health department ☐ To doctor ☐ To manufacturer

Only for children 5 and under

22. Birth weight ____ lb. ____ oz.

23. No. of brothers and sisters

21. Adverse event following prior vaccination (check all applicable, specify)

	Adverse Event	Onset Age	Type Vaccine	Dose no. in series
☐ In patient				
☐ In brother or sister				

Only for reports submitted by manufacturer/immunization project

24. Mfr. / imm. proj. report no.

25. Date received by mfr. / imm. proj.

26. 15 day report? ☐ Yes ☐ No

27. Report type ☐ Initial ☐ Follow-Up

Health care providers and manufacturers are required by law (42 USC 300aa-25) to report reactions to vaccines listed in the Vaccine Injury Table. Reports for reactions to other vaccines are voluntary except when required as a condition of immunization grant awards.

Form VAERS -1

the vaccine, reporting of these occurrences is important because, in conjunction with other reports, they may provide clues to a new or unanticipated adverse reaction.

Reporting of Adverse Reactions

No recommendations can anticipate all possible contingencies, particularly with newly developed vaccines. The physician has an obligation to monitor the results of a vaccine in immunized patients for efficacy and safety. Parents and patients should be questioned concerning possible reactions and side effects after previous immunizations, and physicians should be aware of possible deviations from the expected outcome. Unexpected events occurring soon after administration of any vaccine, particularly those severe enough to require medical attention, should be noted; a detailed description of the occurrence should be recorded; and a report should be made, as described below.

The National Childhood Vaccine Injury Act requires that health care providers report selected events that occur after immunization with most of the routinely administered childhood vaccines* to the U.S. Department of Health and Human Services. Reportable events are listed in Table 5 and include events described in the vaccine package inserts as contraindications to receiving additional doses of vaccine and vaccine-associated events that are compensable (see Federal Vaccine Injury Compensation Table, page 612). The Vaccine Adverse Event Reporting System (VAERS), established by the Department of Health and Human Services to provide a single mechanism for this mandated reporting of vaccine-related adverse events, became operational in November 1990. Reporting forms (see page 26) and instructions have been developed by VAERS and provided to physicians. Reporting forms and related information can be obtained by calling VAERS (800/822-7267).

Significant adverse events occurring after the administration of other vaccines should also be reported to VAERS. This system replaces prior mechanisms for the reporting of vaccine-related adverse events. All reports of suspected adverse events after administration of any vaccine, irrespective of age of the recipient, will be accepted. Submission of a report does not necessarily denote that the vaccine caused the adverse event.

All patient-identifying information will be kept confidential. Written notification that the report has been received is provided to the person submitting the form. VAERS staff will contact these persons for follow-up of the patient's condition at 60 days and at 1 year after serious adverse events.

---

*Routinely administered childhood vaccines are diphtheria, tetanus, pertussis, poliovirus, measles, mumps, and rubella vaccines.

Precautions and Contraindications

Precautions and contraindications are described in specific *Red Book* chapters on vaccine-preventable diseases and in the manufacturers' package; they indicate circumstances in which the physician should be cautious in administering vaccines. In some of these situations, vaccine administration may still be indicated after the benefits and risks to the child have been carefully assessed.

Minor Illness and Fever. Most vaccines are intended for use in healthy individuals or in those whose diseases or conditions are not affected by vaccine. For optimal safety, vaccines should not be used if an undesirable side effect or adverse reaction to the vaccine may be accentuated by an underlying illness. A common situation is the child scheduled for immunizations who has an acute illness. Minor illnesses do not contraindicate the use of vaccines, particularly when a child continually appears to have a minor upper respiratory tract infection or allergic rhinitis. In this situation, no evidence indicates an increased risk from immunization. Deferring immunization of children with this type of minor illness frequently results in unimmunized young children who will need to "catch up" with immunizations at a later age or who develop vaccine-preventable disease.

For the child with an acute, febrile illness, guidelines for immunization are based on the physician's assessment of the child's illness and the specific vaccine the child is scheduled to receive. Although fever per se is not a contraindication to immunizations, if it is associated with other manifestations suggesting a more serious illness, the child should not be vaccinated until he or she has recovered. Other vaccine-specific recommendations are as follows:

- *Live virus vaccines.* Minor illnesses with or without fever do not contraindicate the use of live virus vaccines such as MMR. Such intercurrent illnesses are not known to interfere with the immune response to the vaccines, and no evidence indicates an increased risk from vaccination. Deferring immunization of children in such circumstances frequently results in failure to immunize young children at the desired age.
- *DTP and other vaccines.* Mild illnesses (e.g., upper respiratory illnesses) do not contraindicate administration of DTP or other vaccines. However, a moderate or severe illness with or without fever is a contraindication to administering DTP, as the vaccine may be blamed for the signs and symptoms associated with the illness.
- *Child with frequent febrile illnesses.* In the circumstance of the child who repeatedly has moderate or severe febrile illnesses at the time of scheduled immunizations, the child should be asked to return as soon as the current febrile illness is terminated so that immunization can be completed.

- *Immunocompromised children.* Special consideration needs to be given to immunocompromised children, such as those with congenital immunodeficiencies, AIDS, malignancy, and recipients of immunosuppressive therapy. Immunization of children with these problems is discussed in detail in the section on Immunodeficient and Immunosuppressed Children (see page 47).

Hypersensitivity Reactions to Vaccine Constituents

Hypersensitivity reactions to constituents of vaccines are rare. In some instances, although symptoms appear soon after a vaccine is administered, differentiation between allergic reaction to the vaccine and reaction to some other environmental allergen is impossible.

Four types of hypersensitivity reactions believed related to vaccine constituents are (1) allergic reactions to egg or egg-related antigens, (2) mercury sensitivity in some recipients of immune globulins or vaccines, (3) antibiotic-induced allergic reactions, and (4) hypersensitivity to some component of the infectious agent or other vaccine components.

Allergic Reactions to Egg or Egg-Related Antigens. Current measles, mumps, yellow fever, and influenza vaccines contain only small amounts of egg proteins. Some individuals with history of allergic manifestations after ingesting eggs have no reaction when skin tested with vaccine and tolerate vaccination without incident. However, persons with history of severe egg sensitivity (defined as generalized urticaria, shock, wheezing, or manifestations of upper airway obstruction) after ingesting eggs should not receive vaccines produced in eggs or chick embryos until they have been appropriately skin tested. These precautions should be followed with measles, mumps, influenza, and yellow fever vaccines.

A well-documented report has described a few children sensitive to chicken eggs who developed anaphylaxis after receiving measles vaccine. These patients had positive, immediate reactions to skin tests with measles vaccine and MMR vaccine. IgE antigen-specific antibodies to measles vaccine chicken egg embryo components were identified.

Milder forms of sensitivity to eggs or chicken feathers do not indicate a sensitivity to vaccines made in avian tissues. Persons without anaphylactic symptoms may be given the previously mentioned egg-derived vaccines.

An egg-sensitive individual can be tested with the vaccine before its use in the following manner:

1. *Scratch, prick, or puncture test.* A drop of 1:10 dilution of the vaccine in physiologic saline is applied at the site of a superficial scratch, prick, or puncture of the volar surface of the forearm. The test is read after 15 to 20 minutes. A positive test is a wheal 3 mm larger than that of a control (wheal produced in response to physiologic saline given by scratch, prick, or puncture), usually

with surrounding erythema. If the result of this test is negative, an intradermal test is performed.

2. *Intradermal test.* 0.02 mL of 1:100 dilution of the vaccine in physiologic saline is injected, and the wheal-and-flare reaction is measured after 15 to 20 minutes and compared to a control, as in the scratch, prick, or puncture test. A wheal 5 mm or larger with surrounding erythema is considered a significant reaction.

   Note: Scratch, prick, or puncture tests with other allergens have resulted in fatalities in highly allergic individuals. Although such untoward effects have not been reported for vaccine testing, all skin tests and "desensitization" procedures should be performed by trained personnel familiar with the treatment of acute anaphylaxis. As a minimum, when any skin test is performed in a child, a syringe containing 0.3 mL of 1:1,000 aqueous epinephrine should be within immediate reach.

   "Desensitization." If the child has a history of severe egg sensitivity and has either (1) a positive scratch, prick, or puncture test, or (2) a positive intradermal test to vaccine, the child still may be given the vaccine using a "desensitization" procedure if immunization is imperative. A suggested protocol is subcutaneous administration of the following successive doses of vaccine at 15- to 20-minute intervals:

   1. 0.05 mL of 1:100 dilution in physiologic saline
   2. 0.05 mL of 1:10 dilution
   3. 0.05 mL of full strength
   4. 0.10 mL of full strength
   5. 0.15 mL of full strength
   6. 0.20 mL of full strength

   This type of "desensitization" should be undertaken only with the supervision of a physician experienced in the management of anaphylaxis and with necessary equipment immediately available.

Mercury Sensitivity in Some Recipients of Immune Globulins or Vaccines. Mercury from the organic mercurial preservatives used in the preparation of immune globulin (IG) for intramuscular use can accumulate in individuals given repeated injections. Only one instance of proven mercury sensitivity (acrodynia) has been reported. Immune globulin for intravenous use (IGIV) does not contain preservatives. Reactions to mercury have been suspected in mercury-sensitive individuals exposed to vaccines containing mercurial compounds, but proof of causal association is lacking.

Antibiotic-Induced Allergic Reactions. Antibiotic reactions have been suspected in individuals with known allergies who received vaccines containing trace amounts of antibiotics. Proof of a causal relationship is difficult and often impossible to confirm.

Inactivated poliovirus vaccine (IPV) contains trace amounts of streptomycin and neomycin. Live measles, mumps, and rubella vaccines, singly or in combination (MMR), contain an extremely small amount of neomycin (25 μg). Some persons allergic to neomycin can experience a delayed-type local reaction 48 to 96 hours after administration of MMR or IPV. The reaction consists of an erythematous, pruritic papule. This minor reaction is of little importance when weighed against the benefit of immunization, and should not be considered a contraindication. However, if the individual has a history of anaphylactic reaction to neomycin, neomycin-containing vaccines should not be used.

No currently recommended vaccine contains penicillin or its derivatives.

Hypersensitivity to Some Component of the Infectious Agent, or Other Vaccine Components. DTP (and to a lesser extent cholera, plague, and typhoid vaccines) is associated with local and occasionally systemic reactions, usually of a toxic rather than a hypersensitivity nature. On occasion, urticarial or anaphylactic reactions have occurred in DTP, DT, or Td vaccine recipients. Tetanus and diphtheria antigen-specific antibodies of the IgE type have been identified in some of these patients. Although attributing a specific sensitivity to vaccine components is very difficult, an immediate, severe, or anaphylactic allergic reaction to one of these vaccines is a contraindication to subsequent immunization of the patient with the specific product. A transient urticarial rash, however, unless it occurs immediately after immunization, is not a contraindication to further doses. (For more detailed discussion, see Pertussis, page 358.)

Individuals who have high serum concentrations of tetanus IgG antibody, usually as the result of frequent booster immunizations, can have an increased incidence and severity of reactions to subsequent vaccine administration (see Tetanus, page 465).

Reactions resembling serum sickness have been reported in approximately 6% of patients after a booster dose of human diploid rabies vaccine, probably due to sensitization to human albumin that had been altered chemically by the virus-inactivating agent.

Significant hypersensitivity reactions occurring as a result of pneumococcal or *Haemophilus* b vaccines appear to be extremely rare.

An unusual sensitivity to killed measles virus vaccine (KMV) has been documented. This vaccine has not been available in the last 20 years, but it was received by many patients until 1967 in the United States. A moderate to severe local reaction, occasionally with systemic symptoms, was observed in KMV recipients when live measles virus vaccine was administered months or years later. In some KMV recipients, exposure to natural (wild) measles virus up to 16 years later resulted in atypical measles (often a severe illness with fever, pulmonary infiltrates, polyserositis, and a rash resembling Rocky Mountain spotted fever). Immunologically, the local reaction and atypical illness represent either an Arthus reaction or a delayed hypersensitivity reaction (cell-mediated immune reaction), or both.

Misconceptions Concerning Vaccine Contraindications

Some health care providers inappropriately consider certain conditions or circumstances to be contraindications to vaccination. Conditions most often inappropriately regarded as routine contraindications include the following:

- **Reaction to a previous DTP dose that involved only soreness, redness, or swelling in the immediate vicinity of the vaccination site or temperature of less than 105°F (40.5°C).**
- **Mild acute illness with low-grade fever or mild diarrheal illness in an otherwise well child.**
- **Current antimicrobial therapy or the convalescent phase of illness.**
- **Prematurity**. The appropriate age for initiating immunizations in the prematurely born infant is the usual chronologic age. Vaccine doses should not be reduced for preterm infants (see Preterm Infants, page 46).
- **Pregnancy of mother or other household contact.**
- **Recent exposure to an infectious disease.**
- **Breast-feeding**. The only vaccine virus that has been isolated from breast milk is rubella vaccine virus. No evidence indicates that breast milk from women immunized against rubella is harmful to infants.
- **A history of nonspecific allergies or relatives with allergies.**
- **Allergies to penicillin or any other antibiotic, except anaphylactic reactions to neomycin or streptomycin** (see Hypersensitivity Reactions to Vaccine Constituents, page 29). These reactions occur rarely, if ever. None of the vaccines licensed in the United States contains penicillin.
- **Allergies to duck meat or duck feathers.** No vaccine available in the United States is produced in substrates containing duck antigens.
- **Family history of convulsions in persons considered for pertussis or measles vaccination** (see Children with Personal or Family History of Seizures, page 54).
- **Family history of sudden infant death syndrome in children considered for DTP vaccination.**
- **Family history of an adverse event, unrelated to immunosuppression, following vaccination.**

Passive Immunization

Passive immunization entails administration of preformed antibody to a recipient. It is indicated in the following general circumstances for the prevention or amelioration of infectious diseases:

- When persons are deficient in synthesis of antibody as a result of congenital or acquired B-lymphocyte cell defects, alone or in combination with other immunodeficiencies.
- When a person susceptible to a disease is exposed to it, especially when that person has a high risk of complications from the disease (e.g., a child with leukemia exposed to varicella or measles), or when time does not permit adequate protection by active immunization alone (e.g., some postexposure situations involving measles, rabies, or hepatitis B).
- Therapeutically, when a disease is already present and antibody may ameliorate or aid in suppressing the effects of a toxin (e.g., food-borne or wound [not infant] botulism, diphtheria, or tetanus).

Passive immunization or serotherapy has been accomplished with several different types of products. The choice is dictated by the types of products available, the type of antibody desired, the route of administration, timing, and other considerations. These products include Immune Globulin (Human) and specific ("hyperimmune") Immune Globulins (Human), all of which are intended for intramuscular administration; IGIV (Human); human plasma; and antibodies of animal origin.

Indications for administration of immune globulin other than those relevant to infectious diseases are not reviewed in the *Red Book*. Examples include idiopathic thrombocytopenia purpura and treatment of certain poisonous snake bites.

Immune Globulin (IG)

IG (Human) (often called "gamma globulin") is derived from the pooled plasma of adults by an alcohol-fractionation procedure. It consists primarily of the immunoglobulin fraction (at least 95% IgG and trace amounts of IgA and IgM), is sterile, and is not known to transmit hepatitis, HIV, or any other infectious disease agent. It is a concentrated protein solution (approximately 16.5% and 165 mg/mL).

IG contains specific antibodies in proportion to the infectious and immunization experience of the population from whose serum it was prepared. Large numbers of donors (at least 1,000 donors per lot of final product) are used to ensure inclusion of a broad spectrum of antibodies.

IG is currently recommended for intramuscular administration. Since some recipients of intramuscular IG experience local pain and most feel some local discomfort, IG should be administered deep in a large muscle mass, usually in the gluteal region. Ordinarily no more than 5 mL should be administered in one site in an adult or large child; lesser amounts (1 to 3 mL) should be given to small children and infants. Seldom should more than 20 mL be given at any one time, even to an adult.

Peak serum concentrations of antibodies are usually achieved 48 to 72 hours after intramuscular inoculation. The serum half-life is generally 3 to 4 weeks. Some investigators have used slow subcutaneous administration in immunodeficient patients. Intravenous use of IG is contraindicated; however, intravenous preparations of IG have been developed and are discussed later in this section. IG is not recommended for intradermal use.

Indications for the Use of IG

As Replacement Therapy in Antibody-Deficiency Disorders. The usual dose is 100 mg/kg (equivalent to 0.66 mL/kg) per month. Customary practice is to administer two times this dose initially and to adjust the interval (2 to 4 weeks) between administration of the doses, based on the clinical response (absence of, or decrease in infections). This form of therapy has been, in most cases, replaced by IGIV.

Hepatitis A Prophylaxis. IG can prevent clinical disease resulting from hepatitis A virus in exposed susceptible individuals when given within 14 days of exposure. The usual dose is 0.02 mL/kg, given as soon as possible after exposure. For preexposure use for prolonged travel to countries where hepatitis A is prevalent, a higher dose is warranted (see Hepatitis A, page 236).

Measles Prophylaxis. IG administered to exposed, measles-susceptible individuals will prevent or modify infection if given within 6 days of exposure (see Measles: Care of Exposed Person, page 310). IG is especially indicated for susceptible household or hospital contacts younger than 6 months. If IG is given for this purpose, the individual should receive live measles virus vaccine 3 months later, unless contraindications are present or the individual is not yet 15 months old. A single dose of 0.25 mL/kg (maximum, 15 mL) is given as soon after exposure as possible. If the risk of severe morbidity from the disease is extremely high, as in the immunosuppressed patient, 0.5 mL/kg is given. A child regularly receiving immunoglobulin replacement therapy for antibody immunodeficiency need not receive an additional dose of IG if exposed to measles because the usual dose is probably protective (see Measles: Care of Exposed Person, page 310).

Nonproven Uses of IG

- *Hepatitis B prophylaxis.* IG is prepared from normal adult plasma, whereas Hepatitis B Immune Globulin (HBIG) (Human) is prepared from plasma preselected for high antibody titer against hepatitis B surface antigen (HBsAg). Hence, HBIG should be used for hepatitis B prophylaxis, generally in conjunction with hepatitis B vaccine (see Hepatitis B: Care of Exposed Person, page 249).

- *Hepatitis C.* Results of studies evaluating the prophylactic value of IG have been equivocal. For persons with percutaneous exposure, IG (0.06 mL/kg) may be reasonable to give (see Hepatitis C: Control Measures, page 257).
- *Enterically transmitted non-A, non-B hepatitis.* No evidence indicates that U.S.-manufactured IG will prevent this infection.
- *Asthma or severe allergic diathesis.* No evidence supports the use of IG in these conditions.
- *Burn patients.* Evidence for reduction of infection by IG is contradictory at best. Large doses (1 mL/kg/d for 3 days) of IG resulted in a 50% reduction of infections in one study, but half that dose was nonbeneficial in another investigation.
- *Most acute infections.* Despite the frustration experienced by physicians confronted with severe, even life-threatening, acute bacterial or viral infections, little convincing evidence indicates benefit from IG administration. Of particular note is the lack of efficacy in reduction or modification of undifferentiated, repetitive upper respiratory tract infections.
- *Other clinical circumstances.* IG has not proved beneficial in infants who are septic, debilitated, or malnourished; who are ill because of infection with nonpolio enteroviruses, failure to thrive, or premature; or who have non-B-cell immunodeficiencies.

Precautions in the Use of IG

- IG is recommended for clinical use only in situations where its efficacy has been established.
- IG should be given intramuscularly in a large muscle mass (usually in the gluteal region).
- Caution should be used in giving IG to a patient with a history of adverse reactions to immune globulins.
- Although systemic reactions to IG are rare (see Adverse Reactions to IG), epinephrine and other means of treating acute reactions should be immediately available.
- IG should not be given to patients with severe thrombocytopenia or any coagulation disorder that would preclude intramuscular injection.
- Screening for IgA-deficiency is not routinely recommended for potential recipients of IG (see discussion below in Adverse Reactions to IG).

Adverse Reactions to IG

- The most common problem encountered with the use of IG is discomfort and pain at the site of administration. Less common reactions include flushing, headache, chills, and nausea.
- Serious reactions are uncommon; these may involve chest pain or constriction, dyspnea, or anaphylaxis and systemic collapse. An increased risk of systemic reaction results from inadvertent or deliberate intravenous administration. Persons requiring repeated intramuscular doses have been reported to experience systemic reactions such as fever, chills, sweating, uncomfortable sensations, and shock.
- Because IG contains trace amounts of IgA, persons who are selectively serum IgA deficient can, in rare cases, develop anti-IgA antibodies and react to a subsequent dose of IG, whole blood transfusion, or plasma infusion with systemic symptoms, particularly chills, fever, and shock-like symptoms. In those rare cases when reactions related to anti-IgA antibodies have occurred, use of IgA-depleted preparations will reduce the likelihood of further reactions. Avoidance of anaphylactic reactions, however, may require the use of IG completely devoid of IgA. Because of the rarity of these reactions, screening for IgA-deficiency is not routinely recommended.
- Healthy persons given IG may manufacture antibodies against IgG allotypes that differ from their own. Usually this phenomenon has no clinical significance; on rare occasions a systemic reaction may result.
- One case of acrodynia due to thiomersal in IG has been reported in a young adult who had been receiving IG since early infancy for agammaglobulinemia.
- Careful epidemiologic follow-up of IG recipients, as well as laboratory studies of viral inactivation during preparation of commercial manufacturing products, have demonstrated no evidence of HIV, transmission by IG, specific ("hyperimmune") immune globulins, or immune globulins for intravenous use.

Specific Immune Globulins

Specific immune globulins or "hyperimmune globulins" differ from IG in the selection of donors and the number of donors whose plasma is included in the source from which the pool is prepared. Donors known to have high titers of the desired antibody, either naturally acquired or stimulated by immunization, are selected. These globulins are prepared by the same procedure as IG but contain 10% to 18% protein, whereas IG has approximately 16.5% protein. Specific immune globulins for use in infectious diseases include Hepatitis B Immune Globulin (HBIG) (Human), Rabies Immune Globulin (RIG) (Human), Tetanus Immune Globulin

(TIG) (Human), and Varicella-Zoster Immune Globulin (VZIG) (Human). The products are administered intramuscularly. In addition, Cytomegalovirus Immune Globulin Intravenous (CMV IGIV) (Human) has recently been licensed. Recommendations for use of these globulins are given in the discussion of specific diseases in Part 3.

The precautions and adverse reactions for IG are also applicable to the specific immune globulins.

Immune Globulin Intravenous (IGIV)

Immune Globulin Intravenous (IGIV) (Human) is derived from the pooled plasma of adults by an alcohol-fractionation procedure; it is then modified to be suitable for intravenous use. The donor pool is like that of IG. IGIV consists primarily of the immunoglobulin fraction (more than 95% IgG and trace amounts of IgA and IgM). The protein content varies, depending on the product; both liquid and dried products are available. IGIV does not contain thiomersal and can be used in mercury-sensitive individuals.

Indications for the Use of IGIV

- *Replacement therapy in antibody deficiency disorders.* The usual dose of IGIV in immunodeficiency syndromes is 300 to 400 mg/kg body weight administered once a month by intravenous infusion. Dose or frequency of infusions, however, should be based on the effectiveness in the individual patient, and effective doses have ranged from 200 to 800 mg/kg monthly. Maintenance of a trough IgG concentration of 500 mg/dL has been demonstrated to correlate with clinical response.
- *Kawasaki disease.* IGIV administered within the first 10 days of the illness shortens the duration of fever and decreases the frequency of coronary abnormalities (see Kawasaki Disease, page 284).
- *Low-birth-weight infants.* Results of some clinical trials have indicated that IGIV decreases the incidence of late-onset infections in infants less than 1,500 g in birth weight. Other studies, however, have not confirmed these results. Trials have varied in IGIV dose, time of administration, and other aspects of study design. A National Institutes of Health Consensus Development Panel in May 1990* concluded that while the use of IGIV in the prevention of late-onset infection in preterm neonates had a rational basis, the available data did not support the routine use of IGIV in low-birth-weight infants, including those less than 1,500 g. Additional trials have either

---

*For further information, see NIH Consensus Conference. Intravenous Immunoglobulin: Prevention & Treatment of Disease. *JAMA*. 1990;264:3189-3193.

recently been completed or are in progress, however, and may provide specific indications for IGIV prophylaxis in low- birth-weight infants.

- *Pediatric AIDS.* Some centers have empirically given IGIV to infants and young children with symptomatic HIV infection for the prevention of severe bacterial and viral infections. Small uncontrolled studies have suggested efficacy but no controlled studies have been completed. The National Institutes of Health is currently sponsoring two large controlled trials of IGIV, with and without zidovudine. Pending the results of these trials, no recommendations for the routine use of IGIV in HIV-infected children can be made.*
- *Hypogammaglobulinemia in chronic lymphocytic leukemia.* IGIV in adults with this disease has been demonstrated to reduce the incidence of serious bacterial infections.
- *Bone marrow transplantation.* Results of limited trials in pediatric bone marrow recipients suggest that IGIV may reduce the incidence of infection and death but not acute graft-versus-host disease (GVHD). Studies in adult transplant recipients indicate that IGIV decreases the incidence of interstitial pneumonia (presumably due to cytomegalovirus), may reduce the risk of bacterial infection, and decreases the incidence of GVHD and death, and, in conjunction with ganciclovir (Cytovene†), is effective in the treatment of some patients with cytomegalovirus pneumonia.

Precautions in the Use of IGIV

- IGIV is recommended for clinical use only in situations where its efficacy has been established.
- IGIV should be given only intravenously; other routes have not been evaluated.
- Caution should be used in giving IGIV to a patient with a history of adverse reactions to immune globulins.
- Because systemic reactions to IGIV may occur (see Adverse Reactions to IGIV, page 39), epinephrine and other means of treating acute reactions should be available immediately.
- Adverse reactions can often be alleviated by reducing either the rate or the volume of infusion. For patients with repeated severe reactions unresponsive to these measures, hydrocortisone, 1 to 2 mg/kg intravenously, can be given 30 minutes before infusion.
- Seriously ill patients with compromised cardiac function, who are receiving large fluid volumes of IGIV, may be at increased risk of

---

***In January 1991, while the *Red Book* was in press, one of these trials was terminated, and recommendations were issued by the AAP Task Force on Pediatric AIDS for IGIV treatment of children with symptomatic HIV infection and peripheral CD4 lymphocyte counts of 200/mm^3 or greater.**

†Available from Syntex Laboratories, Inc., Palo Alto, CA

vasomotor or cardiac complications manifested by elevated blood pressure and/or cardiac failure.

- Screening for IgA-deficiency is not routinely recommended for potential recipients of IGIV (for further information, see Adverse Reactions to IGIV).
- As with any biologic or pharmacologic product, the potential for new or previously unrecognized adverse events should be anticipated. With IGIV, these include transmission of blood-borne pathogens, such as hepatitis C virus (**but not HIV**); and with increased dosage or new products, possible immunosuppression.

Adverse Reactions to IGIV

The reported incidence of adverse events associated with the administration of IGIV ranges from 1% to 15%, but usually is less than 5%. Most of these reactions are mild and self limited. Severe reactions occur very infrequently and usually do not contraindicate further IGIV therapy.

Neither HIV nor hepatitis B infection has been transmitted to recipients of products currently licensed in the United States. IGIV is manufactured from large numbers of donors whose plasma is negative for hepatitis B surface antigen and HIV antibody.

Adverse events include the following:

- Pyrogenic reactions marked by high fever and systemic symptoms.
- Minor systemic reactions with headache, myalgia, fever, chills, lightheadedness, nausea, or vomiting.
- Vasomotor or cardiovascular manifestations, marked by changes in blood pressure and tachycardia.
- Hypersensitivity reactions.

Anaphylactic reactions induced by anti-IgA can occur in patients with primary antibody deficiency who have a total absence of circulating IgA and antibodies to IgA. These are extremely rare in panhypogammaglobulinemic individuals and potentially more common in patients with subclass immunoglobulin deficiencies. In those rare instances when reactions related to anti-IgA antibodies have occurred, use of IgA-depleted preparations will reduce the likelihood of further reactions. Avoidance of anaphylactic reactions, however, may require the use of material completely devoid of IgA. Because of the rarity of these reactions, screening for IgA deficiency is not routinely recommended.

Human Plasma

The use of human plasma in the control of infectious diseases should be limited. Human plasma has been administered to burn patients in an attempt to control *Pseudomonas* infections, but the data are insufficient to substantiate this use. Plasma infusions have been useful in treating infants who have protein-losing enteropathy. Plasma infusions have also been substituted for IG in some patients with IgG antibody deficiency when these individuals develop adverse reactions to IG or fail to respond to treatment with IG. However, these immunodeficient patients can be managed with IGIV (or by slow subcutaneous administration of IG).

Whenever human plasma is used, the danger of transmission of hepatitis viruses and other agents must be considered. The "buddy" system has been used for immunodeficient individuals who require repeated infusions; a single healthy donor negative for HBsAg and lacking anti-HBc, HIV, and cytomegalovirus antibodies who has normal serum alanine aminotransferase levels is used for all infusions. Some investigators have found matching of an asymptomatic IgA-deficient donor with an IgA-deficient hypogammaglobulinemic recipient to be beneficial.

Antibodies of Animal Origin

Products of animal origin available in the United States are derived from the serum of horses. Experimental products prepared in other species may also be available. These products are derived by concentrating the serum globulin fraction with ammonium sulfate. Some, but not all, products are also subjected to an enzyme digestion process in an attempt to decrease reactions to foreign proteins.

The use of the following products in infectious disease is discussed in the disease-specific chapters of Part 3:

- Botulism Antitoxin Types A, B, E
- Diphtheria Antitoxin
- Tetanus Antitoxin
- Antirabies Serum

Indications for Use of Animal Antisera

Antibody-containing products prepared from animal sera pose a special risk to the recipient, and the use of such products should be strictly limited to certain indications, in which specific immune globulins of human origin are not available (e.g., diphtheria and botulism).

Reactions to Animal Sera

A careful history must be taken before any animal serum is injected. The patient must be questioned about asthma, hay fever, urticaria, and previous injections of animal sera. Patients with history of asthma, allergic rhinitis, or other allergic symptoms, especially on exposure to horses or other animals, can be dangerously sensitive to the corresponding serum and should be given animal serum only with the utmost caution.

Sensitivity Tests for Reactions to Animal Sera

Each patient who is to be given an animal serum should be tested prior to its administration, as follows:

1. *Scratch, prick, or puncture test.** Apply one drop of a 1:100 dilution of the serum in normal saline to the site of a superficial scratch, prick, or puncture on the volar aspect of the forearm. A positive test is a wheal with surrounding erythema at least 3 mm larger than the reaction to a control test with normal (physiologic) saline, read at 15 to 20 minutes. If the scratch test is negative, an intradermal test is performed.
2. *Intradermal test.** In persons with history of allergy, especially to animals or those who have previously received animal sera, a dose of 0.02 mL of 1:1,000 saline-diluted serum (enough to raise a small intradermal wheal) is administered. If the test is negative, it should be repeated using a 1:100 dilution. In persons with negative history and negative scratch tests, only the 1:100 dilution may be used. Interpretation of the intradermal test is done as with the scratch test.

Whereas intradermal skin tests have resulted in fatalities, the scratch test is usually safe. Therefore, scratch tests should always precede the intradermal tests. These skin tests should always be performed by trained personnel familiar with the treatment of acute anaphylaxis (see Treatment of Anaphylactic Reactions, page 43); a syringe containing 0.3 mL of 1:1,000 aqueous epinephrine must be immediately available.

Positive tests indicate the probability of sensitivity, but a negative skin test is not an absolute guarantee of absence of sensitivity. Therefore, animal sera should be administered with caution, even in individuals whose tests are negative.

If the skin test is positive or if the history for systemic anaphylaxis after previous administration of serum is highly suggestive in a person for whom the need for the serum is unquestioned, "desensitization" can be undertaken (as described below in "Desensitization" for Animal Sera).

If the history and sensitivity tests are negative, the indicated dose of serum can be given intramuscularly. An intravenous injection may be indicated if a high concentration of serum antibody is imperative, such as occurs in the treatment of diphtheria. In these instances, a preliminary dose of 0.5 mL of serum should be diluted in 10 mL of either physiologic saline or 5% glucose solution. This preparation should be given as slowly as possible, and the patient should be observed for 30 minutes for reactions. If no reaction occurs, the remainder of the serum, diluted 1:20, may be given at a rate not to exceed 1 mL/min.

"Desensitization" for Animal Sera

Tables 6 and 7 serve as guides for the "desensitization" procedure for animal sera. Either the intravenous or the intradermal/subcutaneous/intramuscular routes may be chosen. The intravenous route is considered

---

*Antihistamines and decongestants may inhibit reactions in the scratch, prick, or puncture test; eye test; and intradermal allergic skin test. Hence, testing should not be done for at least 12 and preferably 24 hours after receipt of these drugs.

Table 6. "Desensitization" to Serum – Intravenous Route

Dose Number*	Dilution of Serum in Normal Saline	Amount of Injection (mL)
1	1:1,000	0.1
2	1:1,000	0.3
3	1:1,000	0.6
4	1:100	0.1
5	1:100	0.3
6	1:100	0.6
7	1:10	0.1
8	1:10	0.3
9	1:10	0.6
10	undiluted	0.1
11	undiluted	0.2
12	undiluted	0.6
13	undiluted	1.0

*Administer consistently at 15-minute intervals.

safest because it offers better control. The desensitization procedure should be performed by trained personnel familiar with the treatment of anaphylaxis and with appropriate drugs and equipment available, and in controlled conditions. Some physicians advocate the concurrent use of an oral or intramuscular antihistamine (such as diphenhydramine), with or without intravenously administered hydrocortisone or methylprednisolone. If signs of anaphylaxis occur during the procedure, aqueous epinephrine should be administered immediately (see Treatment of Anaphylactic Reactions, page 43). Administration of sera under the protection of a desensitization procedure must be continuous. Once administration is interrupted, protection from desensitization is lost.

Types of Reactions to Animal Serum

The following reactions can occur as the result of animal serum administration. The first two are not mediated by IgE antibodies and, therefore, are not predicted by prior skin testing.

- *Acute Febrile Reactions.* These reactions are usually mild and can be treated with antipyretics. Severe febrile reactions should be treated with antipyretics, tepid water sponge baths, or other available methods to reduce the temperature.
- *Serum Sickness.* Manifestations consist of fever, urticaria, or maculopapular rash (90% of cases); arthritis or arthralgia; and lymphadenopathy, which usually begin 7 to 10 days (occasionally as late as 2 to 3 weeks) after the primary exposure to the foreign protein. Local edema can occur at the serum injection site a few days before the systemic signs and symptoms appear. Angioedema, glomerulonephritis, Guillain-Barré syndrome, peripheral neuritis, and myocarditis can also occur. However, serum sickness may be

Table 7. "Desensitization" to Serum – Intradermal (ID), Subcutaneous (SC), and Intramuscular (IM) Routes

Dose Number*	Route of Administration	Dilution of Serum in Normal Saline	Amount of Injection (mL)
1	ID	1:1,000	0.1
2	ID	1:1,000	0.3
3	SC	1:1,000	0.6
4	SC	1:100	0.1
5	SC	1:100	0.3
6	SC	1:100	0.6
7	SC	1:10	0.1
8	SC	1:10	0.3
9	SC	1:10	0.6
10	SC	undiluted	0.1
11	SC	undiluted	0.2
12	IM	undiluted	0.6
13	IM	undiluted	1.0

*Administer consistently at 15-minute intervals.

mild and resolve spontaneously within a few days to 2 weeks. Persons who have previously received serum injections are at an increased risk after readministration; manifestations in these patients occur shortly (hours to 2 to 3 days) after administration of serum. Drugs that can be helpful in the management of serum sickness include antihistamines (e.g., hydroxyzine or diphenhydramine) for alleviation of pruritus, edema, and urticaria. Fever, malaise, arthralgia, and arthritis can be controlled in most patients by aspirin (30 to 60 mg/kg/d, in four divided doses; maximum single dose, 650 mg) or other anti-inflammatory agents. Corticosteroids may be helpful in controlling serious manifestations that are poorly alleviated by other treatment modalities. Prednisone in therapeutic doses for 7 days is an acceptable approach.

- *Anaphylaxis.* The rapidity of onset and the overall severity of anaphylaxis vary considerably. Usually anaphylaxis begins within minutes of exposure to the etiologic agent, and in general, the more rapid the onset the more severe the overall course. Major manifestations are the following: (1) cutaneous, including pruritus, flushing, urticaria, and angioedema; (2) respiratory, with hoarse voice and stridor, wheeze, dyspnea, and cyanosis; and (3) cardiovascular, with a rapid, weak pulse, hypotension, and arrhythmias. Anaphylaxis is a major medical emergency.

Treatment of Anaphylactic Reactions

Personnel administering biologic products or serum should be prepared to treat anaphylaxis. The necessary medications and equipment to support the patency of the airway and to manage cardiovascular

Table 8. Epinephrine (Adrenalin) in the Treatment of Anaphylaxis*

Subcutaneous or Intramuscular Administration

- Epinephrine 1:1,000 (aqueous): 0.01 mL/kg per dose repeated every 15 to 30 minutes. Usual dose:

  Infants: 0.05 to 0.1 mL
  Children: 0.1 to 0.3 mL

- Long-acting epinephrine suspension (Sus-Phrine): 0.005 mL/kg per dose as a single dose. The usual dose in infants and children is one half that of epinephrine 1:1,000 (see above). This medication should be given for more prolonged effect only after initial management.

Intravenous Administration

- 1 mg (1 mL) of 1:1,000 dilution of epinephrine added to 250 mL of 5% dextrose in water, resulting in a concentration of 4 µg/mL, is infused initially at a rate of 0.1 µg/kg/min, and increased gradually to 1.5 µg/kg/min to maintain blood pressure.

***Maintenance of an airway is critical,** in addition to administering epinephrine.

collapse must be immediately available. Staff should be competent in managing the situation properly.

The emergency treatment of anaphylactic reactions is based on the type of reaction. In all instances, epinephrine is the primary drug. Mild symptoms of pruritus, erythema, urticaria, and angioedema should be treated with epinephrine injected subcutaneously, followed by diphenhydramine, hydroxyzine, or other antihistamine given orally or parenterally (see Tables 8 and 9). Epinephrine administration may be repeated within 15 or 20 minutes in a dose equal to or slightly less than that given initially. If the patient improves with this management, a long-acting epinephrine injection should be given, and oral antihistamines should be taken for the next 24 hours (in three or four doses).

More severe and potentially life-threatening systemic anaphylaxis necessitates additional medications. In the treatment of severe bronchospasm, laryngeal edema, shock, and cardiovascular collapse, intravenous epinephrine may occasionally be indicated. It must always be diluted to 1:10,000 from the 1:1,000 aqueous base using physiologic saline (Table 8). A slow, continuous infusion is preferable to bolus administration. Intravenous aminophylline is indicated for bronchospasm (Table 8). Rapid intravenous infusion of physiologic saline solution or plasma expanders, adequate to maintain blood pressure,

Table 9. Dosages of Commonly Used Secondary Drugs in the Treatment of Anaphylaxis

Drug	Dose*
Antihistamines (H_1 blocking agents)	
Diphenhydramine	Oral, IM, IV: 1 mg/kg every 4-6 hours (50 mg max)
Hydroxyzine	Oral, IM: 10-25 mg every 4-6 hours
H_2 blocking agents (also antihistamines)	
Cimetidine	IV: 5 mg/kg slowly every 8 hours
Ranitidine	IV: 1 mg/kg slowly every 8 hours
Corticosteroids	
Hydrocortisone	IV: 100-200 mg every 4-6 hours
Methylprednisolone	IV: 20-40 mg every 4-6 hours
Prednisone	Oral daily ("burst") dose: 30, 25, 20, 15, 10, and 5 mg (i.e., daily decrease); entire dose given in the morning
Aminophylline	IV: 4-6 mg/kg in 20 mL saline by rapid drip every 6 h

*IM = intramuscular; IV = intravenous.

must be instituted to compensate for the loss of circulating blood volume that occurs.

In some cases, the use of an alpha-adrenergic pressor agent, such as dopamine 200 mg in 250 mL of saline given at a rate of 5 to 50 µg/kg/min, titrated to maintain blood pressure, may be necessary. The combination of H_1 and H_2 blocking agents (Table 9) can be synergistic in their effect and should be used. Airway maintenance measures and oxygen administration should be instituted promptly. Corticosteroids should probably be used in all cases of anaphylaxis except those that are mild and have responded promptly to therapy (Table 9). Corticosteroids do not exert an immediate effect, however, and should not be considered primary drugs.

All patients showing signs and symptoms of anaphylaxis, regardless of severity, should be observed for several hours. Biphasic and protracted anaphylaxis (5 to more than 24 hours) has occurred in spite of adequate initial management. Hence, even patients with apparent remissions of immediate symptoms need careful follow-up.

Anaphylaxis occurring in persons already taking beta-adrenergic blocking agents presents a unique situation. In such individuals, the manifestations are likely to be more profound and significantly less responsive to epinephrine and other beta-adrenergic agonist drugs. More aggressive therapy with epinephrine may be adequate to override the receptor blockade in some patients. The use of intravenous glucagon for cardiovascular manifestations and inhaled atropine for bronchospasm has also been recommended.

Immunization in Special Clinical Circumstances

Preterm Infants

Prematurely born infants should be immunized at the usual chronologic age, even if the infant was very small at birth. Those who had an intraventricular hemorrhage or other neurologic event soon after birth but are clinically stable at age 2 months should also be immunized. Vaccine doses should not be reduced for preterm infants. If an infant is still in the hospital at the time immunizations are scheduled, DTP and *Haemophilus* b conjugate vaccine (HbCV) should be given. To avoid transmission of oral polioviruses in the nursery, the OPV series should be initiated on discharge, or inactivated polio vaccine (IPV) can be given to an infant still in the hospital. The remaining doses of polio vaccine can be completed with OPV after discharge. If the infant is discharged at 2 months of age, DTP, HbCV, and OPV can be given on discharge.

Preterm infants exposed to a mother who is HBsAg-positive should receive HBIG at birth. Vaccine should be initiated as soon as feasible, and within the first month of life (see Hepatitis B, page 249).

Preterm infants who develop chronic respiratory disease should be given influenza immunization at 6 months of age. To protect these infants and those with other chronic conditions before this age, the family and other caretakers should be immunized against influenza (see Influenza, page 278).

Pregnancy

Pregnancy poses special theoretical risks. Although no evidence indicates that vaccines in use today have ill effects on the fetus, for medicolegal reasons pregnant women should receive vaccines only when urgently needed, and the use of vaccines for pregnant women should be limited to a few well-defined situations. The only vaccines routinely recommended for administration during pregnancy in the United States are those for tetanus and diphtheria, provided they are otherwise indicated (either for primary or booster immunization). Influenza immunization can be given if the pregnant woman has a chronic condition that would be adversely affected by this illness. Pregnancy is not a contraindication to hepatitis B vaccination in women for whom the vaccine is indicated. Although data on the safety of hepatitis B vaccines for the developing fetus are not available, no risk should exist because the vaccines contain only noninfectious hepatitis B surface antigen (HBsAg). In contrast, hepatitis B infection in a pregnant woman can result in severe disease in the mother and chronic infection in the newborn.

Pregnancy is a contraindication to administration of all live virus vaccines, except when susceptibility and exposure are highly probable and the disease to be prevented poses a greater threat to the woman or fetus than does the vaccine. Although no evidence for the theoretical risk to the fetus of a live virus vaccine exists, the background rate of anomalies in uncomplicated pregnancies might result in a defect that could be attributed to a vaccine; therefore, live vaccines should be avoided. However, live oral poliovirus vaccine (OPV) may be used if a pregnant woman is expected to have a substantial risk of imminent exposure to wild virus, such as in some circumstances of international travel. Alternatively, inactivated poliovirus vaccine (IPV) can be given if immunization can be completed prior to anticipated exposure. Yellow fever vaccine may be given to susceptible pregnant women who anticipate exposure during their pregnancy and whose travel to endemic areas cannot be postponed.

Vaccines producing severe febrile or systemic reactions can potentially disturb homeostasis, but no evidence indicates that commonly used, inactivated bacterial or viral vaccines have adverse effects on the mother or fetus. Tetanus toxoid is routinely used in pregnancy in areas with high incidence of neonatal tetanus, without evidence of adverse effects.

Efforts should be made to immunize susceptible women before they become pregnant, particularly against rubella, measles, and mumps.

Immunodeficient and Immunosuppressed Children

Experience with vaccine administration in immunodeficient or immunosuppressed children is limited. For many persons, and with most vaccines, theoretical considerations are the only guide because experience with the vaccine in patients with a specific disorder is lacking or because adverse consequences have not been reported. Although the contraindications and lack of efficacy of immunizations in these patients are emphasized in these guidelines, certain immunosuppressed children benefit from immunization with vaccines, such as *Haemophilus*, pneumococcal, meningococcal, and influenza vaccines, and indications for active immunization of the altered host are an important consideration.

Live bacterial and viral vaccines are contraindicated in patients with congenital disorders of immune function. Fatal poliomyelitis, vaccinia, and measles virus infections have occurred in children with these disorders after administration of live virus vaccines. If an inactivated vaccine is available for a given disease (e.g., IPV in poliomyelitis prophylaxis), it is usually preferable and should be administered. Children with deficiency in antibody-synthesizing capacity may be incapable of responding to vaccines; these children receive regular doses of immune globulin which provide passive protection against many infectious diseases. Immune globulins are available for postexposure prophylaxis for other infections (e.g., VZIG for varicella).

Immunologically normal siblings and other household contacts of persons with an immunologic deficiency should not receive oral poliovirus vaccine (OPV) because the vaccine strains are transmissible to the immunocompromised individual. However, these siblings and household contacts can receive live measles, rubella, and mumps vaccines because transmission of these vaccine viruses does not occur.

Inactivated vaccines are not a risk to immunocompromised persons, although their efficacy may be substantially reduced. The ability to develop a quantitatively normal immunologic response usually returns between 3 months and 1 year after discontinuing immunosuppressive therapy.

Because patients with congenital or acquired immunodeficiencies may not have an adequate response to immunizing agents, they may remain susceptible despite having received an appropriate vaccine. If feasible, specific serum antibody titers or other immunologic responses should be determined after immunization to assess immunity and to serve as a guide for management of future exposures and for immunizations.

For the child receiving immunosuppressive therapy, several factors are considered in immunization, including the underlying disease, the specific immunosuppressive regimen (its dose and schedule), and the infectious disease and immunization history of the patient. Live virus vaccines are generally contraindicated because the risk of serious adverse effects cannot be predicted. An exception to this rule appears to be the judicious and cautious use of the live varicella vaccine* in children with cancer, in whom the risk of natural varicella outweighs the risk from the attenuated vaccine virus.

Inactivated vaccines and immune globulins should be used when appropriate. The immune responses of immunosuppressed children to some inactivated vaccines can be inadequate (e.g., DTP and influenza). If possible, influenza vaccine should be given to children with malignancy 3 to 4 weeks after chemotherapy is discontinued and when they have peripheral granulocyte and lymphocyte counts greater than 1,000/mm^3.

Live virus vaccines should generally be administered no less than 3 months after all immunosuppressive therapy has been discontinued. This interval is based on the assumption that immunologic responsiveness

*Investigational vaccine at this time.

will have been restored in 3 months, and that the underlying disease for which the immunosuppressive therapy was given is in remission or under control. However, because the interval may vary with the intensity and type of immunosuppressive therapy, radiation therapy, underlying disease, and other factors, a definitive recommendation for an interval after cessation of immunosuppressive therapy when live virus vaccines can be safely and effectively administered is often not possible.

Patients with leukemia in remission whose chemotherapy has been terminated for at least 3 months may receive live virus vaccines for infections to which they are still susceptible (i.e., those diseases that the child neither had nor was vaccinated against before developing leukemia).

Corticosteroids. Children can become immunocompromised because of corticosteroid therapy. Patients treated with corticosteroids should be categorized as follows:

1. Previously healthy children who are on a short-term (less than 2 weeks), low to moderate, daily maintenance dose of systemic corticosteroids, or on a low or moderate dose, long-term, alternate-day treatment with short-acting systemic corticosteroids for a condition which, in itself, is not associated with a compromised immune system. These patients, who are receiving only maintenance physiologic doses of corticosteroids and who have no underlying immune defects, can receive live virus vaccines. Also, the administration of topical corticosteroids, either on the skin or in the respiratory system or eyes, and intra-articular, bursal, or tendon injections of steroids usually does not result in immunosuppression that would contraindicate live virus vaccines. However, live virus vaccines should be avoided if systemic immunosuppression results from prolonged topical application.
2. Healthy children treated with large amounts of systemic corticosteroids. The exact amount of systemic corticosteroids needed to suppress the immune response in an otherwise healthy child, and the duration of their administration, are not known at this time. However, children in this category should not be given live virus vaccines.
3. Children with a disease which, in itself, is considered to suppress the immune response and who are being treated with either systemic or locally administered corticosteroids. These children are at risk and should not be given live virus vaccine, except under special circumstances.

Hodgkin's Disease. Patients who are 24 months or older, including adults, should be immunized with pneumococcal vaccine. They should also receive *Haemophilus* b conjugate vaccine, according to age-specific recommendations. These patients are at increased risk for invasive pneumococcal infection; most experts believe that they are also at increased risk for invasive *Haemophilus influenzae* type b infection. The antibody response is likely to be best when patients are immunized at least 10 to 14 days before initiation of therapy for Hodgkin's disease. During active chemotherapy and shortly thereafter, the antibody responses to the pneumococcal and *Haemophilus* vaccines are impaired. However, the ability of these patients to respond improves rapidly, and immunization as early as 3 months after the cessation of chemotherapy is reasonable.

Transplant Recipients. A special situation is a child recovering from successful bone marrow transplantation. Many factors can affect the child's immunity to vaccine-preventable diseases, including the donor's immunity, type of transplant, interval since the transplant, receipt of immunosuppressive medications, and graft-versus-host disease (GVHD). Although many of these children acquire the immunity of the donor, some will lose serologic evidence of immunity. Consequently, some experts base the decision to reimmunize against diphtheria and tetanus on serologic titers against tetanus and diphtheria toxoids obtained 1 year after transplantation. Other experts reimmunize all children without serologic evaluation, and some obtain titers to determine the number of doses of diphtheria and tetanus toxoids that should be given. A recent study indicates that reimmunization with three doses of tetanus toxoid is necessary to achieve an adequate immune response. Data on which to base recommendations for reimmunization against *Haemophilus influenzae* type b are not available; until relevant information is available, considerations similar to those for other bacterial vaccines are applicable.

At 2 years after bone marrow transplant, MMR vaccine is often given, since recent data indicate that healthy survivors at that time can receive these live virus vaccines without untoward effects. However, patients with chronic GVHD should not receive MMR vaccine because of concern about resulting chronic latent virus infection that could lead to chronic central nervous system sequelae. A decision to immunize against polio should be based on the child's likelihood of exposure, as determined by reported cases of poliomyelitis in areas where the child resides or will be visiting. Serologic tests for antibody titers against polioviruses are not readily available in commercial or state laboratories. **Only inactivated polio vaccine (IPV) should be given to transplant recipients and their household contacts.**

Other vaccines that should be considered for the bone marrow recipient include pneumococcal and influenza. Data indicate that pneumococcal vaccine is not immunogenic in the first year after marrow transplantation in patients with chronic GVHD, but two or more years after transplantation, patients without GVHD do respond to this polysaccharide vaccine. Similarly, influenza immunization is not effective when given within the initial months after marrow transplantation but does appear to be effective when given later. Thus, vaccination against pneumococcal and influenza infection should be initiated between 12 and 24 months after transplantation.

Children who are scheduled to have a solid organ transplantation and who are older than 12 months should have serologic titers against measles, mumps, and rubella titers. Those who have negative titers should be given MMR vaccine before transplantation. The preferred time to give this vaccine is at least 1 month before transplantation. Measles antibody titers should be measured in all patients 1 and 2 years after transplantation. Information about the use of live virus vaccines in patients after solid organ transplantation is limited. The use of passive immunization with immunoglobulin (IG or IGIV) should be based on negative antibody titers and exposure to disease.

Because of the limited data on immunizations of transplant recipients, immunization schedules vary in different centers. Physicians managing these patients are encouraged to develop immunization protocols and schedules in conjunction with experts in infectious diseases and immunology.

HIV Infection (see also AIDS and HIV Infections, page 115). Data on the use of currently available live viral and bacterial (oral polio, measles, mumps, rubella, and BCG) vaccines in children who are known to be infected with the human immunodeficiency virus (HIV) are limited, but complications, to date, have been reported only after BCG vaccination. Because of reports of severe measles in symptomatic HIV-infected children, including fatalities, measles vaccination (given as MMR) is recommended for these children regardless of clinical status. In accordance with the usual schedule of childhood immunizations, the recommended age of administration is 15 months. If the risk of exposure is high, such as in a measles outbreak, the vaccine can be given at an earlier age (see Measles, page 321). Children with symptomatic HIV infection should receive DTP, influenza, *Haemophilus* b, and pneumococcal vaccines (see Table 22, page 125). **Inactivated polio vaccine (IPV) should be given in place of oral polio vaccine (OPV).** BCG is contraindicated in these patients in the United States. In areas with high incidence of tuberculosis, however, the World Health Organization recommends giving BCG to HIV-infected children who are not symptomatic.

Routine or widespread screening to detect asymptomatic HIV-infected children prior to routine immunization is not recommended. Children without clinical or epidemiologic manifestations of HIV infection should be immunized in accordance with the recommendations for routine childhood immunization.

Household contacts of an adult or child with proven or suspected HIV infection should not receive OPV, since the vaccine virus can spread from person to person, particularly in households. Although no cases of poliovirus vaccine-associated poliomyelitis have been reported, polio immunization of household contacts should be only with IPV,

Asplenic Children

The asplenic state results from the surgical removal of the spleen; from certain diseases, such as sickle-cell disease; or as a congenital asplenia. All asplenic infants, children, and adults, regardless of the reason for the asplenic state, have an increased risk for fulminant bacteremia, which is associated with a high mortality rate. Susceptibility to fulminant bacteremia is influenced considerably by the underlying disease. By comparison with healthy children who have not had splenectomy, the incidence of mortality from sepsis is increased 50-fold in children who have had splenectomy after trauma, approximately 350-fold in sickle-cell disease, and nearly 1,000-fold in thalassemia. The risk of bacteremia may be higher in younger than in older children, and during the initial years after splenectomy. However, long-term follow-up of asplenic children has not been sufficient to conclude that the risk declines substantially with increasing age and time since splenectomy. Fulminant bacteremia has been reported in adults as long as 25 years after splenectomy.

Streptococcus pneumoniae is the most frequent cause of bacteremia in the asplenic child. *Neisseria meningitidis*, *Haemophilus influenzae* type b, and *Escherichia coli* are also important pathogens in asplenic children. Less commonly, causes of bacteremia in these patients include streptococci, *Staphylococcus aureus*, and Gram-negative coliforms such as *Klebsiella* species, *Salmonella* species, and *Pseudomonas aeruginosa*. Persons with an asplenic state are also at increased risk of fatal malaria infections and severe babesiosis. Polyvalent pneumococcal vaccine is recommended for all asplenic children 2 years and older (see Pneumococcal Infections, page 376). Quadrivalent meningococcal polysaccharide vaccine (see Meningococcal Infections, page 326) should also be administered to asplenic children 2 years and older. Immunization against *H influenzae* type b infections should be initiated in infancy, as recommended for otherwise healthy children. Polyvalent pneumococcal vaccine appears to be of value in reducing the risk of fulminant pneumococcal bacteremia in asplenic children. The efficacy of meningococcal and *Haemophilus* vaccines in asplenic children is not certain, although these vaccines are probably as effective as pneumococcal vaccine. No known contraindication exists to giving these vaccines at the same time in separate syringes at different sites.

Daily antimicrobial prophylaxis is also recommended for many asplenic children, irrespective of vaccination status. For infants with sickle-cell disease, oral penicillin prophylaxis against invasive pneumococcal disease should be initiated before 4 months of age (see Pneumococcal Infection, Chemoprophylaxis, page 378). This recommendation is based on a multicenter study demonstrating that oral penicillin V (125 mg twice daily) given to children with sickle-cell disease reduced the incidence of severe bacterial infection by 84% in comparison to that in placebo-treated children. In an earlier study, monthly intramuscular benzathine penicillin tended to lower the number of episodes of pneumococcal bacteremia in children with sickle-cell disease in comparison to children who did not receive penicillin.

Although the efficacy of antimicrobial prophylaxis has been proven only in patients with sickle cell disease, substantial agreement exists that asplenic children with malignancies, thalassemia, and other diseases with particularly high risk for fulminant bacteremia should receive daily chemoprophylaxis; less agreement exists about the need in children who have had splenectomy after trauma. In general, antimicrobial prophylaxis (in addition to vaccination) should be strongly considered for asplenic children younger than 5 years and considered for older children. Some experts continue prophylaxis throughout childhood and in adulthood in particularly high-risk patients with asplenia. The age at which prophylaxis is discontinued in individual patients is an empirical decision, as no studies of this question have been performed.

For antimicrobial prophylaxis, oral penicillin V (125 mg twice daily for children younger than 5 years and 250 mg twice daily for children 5 years and older) is usually recommended. Some experts have recommended amoxicillin (20 mg/kg/d) or trimethoprim-sulfamethoxazole (4 mg to 20 mg/kg/d) for children younger than 5 years.

When antimicrobial prophylaxis is used, its limitations must be stressed to parents and patients; they should recognize that some bacteria, which can cause fulminant bacteremia, are not susceptible to the antimicrobials given for prophylaxis. In all situations, and particularly when continuous prophylaxis is not used, parents should be aware that all febrile illnesses are potentially serious, and that immediate medical attention should be sought because the initial signs and symptoms of fulminant bacteremia can be subtle. When bacteremia is a possibility, the physician should hospitalize the child, obtain samples of blood (and cerebrospinal fluid or other body fluids as indicated) for culture, and immediately treat with intravenous ceftriaxone, cefotaxime, or another antimicrobial regimen effective against *S pneumoniae*, *H influenzae*, and *N meningitidis*. In some clinical situations, other antibiotics such as aminoglycosides may be indicated.

Whenever possible, alternatives to splenectomy should be considered. These include postponement of splenectomy for as long as possible in congenital hemolytic anemias, preservation of accessory spleens and hemisplenectomy during staging for Hodgkin's disease, performance of partial splenectomy for benign tumors of the spleen, and repair rather than removal in traumatic lacerations of the spleen.

Children With Personal or Family History of Seizures

Infants and children with personal and family history of convulsions are at increased risk of having a convulsion after receipt of either pertussis (as DTP) or measles (usually as MMR) vaccine. In most cases, these seizures are brief, self limited, and generalized, and occur in conjunction with fever. These characteristics indicate that such vaccine-associated seizures are usually febrile convulsions. No evidence indicates that these seizures (1) cause permanent brain damage or epilepsy, (2) aggravate neurologic disorders, or (3) affect the prognosis in children with underlying disorders.

In the case of pertussis immunization during infancy, however, administration of DTP may coincide with or hasten the recognition of an inevitable disorder associated with seizures, such as infantile spasms or epilepsy, and cause confusion about the role of pertussis vaccination. Hence, pertussis immunization in infants with recent seizures should be deferred until a progressive neurologic disorder is excluded or the cause of the earlier seizure has been diagnosed. In contrast, measles immunization is given at an age when the cause and nature of the recent convulsion and the child's neurologic status are more likely to be established. This difference and the risk of natural measles provide the basis for the recommendation that measles immunization should not be deferred in children with personal history of one or more convulsions.

A family history of convulsive disorders is not a contraindication to immunization with DTP or measles vaccine, or a reason to defer immunization. Postvaccination seizures in these children are usually febrile in origin, have a generally benign outcome, and are not likely to be confused with manifestations of a previously unrecognized neurologic disorder. In addition, many children have family history of convulsion and would remain susceptible to pertussis and measles if family history were a contraindication to immunization.

Parents whose children may be at increased risk of a seizure after pertussis or measles immunization, either from personal or family history of convulsions, should be informed of the risks and benefits of these immunizations in these circumstances. Advice should be provided about appropriate medical care in the unlikely event of a seizure. Infants and children with personal or family history of convulsive disorders may benefit from antipyretic prophylaxis, especially in the case of DTP immunization.

Additional discussion and recommendations for pertussis and measles immunization of children with personal or family history of convulsions is given in the chapters on measles (see page 320) and pertussis (see page 367). Detailed discussion and recommendations are also provided on pertussis immunization of children with neurologic disorders (see page 368).

Children With Chronic Diseases

Some chronic diseases render children more susceptible to the severe manifestations and complications of common infections. In general, immunizations recommended for healthy children should be given to children with these disorders. However, for children with immunologic disorders, live vaccines are usually contraindicated; exceptions include children with HIV infection (see Immunodeficient and Immunosuppressed Children, page 51). Children with certain chronic diseases (e.g., cardiorespiratory, allergic, hematologic, metabolic, and renal disorders, and cystic fibrosis) may be more susceptible to complications of influenza and pneumococcal infection and should receive influenza and/or pneumococcal vaccines (see Influenza, page 278, and Pneumococcal Infections, page 376).

The appropriateness of administering a live virus vaccine to a specific child with a rare disorder (e.g., galactosemia or renal tubular acidosis) is problematic. The experience in some of these disorders is minimal or nonexistent, and the physician should seek guidance from experts before administering the vaccine(s).

Active Immunization After Exposure to Disease

Since not all susceptible persons receive vaccines before exposure, active immunization in an individual who has been exposed to a specific disease is a consideration in some instances. The following situations are most commonly encountered (see also the chapters on the specific disease in Part 3 for details):

Rabies. Except for those with anticipated high exposure (e.g., veterinarians and animal handlers) who may receive preexposure rabies immunization, postexposure immunization is an essential feature of the immunoprophylaxis of rabies. Most rabies exposures occur because of unanticipated animal contact (bite, scratch, or mucosal contamination). In an unimmunized individual, Rabies Immune Globulin (RIG) (Human) and rabies vaccine should be administered as appropriate for the circumstances of the exposure.

Measles. Live measles virus vaccine given within 72 hours of exposure can be effective in preventing measles because immunity induced by parenterally administered live measles virus vaccine appears more rapidly than that induced by natural measles. Infected individuals can spread measles virus for 3 to 5 days before the appearance of a rash (and 1 to 2 days before the onset of symptoms). Thus, those in continuous contact with such individuals, as in households, day care, and school settings, would have been exposed before the appearance of clinical manifestations.

Measles morbidity is high in children younger than 1 year. Infants (i.e., those younger than 12 months) who have been exposed should receive a preventive dose of IG (0.25 mL/kg) within 6 days; subsequently, when 15 months old, they should receive live measles virus vaccine. Older susceptible children who have been exposed should receive IG between 3 and 7 days after exposure, and then receive live measles virus vaccine 3 months later. Exposed immunodeficient or immunocompromised individuals should receive 0.5 mL/kg of IG (maximal dose, 15 mL); live measles virus vaccine should not be administered subsequently (except in the case of HIV-infected children; see AIDS and HIV Infections, page 124).

Mumps. Exposed susceptible persons are not necessarily protected by postexposure live virus vaccine administration. However, a common practice in mumps exposure is to administer live mumps virus vaccine to presumed susceptible persons so that if mumps does not occur as a result of the current exposure, permanent immunity will be afforded by the immunization. Administration of live mumps virus vaccine is recommended for exposed adults born after 1956 who have not previously had mumps or mumps vaccination.

Rubella. Although rubella may be modified by IG, the benefits are so questionable that IG administration is not recommended for children. Pregnant women exposed to rubella who are presumed or proven to be susceptible and who choose not to undergo therapeutic abortion may be given IG, but congenital rubella can still occur. Postexposure rubella vaccination is not known to be effective.

Hepatitis B. Postexposure vaccination is highly effective if combined with passive antibody. Administration of Hepatitis B Immune Globulin (HBIG) does not inhibit active immunization with the hepatitis B vaccine. For postexposure prophylaxis in an infant whose mother carries hepatitis B surface antigen (HBsAg), hepatitis B vaccination combined with HBIG is essential. For accidental percutaneous or mucosal exposure to HBsAg, combined active and passive immunization is recommended. Children with continuing household contact with a HBsAg carrier should also be vaccinated.

Tetanus. In wound management, the use of Tetanus Immune Globulin (TIG) depends on the nature of the wound and the immunization history of the individual. In addition, unimmunized or incompletely immunized individuals should be given tetanus toxoid immediately (Td, DT, or DTP); the type of vaccine will depend on the patient's age.

Children in Residential Institutions

Children housed together in institutions pose special problems for control of certain infectious diseases. Ensuring appropriate immunization of these children is important because of the risk of transmission within the facility and because the conditions that led to institutionalization may increase the risk of complications from the disease. All children entering a residential institution should have received appropriate routine immunizations for their age; if they have not, arrangements should be made to complete these immunizations as rapidly as possible. Employees should be familiar with procedures for handling contaminated blood and body fluids and accidents involving these fluids, and should be aware of children infected with hepatitis B virus in order to ensure prompt and appropriate management in such circumstances. Specific diseases of concern include the following (see chapters on specific diseases in Part 3 for details):

Measles. Epidemics can occur among susceptible children in institutional settings. Recommendations for managing children in an institutional setting when a case of measles is recognized are as follows: (1) administer live measles virus vaccine immediately to all susceptible children 1 year or older, and (2) administer immune globulin (IG) (0.25 mL/kg, or 0.5 mL/kg for immunocompromised children, 15 mL maximum dose) as soon as possible to all exposed, susceptible children younger than 1 year. These IG recipients will still require live measles virus vaccine at age 15 months.

Mumps. Epidemics may occur among susceptible, nonimmunized children in institutions. The major hazards are disruption of activities and the need for acute nursing care in difficult settings. The occasional serious complication is a hazard for the child and the susceptible adult attendant.

If mumps is introduced into a setting where susceptible persons reside, no prophylaxis is available to limit the spread or modify the disease in an individual. IG is not effective. Although mumps virus vaccine may not be effective after exposure, the vaccine should be administered to susceptible persons to protect against future exposures.

Influenza. This illness can be devastating in a residential or custodial institutional setting. Rapid spread, intensive exposure, and underlying disease may all result in a high risk for severe disease that may affect many residents simultaneously or in close sequence. Current measures useful for control of influenza in institutions include an immunization program with the current influenza vaccine, timed to provide immunity well in advance of possible exposure, and appropriate use of amantadine during influenza A epidemics. Amantadine is not effective in preventing influenza B infection. In considering the use of amantadine, the physician can often obtain information on which strains of influenza are prevalent in the community from local and state health departments.

Pertussis. Since progressive developmental delay is an indication for deferral of pertussis immunization, some children in an institutional setting may not be immunized against pertussis. If pertussis is recognized, patients should be treated with erythromycin, and close contacts of infected patients should receive chemoprophylaxis with erythromycin.

Hepatitis A Virus (HAV). Infection may be a threat to residents and attendants if fecal-oral spread is likely. Symptomatic HAV infection in infants is infrequent. In custodial institutions (e.g., facilities for the developmentally disabled or jails), HAV infection may be readily transmitted. If an outbreak occurs, residents and staff members in close personal contact with patients should receive 0.02 mL/kg of IG.

Hepatitis B. Children living in residential institutions and their caretakers are assumed to be at increased risk of acquiring hepatitis B infection. The high prevalence of hepatitis B virus (HBV) markers among children living in residential institutions for the mentally retarded indicates that HBV infections have the propensity for spread in an institutional setting, presumably by exposure to fluids containing HBV. Factors that can be associated with high prevalence of HBV markers include crowding, high staff-client ratios, and lack of in-service educational programs for the staff. In the presence of such factors, the prevalence of HBV increases with the duration of time spent at the institution. Thus, individuals entering custodial institutions should receive HBV vaccine; screening for HBV markers is probably not cost effective since the prevalence of markers will be low.

After parenteral or sexual exposure to an institutionalized patient recognized to be a hepatitis B surface antigen (HBsAg) carrier, unimmunized, susceptible attendees and/or staff should receive immunoprophylaxis, as described in the section on hepatitis B (page 243).

Haemophilus influenzae type b Infections. These infections can spread within institutions. In outbreaks involving two or more cases, rifampin chemoprophylaxis is indicated. The *Haemophilus* b conjugate vaccine (HbCV) is recommended for routine use for children 2 to 59 months of age.

Varicella. This disease is highly contagious and can occur in a high percentage of susceptible children in an institutional setting. No prophylactic measures are currently recommended unless susceptible children with an underlying disease, rendering them prone to serious complications or death, are exposed. Administration of Varicella-Zoster Immune Globulin (VZIG) is warranted for such high-risk individuals. The availability of varicella vaccine in the future should decrease the need for VZIG.

Other infections that spread in institutions and for which no immunization is currently available include *Shigella*, *Streptococcus pyogenes*, *Staphylococcus aureus*, respiratory viruses, rotaviruses, cytomegalovirus, *Giardia lamblia*, scabies, and lice.

Children in Military Populations

In general, children of active-duty military personnel require the same immunizations as their civilian counterparts. If delay in pertussis immunization is recommended for any reason, parents should be warned that the risk of contracting the disease in countries where pertussis immunization is not routinely given is significantly higher than that in countries where effective vaccine is used. For military dependents going overseas, the risk of exposure to hepatitis B, measles, polio, and rubella may be increased and necessitate additional immunizations. In these instances, the choice of immunizations will be dictated by the country of proposed residence, expected travel and residence, and the age and health of the child. Information on the risk of specific diseases in different countries and preventive measures is provided in the yearly publication of the U.S. Public Health Service, *Health Information for International Travel* (see page 8).

Children susceptible to adverse effects of vaccinia virus (e.g., eczema, immunodeficiency) should be identified and measures taken to avoid contact with their active-duty family members who have active vaccinia lesions. As of 1990, some active-duty United States military personnel were still receiving smallpox vaccine.

Adolescents and College Populations

Teenagers and young adults are the orphans of immunization practices. Reared in an era when new vaccines were introduced and unevenly administered, this group includes individuals who escaped natural infection and who (1) were not immunized with some or all of the recommended vaccines; (2) received relatively ineffective vaccines (e.g., killed measles virus vaccine); (3) received appropriate vaccines but at too young an age (e.g., live measles virus vaccine before 12 months); (4) received incomplete immunization regimens (e.g., only one dose or type of OPV, or incomplete IPV or DTP); or (5) received vaccine by an inappropriate method (e.g., immune globulin mixed in the same syringe with live measles virus vaccine).

Colleges and universities have become major foci of measles outbreaks, impeding efforts to eliminate this disease from the United States. Undue morbidity and cost can continue to result from this situation until an immune cohort enters college. The American College Health Association recommends that colleges and universities implement a Prematriculation Immunization Requirement whereby students are required to present evidence of immunity to measles and other vaccine-preventable diseases as a condition for matriculation. Accordingly, school and college health services should establish a system to obtain immunization histories and to give necessary immunizations as a part of student health services to ensure that all students are protected against measles, mumps, rubella, tetanus, and diphtheria. Documentation of two doses of measles vaccine (preferably as MMR) and appropriate poliovirus vaccine should be required before freshman matriculation, and if it is not available, school health services should be prepared to give immunizations. Epidemic foci of contagious diseases should be identified rapidly by encouraging early reporting and alerting health personnel to the probable occurrence of diseases such as measles, mumps, rubella, and influenza in a school or college.

School immunization laws encourage "catch-up" programs for older adolescents, and many colleges are implementing the American College Health Association recommendations for protection from measles, mumps, rubella, tetanus, diphtheria, and poliovirus. Unfortunately, histories are frequently unreliable, uncertain, or vague, particularly in the teenager or young adult. Physicians should adopt a procedure for systematic assessment of the immunization records of adolescents under their care and provide appropriate immunization. Immunization of adolescent entrants into a practice should have a high priority. The physician should be especially alert to the rubella immunization status of preadolescent girls so that they can be immunized before becoming sexually active. Rubella vaccine should be combined with measles and mumps if the adolescent has received only one prior dose of the latter antigens. Hepatitis B vaccination is recommended for sexually active heterosexuals with multiple sexual partners, those who have had a recent sexually transmitted disease, homosexually active male adolescents, and intravenous drug users (see Hepatitis B, page 246). Td (adult-type tetanus and diphtheria toxoids) should be given if 10 years have elapsed since the last DT, Td, or DTP administration.

Epidemic and endemic influenza can affect any closed population. Physicians responsible for health care in schools and colleges should implement appropriate influenza immunization policies.

Because adolescents and young adults can acquire measles during international travel, immunity against measles in school- and college-aged persons before travel abroad is important (see Foreign Travel, page 64). Unvaccinated individuals 18 years or older should receive inactivated poliovirus vaccine (IPV) if poliovirus protection is necessary for travel and sufficient time is available to induce an immune response (see Poliovirus Infections, page 386). Administration of live poliovirus vaccine (OPV) is generally not recommended in adults, except those who will soon (in less than 4 weeks) be exposed to poliovirus in endemic areas. Those adults can receive a single dose of either OPV or IPV. OPV or IPV can be administered to adults who have previously received a primary course of either polio vaccine and who require an additional dose of vaccine because of increased risk of exposure (e.g., travel to endemic areas).

Pediatricians should assist in distributing information on childhood diseases and immunization to other physicians and health care practitioners caring for adolescents in their communities. Some physicians are unaware of the risks of these diseases in adolescents and young adults, and are not familiar with, or do not give priority to immunization procedures. The pediatrician should take an active role in staff meetings and conferences; in local, state, and regional meetings; and in working with local and state health agencies to heighten awareness of the problem and the need for control measures.

Health Care Professionals

Adults whose occupations place them in contact with patients with contagious diseases are at increased risk of contracting these diseases and, if infected, of transmitting them to their patients. Health care personnel, including physicians, nurses, students, and auxiliary personnel, should protect themselves and susceptible patients by receiving appropriate immunizations, following the usual guidelines for each disease and vaccine. Physicians should play a major role in implementing these policies. Infections of special concern to those involved in the care of children include the following (see the specific diseases in Part 3 for details).

Rubella. Outbreaks of rubella among health care workers have been reported. Although the disease is mild in adults, the risk to the fetus necessitates documentation of rubella immunity in hospital personnel of both sexes. Individuals for whom the risk of rubella infection is heightened include hospital workers in obstetrics and pediatrics, physicians and nurses working in pediatric and obstetric offices and clinics, and all those working in health care areas in which pregnant women are encountered. Persons should be considered immune only on the basis of serologic tests or documented proof of live rubella virus immunization; history is unreliable and should not be used in judging immune status. All susceptible individuals should be immunized with live rubella virus vaccine prior to initial or continuing contact with pregnant patients.

Measles. The ranks of health professionals now and in the immediate future include a proportion of young adults susceptible to measles. Proof of immunity should be established by physician-documented illness, a positive serologic test for antibody, or documented receipt of live measles virus vaccine on or after the first birthday for all health professionals born after January 1, 1957. Physicians should be aware of the requirement of a second dose of measles vaccine for health care workers in hospitals.

Hepatitis B. Personnel who come in frequent contact with blood, such as laboratory workers or emergency room personnel, are at risk for acquiring hepatitis B. Hepatitis B vaccine is recommended for all health care personnel (including physicians) who are likely to be exposed to the blood of hepatitis B surface antigen (HBsAg) carriers. Among physicians caring for children, 10% to 20% have evidence of prior hepatitis B infection.

Influenza. Certain groups of patients, such as those with chronic cardiovascular or pulmonary disease, are at high risk for serious or complicated influenza infection. Because medical personnel can transmit influenza to their patients, and because nosocomial outbreaks can occur, influenza immunization programs for hospital workers and other health care professionals should be organized each fall. Infants younger than 6 months cannot be protected by immunization; therefore, vaccination of personnel working in nurseries and infant wards is highly advised.

Varicella. The virus can spread readily in hospitals, and varicella can be a devastating disease in immunosuppressed children or in adults. To facilitate varicella infection control, some experts advise that immune status to varicella should be determined on all patient-care hospital personnel with negative histories of disease (see Varicella-Zoster Infections, page 519). A minority of these persons will be seronegative. If a patient with varicella or zoster is admitted, previously identified susceptible personnel can be excluded from contact. When a licensed varicella vaccine becomes available, immunization of susceptible personnel should be possible.

Refugees

Prevention of infectious diseases in refugee children presents special problems because of the diseases to which these children have been exposed and the immunization practices unique to their native countries. Whereas most of these children will be free of contagious diseases, certain infections are more common in refugees than in residents of the United States (see Table 19, page 110).

Experience with the thousands of southeast Asian refugees who have resettled in the United States illustrates the generic issues of refugees. Usually these children who come from refugee camps will have received DTP, OPV, and MMR vaccines as appropriate for their ages before entry into the United States. However, some children may not have been completely immunized before arrival. For these children, OPV, DTP (or DT or Td), MMR, and *Haemophilus* b conjugate vaccines should be administered simultaneously, as indicated for their ages, particularly when follow-up care is likely to be disrupted by relocation.

Tuberculosis is the most important public health problem of southeast Asian refugees. Approximately 1% to 2% of refugees have had active tuberculosis on entry into the United States, and about half the refugees have positive tuberculin skin tests. The number who have received BCG vaccination is unknown. All refugee children should be skin tested with tuberculin at the time of the first visit and 3 months later to identify recently acquired infection. Prior BCG vaccination is not a contraindication to skin testing, although a vaccinated individual may have a positive tuberculin skin test. However, since tuberculin hypersensitivity due to BCG is neither great nor persistent, a positive skin test should not be attributed to BCG except in unusual circumstances (see Tuberculosis, page 506). A chest roentgenogram is usually indicated if the skin test is positive in BCG-vaccinated infants or children.

The physician should be aware of the presence of tuberculosis in refugee families and resulting disease classification (Class A or B) as identified by immigration authorities. Before entry into the United States, refugees with active or suspected active tuberculosis (Class A) are supposed to receive treatment until their disease is no longer contagious. Refugees with inactive tuberculosis (Class B) are referred for medical evaluation on arrival in the United States. Medical examination forms must specify if the individual has Class A or Class B disease, give the results of roentgenographic and bacteriologic studies, and detail the treatment. This information is provided to the local health department and the refugee. Bacteriologic studies should be performed in the United States as part of the medical evaluation of children with tuberculosis. Management of tuberculosis in southeast Asian refugees necessitates anticipation of drug resistance (see Tuberculosis, page 497).

Malaria should be suspected in refugees with fever, chills, headache, anemia, or splenomegaly. The diagnosis is made by identification of the parasite in blood smears. Parasitemia almost always accompanies a clinical attack of malaria, but malaria can also occur in the absence of significant symptoms. Chloroquine-resistant *Plasmodium falciparum* malaria is endemic in Southeast Asia, so alternative drug regimens are indicated for ill patients from this area with suspected *P falciparum* malaria (see Malaria, page 302).

Enteric helminths and protozoa are common intestinal parasites in southeast Asian and other refugees. Infections with these parasites do not present a significant public health hazard as adequate sewage disposal interrupts helminth transmission, and adequate hygienic practices minimize the risk of transmission of protozoa.

The prevalence of hepatitis B surface antigen (HBsAg) carriers in eastern Asian refugees is estimated to be 10% to 15%. Most of these persons are asymptomatic, and transmission can be limited by appropriate hygienic practices and administration of hepatitis B vaccine to susceptible household contacts. Screening of pregnant refugee women is particularly important for the prevention of perinatal transmission. The newborn infant of a carrier mother should be given Hepatitis B Immune Globulin (HBIG) promptly after birth (preferably in the delivery room), followed by the first dose of hepatitis B vaccine before discharge (see

Hepatitis B, page 249). Arrangements should be made to ensure completion of the three-dose vaccine series.

Most recently, universal hepatitis B vaccination of infants living in areas in which infection is highly endemic has been recommended. Refugees from endemic areas, particularly eastern Asia and Africa, should be serologically screened for HBsAg; if a carrier is found, all susceptible household contacts should be vaccinated. Even if no carriers are found within a family, vaccination should be considered for susceptible children younger than 7 years. Spread of this infection has been documented without the presence of a known carrier in the family.

Typhoid fever is relatively common in Southeast Asia. Some 3% to 5% of infected individuals become stool carriers and are potential sources of imported disease, particularly within their families. Because *Salmonella typhi* from Southeast Asia may be resistant to chloramphenicol and/or ampicillin, trimethoprim-sulfamethoxazole should be used for initial therapy until in vitro antimicrobial susceptibility test results are available.

Melioidosis, caused by *Pseudomonas pseudomallei*, is endemic in Southeast Asia. The disease may present as a localized suppurative infection, acute or chronic pulmonary disease, or fulminating septicemia. Most often melioidosis simulates pulmonary tuberculosis, with a long latent period and a chronic course.

Foreign Travel

The best source for comprehensive information is the annually revised booklet *Health Information for International Travel* (see page 8). The Centers for Disease Control (CDC) also publishes throughout the year the *Summary of Health Information*, the "blue sheet," which lists areas infected with yellow fever and cholera, and outlines changes in the official recommendations for entry to certain countries. Local and state health departments can be consulted for updated information prior to travel. Information is also available from CDC through the Disease Information Hotline (404/639-1610).

Special attention should be given to ensure that infants and children embarking on international travel receive routine immunizations appropriate for their ages. Some immunizations may have to be given at an accelerated rate before departure to ensure immunity (see Tables 2 and 3, pages 17 and 18). Infants 6 to 15 months traveling to geographic areas where polio is endemic should receive a third dose of OPV before departure. Depending on destination and length of stay, required or recommended travel immunizations can include vaccines against yellow fever, cholera, meningococcal disease, typhoid, and hepatitis B. Health authorities at the destination should be consulted if a prolonged stay is contemplated.

Table 10. Recommendations for Travelers to Developing Countries*

Preventive Measures	Length of Travel†		
	Brief (< 2 wk)	Intermediate (2 wk to 3 mo)	Long-Term Residential (> 3 mo)
Immunizations			
Routine review and update	+	+	+
DTP and OPV given at shorter intervals‡ than routinely recommended	+	+	+
OPV: extra dose given if 6 to 14 months old	+	+	+
Measles: extra dose given if 6 to 11 months old	±	+	+
Hepatitis B	–	±	+
Typhoid fever	–§	±§	+
Yellow fever‖	+	+	+
Cholera¶	–	–	–
Japanese encephalitis**	–	±	+
Rabies	–††	–††	+
Immune globulin for hepatitis A	–§	0.02 mL/kg	0.06 mL/kg every 5 mo.
Chemoprophylaxis for malaria#	+	+	+

*See specific disease chapters in Part 3 for details. Also, for further information, call CDC (404/639-1610).

† " + " = recommended; " ± " = consider; " – " = not recommended.

‡DTP and OPV can be given at 4- and 6-week intervals, respectively, to accelerate completion of schedule.

§Indicated for travelers who will consume food at nontourist facilities.

‖For endemic regions of Africa and South Africa (see *Health Information for International Travel*, page 8).

¶See *Health Information for International Travel* (page 8) for country requirements. One dose or a medical exemption letter will satisfy entry requirements in most countries.

**Not currently available in U.S. Vaccine is available in endemic Asian countries for individuals who will be in rural areas.

††Rabies vaccine may be indicated for individuals with high risk of wild animal exposure and for spelunkers.

#See Malaria (page 305) and *Health Information for International Travel* (page 8) for recommendations for specific countries.

Some cases of measles in the United States result from exposure to the disease in foreign countries, so persons traveling abroad should be immune to measles (see Measles, page 315). Unless a contraindication exists, consideration should be given to providing a dose of measles vaccine for all persons born after 1956 traveling abroad who have not already received two doses of vaccine or have no other proof of immunity. For children traveling to areas in which measles is present, the age for measles vaccination should be lowered. Infants 6 to 11 months should receive a dose of monovalent measles; those 12 to 14 months should receive MMR prior to departure. MMR should be given at 15 months to those vaccinated before 12 months.

Recommendations for prophylaxis of infection for travelers to developing countries are listed in Table 10 (see specific disease chapters in Part 3 for details). Of all the diseases, malaria is probably the greatest threat. Prophylaxis requires taking daily or weekly doses of antimalarial drugs (see Malaria, page 305). Immune globulin may be indicated to prevent hepatitis A if food and water will be consumed in nontourist facilities or extended periods of travel are planned. Hepatitis B vaccine is indicated for persons who will reside for more than 6 months in areas in which the infection is highly endemic and who will have close contact with the local population; it should also be considered for short-term travelers who are likely to have contact with blood, or sexual contact with residents of these areas. Rabies immunization should be considered if children will be living in areas where they may encounter rabid animals. Preventive measures for yellow fever (vaccination) and dengue (prevention of mosquito bites) should be recommended for travel to those areas where these diseases are present. The currently available cholera vaccine has limited prophylactic value, but the vaccine or a letter documenting medical exemption may be required to allow entry to certain countries. Typhoid vaccine should be given only to those who expect to consume food and water at nontourist facilities and to children who will reside in endemic areas. A new oral typhoid vaccine is now available (see Salmonellosis, page 421). Meningococcal C vaccine should be considered for travelers to endemic areas in central Africa and Brazil and in countries with current meningococcal A or C epidemics.

Prevention of mosquito bites is important in minimizing the risk of dengue and malaria. Wearing long-sleeved cotton clothing, the use of screens and bednets, and judicious use of repellents are appropriate in high-risk areas.

Traveler's diarrhea is a significant problem that may be mitigated by attention to the foods and beverages ingested. Chemoprophylaxis is not recommended for general use, but provision of an antibiotic for the treatment of traveler's diarrhea is a useful precaution (see *Escherichia coli* Diarrhea, page 207). Giardiasis is common in some areas.

PART 2

RECOMMENDATIONS FOR CARE OF CHILDREN IN SPECIAL CIRCUMSTANCES

Children in Day Care*

Infants and young children who are brought together in groups for care have a potential for exposure to infectious disease agents analogous to that of a large family. Prevention and control of infection in out-of-home child care settings is influenced by the caregivers' practice of personal hygiene and environmental sanitation, food handling procedures, the ages of the children, the ratio of children to caregiver, and the physical space and quality of the facilities.

Public health agencies alone cannot provide all the services needed to ensure infectious disease prevention and control in child care, and licensing agencies are often ill-equipped to provide solutions. To adequately address the problems of infection control in child care settings requires the collaborative efforts of public health officials, licensing agencies, child caregivers, physicians, nurses, parents, and employers.

Child care programs should require that all children receive needed immunizations and routine health care. Many of these programs give young, inexperienced parents day-to-day instruction in child development, hygiene, appropriate nutrition, and management of minor illnesses.

Classification of Care Service

Child care services are commonly classified by the type of setting, the number of children in care, age of the children, and their health status. **Family child care** is out-of-home care provided in a private residence where a homemaker cares for a small number of unrelated children. These programs usually provide care only for well children. **Group child**

*This section is based on the recommendations formulated by a joint committee of the American Academy of Pediatrics (AAP) and the American Public Health Association (APHA). The recommendations will be included in the national standards for out-of-home child care programs developed by the AAP/APHA joint project and will be published in 1991.

care is also provided in a private residence and consists of seven to 12 children. These programs usually provide care only for well children. **Center child care** is provided in a nonresidential facility to 13 or more children in a part-day or full-day program. These programs may be structured to provide care for well and for mildly ill children. **Sick child care** describes specialized programs designed to provide care for mildly ill children who are excluded from regular child care programs. All 50 states license out-of-home child care; however, licensing is directed toward center-based child care; few states or municipalities license family, group, or sick child care programs.

When children are grouped by age, these age groupings are **infant** (birth to 12 months), **toddler** (13 to 35 months), **preschooler** (36 to 59 months), and **school-aged** (5 to 12 years).

Infants and young children require diapering or assistance in toileting, they explore the environment with their mouths, and they are careless about their secretions. Therefore, day care programs that provide infant and toddler care need to give special attention to measures for infection control.

Management and Prevention of Illness

The major pathogens that potentially can be transmitted within child care settings are listed in Table 11. Studies are in progress to evaluate the specific characteristics or practices that promote or inhibit transmission of infection. In most instances, the risk of introducing a particular infectious agent into a child care group is directly related to its prevalence in the population and to the number of susceptible children in that group. Transmission of the agent within the group depends partly on its characteristics, such as mode of spread, infective dose, and survival in the environment; the frequency of unrecognized, asymptomatic infection or carrier state; and immunity to the respective pathogen. Transmission can also be affected by characteristics of the child care center, particularly hygienic aspects of child handling, environmental practices, and ages of the children in the group. Infected children in a child care group can subsequently transmit infection not only within the group but also within their households and the community.

The major options for management of ill or infected children in child care and for controlling spread of infection include antimicrobial treatment or prophylaxis when available, exclusion of the ill or infected child from the facility, provision of alternative care at a separate site, cohorting (i.e., inclusion of infected children in a group with separate staff and facilities), and, rarely, closing the facility. Specific recommendations for control of the spread of specific infectious agents differ according to the epidemiology of specific pathogens (see chapters on specific diseases in Part 3).

Table 11. Pathogens and Infections That Can Be Transmitted in Day Care

Mode of Transmission	Bacteria	Viruses	Parasites
Fecal-oral	*Campylobacter* *Escherichia coli* *Salmonella* *Shigella*	Enteroviruses Hepatitis A Rotaviruses	*Cryptosporidium* *Entamoeba histolytica* *Enterobius vermicularis* *Giardia lamblia*
Respiratory	*Haemophilus influenza* type b *Neisseria meningitidis* Pertussis Tuberculosis	Adenovirus Influenza A & B Measles Parainfluenza Parvovirus B19 Respiratory syncytial virus Rhinoviruses Varicella	
Person-to-person via skin contact	Group A streptococci *Staphylococcus aureus*	Herpes simplex	Pediculosis Scabies
Contact with blood, urine, or saliva		Cytomegalovirus Hepatitis B Herpes simplex	Tinea capitis Tinea corporis

Certain general and disease-specific infection control procedures in child care programs reduce the acquisition and transmission of communicable diseases within and outside the programs. Among these procedures are the following: acquisition of child and employee illness records and current immunization records for children and staff; hygienic and sanitary procedures for toileting and toilet training; hand washing procedures (the single most important measure for preventing infection); environmental sanitation; personal hygiene for children and staff; sanitary handling of food; and management of pets. Specific staff policies—including training procedures for full- and part-time employees, periodic licensing evaluations, and staff illness exclusion policies—also aid in infectious disease control. Health departments should have plans for responding to reportable and nonreportable communicable diseases in child care programs, and they should provide training, written information, and technical consultation to child care programs. Each day, upon entry of the child at the site, and during continual observation of the child at play, a health screening of each child should be performed by a qualified staff member. Parents should be encouraged to share information about their child's health with child care staff.

Recommendations for Inclusion or Exclusion

Mild illness is very common among children, and most children should not be excluded from their usual source of care for common respiratory and gastrointestinal illnesses of mild severity. Infectious disease prevention and control strategies are often influenced by the fact that asymptomatically infected persons can transmit certain infectious microorganisms to others. Parents of children in child care and adult child caregivers should be educated as to the infectious disease risks of child care. Much illness risk can be reduced by following common-sense hygienic practices.

Exclusion of children from out-of-home child care settings has been recommended for illnesses known to be transmitted among, by, and to children when exclusion of the child or adult has a potential for reducing the likelihood of secondary cases. Exclusion has also been recommended in cases of serious illness for which a hypothetical risk of transmission exists but for which data at present are insufficient to quantitate the risk. In many situations, the expertise of the program's medical consultant and the responsible local and state public health authorities are helpful in determining the benefits and risks of excluding children from their usual care program.

Child- and caregiver-specific exclusion policies reflect the present state of knowledge. Children need not be excluded for a minor illness unless any of the following exists:

- The illness prevents the child from participating comfortably in program activities.
- The illness results in a greater care need than the child care staff can provide without compromising the health and safety of the other children.
- The child has any of the following conditions: fever; unusual lethargy, irritability, persistent crying, difficult breathing, or other signs of possible severe illness.
- Diarrhea (defined as an increased number of stools compared with the child's normal pattern, with increased stool water and/or decreased form) that is not contained by diapers or toilet use.

- Vomiting two or more times in the previous 24 hours unless the vomiting is determined to be due to a noncommunicable condition and the child is not in danger of dehydration.
- Mouth sores associated with an inability of the child to control his/her saliva, unless the child's physician or local health department authority states that the child is noninfectious.
- Rash with fever or behavior change until a physician has determined the illness not to be a communicable disease.
- Purulent conjunctivitis (defined as pink or red conjunctiva with white or yellow eye discharge, often with matted eyelids after sleep and eye pain or redness of the eyelids or skin surrounding the eye), until examined by a physician and approved for readmission, with or without treatment.
- Tuberculosis, until the child's physician or local health department authority states that the child is noninfectious.
- Impetigo, until 24 hours after treatment has been initiated.
- Streptococcal pharyngitis, until 24 hours after treatment has been initiated, and until the child has been afebrile for 24 hours.
- Head lice (pediculosis), until the morning after the first treatment.
- Scabies, until after treatment has been completed.
- Varicella, until the sixth day after onset of rash or sooner if all lesions have dried and crusted (see Varicella-Zoster Infections, page 520).
- Pertussis (which is confirmed by laboratory or suspected based on symptoms of the illness or because of cough onset within 14 days of having face-to-face contact with a person in a household or classroom who has a laboratory-confirmed case of pertussis) until 5 days of appropriate antibiotic therapy (currently, erythromycin) has been completed (total course of treatment is 14 days).
- Mumps, until 9 days after onset of parotid gland swelling.
- Hepatitis A virus infection until one week after onset of illness and jaundice, if present, has disappeared or until passive immunoprophylaxis (immune serum globulin) has been administered to appropriate children and staff in the program, as directed by the responsible health department.

Certain conditions do not constitute an a priori reason for excluding a child from child care unless the child would be excluded by the above criteria or the disease is determined by a health authority to contribute to transmission of the illness at the program. These conditions include the following: asymptomatic excretion of an enteropathogen; nonpurulent conjunctivitis (defined as pink conjunctiva with a clear, watery eye discharge and without fever, eye pain, or eyelid redness); rash without fever and without behavior change; cytomegalovirus infection; hepatitis B virus carrier state; and HIV infection.

During the course of an identified outbreak of any communicable illness at the child care setting, a child may be excluded if it is determined that she or he is contributing to the transmission of the illness at the program. The child may be readmitted when the risk of transmission is determined to be no longer present.

Infectious Diseases - Epidemiology and Control (see also chapters on specific diseases in Part 3)

Enteric Diseases

The close, personal contact and poor hygiene of young children provide ready opportunities for the spread of enteric bacteria, viruses, and parasites in day care groups. Although many enteropathogens can cause diarrhea among children in child care, rotavirus, *Giardia lamblia, Shigella,* and *Cryptosporidium* have been the principal organisms implicated in outbreaks; infrequently, *Salmonella* and *Campylobacter jejuni* have been problems in child care.

The most important aspect of child care associated with increased frequencies of enteric illness and hepatitis A is the presence of young children who are not toilet trained. Fecal contamination of the environment is frequent in child care programs and is highest in infant and toddler areas where enteric disease and hepatitis A are known to occur most often. Enteropathogens can be spread fecally or orally either directly, by person-to-person transmission, or indirectly, by toys and other objects, environmental surfaces, and food. The risk of food contamination may be increased when staff caring for diapered children also prepare or serve the food. Several important enteric pathogens, including rotavirus, hepatitis A virus, and *Giardia* cysts, survive on environmental surfaces for periods ranging from hours to weeks.

Child care programs can be a major source of hepatitis A spread within the community. This infection differs from most other diseases in child care centers in that symptomatic illness occurs primarily among adult contacts of infected, asymptomatic children. To recognize outbreaks and take appropriate control measures (i.e., administration of immune globulin), health care personnel and staff need to be aware of this epidemiologic characteristic (see Hepatitis A, page 236).

Procedures to minimize fecal or oral transmission can reduce the frequency of enteric illness in child care. The single most important procedure is frequent hand washing. Staff training and weekly monitoring of staff procedures also reduce spread of enteric illness. A child who develops acute diarrhea (as defined above) or jaundice while in child care should be moved to a separate area away from contact with other children until the child can be removed by a parent or guardian. Exclusion for acute diarrhea should continue until the diarrhea ceases; children with shigellosis should also receive antimicrobial therapy before readmission. The jaundiced child with hepatitis A should be excluded until 1 week after the onset of the jaundice. Specialized child care facilities could be provided for children with enteric illness and hepatitis A. Asymptomatic children without diarrhea who excrete enteropathogens do not require treatment nor exclusion from child care unless there are specific public health indications.

Respiratory Diseases

Diseases spread by the respiratory route include those causing acute upper respiratory tract infections or invasive diseases caused by pathogens such as *Haemophilus influenzae* type b, *Neisseria meningitidis, Bordetella pertussis,* and *Mycobacterium tuberculosis.* Possible modes of spread of respiratory viruses include aerosols, respiratory droplets, direct hand contact with infected secretions, toys, and other objects. The viral pathogens responsible for respiratory tract disease in child care settings are those causing disease in the community and include respiratory syncytial virus, parainfluenza virus, influenza virus, and rhinovirus. The incidence of these respiratory virus infections is increased in child care settings, and outbreaks can occur.

No evidence indicates that the incidence of acute common respiratory disease can be reduced among children in child care by any specific intervention including exclusion from the program. Therefore, children with respiratory illness symptoms of mild or moderate severity without fever associated with the common cold, croup, bronchitis, pneumonia, and otitis media need not be excluded from child care. Moreover, such children need not be separated from other children in the program unless their illness is characterized by one or more of the following conditions: (1) it has a specified etiology, which requires exclusion; (2) it limits the child's comfortable participation in child care activities; or (3) it results in a greater care need than can be provided by the staff without compromising the health and safety of other children.

Transmission of *H influenzae* type b is likely among young children in group child care who are susceptible to primary disease, especially those younger than 24 months. Transmission can originate from either asymptomatic or symptomatic carriers. Children should be immunized with *H influenzae* type b conjugate vaccine according to current recommendations. In an outbreak of invasive *H influenzae* disease in attendees, defined as two or more cases within 60 days, rifampin prophylaxis is indicated for all children and personnel; the need for rifampin after a single case is controversial (see *Haemophilus influenzae* Infections, page 223).

Infections caused by *N meningitidis* occur in all age groups. The highest attack rates occur in children younger than 1 year. Close contact, for an extended time, of children and staff exposed to an index case of meningococcal disease predisposes to secondary transmission, and outbreaks have occurred. Thus, rifampin chemoprophylaxis is indicated for child care contacts.

Group A streptococcal infection among children in child care generally has not been an important problem, but child care outbreaks of streptococcal pharyngitis have been reported. A child with proven group A streptococcal infection should be excluded from classroom contact until 24 hours after initiation of antibiotic therapy.

Infants and young children with tuberculosis are not usually contagious, do not require isolation precautions, and, if approved by health officials, may attend a day care group after chemotherapy is begun. Because an adult with tuberculosis poses a particular hazard to children in a child care group, tuberculin screening of child care workers and volunteers with a Mantoux skin test is strongly recommended before they begin work. The need for periodic, repeat tuberculin testing of persons without clinically important reactions should be based on their risk of acquiring new infection and local health department recommendations.

Vaccine-Preventable Diseases

Routine immunization at the appropriate age is particularly important for children in day care because preschool-aged children currently have the highest age-specific incidence of measles, rubella, *H influenzae* type b disease, and pertussis.

All children enrolling in child care should provide written documentation of satisfactory immunization appropriate for age. Unless contraindications exist, children should demonstrate the following:

- One dose of DTP vaccine by 3 months, two doses by 5 months, three doses by 7 months, and four doses by 19 months.
- One dose of trivalent poliomyelitis vaccine, either OPV or IPV, by 3 months, two doses by 5 months, and three doses by 19 months.
- One dose of MMR vaccine by 16 months.
- One or more doses of *Haemophilus* b conjugate vaccine according to the age-appropriate recommendations (see Tables 2 and 3, pages 17 and 18, and *Haemophilus influenzae* Infections, page 227).*

Children who have not been immunized in an age-appropriate manner before enrollment should have their immunization series initiated as soon as possible, and no later than within one month, and completed according to Tables 2 and 3 (pages 17 and 18). In the interim, unimmunized or underimmunized children should be allowed to attend child care unless a vaccine-preventable disease to which they are susceptible is present in the child care program. In such a situation, all underimmunized children should be excluded for the duration of possible exposure or until after they have completed their immunizations.

---

*Recommendations as of October 1990. These will be revised with approval of an additional *Haemophilus* b conjugate vaccine for use in children younger than 15 months.

Child caregivers should be current for all immunizations routinely recommended for adults. All staff should have completed a primary series for tetanus and diphtheria, and should receive boosters every 10 years. All staff should have been immunized against measles, mumps, rubella, and poliomyelitis, according to the guidelines for adult immunization of the Immunization Practices Advisory Committee (ACIP) of the U.S. Public Health Service and the American College of Physicians Task Force on Adult Immunizations.

Measles is highly contagious, and the highest incidence occurs among preschool-aged children. Outbreaks of mumps in child care settings have not been reported, but any cluster of susceptible persons can sustain transmission. Outbreaks of pertussis in child care settings can occur, particularly in centers with large numbers of children inadequately immunized with DTP, and have been reported in Canada. Because the highest age-specific incidence of rubella now occurs in preschoolers, children and staff members in child care programs are probably at higher risk of exposure than the general population. Of particular concern are susceptible women of childbearing age (staff members and mothers of young children) who might deliver an infant with congenital rubella if infected while pregnant. Child caregivers who have not been immunized against poliomyelitis and who will be caring for infants and children receiving oral polio vaccine (OPV) may become infected and have a very small risk of vaccine-associated paralytic poliomyelitis.

Varicella-Zoster Virus, Herpes Simplex Virus, and Cytomegalovirus Infections

Children with varicella-zoster virus (VZV) who have been excluded from day care may return on the 6th day after the onset of the rash; in mild cases with only a few lesions and rapid resolution, an otherwise healthy child may return sooner (see Recommendations for Inclusion or Exclusion, page 70). All staff members and parents should be notified when a case of chicken pox occurs; they should be informed concerning the greater likelihood of serious infection in susceptible adults and of the potential for fetal damage if infection occurs during pregnancy. Approximately 5% to 10% of adults will be susceptible to VZV; susceptible child care staff who are pregnant and exposed to children with chicken pox should be referred to qualified physicians or other professionals for counseling and management within 24 hours of the exposure.

Exclusion of staff members or children with herpes zoster (shingles) whose lesions cannot be covered should be based on similar criteria to those for varicella. Lesions that can be covered pose little risk to susceptible persons. They should be covered by clothing or a dressing until lesions have crusted.

Children with herpes simplex virus (HSV) gingivostomatitis, who do not have control of oral secretions, should be excluded from child care during the time of active lesions. In selected situations, a child with mild disease who is in control of his or her mouth secretions may not require exclusion. Although HSV can be transmitted from mother to fetus or newborn, maternal HSV infections that are a threat to offspring are sexually transmitted, genital infections; therefore, maternal exposure to HSV in a child care setting carries little, if any, risk for the fetus.

Caregivers should be instructed in the importance of hand washing and other measures aimed at limiting the transfer of infected material for children with VZV or HSV infection (e.g., saliva, tissue fluid, or fluid from a skin lesion).

The risk of spread of cytomegalovirus (CMV) from asymptomatic infected children in child care to their mothers or to child caregivers is the most important consequence of child-care-related CMV infection (see Cytomegalovirus Infections, page 187). Children enrolled in child care programs are more likely to acquire CMV than those cared for primarily at home. The highest rates of viral excretion (as high as 70%) occur in children between 1 and 3 years of age, and excretion often continues for years. Evidence indicates that young children can transmit CMV to their parents and other caregivers. Studies of CMV seroconversion among child care workers have shown annualized seroconversion rates of 14% to 20%. Exposure to CMV with the increased rate of acquisition that occurs in child care staff most likely leads to an increased rate of gestational CMV infection in seronegative staff and an increased risk of congenital CMV infection in their offspring. Women who are seropositive before pregnancy have a negligible risk of having a baby damaged by congenital CMV infection.

Transmission of CMV appears to require direct contact with virus-containing secretions. Therefore, careful attention to hygiene, specifically hand washing and avoiding contact with secretions, is recommended to prevent infection in child caregivers. However, the effectiveness of these measures in an environment where CMV is ubiquitous has not been determined. Because CMV excretion is so prevalent, attempts at isolation or segregation are impractical and inappropriate. Similarly, testing of children to detect CMV excretion is inappropriate because excretion is often intermittent, and results of testing can be misleading.

In view of the risk of CMV infection in child care staff and potential consequences of gestational CMV infection, child care staff should be counseled regarding risks. Serologic testing for CMV is available in nearly all communities in the United States.

Blood-Borne Virus Infections — Hepatitis B (HBV) and Human Immunodeficiency Viruses (HIV)

Possible transmission of HBV in the child care setting is an increasing concern to public health authorities due to the increasing number of children known to be HBV carriers (hepatitis B surface antigen [HBsAg] positive) in child care. HBV transmission in a child care setting is most likely to occur through direct exposure from bites or scratches which break the skin and introduce blood or body secretions from the HBV carrier into the victim. Indirect transmission through environmental contamination with blood or saliva is possible but has not been documented in the child care setting in the United States. Because saliva contains much less virus than blood, the potential infectivity of saliva is low. Infectivity of saliva has been demonstrated only when inoculated through the skin of gibbons and chimpanzees; it has not caused infection when administered by aerosol through the nose or mouth, ingestion through the mouth, or by toothbrush on the gums.

Based on available, albeit limited data, the risk of disease transmission from an HBV carrier child or staff with normal behavior and without generalized dermatitis or bleeding problems is negligible. This extremely low risk does not justify exclusion of an HBV carrier child from day care or hepatitis B vaccination of day care contacts. The routine screening of children for HBV carriage before admission to child care is also not justified. Admission of HBV carrier children with risk factors (e.g., biting, frequent scratching, generalized dermatitis, and bleeding problems) should be assessed on an individual basis by the child's physician, the program director, and the responsible public health authorities. Regular assessment of behavioral risk factors and medical conditions of enrolled HBV carrier children is necessary, and it requires that the center director and primary caregivers are informed about a known HBV carrier child.

Children who bite pose an additional concern. Existing data in humans suggest a small risk of HBV transmission from the bite of an HBV carrier. Several episodes and one outbreak have been reported in which the most likely pathway of HBV transmission was through bites by HBV carriers. The risk of transmission from a bite, however, has not been quantified. For victims of bites by HBV carriers, hepatitis B immune globulin (HBIG) prophylaxis is recommended (see Hepatitis B, page 252).

The risk of HBV acquisition when a susceptible child bites an HBV carrier is not known. A theoretical risk exists if HBsAg-positive blood enters the oral cavity of the biter, but transmission by this route has not been reported. In animal studies in which infectious material was applied to the oral mucosa, transmission occurred only under circumstances of oral manipulation or trauma, such as tooth brushing. Although the data on risks of transmission are limited, most experts would not give HBIG to the susceptible biting child who does not have oral mucosal disease when the amount of blood transferred is small.

In the common circumstance in which the HBsAg status of both the biting child and the victim is unknown, the risk of HBV transmission is extremely low because of the expected low seroprevalence of HBsAg in most groups of preschool-aged children and the low efficiency of disease transmission by bite exposure. Since a bite in this situation is extremely unlikely to involve an HBsAg-positive child, screening and immunoprophylaxis is not warranted.

Efforts to reduce risk of disease transmission in child care through hygienic and environmental standards in general, and particularly when a known HBV carrier child is enrolled, should focus primarily on precautions in blood exposures and limiting potential saliva contamination of the environment. Toothbrushes should not be shared among children. Accidents which lead to bleeding or contamination with blood-containing body fluids by any child should be handled as follows: (1) the area should be disinfected with a freshly prepared solution of 1:64 household bleach (1/4 cup diluted in one gallon of water); (2) disposable gloves should be used unless the amount of blood or body fluid is so small that it can be easily contained by the material used for cleaning; (3) persons involved in cleaning contaminated surfaces should avoid exposure of open skin lesions or mucous membranes to blood or blood-containing body fluids and to wound or tissue exudates; (4) hands should be washed thoroughly after exposure to blood or blood-containing body fluids; (5) optimally, disposable towels or tissues should be used and properly discarded, and mops should be rinsed in the disinfectant; and (6) blood-contaminated material and diapers should be disposed of in a plastic bag with a secure tie.

No reported cases of HIV infection are known to have resulted from transmission in out-of-home child care. Although the risk of transmission of HIV infection to children in the child care setting appears to be extremely low, data do not exist that directly address this issue. Since HIV-infected children whose status is unknown can be attending day care, routine procedures should be adopted for handling spills of blood and blood-containing body fluids and wound exudates of all children, as previously described.

HIV-infected children should be admitted to child care if their health, neurologic development, behavior, and immune status are appropriate. This decision is best made on an individual basis by qualified persons, including the child's physician, who are able to evaluate whether the child will receive optimal care in the program, and whether an HIV- infected child poses a potential threat to others. Information regarding a child who has immunodeficiency, whatever its etiology, should be available to those caretakers who need to know to help protect the child against other infections. For example, immunodeficient children exposed to measles or varicella should immediately receive postexposure immunoprophylaxis (see Measles, page 310, and Varicella, page 520).

Currently available data give no reason to believe that HIV-infected adults will transmit HIV to children in the course of their normal duties. Therefore, asymptomatic HIV-infected adults who do not have open, uncoverable skin lesions or other conditions that would allow contact with their body fluids, may care for children in child care programs. However, immunosuppressed adults with AIDS may be more likely to acquire infectious agents from children and should consult with their physicians regarding the safety of their continuing child care work.

General Practices

The following practices are recommended to reduce the transmission of infectious agents in a day care setting without losing the developmentally desirable features of child care:

- Each day care facility should have **written policies** for managing child and employee illness in child care.
- **Toileting and toilet training equipment** should be maintained in a sanitary condition. **Diaper changing surfaces** should be nonporous and sanitized between uses for different children. Alternately, the diaper changing surface should be covered with a paper pad, which is discarded after each use. If the surface becomes wet or soiled, it should be cleaned and sanitized.
- **Diaper changing procedures** should be posted at the changing area. Soiled disposable diapers, or soiled disposable wiping cloths, should be disposed of in a secure, foot-activated, plastic-lined container. Diapers should be able to contain urine and stool and minimize fecal contamination of the children, providers, and environmental surfaces and objects in the child care program. The diaper should have an absorbent inner lining attached to an outer covering made of waterproof material that prevents escape of feces and urine. Outer and inner linings must be changed as a unit and not reused unless both are cleaned and disinfected. Only modern disposable paper diapers with absorbent gelling meet these requirements. Fecal contents may be placed in a toilet, but diapers should not be rinsed.
- **Diaper changing areas should never be located in food preparation areas, and should never be used for temporary placement of food.**
- The use of **child-sized toilets** or access to steps and modified toilet seats, which provide for easier maintenance, should be encouraged in child care programs; the use of potty chairs should be discouraged. If potty chairs are used, they should be emptied into a toilet, cleaned in a utility sink, and disinfected after each use. Staff should sanitize potty chairs, flush toilets, and diaper changing areas

with a freshly prepared solution of 1:64 household bleach (1/4 cup diluted in one gallon of water).

- Written procedures for **hand washing** (the single most important measure for preventing infection) that foster routine hand washing should exist. Hand washing sinks should be adjacent to each diapering and toileting area; they should be washed and disinfected at least daily and when soiled; they should not be used for food preparation; and they should not be used for rinsing soiled clothing or for cleaning potty chairs.
- Written **personal hygiene policies** for staff and children are necessary.
- Written **environmental sanitation policies and procedures** should include floor cleaning and disinfecting, covering sandboxes, cleaning and sanitizing play tables, and cleaning/disinfecting spills of blood, body fluids, and wound or tissue exudates. In general, routine housekeeping procedures using a freshly prepared solution of commercially available cleaner (detergents, disinfectant-detergents, or chemical germicides) compatible with most surfaces are satisfactory for cleaning spills of vomitus, urine, and feces. For spills of blood or blood-containing body fluids, and of wound and tissue exudates, the previously described procedures should be used.
- Each item of **sleep equipment** should be used only by the child while enrolled in the program, and should be cleaned and sanitized prior to assigning to another child. Crib mattresses should be cleaned and sanitized when soiled or wet. Sleeping mats should be stored so that contact with the sleeping surface of another mat does not occur. Bedding (sheets and blankets) should be assigned to each child and cleaned when soiled or wet.
- Optimally, **toys** which are placed in children's mouths should be cleaned with water and detergent, disinfected, and rinsed before handling by another child. All frequently touched toys in rooms in which infants and toddlers are cared for should be cleaned and disinfected daily. Toys in rooms in which older children (nondiapered) are cared for should be cleaned weekly and when soiled. The use of soft, nonwashable toys in infant/toddler areas of child care programs should be discouraged.
- **Food** should be handled in a safe and careful manner to prevent the growth of bacteria, viruses, fungi, and parasites, and to prevent its contamination by insects or rodents. Tables and counter tops used for food preparation and food service should be cleaned and sanitized between uses, and before and after eating. No one who has signs or symptoms of illness, including vomiting, diarrhea, and infectious skin lesions which cannot be covered, or who is infected with potential food-borne pathogens, should be responsible for food handling. Hands should be washed before handling food. Because of their fre-

quent exposure to feces and children with enteric diseases, staff who work with diapered children, whenever possible, should not prepare food for others. Caregivers who prepare food for infants should be especially aware of the importance of careful hand washing. No unpasteurized milk or milk products should be served.

- The living quarters of **pets** should be enclosed and kept clean of waste to reduce the risk of human contact with this waste. Hands should be washed after handling animals or animal wastes. Animals should be handled by children only under close staff supervision. Dogs and cats should be kept away from child play areas and should be handled only with staff supervision.
- Written policies, which comply with local and state regulations, for filing and regularly updating each child's **immunization records** should be maintained.
- Each child care program should use the services of a **health consultant** to assist in the development and implementation of written policies for the prevention and control of communicable diseases and in providing related health education to children, staff, and parents.
- The child care program should, upon registration of each child, **inform parents of the need to share information about illness,** which can be of a communicable nature, in the child or in any member of the immediate household to facilitate prompt reporting of disease. The program director, after consulting with the program's health consultant or the responsible public health authority, should follow the recommendations of the consultant or authority regarding **notification of parents of children** who attend the program about exposure of their child to a communicable disease.

Infection Control for Hospitalized Children

Isolation Precautions

Nosocomial infections are a major cause of morbidity and mortality in hospitalized children, particularly those in intensive care units. Procedures and policies for prevention of these infections include routine hygienic practices used in the care of all patients, such as hand washing and isolation precautions for patients known to be potential sources of transmission of infection. Hand washing before and after each patient contact remains the single most important routine practice in the control of nosocomial infections.

Recommendations for the isolation of hospitalized patients are most commonly based on the guidelines of the Centers for Disease Control (CDC)*,† These guidelines recommend either of two systems of isolation—category-specific or disease-specific. For category-specific precautions, six categories—Strict, Contact, Respiratory, Tuberculosis (AFB), Enteric, and Drainage/Secretion—currently exist (see Categories of Isolation Precautions, page 83). The CDC has deleted the category of Blood/Body Fluids and now recommends these precautions for all patients (see Universal Precautions).‡ The disease-specific recommendations constitute an alternative system that allows individualization of infection control measures for the disease in question, but the recommendations, as a result, are more complex for hospital personnel to implement.

Recommendations in the *Red Book* are primarily category specific.

Universal Precautions

Since medical history and examination cannot reliably identify all patients infected with the human immunodeficiency virus (HIV) or other blood-borne pathogens, such as the hepatitis B virus (HBV), the CDC recommends that blood and body fluid precautions be used for all patients, especially those in emergency care settings in which the risk of blood exposure is increased and the infection status of the patient is unknown.‡ These precautions apply to blood, certain other body fluids (amniotic fluid, pericardial fluid, peritoneal fluid, pleural fluid, synovial fluid, cerebrospinal fluid, and semen and vaginal secretions), or any other body fluid visibly contaminated with blood. Since HIV and HBV transmission has not been documented from exposure to other body fluids (feces, nasal secretions, sputum, sweat, tears, urine, and vomitus), universal precautions do not apply to these fluids. Universal precautions also do not apply to saliva, except in dental settings where saliva is likely to be contaminated with blood.

All hospitalized children, thus, should be treated as potentially carrying infections communicable by blood or blood-contaminated body fluids. Gloves should be worn for contact with blood or blood-containing fluids and for any procedures entailing exposure to blood, as listed on Table 12. Exposure to non-blood-contaminated fluids, such as urine, nasal secretions, and stool, does not require gloves. However, if such an excretion contains blood, gloves are warranted.

---

*Garner JS, Simmons BP. Guidelines for isolation precautions in hospitals. *Infect. Control.* 1983;4(suppl.):245-325.

†Centers for Disease Control. Risks associated with human parvovirus B-19 infection. *MMWR*. 1989;38:81-88,93-97.

‡Centers for Disease Control. Guidelines for prevention of transmission of human immunodeficiency virus and hepatitis B virus to health-care and public safety workers. *MMWR*. 1989;38;No. S-6:9-10.

Table 12. Infection Control Recommendations for Exposure to Blood and Body Fluids

HAND WASHING IS NECESSARY AFTER PHYSICAL CONTACT WITH ALL PATIENTS

Body fluids and procedures for which gloves are recommended (barrier eye protection should also be used whenever spattering is likely):

Blood
Blood-contaminated fluids
Intubation
Endoscopy
Dental procedures
Wound irrigation
Phlebotomy
Arterial puncture
Vascular catheter placement
Tracheostomy suctioning
Rinsing of used instruments
Lumbar puncture
Puncture of other cavities (e.g., pleural or peritoneal)

Body fluids and procedures for which only hand washing is recommended:

Urine
Stool
Vomitus
Tears
Nasal secretions
Oral secretions
Diaper change

Categories of Isolation Precautions

The specifications for the categories of isolation precautions are summarized in Table 13. Color-coded cards that give these specifications and help to draw attention to the precautions in effect have been designed (see sample instruction cards, page 86). For patients in different categories of isolation, the appropriate card should be posted conspicuously in the immediate vicinity of the patient. **Signs for blood and body fluid precautions should not be posted, however, since these precautions apply to all patients and the signs could lead to the inference that the patient is HIV-infected.**

Table 13. Recommendations for Category-Specific Isolation Precautions for Hospitalized Patients*

Category of Precautions	Hand Washing for Patient Contact	Single Room	Masks	Gowns	Gloves	Other†
Strict isolation	Yes	Yes	Yes	Yes	Yes	------
Contact isolation	Yes	Yes‡	Yes, for those close to patient	Yes, if soiling likely	Yes, for touching infective material	------
Respiratory isolation	Yes	Yes‡	Yes, for those close to patient	No	No	------
Tuberculosis (AFB) isolation	Yes	Yes, with special ventilation	Yes, if patient is coughing and does not cover mouth	Only if needed to prevent gross contamination of clothing	No	------
Enteric precautions	Yes	Only if patient hygiene is poor‡	No	Yes, if soiling likely	Yes, for touching infective material	------

Drainage/ secretion precautions	Yes	No	No	Yes, if soiling likely	Yes, for touching infective material	------
Blood/blood-containing body fluid precautions§	Yes (immediately), if potentially contaminated with blood or body fluids	No	No	Yes, if soiling with blood or body fluids is likely	Yes, for touching blood or body fluids	Avoid needle-stick injuries; clean up blood spills promptly wirh diluted bleach

*Based on recommendations of the Centers for Disease Control (see page 82).
†In each case, articles contaminated with infective material should be discarded or bagged and labeled before being sent for decontamination and reprocessing.
‡Cohorting allowed.
§Recommended for all patients (see Universal Precautions, page 82).

SAMPLE INSTRUCTION CARDS FOR CATEGORY-SPECIFIC ISOLATION PRECAUTIONS

(Front of Card)

Strict Isolation

Visitors—Report to Nurses' Station Before Entering Room

1. Masks are indicated for all persons entering room.
2. Gowns are indicated for all persons entering room.
3. Gloves are indicated for all persons entering room.
4. HANDS MUST BE WASHED AFTER TOUCHING THE PATIENT OR POTENTIALLY CONTAMINATED ARTICLES AND BEFORE TAKING CARE OF ANOTHER PATIENT.
5. Articles contaminated with infective material should be discarded or bagged and labeled before being sent for decontamination and reprocessing.

(Back of Card)

Diseases Requiring Strict Isolation*

Diphtheria, pharyngeal
Lassa fever and other viral hemorrhagic fevers, such as Marburg virus disease§
Plague, pneumonic
Smallpox§
Varicella (chickenpox)
Zoster, localized in immunocompromised patient, or disseminated

*A private room is indicated for Strict Isolation; in general, however, patients infected with the same organism may share a room. See Guideline for Isolation Precautions in Hospitals for details and for how long to apply precautions.
§A private room with special ventilation is indicated.

(Front of Card)

Contact Isolation

Visitors—Report to Nurses' Station Before Entering Room

1. Masks are indicated for those who come close to patient.
2. Gowns are indicated if soiling is likely.
3. Gloves are indicated for touching infective material.
4. HANDS MUST BE WASHED AFTER TOUCHING THE PATIENT OR POTENTIALLY CONTAMINATED ARTICLES AND BEFORE TAKING CARE OF ANOTHER PATIENT.
5. Articles contaminated with infective material should be discarded or bagged and labeled before being sent for decontamination and reprocessing.

(Back of Card)

Diseases or Conditions Requiring Contact Isolation*

Acute respiratory infections in infants and young children, including croup, colds, bronchitis, and bronchiolitis caused by respiratory syncytial virus, adenovirus, coronavirus, influenza viruses, parainfluenza viruses, and rhinovirus
Conjunctivitis, gonococcal, in newborns
Diphtheria, cutaneous
Endometritis, group A *Streptococcus*
Furunculosis, staphylococcal, in newborns
Herpes simplex, disseminated, severe primary or neonatal
Impetigo
Influenza, in infants and young children
Multiply-resistant bacteria, infection or colonization (any site) with any of the following:

1. Gram-negative bacilli resistant to all aminoglycosides that are tested. (In general, such organisms should be resistant to gentamicin, tobramycin, and amikacin for these special precautions to be indicated.)
2. *Staphylococcus aureus* resistant to methicillin (or nafcillin or oxacillin if they are used instead of methicillin for testing)
3. *Pneumococcus* resistant to penicillin
4. *Haemophilus influenzae* resistant to ampicillin (beta-lactamase positive) and chloramphenicol
5. Other resistant bacteria may be included in this isolation category if they are judged by the infection control team to be of special clinical and epidemiologic significance.

Pediculosis
Pharyngitis, infectious, in infants and young children
Pneumonia, viral, in infants and young children
Pneumonia, *Staphylococcus aureus* or group A *Streptococcus*
Rabies
Rubella, congenital and other
Scabies
Scalded skin syndrome (Ritter's disease)
Skin, wound, or burn infection, major (draining and not covered by a dressing or dressing does not adequately contain the purulent material), including those infected with *Staphylococcus aureus* or group A *Streptococcus*
Vaccinia (generalized and progressive eczema vaccinatum)

*A private room is indicated for Contact Isolation; in general, however, patients infected with the same organism may share a room. During outbreaks, infants and young children with the same respiratory clinical syndrome may share a room. See Guideline for Isolation Precautions in Hospitals for details and for how long to apply precautions.

(Front of Card)

Respiratory Isolation

Visitors—Report to Nurses' Station Before Entering Room

1. Masks are indicated for those who come close to patient.
2. Gowns are not indicated.
3. Gloves are not indicated.
4. HANDS MUST BE WASHED AFTER TOUCHING THE PATIENT OR POTENTIALLY CONTAMINATED ARTICLES AND BEFORE TAKING CARE OF ANOTHER PATIENT.
5. Articles contaminated with infective material should be discarded or bagged and labeled before being sent for decontamination and reprocessing.

(Back of Card)

Diseases Requiring Respiratory Isolation*

Epiglottitis, *Haemophilus influenzae*
Erythema infectiosum
Measles
Meningitis
  Bacterial, etiology unknown
  Haemophilus influenzae, known or suspected
  Meningococcal, known or suspected
Meningococcal pneumonia
Meningococcemia
Mumps
Pertussis (whooping cough)
Pneumonia, *Haemophilus influenzae*, in children (any age)

*A private room is indicated for Respiratory Isolation; in general, however, patients infected with the same organism may share a room. See Guideline for Isolation Precautions in Hospitals for details and for how long to apply precautions.

(Front of Card)

AFB Isolation

Visitors—Report to Nurses' Station Before Entering Room

1. Masks are indicated only when patient is coughing and does not reliably cover mouth.
2. Gowns are indicated only if needed to prevent gross contamination of clothing.
3. Gloves are not indicated.
4. HANDS MUST BE WASHED AFTER TOUCHING THE PATIENT OR POTENTIALLY CONTAMINATED ARTICLES AND BEFORE TAKING CARE OF ANOTHER PATIENT.
5. Articles should be discarded, cleaned, or sent for decontamination and reprocessing.

(Back of Card)

Diseases Requiring AFB Isolation*

This isolation category is for patients with current pulmonary TB who have a positive sputum smear or a chest X-ray appearance that strongly suggests current (active) TB. Laryngeal TB is also included in this category. In general, infants and young children with pulmonary TB do not require isolation precautions because they rarely cough and their bronchial secretions contain few AFB compared with adults with pulmonary TB. To protect the patient's privacy, this instruction card is labeled AFB (acid-fast bacilli) Isolation rather than Tuberculosis Isolation.

*A private room with special ventilation is indicated for AFB isolation. In general, patients infected with the same organism may share a room. See Guideline for Isolation Precautions in Hospitals for details and for how long to apply precautions.

(Front of Card)

Enteric Precautions

Visitors—Report to Nurses' Station Before Entering Room

1. Masks are not indicated.
2. Gowns are indicated if soiling is likely.
3. Gloves are indicated for touching infective material.
4. HANDS MUST BE WASHED AFTER TOUCHING THE PATIENT OR POTENTIALLY CONTAMINATED ARTICLES AND BEFORE TAKING CARE OF ANOTHER PATIENT.
5. Articles contaminated with infective material should be discarded or bagged and labeled before being sent for decontamintion and reprocessing.

(Back of Card)

Diseases Requiring Enteric Precautions*

Amebic dysentery
Cholera
Coxsackievirus disease
Diarrhea, acute illness with suspected infectious etiology
Echovirus disease
Encephalitis (unless known not to be caused by enteroviruses)
Enterocolitis caused by *Clostridium difficile* or *Staphylococcus aureus*
Enteroviral infection
Gastroenteritis caused by
- *Campylobacter* species
- *Cryptosporidium* species
- *Dientamoeba fragilis*
- *Escherichia coli* (enterotoxic, enteropathogenic, or enteroinvasive)
- *Giardia lamblia*
- *Salmonella* species
- *Shigella* species
- *Vibrio parahaemolyticus*
- Viruses—including Norwalk agent and rotavirus
- *Yersinia enterocolitica*
- Unknown etiology but presumed to be an infectious agent

Hand, foot, and mouth disease
Hepatitis, viral, type A
Herpangina
Meningitis, viral (unless known not to be caused by enteroviruses)
Necrotizing enterocolitis
Pleurodynia
Poliomyelitis
Typhoid fever (*Salmonella typhi*)
Viral pericarditis, myocarditis, or meningitis (unless known not to be caused by enteroviruses)

*A private room is indicated for Enteric Precautions if patient hygiene is poor. A patient with poor hygiene does not wash hands after touching infective material, contaminates the environment with infective material, or shares contaminated articles with other patients. In general, patients infected with the same organism may share a room. See Guideline for Isolation Precautions in Hospitals for details and for how long to apply precautions.

(Front of Card)

Drainage/Secretion Precautions

Visitors—Report to Nurses' Station Before Entering Room

1. Masks are not indicated.
2. Gowns are indicated if soiling is likely.
3. Gloves are indicated for touching infective material.
4. HANDS MUST BE WASHED AFTER TOUCHING THE PATIENT OR POTENTIALLY CONTAMINATED ARTICLES AND BEFORE TAKING CARE OF ANOTHER PATIENT.
5. Articles contaminated with infective material should be discarded or bagged and labeled before being sent for decontamination and reprocessing.

(Back of Card)

Diseases Requiring Drainage/Secretion Precautions*

Infectious diseases included in this category are those that result in production of infective purulent material, drainage, or secretions, unless the disease is included in another isolation category that requires more rigorous precautions. (If you have questions about a specific disease, see the listing of infectious diseases in Guideline for Isolation Precautions in Hospitals, Table A, Disease-Specific Isolation Precautions.)

The following infections are examples of those included in this category provided they are *not* a) caused by multiply-resistant microorganisms, b) major (draining and not covered by a dressing or dressing does not adequately contain the drainage) skin, wound, or burn infections, including those caused by *Staphylococcus aureus* or group A *Streptococcus*, or c) gonococcal eye infections in newborns. See Contact Isolation if the infection is one of these 3.

Abscess, minor or limited
Burn infection, minor or limited
Conjunctivitis
Decubitus ulcer, infected, minor or limited
Skin infection, minor or limited
Wound infection, minor or limited

*A private room is usually not indicated for Drainage/Secretion Precautions. See Guideline for Isolation Precautions in Hospitals for details and for how long to apply precautions.

Intensive Care Units

Infection control practices in neonatal and pediatric intensive care units (ICUs) frequently must be modified to accommodate special circumstances, particularly those pertaining to isolation in a private room. Separate isolation rooms are often not available in ICUs, and newborn nurseries may not be desirable for the optimal care of critically ill patients. If air-borne transmission is not likely, an isolation area can be defined within the ICU by curtains, partitions, or other markers.

For newborn infants, separate isolation rooms are not necessary if the following conditions are met:

- The number of nursing and medical personnel is adequate and sufficient time for appropriate hand washing is available.
- Sufficient space is available for a 4- to 6-foot aisle or area between newborn infant stations.
- An adequate number of sinks for hand washing are available in each nursery room and area.
- Continuing instruction is given to personnel about the mode of transmission of infections.

When a private room is mandated by the possibility of air-borne transmission (e.g., an infant with chickenpox), a forced-air incubator is not a substitute for a private room because these incubators do not filter the air discharged into the environment. Another modification that may be necessary for newborn infants and children during outbreaks is the cohorting of patients and personnel. Decisions of this type should be made in conjunction with the hospital's infection control and nursery directors. In all instances, appropriate hand washing between patient contacts is mandatory.

Personnel Health

Prevention of the transmission of infectious agents between pediatric patients and health care personnel is particularly important in the care of children. Some infections pose increased risks for pregnant health care workers, and especially their fetuses, or for immunocompromised personnel; these include varicella, tuberculosis, parvovirus B19, cytomegalovirus, rubella, and herpes simplex virus. The consequences to pediatric patients of acquiring infections from infected adults are also significant. Mild and severe illness in the adults, such as viral gastroenteritis, upper respiratory tract viral infection, varicella, pertussis, herpes simplex infection, and tuberculosis can cause life-threatening disease in children. Those at greatest risk are premature infants, children who have heart disease or chronic pulmonary disease, and immunocompromised patients. Since children often lack immunity to many common viruses and bacteria, they are a highly susceptible population.

The transmission of infectious agents within hospitals is facilitated by the close contact between patients and health care providers, which the care of children requires. In addition, children do not routinely have good hygienic practices, and, in comparison to adults, have an increased incidence of infections.

To limit the risks for both children and caretakers, hospitals should have established employee health policies and services. All employees should be interviewed and immunity, either from history of disease or immunization, should be documented for rubella, measles, mumps, varicella, hepatitis B, pertussis, and polio. Vaccines should be administered as indicated (see Health Care Professionals, p. 61). For nonvaccine-preventable infections, employees should be counseled about exposures and possible need for leave if they are exposed to a specific infectious agent.

Employees should be screened by Mantoux skin testing for tuberculosis. Those with common infections, such as gastroenteritis, dermatitis, or upper respiratory infections should be evaluated to determine the resulting risk of transmission to their patients.

Pregnant personnel should be counseled about the risks of caring for children with potentially contagious diseases. Specific concerns include exposure to rubella, varicella, cytomegalovirus, and parvovirus B19 infection.

Employee education is of paramount importance in infection control. Pediatric health care providers should be knowledgeable about the modes of transmission of infectious agents, proper hand washing technique, and the potential serious risks to children of certain mild infections in adults.

Sibling Visits

Sibling visits to birthing centers, postpartum rooms, pediatric wards, and intensive care units are encouraged. Newborn intensive care, with its increasing sophistication in medical care, often results in long hospital stays for the sick newborn, making family visits an important part of neonatal care. Studies to date indicate that sibling visits in newborn intensive care units are favorably received by parents, and bacterial colonization or subsequent infection is not increased in either the sick or well newborn who has been visited by his or her brothers or sisters. Since these studies are limited by small numbers, the concept of sibling visits, however, needs continued evaluation.

Guidelines for sibling visits should be established in an effort to maximize opportunities for visiting and to minimize the risks of nosocomial spread of pathogens brought into the hospital by these young visitors. The following guidelines for sibling visits to pediatric patients are provided; they may need to be modified by local nursing, pediatric, obstetric, and infectious disease staffs to address specific issues in their hospital settings:

- Sibling visits should be encouraged in both the normal infant and newborn intensive care nurseries, for chronically and critically ill children as well as for other hospitalized children.
- Prior to the visit, a nurse or physician should interview the parents to assess the current health of each sibling. No child with fever or symptoms of an acute illness, including an upper respiratory tract infection, gastroenteritis, or dermatitis, should be allowed to visit. Siblings who have recently been exposed to a known communicable disease (e.g., chickenpox) should not be allowed to visit. These interviews should be documented in the patient's record, and approval for each sibling visit should be noted.
- Adequate observation and monitoring of all visitors by the medical and nursing staff should occur.
- The visiting sibling should visit only his or her sibling.
- Children should carefully wash their hands prior to patient contact, especially in the case of neonatal and immunocompromised siblings.
- Throughout the visit, sibling activity should be supervised by parents or a responsible adult and limited to the mother's or patient's private room and/or other designated areas.

Sexually Transmitted Diseases

Sexually transmitted diseases (STDs), including HIV infections, are a major and growing problem in children, adolescents, and young adults. Since the early 1970s, health care professionals have been alarmed by the increasing incidence of these diseases. Among other factors, the increase has been associated with declining age at first intercourse.

Physicians should be aware of the increasing prevalence of STDs, the potential seriousness of their sequelae for adolescents and their offspring, implications of the diagnosis of an STD in prepubescent children with regard to child abuse, and the notable increase in the number of recognizable agents. The traditional STDs (e.g., syphilis, gonorrhea, chancroid, and lymphogranuloma venereum) presently account for only a fraction of the currently recognized sexually transmitted pathogens (see Tables 14 and 15). For example, hepatitis B is now recognized as a major STD, as both heterosexual and homosexual activity are important modes of transmission of the hepatitis B virus.

Table 14. Sexually Transmitted Diseases: Factors and Features Related to Etiologic Agents

Agents	Diseases/Syndromes	Laboratory Tests	Antimicrobial Choices
Bacterial Agents			
*Calymmatobacterium granulomatis**	Granuloma inguinale	Stained scraping or crushed preparation of lesion (Donovan bodies)	Tetracycline,† trimethoprim-sulfamethoxazole
Campylobacter fetus‡	Enteritis, proctitis (primarily in homosexual males)	Culture stool (with special technique)	Erythromycin
Chlamydia trachomatis	Urethritis, cervicitis, proctitis, bartholinitis, endometritis, salpingitis, epididymitis, perihepatitis, pelvic inflammatory disease, pharyngitis, conjunctivitis, infant pneumonia, trachoma, lymphogranuloma venereum, Reiter's syndrome	Tissue-cell culture, smears for intracytoplasmic inclusions; antigen detection tests (direct fluorescence, EIA)	Tetracycline,† erythromycin, sulfisoxazole
Gardnerella vaginalis (in association with anaerobic Gram-negative rods)*	Vaginosis	Wet mount of vaginal discharge to look for "clue cells" (> 20%); pH of discharge > 4.5; "fishy" odor when 10% KOH added	Metronidazole; possibly clindamycin, amoxicillin, or ampicillin

*Diagnosis in prepubertal child indicates need to consider sexual abuse.
†Not given to children younger than 9 years if acceptable alternative drug is available.
‡Agent occasionally transmitted sexually.

Table 14. Sexually Transmitted Diseases: Factors and Features Related to Etiologic Agents *(continued)*

Agents	Diseases/Syndromes	Laboratory Tests	Antimicrobial Choices
*Haemophilus ducreyi**	Chancroid (genital ulcers)	Culture purulent exudate from ulcer	Ceftriaxone, erythromycin, trimethoprim-sulfamethoxazole
*Mycoplasma hominis**,§	Pelvic inflammatory disease, postpartum fever, pyelonephritis	Culture	Clindamycin, tetracycline†
*Neisseria gonorrhoeae**	Vaginitis (prepuberty), urethritis, cervicitis, pelvic inflammatory disease, proctitis, pharyngitis, conjunctivitis, bartholinitis, endometritis, amnionitis, epididymitis, perihepatitis, tenosynovitis, dermatitis, meningitis, arthritis, endocarditis, neonatal ophthalmia, and invasive infections	Gram stain of exudative materials, cultures using selective media, antimicrobial susceptibility testing	Ceftriaxone, ampicillin, or amoxicillin with probenecid, penicillin G (IM), ciprofloxacin,‖ spectinomycin, cefoxitin, cefotaxime, tetracycline†
*Treponema pallidum**	Syphilis	Darkfield examination, direct fluorescent antibody, serology (VDRL, RPR, FTA-ABS)	Penicillin G (IM); alternatives: tetracycline,† erythromycin
Nontyphoidal *Salmonella* species‡	Enteritis (mainly in homosexual males)	Stool culture	None (except in invasive infection)

Shigella	Enteritis (primarily in homosexual males)	Stool culture	Trimethoprim-sulfamethoxazole, ampicillin
Ureaplasma urealyticum	Urethritis in males, chorioamnionitis, infant pneumonia, neonatal meningitis	Culture of discharge	Tetracycline,† erythromycin
	Viral Agents		
Cytomegalovirus	Infectious mononucleosis syndrome, congenital infection	Viral culture	None
Hepatitis A virus‡	Hepatitis (especially homosexual males)	Serology (anti-HAV, IgM anti-HAV)	None (IG for contacts)
Hepatitis B virus	Acute, chronic, and fulminant disease; hepatocellular cancer (late sequelae)	Serology (e.g., HBsAg, anti-HBs, anti-HBc)	None (HBIG and/or HBV vaccine for contacts)
Herpes simplex* (usually type 2)	Primary and recurrent genital herpes (including urethritis and cervicitis), meningoencephalitis, neonatal infection	Viral culture, Papanicolaou smear, Tzanck preparation, rapid diagnostic tests, brain biopsy (encephalitis)	Acyclovir, vidarabine
Human immunodeficiency virus (HIV)	AIDS and other HIV infections	Serology, immunologic studies	Zidovudine¶ and treatment of opportunistic infections

*Diagnosis in prepubertal child indicates need to consider sexual abuse.
†Not given to children younger than 9 years if acceptable alternative drug is available.
‡Agent occasionally transmitted sexually.
§Some experts question the importance of this organism in STD.
‖Only for adults (≥ 21 years).
¶Formerly termed azidothymidine (AZT).

Table 14. Sexually Transmitted Diseases: Factors and Features Related to Etiologic Agents *(continued)*

Agents	Diseases/Syndromes	Laboratory Tests	Antimicrobial Choices
Molluscum contagiosum virus	Umbilicated papules, furuncle-like lesion on genitalia	Stain lesion material for intracytoplasmic inclusions	None (mechanical removal)
Papillomavirus*	Condylomata acuminata (genital warts), laryngeal papilloma in infants; squamous cell carcinoma (late)	Biopsy, Papanicolaou smear, DNA hybridization probes	None (local treatment with cryotherapy, see Papillomaviruses, page 340)
Protozoan Agents			
*Cryptosporidium**	Enteritis (especially homosexual males)	Stained stool or biopsy	None
Entamoeba histolytica‡	Enteritis, amebiasis, liver abscess (especially homosexual males)	Stool examination, sigmoidoscopy, swabs (via endoscopy), serology	See Amebiasis (page 135)
Giardia lamblia‡	Enteritis (especially homosexual males	Stool examination, duodenal aspirate (or "string test")	Quinacrine; alternatives: furazolidone, metronidazole
*Trichomonas vaginalis**	Vaginitis, urethritis	Saline wet mount of vaginal discharge, Papanicolaou smear, vaginal or urethral culture	Metronidazole, clotrimazole

Miscellaneous Agents			
Candida albicans	Vulvovaginitis, cystitis, thrush, esophagitis, invasive disease (immunocompromised hosts)	KOH wet mount, culture of discharge on special media	Nystatin, clotrimazole, miconazole, ketoconazole, amphotericin B
Phthirus pubis	Pubic lice infestation	Identify eggs, nymphs, or lice with naked eye or hand lens	1% permethrin, pyrethin-based products, 1% lindane shampoo
Sarcoptes scabiei, subspecies *hominis*‡	Scabies	Examine scrapings of affected skin for mites	5% permethrin; alternatives: lindane, 10% crotamiton

*Diagnosis in prepubertal child indicates need to consider sexual abuse.
‡Agent occasionally transmitted sexually.

Table 15. Major Syndromes Caused by Sexually Transmitted Agents

Syndrome	Agents
AIDS/ARC	Human immunodeficiency virus (HIV)
Amnionitis	*Neisseria gonorrhoeae* *Ureaplasma urealyticum* Herpes simplex Group B *Streptococcus*
Arthritis	*Neisseria gonorrhoeae* *Chlamydia trachomatis* *Salmonella* species
Bartholinitis	*Neisseria gonorrhoeae* *Chlamydia trachomatis* *Mycoplasma hominis*
Cervicitis	*Neisseria gonorrhoeae* *Chlamydia trachomatis* Herpes simplex
Conjunctivitis	*Neisseria gonorrhoeae* *Chlamydia trachomatis*
Endocarditis	*Neisseria gonorrhoeae*
Endometritis	*Neisseria gonorrhoeae* *Chlamydia trachomatis*
Enteritis (primarily homosexual)	*Giardia lamblia* *Entamoeba histolytica* *Shigella* species *Salmonella* species Cryptosporidia *Enterobius vermicularis* *Campylobacter fetus* *Mycoplasm hominis* *Ureaplasma urealyticum* *Chlamydia trachomatis*, LGV subtypes
Epididymitis	*Neisseria gonorrhoeae* *Chlamydia trachomatis*
Exanthems	*Treponema palladium* (secondary) *Phthirus pubis* (pubic lice) *Sarcoptes scabiei*, subspecies *hominis* *Candida* species

Table 15. Major Syndromes Caused by Sexually Transmitted Agents *(continued)*

Syndrome	Agents
Genital ulcers	Herpes simplex *Treponema pallidum* *Chlamydia trachomatis* (LGV subtypes) *Haemophilus ducreyi* (chancroid) *Calymmatobacterium granulomatis* (granuloma inguinale)
Genital warts	Human papillomavirus
Hepatitis	Hepatitis B Hepatitis A *Treponema pallidum* Cytomegalovirus Herpes simplex
Meningitis	*Neisseria gonorrhoeae*
Meningoencephalitis	*Treponema pallidum* Herpes simplex HIV
Pelvic inflammatory disease	*Neisseria gonorrhoeae* *Chlamydia trachomatis* *Mycoplasma hominis* *Ureaplasma urealyticum* Anaerobic bacteria
Perihepatitis	*Neisseria gonorrhoeae* *Chlamydia trachomatis* *Treponema pallidum*
Pharyngitis	*Neisseria gonorrhoeae* *Chlamydia trachomatis* *Treponema pallidum*
Pneumonia (infant)	*Chlamydia trachomatis* *Ureaplasma urealyticum*
Proctitis	*Neisseria gonorrhoea* *Chlamydia trachomatis* Herpes simplex *Campylobacter fetus*
Urethritis	*Neisseria gonorrhoeae* *Chlamydia trachomatis* *Ureaplasma urealyticum* *Trichomonas vaginalis* Herpes simplex

Table 15. Major Syndromes Caused by Sexually Transmitted Agents *(continued)*

Syndrome	Agents
Vaginitis	*Candida albicans* *Trichomonas vaginalis* Anaerobic Gram-negative bacteria *Gardnerella vaginalis* (bacterial vaginosis) *Mycoplasma hominis*

Management

Physicians need to identify patients at risk for STD and to diagnose and appropriately treat infections caused by sexually transmitted pathogens. Screening by history, physical examination, and appropriate laboratory tests, and patient education are indicated for high-risk groups. These include the following:

- Adolescents who are heterosexually or homosexually active.
- Pregnant adolescents and their sexual contacts.
- Adolescents undergoing a therapeutic abortion.
- Adolescents with symptoms compatible with STD, such as cervical or urethral discharge, lower abdominal or right upper quadrant pain in a female, testicular tenderness, tenesmus, rectal pain or rectal discharge.
- Prepubescent children with genital, anal, or perineal ulcers; perineal pruritus; condyloma acuminata; or vaginitis and dysuria.
- Adolescents living in group homes or in detention homes.
- Any child or adolescent suspected of being a victim of sexual abuse, rape, or incest.
- Adolescent prostitutes.
- Street youth.
- Intravenous drug abusers.

Because more than one STD frequently coexists in the same patient, the detection of one infection should lead to a search for others, regardless of the presenting symptoms. A careful physical examination, including examination of the oropharynx, rectum, genitalia, and skin, should be performed. Relevant laboratory studies include urinalysis, appropriate serologic tests, Gram stains of cervical or urethral discharge, wet mounts of vaginal secretions, rapid diagnostic tests (DFA or ELISA) for *Chlamydia trachomatis* on cervical or urethral specimens, and/or gonococcal cultures of the oropharynx, rectum, and cervix, or penile urethra in individual circumstances.

The diagnosis of a primary case of an STD incurs additional major responsibilities for public health reporting, evaluation for possible sexual abuse (see Sexual Abuse, page 103), contact tracing, and patient education. Patients who have an STD or who have multiple sexual partners should receive hepatitis B vaccine (see Hepatitis B, page 246). The physician should report diseases to the responsible health department to facilitate partner notification and should explain to the patient the importance of examining partners as well as the route of transmission of these infections. The potential long-term sequelae of disease(s) should be emphasized. Whereas control through partner notification and identification of secondary spread frequently is best coordinated by public health departments, the patient's physician is responsible for education and appropriate treatment. If no private physician is identified, the public health or STD clinic should assume this task.

Sequelae

Major sequelae of STDs in adolescent females include ectopic pregnancies, infertility, chronic hepatitis, and carcinoma of the cervix. STDs also cause risks for neonatal infections, and these risks are increased in adolescent pregnancies. Failure to consider the possibility of an STD in the mother can result in delay or omission of neonatal therapy and lead to serious consequences. Hence, screening and treatment in pregnancy and early diagnosis and treatment of the infant are essential. Neonatal consequences of certain maternal STDs are listed in Table 16.

STD Prevention

Adolescents consider health care providers to be accurate and confidential sources of information about STD, including HIV infection. Physicians caring for adolescents not only need to be knowledgeable about the diagnosis and management of STDs but also need to educate adolescents about STDs and their prevention. Providing information about STDs, including the proper use of condoms (see Table 17), can help to overcome many myths and negative beliefs, and can reduce the patient's risks of acquisition of a sexually transmitted pathogen.

STDs are a major and growing source of morbidity in children and adolescents. Active cooperation and involvement of both public and private sectors of medicine are necessary to control this significant problem.

Sexual Abuse

Some infections known to be sexually transmitted in adults are similarly spread to children. If sexual abuse is considered to be chronic or to have occurred more than 72 hours before evaluation, specimens can be

Table 16. Neonatal Consequences of Certain Maternal Sexually Transmitted Pathogens

Maternal Infection	Neonatal Consequences	Prevention	Neonatal Treatment
Candida albicans	Thrush, dermatitis	None known	Nystatin
Chlamydia trachomatis	Conjunctivitis, pneumonia	Screen and treat mother and her sexual partner; neonatal ocular prophylaxis of some value	Erythromycin
Cytomegalovirus	Congenital infection	None known	None
Hepatitis B	Development of chronic carriage, hepatitis	Screen mother	HBIG and HBV vaccine (for prevention)
HIV	AIDS	Screen mother; if negative, counsel regarding prevention; if positive, consider abortion	None (zidovudine* is not approved for use in young infants)
Herpes simplex, type 2	Central nervous system disease, disseminated infection, spontaneous abortion, premature delivery	Cesarean section	Acyclovir (alternative: vidarabine)

Neisseria gonorrhoeae	Conjunctivitis, arthritis, sepsis, meningitis, premature delivery	Screen and treat mother and her sexual partner; ocular silver nitrate, erythromycin, or tetracycline	Ceftriaxone (or penicillin G if susceptible)
Syphilis	Stillbirth, low birth weight, premature delivery, congenital infection	Screen mother and her sexual partner and treat	Penicillin G
Ureaplasma urealyticum	Pneumonia, meningitis	None known	Erythromycin

*Formerly termed azidothymidine (AZT).

Table 17. Recommendations for Use of Condoms*

1. Latex condoms should be used because they may offer greater protection against HIV and other viral STDs than natural membrane condoms.
2. Condoms should be stored in a cool, dry place out of direct sunlight.
3. Condoms in damaged packages or those that show obvious signs of age (e.g., those that are brittle, sticky, or discolored) should not be used. They cannot be relied upon to prevent infection or pregnancy.
4. Condoms should be handled with care to prevent puncture.
5. The condom should be put on before any genital contact to prevent exposure to fluids that may contain infectious agents. Hold the tip of the condom and unroll it onto the erect penis, leaving space at the tip to collect semen, yet ensuring that no air is trapped in the tip of the condom.
6. Only water-based lubricants should be used. Petroleum- or oil-based lubricants (such as petroleum jelly, cooking oils, shortening, and lotions) should not be used because they weaken the latex and may cause breakage.
7. Use of condoms containing spermicides may provide some additional protection against STDs. However, vaginal use of spermicides along with condoms is likely to provide still greater protection.
8. If a condom breaks, it should be replaced immediately. If ejaculation occurs after condom breakage, the immediate use of spermicide has been suggested. However, the protective value of postejaculation application of spermicide in reducing the risk of STD transmission is unknown.
9. After ejaculation, care should be taken so that the condom does not slip off the penis before withdrawal; the base of the condom should be held throughout withdrawal. The penis should be withdrawn while still erect.
10. Condoms should never be reused.

*From Centers for Disease Control. 1989 Sexually Transmitted Diseases Treatment Guidelines, *MMWR.* 1989;38:ix

Table 18. Testing for Sexual Abuse

	Organism	Specimens
All children	*Neisseria gonorrhoeae*	Rectal, throat, vaginal, and/or endocervical culture(s)
	Chlamydia trachomatis	Throat, rectal, and/or vulvovaginal culture(s)
	Syphilis	Darkfield exam of chancre fluid, if present; blood for serologic tests
Selected cases	HIV	Serology of abuser if possible), serology of child at time of abuse and 12 weeks later
	Hepatitis B	Serology of abuser
	Herpes simplex	Culture of lesion
	Gardnerella vaginalis	Wet mount of vaginal discharge
	Papillomavirus	Biopsy of lesion
	Trichomonas vaginalis	Wet mount of vaginal discharge, culture of discharge

collected for evaluation of STDs. If the abuse was more recent, appropriate forensic specimens should be collected but the collection of specimens for evaluation of STD should be delayed. Antimicrobial treatment should be considered if the attacker was known to be infected with an STD, more than one assailant was involved, the patient is unlikely to return for follow-up, or the patient is very anxious about the possibility of acquiring an STD. When evaluating a child for possible sexual abuse, appropriate tests for the three organisms described below should be obtained (see also Table 18). Specimens must be properly evaluated for both medical and legal reasons, given the implications of a positive test.

1) *Neisseria gonorrhoeae*. Swabs of the throat, rectum, and vagina should be obtained and placed immediately into commercially available transport media for *N gonorrhoeae* or plated immediately on Thayer-Martin and chocolate agar and incubated inactivated in a CO2-enriched atmosphere. Isolates should be confirmed by carbohydrate utilization and fluorescent antibody or coagglutination techniques, preferably using at least two confirmatory techniques.

   Rapid detection techniques applied directly to patient specimens should not be used. If a Gram stain of discharge is suggestive of *N gonorrhoeae* in the presence of a negative culture, the culture should be repeated. The presence of culture-proven *N gonorrhoeae* after one year of age is due to sexual contact in almost all cases.

2) *Chlamydia trachomatis.* Specimens should be obtained from the throat, rectum, and vagina for culture. Rapid detection techniques should not be used since fecal flora may give a false positive reaction. Vaginal chlamydial infection after two years of age is usually due to sexual contact. Rectal and pharyngeal infection may be found in children without sexual contact.
3) *Syphilis.* Darkfield microscopy should be obtained to study fluid from a chancre, if present. Serology for syphilis (VDRL, RPR, or FTA-ABS) should be obtained as part of an evaluation for sexual abuse. If not congenitally acquired, a positive serology is highly suggestive of sexual contact.

Other infectious agents can be found in sexually abused children. In selected situations screening for one or more of the following organisms may be desirable:

Human immunodeficiency virus (HIV). If possible, serologic evaluation of the abuser should be performed. The child should be tested serologically at the time of abuse and at 12 and 24 weeks after sexual contact with an assailant likely to be HIV infected. Counseling of the child and family needs to be provided. The risk of transmission of HIV is small.

Hepatitis B. If the abuser is a known or suspected carrier of hepatitis B surface antigen (HBsAg), the victim should receive hepatitis B immune globulin within 14 days and should be tested at that time and 3 months later for HBsAg.

Herpes simplex virus (HSV). Type 1 HSV may be spread sexually or nonsexually, but type 2 HSV suggests sexual transmission. Viral culture of lesions should be done. Routine cultures in the absence of lesions are not recommended.

Bacterial vaginosis (nonspecific vaginitis or *Gardnerella*-associated vaginalis). Nonspecific vaginitis is more common in children who have had sexual contact. Clue cells may be seen in a wet preparation obtained from a vaginal discharge or a vaginal wash, and a fishy odor develops after 10% KOH is added to vaginal fluid.

Human papillomavirus (HPV). Genital or rectal warts (condyloma acuminata) that develop 3 months or later after sexual abuse may be biopsied. Neonatally acquired disease can appear as genital or rectal warts several years after birth. A Papanicolaou smear of the cervix will detect some subclinical HPV infections and can be used in postpubertal children.

Trichomonas vaginalis. A wet mount preparation of vaginal secretion can be performed. Although infection has been reported to be spread between mother and infant, most infections in prepubertal girls are probably caused by sexual abuse.

Several organisms usually thought to be sexually transmitted can be seen in children where sexual abuse does not appear likely. Although infection with *Gardnerella vaginalis, Mycoplasma hominis, Ureaplasma urealyticum, Haemophilus ducreyi,* and *Calymmatobacterium granulomatis* can be seen in sexually abused children, their presence does not necessarily indicate sexual abuse.

In addition to the medical evaluation, counseling of the child and family is essential.

Medical Evaluation of Internationally Adopted Children

More than 10,000 orphans from abroad are adopted each year by families in the United States. Asian nations (such as Korea, India, and the Philippines) and Central and Latin American countries account for nearly 90% of these international adoptees. However, increasing numbers of adoptees are coming from Haiti, other areas in the Caribbean, and African nations. The diverse origins of these children, their unpredictable backgrounds prior to adoption, and vagaries of health care in developing countries make the appropriate medical evaluation of internationally adopted children an important task.

Internationally adopted children differ from refugee children in several ways. International adoptees, regardless of country of origin, are seldom appropriately screened for medical illness. Preventive health care, such as immunizations, may be delayed or omitted. Moreover, the results of medical testing performed in the country of origin are often inaccurate or incomplete. Thus, a thorough medical evaluation should be initiated after the child's arrival in the United States.

In prospective studies of internationally adopted children, infectious diseases have constituted most medical diagnoses and have been found in nearly 60% of international adoptees (see Table 19). These infections are often subclinical. The straightforward application of screening tests designed to determine the presence of certain illnesses is a cost-effective step toward preventive health care for these children.

Infectious diseases of special importance in internationally adopted children are as follows:

1. *Hepatitis B.* The prevalence of hepatitis B markers ranges from 5% to 20% in internationally adopted children, depending on the country of origin. These children should be tested for serum hepatitis B surface antigen (HBsAg). The prevalence of chronic hepatitis B (defined by the persistence of HBsAg for more than 6 months) is high. Liver function tests should be performed on these HBsAg-positive patients, and susceptible household contacts should be immunized (see Hepatitis B, page 246). Some experts

Table 19. Infectious Diseases of Importance in International Adoptees and Refugees

Bacteria	Viruses	Protozoa	Helminths	Arthropoda
Campylobacter	Cytomeg-alovirus	Amebiasis	Ascariasis	Lice
Melioidosis*	Hepatitis A	Giardiasis	Filariasis*	Scabies
Salmonella	Hepatitis B	Malaria*	Hookworms	
Shigella	HIV		Liver flukes*	
Syphilis			Lung flukes*	
Tuberculosis*			Schisto-somiasis*	
Typhoid Fever*			Strongy-loidiasis	
Yersinia			Tapeworms	
			Trichuriasis	

*More commonly encountered in refugee children than in international adoptees.

recommend additional hepatitis B serologic testing as the presence of antibodies to the hepatitis B surface and core antigens may identify additional children at risk for chronic hepatitis.

2. *Hepatitis A.* Since current diagnostic tests detect antibodies formed in response to acute infection, and the child is not infectious once these antibodies are present, routine serologic screening for hepatitis A antibodies is not recommended. Many internationally adopted children acquire hepatitis A early in life; thus, acute infections after adoption are rare and chronic hepatitis A does not occur.
3. *Cytomegalovirus.* Cytomegalovirus (CMV) is excreted by approximately one fourth of internationally adopted children, who typically acquired the virus perinatally and suffer no adverse consequences. Instructions on the value of good hand-washing after contact with urine, diapers, and respiratory secretions should be given to the adoptive parents. Routine screening for CMV infection is not recommended.
4. *Intestinal pathogens.* Fecal examination for ova and parasites, when performed by an experienced laboratory, uncovers a pathogen in nearly 50% of internationally adopted children. Although parasitic infection is rare among children from Korean foster homes, children from India and Central or South America, and any child abandoned before adoption, are at risk for parasites. In addition, children with diarrhea, especially those from India, may also need stool cultures for *Salmonella, Shigella, Yersinia,* and *Campylobacter.* Because of the recognition of additional parasites after treatment of the primary infestation, follow-up stool examinations for ova and parasites should be obtained until all pathogens have been eliminated.

5. *Tuberculosis.* Although less common in international adoptees than in refugee children from Indochina, tuberculosis is still frequently encountered. Screening for tuberculosis should include the placement of the Mantoux test (5TU PPD) (see Tuberculosis, page 490). In addition, in children younger than 2 years and those of poor nutritional status, the simultaneous placement of a *Candida* skin test or other test of delayed hypersensitivity is helpful in differentiating anergy from lack of exposure to *M tuberculosis.* Routine chest roentgenograms are not warranted in asymptomatic children with negative PPD tests. The application of the PPD should not be deferred because of the suspicion of BCG vaccination, and a positive PPD test (10 mm or more of induration) should not be attributed to BCG without further investigation (see Tuberculosis, page 506). In refugees and international adoptees found to have active tuberculosis, efforts to isolate the responsible organism must be diligently pursued because of the high prevalence of drug resistance in many foreign countries.
6. *Syphilis.* Congenital syphilis, especially with involvement of the central nervous system, is sometimes undiagnosed and often inadequately treated in many developing nations. The importance of reliable serologic testing for syphilis cannot be overemphasized.
7. *HIV infection.* The risk of HIV infection in internationally adopted children depends on the country of origin. Recent data from the World Health Organization indicate that India, Korea, and most Central and South American countries still have only small numbers of patients identified with AIDS, whereas countries such as Brazil, Venezuela, Haiti, Honduras, and tropical African nations have a substantially greater frequency of infection. Testing for HIV infection in individual children should be based on the child's history, physical examination, and country of origin. Transplacentally acquired maternal antibody in the absence of infection in the child can be present in the child younger than 15 months. Hence, positive serologic tests in asymptomatic children of this age require follow-up testing and clinical evaluation. As the international epidemiology of HIV infection changes, screening for HIV infection may become routine for all internationally adopted children.
8. *Other infectious diseases.* Diseases such as typhoid fever or melioidosis are infrequently encountered in internationally adopted children, except those of southeast Asian origin. Routine screening for malaria is not indicated. However, malaria can occur, typically in children from rural India. In symptomatic children with fever of unknown etiology, anemia, or splenomegaly, thick smears of peripheral blood with Giemsa staining should be obtained.

Apart from vision and hearing testing in all children, which often detects unsuspected deficits, especially in the young infant, the use of other tests in specific groups of children is warranted. For example, screening for sickle hemoglobinopathies may be appropriate in children of mixed parentage from India, Central America, or South America; hemoglobin E can be found in children from Southeast Asia. In young children with sickle-cell disease, penicillin prophylaxis is recommended (see Pneumococcal Infections, page 378). Screening for glucose-6-phosphate dehydrogenase deficiency should be considered in children of Mediterranean or African origin before administering sulfa-containing antibiotics.

Control Measures for Prevention of Tick-Borne Infections

Tick-borne infectious diseases in children that can occur in the United States include Lyme disease, Rocky Mountain spotted fever, and tularemia. The control of these and other tick-borne diseases, such as babesiosis, relapsing fever, and typhus, requires preventing or at least minimizing opportunity for infected ticks to bite and engorge on humans. Control of the tick population in the field is not a practical public health measure. Specific control measures for prevention are as follows:

- Physicians, parents, and children, whenever possible, should be aware of ticks and the possibility of acquisition of disease.
- Tick-infested areas should be avoided whenever possible.
- If a tick-infested area is entered, protective clothing that covers the arms, legs, and other exposed areas should be worn. Other measures include tucking the pants into boots or socks and buttoning long-sleeved shirts at the cuff. In addition, permethrin is effective in decreasing tick attachment and can be sprayed onto clothes.
- Tick/insect repellents,* such as "deet" (N,N-diethyl-m-toluamide), applied to the skin, provide additional protection but require reapplication every 1 to 2 hours for effectiveness. If "deet" is used, and because seizures in young children have been reported coincident with its application, it should be applied sparingly and only to exposed skin, it should not be applied on a child's hands or irritated or abraded skin, and it should be washed off after the child comes indoors.
- Persons should be taught to inspect themselves and their children's bodies and clothing daily after possible tick exposure, such as in the woods during the tick season. Special attention should be given to the exposed hairy regions of the body where ticks often sequester.

*For further information, see Insect repellents, *The Medical Letter.* 1989;31:45-47.

- Ticks should be removed promptly. Care should be taken to avoid squeezing the body of the tick because transmission of infection can result. The tick should be grasped with a fine tweezer close to the skin and removed by gentle pulling. If fingers are used to remove ticks, they should be protected with facial tissue and washed afterwards.
- Daily inspection of pets and removal of ticks is indicated.

PART 3

SUMMARIES OF INFECTIOUS DISEASES

AIDS and HIV Infections

Clinical Manifestations: Human immunodeficiency virus (HIV) infection in children causes a broad spectrum of disease manifestations and a varied clinical course. Acquired immunodeficiency syndrome (AIDS) represents the most severe end of the clinical spectrum. The current Centers for Disease Control (CDC) surveillance definition for AIDS is given in Table 20. Patients meeting these criteria for AIDS must be reported to the appropriate public health department. The spectrum of HIV infection in children also includes indeterminate and asymptomatic infections as well as diverse symptomatic illness. To define and categorize HIV infection in children younger than 13, the CDC has also established a pediatric classification system (Table 21).

HIV affects multiple organ systems. Manifestations are diverse and include nonspecific findings, progressive neurologic disease, lymphoid interstitial pneumonia, recurrent invasive bacterial infection, opportunistic infections, and specified malignancies (Table 20). Other common clinical manifestations include generalized lymphadenopathy, hepatosplenomegaly, failure to thrive, recurrent diarrhea, and parotitis. Cardiomyopathy, hepatitis, and nephropathy can also occur. Craniofacial abnormalities in infants with prenatally acquired HIV infection have been reported, but whether these are caused by HIV infection or by other factors, such as maternal drug use or genetic characteristics, is controversial.

Pediatric AIDS patients often have recurrent serious infections caused by common bacteria such as *Streptococcus pneumoniae, Haemophilus influenzae* type b, *Staphylococcus aureus,* and *Salmonella* species. Lymphoid interstitial pneumonitis (LIP) occurs in 30% to 50% of children with AIDS. Developmental delay and failure to thrive are common, and a progressive or static encephalopathy develops in many HIV-infected children.

Pneumocystis carinii pneumonitis (PCP) is the most common opportunistic infection in children with AIDS, and is associated with high mortality. It occurs frequently between 4 and 8 months of age in infants whose infection was acquired before or at birth. Other common opportunistic infections include *Candida* esophagitis, disseminated primary or reactivated latent cytomegalovirus infection (onset after 1 month of age), chronic or disseminated herpes simplex virus infection (onset after 1 month of age), *Mycobacterium avium-intracellularae* (MAI) complex infection, chronic enteritis due to *Cryptosporidium* or other agents, and rarely disseminated or central nervous system cryptococcal infection.

Malignancies in pediatric HIV infection are uncommon, but certain lymphomas, including those of the central nervous system and non-Hodgkin's B-cell lymphomas of the Burkitt type, have occurred. Lymphadenopathic Kaposi's sarcoma is very rare.

Characterization of the natural history of HIV infection in children is still emerging. The development of opportunistic infections, particularly PCP, progressive neurologic disease, or severe wasting is associated with a poor prognosis. Survival also tends to be poor in children infected perinatally who become symptomatic in the first year of life. In contrast, median survival in children with lymphoid interstitial pneumonitis is longer.

Etiology: The cause of AIDS is an RNA cytopathic human retrovirus, human immunodeficiency virus, type 1 (HIV-1). A second virus, HIV-2, is serologically distinct from HIV-1, but causes clinically indistinguishable AIDS in Africa. These viruses are particularly tropic for T-helper (CD4) lymphocytes and macrophages. Since retroviruses integrate into the target cell genome as proviruses and the viral genome is copied during cell replication, the virus persists in infected individuals for life. The role of cofactors (such as simultaneous infection with other viruses, particularly cytomegalovirus or Epstein-Barr virus, or malnutrition) in the natural history of infection is not known.

Epidemiology: Humans are the only known reservoir of HIV. The modes of HIV transmission include intimate homosexual or heterosexual contact; sharing of contaminated needles for injection; transfusion of blood or blood components and clotting factor concentrates; and from mother to infant before or around the time of birth. As of October 1990, transmission of HIV has not been documented to occur by casual contact in families or households, in schools or day care settings, or with routine care in hospitals or clinics in the absence of parenteral or mucous membrane blood contact. HIV has been isolated from blood (including lymphocytes,

Table 20. Centers for Disease Control Surveillance Definition for AIDS – Diagnoses Indicative of AIDS

Candidiasis of the esophagus*,†
Candidiasis of the trachea, bronchi, or lungs*
Coccidioidomycosis, disseminated or extrapulmonary‡
Cryptococcosis, extrapulmonary*
Cryptosporidiosis, chronic intestinal*
Cytomegalovirus disease (other than liver, spleen, nodes), onset at > 1 month of age*
Cytomegalovirus retinitis (with loss of vision)*,†
Herpes simplex ulcer, chronic (> 1 month duration) or pneumonitis or esophagitis, onset at > 1 month of age*
HIV encephalopathy‡
Histoplasmosis, disseminated or extrapulmonary‡
Isosporiasis, chronic intestinal (> 1 month duration)‡
Kaposi's sarcoma*,†
Lymphoid interstitial pneumonitis*,†
Lymphoma, primary brain*
Lymphoma (Burkitt's, or immunoblastic sarcoma)‡
Multiple or recurrent bacterial infections‡
Mycobacterium avium complex or *M kansasii*, disseminated or extrapulmonary*
M tuberculosis or acid-fast infection (species not identified), disseminated or extrapulmonary‡
Pneumocystis carinii pneumonia*,†
Progressive multifocal leukoencephalopathy*
Toxoplasmosis of brain, onset at > 1 month of age*,†
Wasting syndrome due to HIV‡

*If indicator disease diagnosed definitively (e.g., biopsy or culture) and no other cause of immunodeficiency, laboratory documentation of HIV infection is not required.

†Presumptive diagnosis of indicator disease is accepted, if laboratory evidence of HIV infection.

‡Requires laboratory evidence of HIV infection.

macrophages, and plasma), other internal body fluids such as cerebrospinal fluid and pleural fluid, human milk, semen, cervical secretions, saliva, urine, and tears. However, only blood, semen, cervical secretions, and human milk have been implicated epidemiologically in the transmission of infection.

Accidental exposure of health care personnel to the virus, such as from needlestick injuries, has rarely resulted in HIV infection, occurring in less than 0.5% of cases. Many of the cases might have been prevented by careful adherence to infection control measures, especially during emergencies.

AIDS in children and adolescents currently accounts for 2% of all reported cases of AIDS in the United States. However, the total number of reported cases continues to increase. HIV acquisition during adolescence contributes to the increased number of cases in young adults. Adolescent risk factors for HIV infection become similar to those for adults as children approach adulthood, i.e., engage in intimate heterosexual contact, male homosexual contact, intravenous drug abuse, and transfusion of contaminated blood or blood components. In 13- to 15-year-olds, transfusion is the major cause of infection but it decreases markedly by age 19 years.

Of infected children younger than 13 years in the United States, 80% have been born to families in which one or both parents have a risk factor for HIV infection and AIDS. The remainder received contaminated blood or its components, or clotting factor concentrates (11%), including patients with hemophilia or other coagulation disorders (5%). Approximately 3% have no identifiable risk factor, but on investigation, nearly all can be attributed to one of the established risk factors.

Transplacental transmission from an infected mother to her infant has been demonstrated, and intrapartum transmission is presumed. Most evidence suggests that transmission is predominantly in utero. The risk of infection for an infant born to an HIV-seropositive mother is estimated to be 30% to 35% and could be as high as 50%. In women who have previously delivered an HIV-infected infant, the risk of infection in subsequent infants can be as high as 50%. The factors responsible for transmission have not been identified. Some studies suggest higher rates of infection in women who have AIDS. It is not known whether delivery by cesarean section prevents transmission.

The HIV genome has been detected in cell-free extracts of human breast milk, and breast milk has been implicated in the transmission of HIV infection to at least eight infants. Most of these mothers had blood transfusions postpartum and breast-fed their infants. The blood donors later developed clinical evidence of HIV infection, and mothers and infants, on subsequent testing, were seropositive. These

Table 21. Classification System for HIV Infection in Children Younger Than 13 Years*

Class P-0. Indeterminate Infection. Includes perinatally exposed infants and children younger than 15 months who cannot be classified as definitely infected according to the above definition but who have antibody to HIV, indicating exposure to a mother who is infected.

Class P-1. Asymptomatic Infection.

- Subclass A. Normal immune function
- Subclass B. Abnormal immune function
- Subclass C. Immune function not tested

Class P-2. Symptomatic Infection.

- Subclass A. Nonspecific findings
- Subclass B. Progressive neurologic disease
- Subclass C. Lymphoid interstitial pneumonitis
- Subclass D. Secondary infectious disease
  - Category D-1. Specified secondary infectious diseases listed in the CDC surveillance definition for AIDS
  - Category D-2. Recurrent serious bacterial infections
  - Category D-3. Other specified secondary infectious diseases
- Subclass E. Secondary cancers
  - Category E-1. Specified secondary cancers listed in the CDC surveillance definition for AIDS
  - Category E-2. Other cancers possibly secondary to HIV infection
- Subclass F. Other diseases possibly due to HIV infection. Includes children with other conditions possibly due to HIV infection not listed in the above subclasses, such as hepatitis, cardiopathy, nephropathy, hematologic disorders (anemia, thrombocytopenia), and dermatologic diseases.

---

*From Centers for Disease Control: Classification for human immunodeficiency virus (HIV) infection in children under 13 years of age. *MMWR.* 1987;36(15):225-230, 235-236.

women possibly represent a unique situation in which the mother has high concentrations of virus shortly after acquiring the infection. However, the HIV-infected infant born to a mother who was infected before pregnancy or early in gestation is much more common. The additional risk, if any, of transmission of the virus to an infant through breast-feeding appears to be small compared to the risk of transplacental or intrapartum transmission.

The **incubation period** of disease is variable, ranging from months to years. Infants infected prenatally (in utero) or perinatally often exhibit signs and symptoms of infection during the first year of life and most are symptomatic before 2 years of age. However, some may not manifest symptoms until they are older than 5 years and a few children have been diagnosed at as late as 11 years of age. The median age of onset of symptoms is estimated to be 3 years or older. In transfusion-associated cases in young children, the incubation period for onset of clinical disease has an estimated median of 3.5 years, but has considerable individual variability. Infection acquired in adolescence may not become clinically apparent until young adulthood. Other than infants born of infected mothers, persons infected with HIV usually develop serum anti-HIV antibody 6 to 12 weeks after infection.

Diagnostic Tests: Diagnosis of HIV infection is usually made by serologic tests. In infants with inconclusive serologic test results, primary immunodeficiency diseases or secondary immunodeficiency associated with immunosuppressive therapy, lymphoreticular malignancy, or malnutrition should be excluded. Diagnostic testing is indicated for children who have clinical and epidemiologic features suggestive of HIV infection. Epidemiologic features include receipt of multiple blood or blood product transfusions between 1978 and 1985, male homosexuality or bisexuality, intravenous drug abuse, having a mother who is HIV infected, or being at increased risk of HIV infection and sexual abuse (for children or adolescents). Because HIV infection should be considered in the differential diagnosis of many presenting illnesses, serologic HIV testing is often indicated in circumstances in which a positive result is unlikely. The interests of the child are paramount.

Multiple diagnostic tests, including serologic antibody assays and HIV detection techniques, have been developed. The serologic HIV antibody tests currently licensed are enzyme-linked immunosorbent assays (ELISA). These tests are highly sensitive and specific, but nonspecific test results have been reported in a small percentage of cases. Repeat ELISA testing of initially reactive specimens is required to reduce the likelihood of laboratory error; repeatedly reactive tests are highly reliable. Western blot and immunofluorescent antibody tests are used for confirmation of ELISA test results. They are available in an increasing number of medical centers, large commercial laboratories, and public health department laboratories, but only one Western blot test is currently licensed. Assays for the detection of HIV-specific IgM and IgA antibodies are currently experimental and require further development. Viral culture for HIV is not widely available. A test for detection of HIV p24 antigen in serum is commercially available but this test is relatively insensitive in the diagnosis of HIV infection in infants and children. Amplification of HIV proviral DNA by polymerase chain reaction (PCR) is a newer technique that holds promise for earlier diagnosis of infection in infants.

Serum antibodies to HIV are present in virtually all infected persons, although some patients with AIDS become seronegative late in disease. Some patients develop antibodies long after infection is proven by culture techniques. Some children with HIV infection have hypogammaglobulinemia and may be unable to produce antibody. In addition, a small percentage of HIV-infected children are antibody negative by ELISA testing but are positive on Western blot testing for anti-HIV antibody or are found to be infected by HIV p24 antigen tests and/or cultures for HIV.

Infants born to HIV-seropositive women pose a special diagnostic challenge since they are usually seropositive at birth due to passive transfer of maternal antibody, irrespective of HIV infection, and serum HIV antibodies can persist in the infant for as long as 15 months. Sequential HIV antibody testing should be done in these infants to determine whether the antibody is of infant or maternal origin. In a child younger than 15 months, HIV infection can be diagnosed by a positive blood or body fluid culture for HIV; the presence of clinical manifestations (see Tables 20 and 21) with HIV seropositivity and evidence of cellular and humoral immune deficiency; a quantitative increase in serum HIV antibody; or the development of a new antibody to a specific viral protein. A positive PCR test for HIV proviral DNA in blood or other body fluid also indicates infection but this test is currently investigational. On the basis of present knowledge, a positive antibody test for HIV in a child older than 15 months is usually indicative of infection, but rare instances in which detectable maternal antibody has persisted in an infant for 18 months have occurred.

Other laboratory tests yield characteristic findings. The most notable finding, particularly as the disease progresses, is a profound loss of T-cell immunity. Initially, the peripheral blood lymphocyte count can be normal, but eventually lymphopenia develops because of a decrease in the total circulating T-lymphocytes. The cells most affected are the T-helper (CD4) lymphocytes. The T-suppressor

(CD8) lymphocytes are not depleted until late in the course of the infection. These changes in cell population result in inversion of the normal T-helper to T-suppressor cell ratio to less than 1.0. This nonspecific finding, while typical of HIV infection, also occurs with other acute viral infections, such as those caused by cytomegalovirus or Epstein-Barr virus.

In contrast to adults, HIV-infected infants and young children with CD4 cell counts of more than 400/mm^3 can have significant disease manifestations, especially *Pneumocystis carinii* infection. B-lymphocytes remain normal or are increased in number. The serum IgG concentration is frequently elevated, and IgM and IgA concentrations can be normal or elevated. A few patients will develop a panhypogammaglobulinemia. Specific antibody response to new antigens may be abnormal. Response of T-lymphocytes to plant lectin mitogens (phytohemagglutinin, concanavalin A, and particularly pokeweed) are decreased or absent, and patients may be anergic to skin test antigens such as mumps, *Candida, Trichophyton,* tetanus, and tuberculin PPD.

Informed Consent for HIV Serologic Testing. Testing for HIV infection is unlike routine blood testing in that substantial psychosocial risks can be incurred. When testing of an infant or child is undertaken, parents or other primary caretakers, and patients, if old enough to comprehend, should be counseled about the possible risks and benefits of testing and consequences of HIV infection. Oral consent should be obtained from the parent or legal guardian and recorded in the patient's chart. Special written consent procedures for HIV testing should be discouraged as they can inhibit the performance of testing without adding significant benefit. Nevertheless, state and local laws and hospital regulations should be considered in deciding whether written consent is required. The necessity for counseling and consent should not deter the undertaking of appropriate testing for the diagnosis of HIV infection, and refusal to give consent should be considered analogous to other instances in which parents or guardians refuse necessary diagnostic tests. If the physician believes that testing is essential to the child's health, refusal constitutes medical neglect, and authorization for testing may need to be obtained by other means. The results of serologic tests should be discussed in person with the family, primary caretaker, and, if appropriate according to age, the patient; if positive, appropriate counseling and subsequent follow-up care must be provided. Confidentiality in all cases is essential to preserving patient and parent trust and consent.

Treatment: Adults and children treated with zidovudine (formerly termed "azidothymidine" or "AZT") have shown clinical and immunologic improvement, and trials to determine the effect of this drug on morbidity and mortality are ongoing. Oral zidovudine has been licensed for use in children, adolescents, and adults, and it is now the recommended therapy for HIV-infected adults and for adolescents with symptomatic HIV infection or with CD4 lyphocyte cell counts of less than 500/mm^3. For children with AIDS, zidovudine in a dose of 180 mg/m^2 every 6 hours is recommended (see Antiviral Drugs, page 580). It appears to be well tolerated in children, although hematologic toxicity has occurred. Zidovudine is also approved for HIV-infected children who are asymptomatic but have laboratory evidence of HIV-related immunosuppression. Trials of other antiretroviral drugs with in vitro activity against HIV, such as dideoxycytidine (DDC), dideoxyinosine (DDI), and soluble CD4, are currently in progress in symptomatic HIV-infected infants and children.

Further information on drug trials in HIV-infected children can be obtained from the Pediatric Clinical Trials Group (800/TRI-ALSA) or the Pediatric Branch, National Cancer Institute, Bethesda, MD (301/496-4250).

The benefit of, and need for monthly or biweekly administration of intravenous immune globulin (IGIV) to HIV-infected children has been controversial. Some centers have advocated treating all infected children with IGIV. Studies of the efficacy of IGIV in preventing bacterial infections in infected infants and children are in progress.* IGIV treatment may be beneficial in combination with an antiviral agent for children with recurrent bacterial infections, significant B-cell defects, or those who fail to form antibodies to common antigens.

Early diagnosis and aggressive treatment of opportunistic infections may prolong survival. Because death is frequently caused by *P carinii* pneumonia (PCP), chemoprophylaxis should be given to HIV-infected children at risk of PCP. Indications in children younger than 13 years include prior PCP, T-helper (CD4) lymphocyte count less than 400 cells/mm^3, or age less than 1 year. Since PCP may be an early complication of perinatally acquired HIV infection, most experts recommend prophylaxis for infants younger than 1 year who are known to be infected. In children, data on efficacy and safety of prophylactic regimens are insufficient to provide a basis for scientifically validated guidelines. Based on trials in pediatric cancer patients, trimethoprin-sulfamethoxazole (TMP-SMX) is the drug of choice for prophylaxis. Although the reported incidence of adverse reactions to TMP/SMX has been high in adults with AIDS, these

***In January 1991, while the *Red Book* was in press, one of these studies was terminated, and recommendations were issued by the AAP Task Force on Pediatric AIDS for IGIV treatment of children with symptomatic HIV infection and peripheral CD4 lymphocyte counts of 200/mm^3 or greater.**

findings have not been confirmed in young children. For adults and adolescents 13 years or older, aerosolized pentamidine or oral TMP-SMX appear to be effective. For further information, see *Pneumocystis carinii*, page 380.

Immunization Recommendations (see also Table 22).

Children With Symptomatic HIV Infection. In general, live virus (e.g., oral poliovirus) vaccines and live bacterial (e.g., BCG) vaccines should not be given to patients with AIDS or other clinical manifestations of HIV infection and who are therefore immunosuppressed. The exception is MMR. For routine immunizations, DTP, inactivated poliovirus vaccine (IPV), and *Haemophilus* b conjugate vaccine should be given according to the usual immunization schedule (see Tables 2 and 3, pages 17 and 18). Pneumococcal vaccine at 2 years of age and yearly influenza vaccination beginning at age 6 months are also recommended.

Measles and MMR. The occurrence of severe measles in symptomatic HIV-infected children and the lack of reported serious or unusual reactions to immunization with MMR vaccine have led to the recommendation for measles immunization of HIV-infected children, regardless of symptoms, with MMR vaccine. MMR should be given at age 15 months according to recommendations for routine administration of measles vaccine; and, if the risk of exposure to measles is increased, such as during an outbreak, these children should receive vaccine at younger ages (see Measles Vaccine Recommendations, page 312).

In general, children with symptomatic HIV infection have poor immunologic responses to vaccines. Hence, such children, when exposed to a vaccine-preventable disease such as measles or tetanus, should be considered susceptible regardless of the history of vaccination, and should receive, if indicated, passive immunoprophylaxis (see Passive Immunization of Children With HIV Infection, page 51).

Children With Asymptomatic HIV Infection. Children with asymptomatic HIV infection should receive DTP, IPV, HbCV, and MMR vaccines according to the usual immunization schedules (see Tables 2 and 3, pages 17 and 18). Although oral poliovirus vaccine (OPV) has been given to this group without adverse effect, IPV is recommended because family members of such children can be immunocompromised due to symptomatic HIV infection and, therefore, are at risk for vaccine-associated paralytic poliomyelitis from acquisition of the vaccine virus.

Pneumococcal vaccination is indicated for children 2 years and older in view of the high incidence of invasive pneumococcal infection when HIV-infected children become symptomatic. Yearly

Table 22. Recommendations for Routine Immunization of HIV-Infected Children in the United States*

Vaccine†	Known Asymptomatic HIV Infection	Symptomatic HIV Infection
DTP	Yes	Yes
OPV	No	No
IPV	Yes	Yes
MMR	Yes	Yes
Haemophilus b	Yes	Yes
Pneumococcal	Yes	Yes
Influenza	Should be considered	Yes

*See text for age at which specific vaccines are indicated.
†DTP = diphtheria and tetanus toxoids and pertussis vaccine; OPV = oral poliovirus vaccine; IPV = inactivated poliovirus vaccine; MMR = live virus measles, mumps, and rubella.

influenza vaccination should be considered for those 6 months or older.

In the United States and in areas of low tuberculosis prevalence, BCG vaccine is contraindicated. However, in areas where the prevalence is high, the World Health Organization recommends that BCG should be given to asymptomatic infants who are suspected to be HIV infected at birth or as soon as possible thereafter.

Seronegative Children Residing in the Household of a Patient With Symptomatic HIV Infection. In a household with an adult or child immunocompromised due to HIV infection, seronegative children should receive IPV vaccine because the live poliovirus in OPV can be excreted and transmitted to immunosuppressed contacts. MMR vaccine may be given because MMR vaccine viruses are not transmitted. To reduce the risk of transmission of influenza to patients with symptomatic HIV infection, yearly influenza vaccination is indicated for their household contacts (see Influenza, page 277).

Passive Immunization of Children With HIV Infection.

- *Measles* (see Measles, Care of Exposed Persons, page 310).
  1) Symptomatic HIV-infected children who are exposed to measles should receive immune globulin (IG) prophylaxis (0.5 mL/kg, maximum 15 mL) regardless of vaccination status.
  2) Exposed, asymptomatic HIV-infected patients who are susceptible should also receive IG; the recommended dose is 0.25 mL/kg.
  3) Children who have received intravenous immunoglobulin (IGIV) within 2 weeks of exposure do not require additional passive immunization.

- *Tetanus.* In the management of wounds classified as tetanus-prone, children with AIDS should receive Tetanus Immune Globulin (TIG) regardless of vaccination status.
- *Varicella.* HIV-infected children who are exposed to varicella or zoster and who are susceptible should receive Varicella-Zoster Immune Globulin (VZIG) (see Varicella-Zoster Infections, page 520).

Isolation of the Hospitalized Patient: The routinely recommended blood and body fluid precautions for all patients (see Isolation Precautions, page 81) should be scrupulously followed for patients with HIV infection. The risk to health care personnel of acquiring HIV infection from a patient is minimal, even after accidental exposure from a needle-stick injury. Nevertheless, every effort should be made to avoid exposures to blood and other body fluids that could contain HIV (see Table 12, page 83).

Control Measures:

Exposed Health Care Workers. Management of the health care worker who has had a parenteral or mucous membrane exposure to blood or bloody secretions from an HIV-positive patient should include the following:

1. Confirm that the patient is HIV-positive.
2. Evaluate the health care worker clinically and serologically for evidence of HIV infection as soon as possible after the exposure. If the health care worker is seronegative, he or she should be retested at 6 weeks, 3 months, and 6 months after exposure to determine whether transmission has occurred. Most exposed individuals who have been infected will seroconvert during the first 12 weeks after exposure.
3. The exposed health care worker should immediately be informed of any possibly effective chemoprophylaxis, and such therapy should immediately be instituted if the worker wishes to do so. Recommendations from the Centers for Disease Control for zidovudine in these circumstances have been recently promulgated. The dose is 200 mg every 4 hours for 4 to 6 weeks.
4. Counseling should be provided.

Guidelines for Infection Control of HIV in Hospital and Other Medical Settings. Universal blood and body fluid precautions should be implemented in all pediatric health care facilities. (For further discussion, see Isolation Precautions, page 81.*)

*For additional information, see Centers for Disease Control. Guidelines for prevention of transmission of human immunodeficiency virus and hepatitis B virus to health-care and public safety workers. MMWR 1989;38;No. S-6:9-10.

Adolescent Education. Adolescents should be educated about risk factors for HIV infection, including sexual transmission, injecting drugs, and sharing needles or syringes. Sexual contact with multiple partners or with those who have multiple partners increases the risk of infection. If adolescents are sexually active, they should be counseled about the correct and consistent use of condoms to reduce the risk of infection (see Sexually Transmitted Diseases, page 94).

School Attendance. HIV infection is not acquired through casual person-to-person contact, such as occurs in a school setting, and transmission through saliva or tears has not been documented in any setting. The determination of whether a child with HIV infection should be allowed to attend school or day care should take into consideration the risks, which are severe, to the affected child of acquiring infections, and the theoretical risk of possible transmission of HIV to the staff and other children.

Specific recommendations concerning school attendance of children and adolescents with HIV infection are the following:

- Most school-aged children and adolescents infected with HIV should be allowed to attend school without restrictions, provided the child's physician gives approval.
- Some infected students may pose an increased risk to others in school. For students who display biting behavior or who have exudative, weeping skin sores that cannot be covered, a more restricted school environment is recommended, pending more information about the transmission of HIV in these circumstances. Special education must be provided for children who are unable to attend regular school classes.
- No one besides the child's physician has an absolute need to know the child's primary diagnosis. The number of personnel aware of the child's condition should be kept to the minimum needed to ensure proper care of the child. The family has the right to inform the school. Persons involved in the care and education of an infected student must respect the student's right to privacy. Confidential records should be maintained.
- All schools should adopt routine procedures for handling blood or blood-contaminated fluids, including the disposal of sanitary napkins, regardless of whether students with HIV infection are known to be in attendance. School health care workers, teachers, administrators, and other employees should be educated about procedures (see Housekeeping Procedures for Blood and Body Fluids). For example, soiled surfaces should be promptly cleaned with disinfectants, such as a freshly prepared solution of dilute (1:64) household bleach (1/4 cup diluted in one gallon of water).
- Children infected with HIV develop progressive immunodeficiency, which increases their risk of experiencing severe complica-

tions from infections such as varicella, tuberculosis, measles, cytomegalovirus, and herpes simplex virus. The child's physician should regularly assess the risk of an unrestricted environment on the health of the HIV-infected student, including evaluation of possible contagious diseases in the school (e.g., adult tuberculosis).
- Routine screening of schoolchildren for HIV infection is not recommended.

Day Care* and Foster Care. Acquisition of HIV infection in day care from infected children or adults has not been reported, and foster parents have not acquired disease by caring for HIV-infected children. In view of these findings, current recommendations for day care and foster care personnel are as follows:

- The decision as to whether a child who has known HIV infection may attend day care or may be placed in foster care should be made on an individual, case-by-case basis. This decision is best made by qualified individuals, including the child's physician, who can evaluate (1) whether the child will receive optimum care in the setting under consideration and (2) whether an infected child poses a potential threat of HIV transmission to others. Most infected children do not pose risks to others. Although HIV-infected children who repeatedly bite other children or who have exudative skin lesions theoretically might transmit the virus, transmission in these circumstances has never been conclusively demonstrated. Hence, even in the presence of these factors, a foster family whose members have been appropriately counseled can care for an HIV-infected child.
- The decision to enroll a child in day care or foster care or to continue enrollment of a child who is subsequently found to be infected with HIV should also be made according to the preceding guidelines. Only persistent biting behavior or the presence of exudative skin lesions is an acceptable reason for exclusion for the purpose of protection of day care contacts. Decisions regarding notification and management of staff, parent(s), and child contacts in the day care or foster care setting should be made by the child's parents in concert with the child's physician and the director of the day care center. If parents of attendees are to be notified, they should be aware that transmission of HIV to other children in these conditions is extremely unlikely.
- Widespread screening of children in day care for the presence of HIV antibody is not warranted or recommended, as the risk of HIV transmission in the day care setting is only hypothetical at present.

---

*For additional discussion of recommendations for day care, see Children in Day Care, Blood-Borne Virus Infections, page 76.

- Some children are unknowingly infected with HIV or other infectious agents, such as hepatitis B virus, that may be present in blood or body fluids. Thus, all day care and foster care services, regardless of whether children with HIV infection are known to be in attendance, should adopt routine procedures for handling blood and blood-contaminated body fluids (see Housekeeping Procedures for Blood and Body Fluids). All child care personnel should be informed about these procedures. For example, soiled surfaces should be promptly cleaned with disinfectants, such as dilute (1:64), freshly prepared household bleach.
- Children infected with HIV develop progressive immunodeficiency, which increases their risk of severe complications from infections such as varicella, tuberculosis, measles, cytomegalovirus, and herpes simplex virus. Children may have a greater risk of encountering these infectious agents in child day care than at home. The risk to the immunodeficient child of attending day care in an unrestricted setting is best assessed by a physician who is aware of the child's immune status.
- Persons involved in the care and education of a preschool-aged, HIV-infected child should respect the child's and family's right to privacy. Records of HIV status should be kept only if strict confidentiality can be maintained. Only the child's family has the right to inform about the child's condition, and the number of informed personnel should be restricted to those needed to ensure proper care of the child and to detect situations in which the potential for transmission may change.

Adults With HIV Infection Working in Day Care or Schools. Asymptomatic HIV-infected adults may care for children in school or day care settings provided that they do not have exudative skin lesions or other conditions that would allow contact with their body fluids. No data indicate that HIV-infected adults have transmitted HIV in the course of normal day care or school responsibilities.

Adults with symptomatic HIV infection are immunocompromised and at increased risk from infectious diseases of young children. They should consult their physicians regarding the safety of their continuing work.

Housekeeping Procedures for Blood and Body Fluids. In general, routine housekeeping procedures using a commercially available cleaner (detergents, disinfectant-detergents, or chemical germicides) compatible with most surfaces are satisfactory for cleaning spills (e.g., vomitus, urine, and feces). For large spills involving blood or other human secretions or excretions, a freshly prepared solution of dilute (1:64) household bleach (1/4 cup diluted in one gallon of water) or other chemical germicide is useful as a disinfectant. Reusable rubber gloves may be useful for cleaning large spills to avoid contamination of the hands of the person cleaning the spill, but gloves are not essential for cleaning up small amounts of blood that can be contained easily by the material used for cleaning. Persons involved in cleaning contaminated surfaces should avoid exposure of open skin lesions or mucous membranes to blood or bloody fluids. Whenever possible, disposable towels or tissues should be used and properly discarded, and mops should be rinsed in the disinfectant.

Management and Counseling of Families. Infection acquired by children before or during birth is a disease of the family. Serologic screening of siblings and parents is recommended. In each case, the physician needs to provide education and ongoing counseling regarding HIV and its transmission, and to outline precautions to be taken within the household and the community to prevent spread of this virus.

Infected women need to be made aware of the risks of having an infected child if they become pregnant, and they should be referred for family planning counseling. Infected individuals should not donate blood, plasma, sperm, organs, corneas, bone, or breast milk.

The infected child should be taught good hygiene and behavior. How much he or she is told about the illness will depend on age and maturity. Older children, in particular, should be made aware that the disease can be transmitted sexually, and should be provided with appropriate counseling. Most families are not willing to share the diagnosis with others, since it can create social isolation. Feelings of guilt are common. Family members, including children, can become clinically depressed and require psychiatric counseling.

Breast-feeding. The risks of HIV transmission by breast milk are small. In the United States, where alternative effective sources of feeding are available, an HIV-infected woman should be counseled not to breast-feed her infant or donate to milk banks.

Sexual Abuse. Following sexual abuse by a person with or at risk for HIV infection, the child should be tested serologically at the time of abuse and at 12 and 24 weeks after sexual contact for anti-HIV. If possible, serologic evaluation of the abuser for HIV infection should be obtained. Counseling of the child and family needs to be provided. The risk of HIV transmission, however, is low.

Blood, Blood Components, and Clotting Factors. Screening blood and plasma for HIV antibody has dramatically reduced the risk of infection. Nevertheless, careful scrutiny of the requirements of each patient for blood, its components, or clotting factors is prudent.

The treatment of hemophiliacs has undergone extensive change in recent years. All factor VIII and factor IX concentrates available in the United States are now manufactured from plasma screened for HIV antibody, and the concentrates are heated or treated with solvents or detergents for inactivation of HIV (as well as hepatitis B and hepatitis C viruses) and are safe. Cryoprecipitate from single or pooled donor plasma is screened for anti-HIV antibody but does not undergo any process to inactivate HIV or other viruses. Patients with hemophilia should be managed in consultation with specialists familiar with current aspects of treatment, such as desmopressin for the treatment of individuals with mild or moderate factor VIII deficiency.

Actinomycosis

Clinical Manifestations: The three major types of clinical disease are cervicofacial, thoracic, and abdominal. Cervicofacial lesions frequently occur after tooth extraction or facial trauma, or are associated with carious teeth. Localized pain and induration progress to "woody hard" nodular lesions that terminate in draining sinus tracts. The infection usually spreads by direct invasion of adjacent tissues. Thoracic disease is primarily pneumonic, with development of abscesses, empyema, and pleurodermal sinuses. In abdominal infection, the appendix and cecum are the most frequent sites, and symptoms simulate those of appendicitis. Intra-abdominal abscesses and peritoneal-dermal draining sinuses eventually develop.

Etiology: *Actinomyces israeli* is the usual cause. *A israeli* and other *Actinomyces* and *Arachnia* (a related genus) species are slow-growing, Gram-positive bacteria that grow anaerobically.

Epidemiology: *Actinomyces* species are worldwide in distribution. Infection is rare in infants and children and occurs sporadically. The organisms are components of the endogenous flora; disease results from autoinfection and, rarely, from a human bite. Actinomycosis is not contagious.

Diagnostic Tests: A demonstration of beaded, branching, Gram-positive rods in pus suggests the diagnosis. A Gram stain of sulfur granules discloses a dense reticulum of filaments; the ends of individual filaments may project around the periphery of the granule, with or without radially arranged hyaline clubs. Specimens must be cultured anaerobically on selective media in the presence of carbon dioxide.

Treatment: Penicillin, erythromycin, clindamycin, chloramphenicol, and tetracycline (which should not be given to children younger than 9 years) are usually effective. Penicillin is preferred. High doses of antimicrobials for periods of 6 months or longer are commonly required to effect a cure. Surgical drainage may be necessary.

Isolation of the Hospitalized Patient: No special precautions are recommended.

Control Measures: Good oral hygiene, adequate regular dental care, and careful cleansing of wounds after a human bite can prevent infection.

Adenovirus Infections

Clinical Manifestations: The major clinical syndromes caused by adenovirus are upper respiratory tract symptoms accompanied by moderate systemic manifestations in children and adolescents. Severe pneumonia, which is occasionally fatal, can occur in younger infants and, less commonly, in older children and adolescents. Disease is often more severe in immunocompromised patients. Conjunctivitis is common, either alone or in combination with pharyngitis and other respiratory symptoms. Adenoviruses are infrequent causes of a pertussis-like syndrome, croup, bronchiolitis, and hemorrhagic cystitis. Adenoviruses have also been associated with gastroenteritis. The illness is similar to, although less common than that caused by rotavirus.

Etiology: Adenoviruses are DNA viruses; 47 distinct serotypes cause human infections. Types 40 and 41 have been incriminated as causes of gastroenteritis.

Epidemiology: Infection occurs throughout the pediatric age range. Adenoviruses causing respiratory infection are transmitted by person-to-person contact, usually through respiratory spread. Enteric strains of adenoviruses can be transmitted by the fecal-oral route. Other routes have not been clearly defined and may vary with age, type of infection, and environmental or other factors. The eyes may provide a portal of entry; e.g., infections have resulted from direct introduction of virus by the use of contaminated ophthalmologic instruments. Epidemics attributed to contaminated swimming pools have occurred. Shared towels and direct inoculation by fingers are involved in epidemic keratoconjunctivitis. Epidemics in military and educational institutions, or those resulting from a common source, have occurred. Nosocomial outbreaks of adenoviral respiratory and gastrointestinal infections have been documented. The incidence of adenovirus-induced respiratory disease is slightly increased in late winter, spring, and early summer. Enteric disease occurs during most of the year. Infections are most communicable during the first few days of an acute illness. Asymptomatic infections are common.

The **incubation period** varies from 2 to 14 days. For gastroenteritis, it is 3 to 10 days.

Diagnostic Tests: Adenoviruses can be isolated from pharyngeal secretions, eye swabs, and feces by inoculation of specimens into a variety of cell cultures. A pharyngeal isolate is more suggestive of recent infection than a fecal isolate, which may indicate either prolonged carriage or recent infection. Adenovirus antigen has been detected in body fluids of infected patients by immunoassay techniques. These techniques are especially useful in the diagnosis of diarrheal disease, as the enteric adenovirus strains usually cannot be isolated in standard tissue cultures. Enteric adenoviruses can also be identified by electron microscopy of stool specimens. Multiple serologic tests, including fluorescent antibody and enzyme immunoassay, are now commercially available for antibody testing. By complement fixation enzyme immunoassay tests that detect antibody to a common adenovirus antigen, a fourfold or greater rise in antibody titer in paired acute and convalescent sera is diagnostic of recent infection. Type-specific antibodies are detectable by hemagglutination inhibition or neutralization techniques or, for types 40 and 41, by enzyme immunoassays.

Treatment: Supportive.

Isolation of the Hospitalized Patient: For young children with respiratory adenoviral infection, contact isolation is advised for the duration of hospitalization. For patients with conjunctivitis, drainage/secretion precautions are recommended. Enteric precautions are advisable for patients with adenoviral gastroenteritis.

Control Measures: Live, attenuated adenovirus vaccines containing types 4, 7, and 21 have been used successfully to reduce acute respiratory disease in military personnel, but these vaccines are not available for civilian use.

Adequate chlorination of swimming pools is recommended to prevent pharyngoconjunctival fever. Appropriate hand washing before and after administering eye medications is required to prevent spread of keratoconjunctivitis. Ophthalmologic instruments should be decontaminated after use in infected patients.

Amebiasis

Clinical Manifestations: Persons with amebiasis are most commonly asymptomatic, or have nonspecific or mild intestinal symptoms, such as abdominal distention, flatulence, constipation, and, occasionally, loose stools. The usual clinical presentation is an acute diarrhea with some cramps. Less frequently, amebiasis can cause dysentery with bloody and mucoid stools, abdominal pain, fever, headache, and chills. Ulcerative lesions can lead to perforation of the colon and, therefore, peritonitis. Hepatic abscess develops by metastasis to the liver via the portal vein. Lesions in other locations, such as the lung, brain, and skin, arise by contiguous or hematogenous spread from a liver abscess or primary site in the colon. A granulomatous ameboma resembling an adenocarcinoma can develop in the colon.

Etiology: *Entamoeba histolytica* is a protozoan that is excreted as cysts and/or trophozoites in the feces of carriers. Each ingested cyst ultimately results in eight trophozoites, which continue to multiply by binary fission. Trophozoites can cause invasive disease.

Epidemiology: Infection occurs by ingestion of cysts in fecally contaminated material. Ingested trophozoites are not infectious because they are destroyed by the acidity of the stomach and by intestinal enzymes. The usual mode of transmission in the United States is by person-to-person spread and occasionally through contaminated food or drink. A patient is infectious intermittently and for prolonged periods, if untreated. Infection and reinfections are common in male homosexuals. The disease is worldwide in distribution, although prevalence is higher in areas with poor sanitary practices.

The **incubation period** is extremely variable, ranging from a few days to several months or years; commonly it is 2 to 4 weeks.

Diagnostic Tests: Diagnosis is made by identification of the organism in the stool or in tissues obtained from lesions. Cysts are shed intermittently in asymptomatic and mild infections, and multiple stool specimens may be needed to demonstrate the organism. Liquid stools are more likely than formed stools to contain trophozoites. Unless preserved promptly in fixative, trophozoites deteriorate rapidly after passage. When rapid transport of the specimen to the laboratory is not feasible, diagnosis is facilitated by take-home stool collection kits with childproof containers of 10% formalin and polyvinyl alcohol fixative. Fresh stool, sigmoidoscopic scrapings, or biopsy tissue can be examined by wet mount, but permanently stained smears or sections always should be made to confirm the diagnosis and for future reference. Aspirates of abscesses rarely contain amebae, but organisms sometimes can be identified in sections from abscess walls. Multiple serologic tests are available, including double diffusion, indirect immunofluorescence, countercurrent electrophoresis, ELISA, and indirect hemagglutination (IHA), which is one of the most commonly used. IHA is helpful in detecting invasive disease. Although only about 10% of asymptomatic carriers and fewer than 50% of those with amebic diarrhea will have IHA titers greater than or equal to 1:256; 85% with invasive (ulcerative) amebic dysentery and 95% with liver abscess will have serologic titers of this magnitude or greater.

Treatment: **Asymptomatic infections** and **mild intestinal disease** without dysentery or ulcerations should be treated with iodoquinol. The alternative drugs are diloxanide furoate* and paromomycin. **Moderate and severe intestinal disease** and **extraintestinal amebiasis,** such as **hepatic abscess,** should be treated with metronidazole followed by iodoquinol. However, the safety of metronidazole has not been established in children. Metronidazole ordinarily should not be prescribed for pregnant patients because of evidence that it is mutagenic in bacteria and carcinogenic in experimental animals. However, in life-threatening disease, its benefit may well outweigh the theoretical danger. A hepatic abscess should not be aspirated unless it keeps enlarging despite treatment or is so large and tense that spontaneous perforation is a danger. Patients with the diagnosis of amebic abscess confirmed by laboratory tests who do not respond to metronidazole may be treated with emetine or dehydroemetine,* followed by chloroquine phosphate plus iodoquinol.

Isolation of the Hospitalized Patient: Enteric precautions are recommended for patients with dysentery.

Control Measures: Measures to control spread of the disease include good hand washing after defecation and before eating, avoidance of sources of fecal contamination, sanitary disposal of feces, and provision of unpolluted drinking water. Persons in close physical contact with infected individuals can be screened for asymptomatic infection.

---

*Available from the Drug Service of the Centers for Disease Control (see Services of the Centers for Disease Control, page 622).

Primary Amebic Meningoencephalitis

(Naegleria fowleri, Acanthamoeba)

Clinical Manifestations: *Naegleria fowleri* causes an acute, progressive, fatal meningoencephalitis affecting children and young adults. Early symptoms include severe headache, fever, and sometimes rhinitis; these symptoms may progress to vomiting, nuchal rigidity, confusion, and delirium. Coma, seizures, and death ensue within 2 to 12 days.

Infection with *Acanthamoeba* species causes a granulomatous encephalitis that develops insidiously during a period of months, with progressive neurologic signs. These can include mental status abnormalities such as confusion, irritability, somnolence, seizures, hemiparesis, and other focal motor deficits. Nonspecific symptoms and signs, such as headache, fever, nausea, and vomiting, can also occur. Coma and death are invariable.

Etiology: *N fowleri* and *Acanthamoeba* species are free-living amoebae.

Epidemiology: The causative amebic species are most common in freshwater and moist soil. *Acanthamoeba* species have also been isolated from air-borne dust, hot tubs, brackish water, and sea water. Despite worldwide distribution of these amebic organisms, however, systemic infections are extremely rare. Fewer than 200 cases have been reported, but they have occurred on all inhabited continents and in a wide range of climatic zones.

N fowleri is normally acquired by swimming and diving in infested freshwater. The organism is ubiquitous and tends to thrive in waters with a temperature above 32°C (89.6°F), especially in the presence of coliform bacteria, on which it feeds. Disease in the United States occurs in summer and is acquired predominantly from infested lakes, ponds, swimming holes, and hot spring water in the southeastern and southwestern states, including Florida, Virginia, California, Texas, Georgia, South Carolina, Arkansas, Louisiana, and Mississippi. Children and young adults are usually affected. Infection occurs through the nose, along the olfactory nerves via the cribriform plate.

The **incubation period** is within 1 to 2 weeks after exposure to water harboring the organism.

Acanthamoeba infections frequently, although not exclusively, occur in immunocompromised or debilitated patients, such as those with neoplastic disease, diabetes, or alcoholism. They have also occurred in pregnant women. The modes of transmission are only partially identified. Organisms are not transmitted from person to person. Contaminated homemade saline solutions used to clean contact lenses have been associated with dendritic keratitis caused by *Acanthamoeba.* Infection of the central nervous system appears to result from hematogenous dissemination from a portal of entry in the skin, eye, lung, or kidney.

The **incubation period** is not known.

Diagnostic Tests: *Naegleria* infection is diagnosed by identification in unstained sediment of cerebrospinal fluid of the characteristic trophozoites, which can be confused with motile leukocytes. A Wright stain, but not a Gram stain, can help to distinguish leukocytes from trophozoites. Serologic tests are available on special request from the Centers for Disease Control (CDC). Culture methods using coliform-seeded, nonnutrient agar can be performed. The CDC can provide 24-hour assistance in the management of suspected cases, including confirmation of the diagnosis in cerebrospinal fluid and testing of serum specimens (shipped by air express). Specimens should be stored and transported at room temperature to maintain the viability of the amoebae.

In *Acanthamoeba* infections, organisms are rarely visualized in the cerebrospinal fluid. Diagnosis can be made only histologically by brain biopsy or at postmortem examination.* Serologic tests can be performed by special request at the CDC.

Treatment: Treatment of suspected *Naegleria* infection should not be delayed while waiting for confirmation of the diagnosis. The drug of choice is amphotericin B, given intravenously and intrathecally, and at maximum doses when therapy is initiated (see Systemic Treatment With Amphotericin B, page 574). The only documented survivor of this disease in the United States was treated with amphotericin B and miconazole, both given intravenously and intrathecally, and with oral rifampin.

Effective treatment for *Acanthamoeba* central nervous system infection has not been established.† Although these organisms are susceptible to a variety of agents in vitro, most antimicrobials have been clinically ineffective. Sulfadiazine was found to protect mice experimentally infected with *Acanthamoeba cullbertsoni,* and a Nigerian patient partially recovered after therapy with sulfametha-

---

*Corneal infections can be diagnosed by culture or histology.

†Acanthamoeba keratitis has been successfully treated with 0.1% propamidine isethionate eye drops (available only as an investigational drug in the United States; for information, contact the Food and Drug Administration, 301/295-8012) and polymyxin B/neomycin. In some cases, 1% clotrimazole (ocular formulation available only as an investigational drug in the United States) has been added to this combination.

zine. The efficacy of miconazole is under study. The simultaneous use of amphotericin B and sulfamethazine has been recommended by some experts.

Isolation of the Hospitalized Patient: No special precautions are recommended.

Control Measures: The public should be warned about the risk of swimming in infected, warm, polluted freshwater.

Anthrax

Clinical Manifestations: The spectrum of illness includes cutaneous (malignant pustule), inhalation (woolsorter's disease), gastrointestinal, septicemic, and meningeal anthrax. Cutaneous anthrax, which accounts for 95% of the cases of anthrax in the United States, is characterized by a painless lesion that progresses from a papule to a vesicle, to necrosis, and eventually to eschar formation. In inhalation anthrax, mild upper respiratory tract symptoms occur initially; approximately 2 to 5 days later, severe dyspnea, cyanosis, tachycardia, tachypnea, diaphoresis, fever, rales, and, usually, death occur. Gastrointestinal disease is characterized by abdominal pain and distention, vomiting, bloody diarrhea, and, frequently, toxemia and shock. Pharyngeal anthrax with profound submental swelling has also been reported. Septicemia and hemorrhagic meningitis are secondary manifestations of cutaneous, inhalation, or gastrointestinal anthrax. Disease manifestations are similar in adults and children.

Etiology: *Bacillus anthracis* is a Gram-positive, encapsulated, spore-forming, nonmotile rod.

Epidemiology: Anthrax is endemic in many agricultural regions of the world and is common in developing countries, but is rarely reported in the United States. Spores of *B anthracis* are found on hides, carcasses, hair, wool, bone meal, and other animal byproducts of domesticated and wild animals, such as goats, sheep, cattle, swine, horses, buffalo, and deer. Imported dolls and toys decorated with infected hair or hides have been a source of infection. Spore forms of the organism have been found in soil in rural farming regions in several areas of the United States. Spores can remain viable for 40 years or more.

Cutaneous anthrax, which occurs principally in agricultural and industrial employees, results from contact with infected animals, carcasses, hair (especially goat hair), wool, hides, or, rarely, soil. Pulmonary anthrax results from inhalation of spores resulting from industrial processing of animal by-products or laboratory work with *B anthracis*. In gastrointestinal anthrax, ingestion of contaminated, undercooked meat is the mode of acquisition. Biting flies and other insects may also serve as mechanical vectors. Discharges from cutaneous lesions are potentially infectious; accidental infections have occurred in laboratory workers. *B anthracis* is not known to be transmitted from person to person.

The **incubation period** is 1 to 7 days; most cases occur within 2 to 5 days of exposure.

Diagnostic Tests: The following procedures have been used for diagnosis: (1) microscope visualization of *B anthracis* on direct Gram-stained smears and/or cultures on blood agar of lesions or discharges; (2) fluorescent antibody identification of the organisms in vesicle fluid, cultures, or tissue sections; (3) detection of antibody to *B anthracis* toxin by immunoblot; or (4) a fourfold or greater titer rise in serum antibody by an ELISA test between acute and convalescent sera.

Treatment: Penicillin is the antimicrobial of choice and is given for 5 to 7 days. Erythromycin, tetracycline, and chloramphenicol are also effective. Combined penicillin and streptomycin should be used for treating meningitis or inhalation anthrax.

Isolation of the Hospitalized Patient: For patients with cutaneous or inhalation anthrax, drainage/secretion precautions are indicated until antibiotic therapy is completed and lesions have begun to heal. Gloves should be worn for touching infective material; gowns should be worn if soiling is likely. Contaminated dressings and bedclothes should be burned or steam sterilized to destroy spores.

Control Measures: A cell-free vaccine* is available for persons at significant ongoing risk of acquiring anthrax. The vaccine is at least 90% effective in adults and produces minimal adverse effects. No data on vaccine effectiveness or adverse reactions in children are available.

Surveillance and control of industrial and agricultural sources of *B anthracis* by public health authorities is important.

---

*Available from the Drug Service of the Centers for Disease Control (see Services of the Centers for Disease Control, page 622).

Arboviruses

Clinical Manifestations: Some arboviruses cause principally a central nervous system infection. Others produce an undifferentiated febrile illness, fever with rash, hemorrhagic manifestations, hepatitis, myalgia, or polyarthritis; other organ systems can also be involved.

Etiology: Approximately 530 arthropod-borne viruses, commonly referred to as arboviruses, have been identified. Although they originally were grouped together because of their common mode of transmission, the members belong to a variety of taxonomic groups (Table 23). Most arboviruses belong to the families Bunyaviridae, Togaviridae, or Flaviviridae. Of the more than 230 recognized arboviruses in the Western hemisphere, more than 30 have been shown to be responsible for human disease.

Epidemiology: Most arboviruses are maintained in nature through cycles of transmission among birds or small mammals by arthropod vectors, such as mosquitoes, ticks, and phlebotomine flies. Humans and domestic animals are infected incidentally as "dead-end" hosts. Direct person-to-person spread does not occur; however, infected vectors may spread dengue, yellow fever, and chikungunya viruses from person to person. Colorado tick fever has been transmitted through transfusion. During epidemics, individuals of all ages may be infected, but most infections do not cause disease. St. Louis encephalitis and Western equine encephalitis are more likely to produce clinical manifestations in the elderly than in children, whereas California encephalitis (LaCrosse virus) infections occur almost exclusively in children younger than 15 years. The prevalence of different arboviral diseases is related to ecologic conditions that affect the prevalence of infected vectors. Mosquito-borne arbovirus infections usually occur during the late summer in the United States.

The geographic distribution and **incubation periods** for the principal infections occurring in the Western hemisphere are given in Tables 24 and 25.

Diagnostic Tests: A definitive diagnosis can be made only by serologic testing or by virus isolation, techniques for which are available only in research and some reference laboratories. In some infections, particularly dengue, yellow fever, Colorado tick fever, sandfly fever, and Venezuelan equine encephalitis, virus may be isolated from blood obtained in the acute phase of illness. In cases of encephalitis, an attempt should be made to recover virus from biopsy or postmortem brain tissue. Virus-specific IgM antibodies in serum appear early

Table 23. Classification of Major Arthropod-Borne Virus Groups

Family	Genus	Representative Agents
Bunyaviridae	*Bunyavirus*	California serogroup viruses
	Phlebovirus	Sandfly fever
Togaviridae	*Alphavirus*	Western equine encephalitis virus Eastern equine encephalitis virus Venezuelan equine encephalitis virus Mayaro virus (South America) Chikungunya virus (Africa, India, Asia)
Flaviviridae	*Flavivirus*	St. Louis encephalitis virus Japanese B encephalitis virus Dengue viruses (types 1-4) Yellow fever virus Tick-borne encephalitis virus Russian summer-spring encephalitis virus Murray Valley encephalitis virus West Nile virus Powassan virus
Reoviridae	*Orbivirus*	Colorado tick fever
Rhabdoviridae	*Rhabdovirus*	Vesicular stomatitis virus

in disease. Although the presence of specific IgM may be a clue to recent infection, serologic tests of paired sera are necessary to confirm the diagnosis. Identification of virus-specific IgM in cerebrospinal fluid is diagnostic.

Treatment: Supportive.

Isolation of the Hospitalized Patient: For patients with dengue, yellow fever, and Colorado tick fever, the routinely recommended blood/body fluid precautions (see Isolation Precautions, page 81) should be scrupulously followed.

Control Measures:

Active Immunization.

Yellow Fever. The vaccine is a live attenuated vaccine preparation. Immunization is recommended for all individuals 9 months or older living in or traveling to endemic areas (contact local health authorities for information about vaccine availability). For immunization, a single dose of vaccine is given subcutaneously. Infants younger than 4 months should not be immunized because they are more suscep-

Table 24. Arbovirus Infections of the Central Nervous System Occurring in the Western Hemisphere

Disease (Causal Agent)*	Geographic Distribution of Virus	Incubation Period (days)
California encephalitis (several California serogroup viruses)	Widespread in the U.S. and Canada, including the Yukon and Northwest Territories; most prevalent in upper Midwest	5-15
Eastern equine encephalitis (Eastern equine encephalitis virus)	Central and eastern seaboard and Gulf states of the U.S.; Canada; South and Central America	5-15
Powassan encephalitis (Powassan virus)	Canada; northeastern and north central U.S.	4-18
St. Louis encephalitis (St. Louis encephalitis virus)	Widespread: central, southern, northeastern, and western U.S.; Manitoba and Southern Ontario; Caribbean area; South America	4-21
Venezuelan equine encephalitis (Venezuelan equine encephalitis virus)	Texas, Florida; Mexico; Central and South America	2-5
Western equine encephalitis (Western equine encephalitis virus)	Central and western U.S.; Canada; South America	5-10

*All are mosquito-borne except Powassan encephalitis, which is tick-borne.

tible to encephalitis temporally associated with yellow fever vaccination than older children. The decision to immunize children between 4 and 9 months of age should be based upon estimates of the risk of exposure (e.g., infants older than 4 months traveling to an area of epidemic activity should receive the vaccine). If possible, cholera vaccine should not be given concurrently with yellow fever vaccine; ideally, these vaccinations should be separated by at least 3 weeks. Since yellow fever vaccine is prepared in embryonated eggs and contains egg protein, which may cause allergic reactions, persons who have experienced signs or symptoms of anaphylactic reaction after eating eggs should not receive the vaccine. Pregnant women should

Table 25. Acute, Febrile Diseases and Hemorrhagic Fevers Caused by Arboviruses That Are Not Characterized by Encephalitis

Disease (Causal Agent)*	Geographic Distribution of Virus	Incubation Period (days)
Yellow fever (Yellow fever virus)	Tropical areas of South America and Africa	3-6
Dengue fever (Dengue virus types 1 to 4)	Tropical areas worldwide: Caribbean, Central and South America, Asia, India, Australia, Oceania, Africa	3-12
Mayaro fever (Mayaro virus)	Caribbean area, Central and South America	4-11
Colorado tick fever (Colorado tick fever virus)	Rocky Mountain area and Pacific Northwestern U.S., Western Canada	3-6

*All are mosquito-borne except California tick fever, which is tick-borne.

not be vaccinated except in high-risk areas. The decision to immunize immunocompromised patients should be based upon the individual patient's risk of exposure and clinical status.

Japanese B Encephalitis and Other Arbovirus Vaccines. Inactivated vaccines for tick-borne encephalitis and Japanese B encephalitis are licensed in various countries in Europe and Asia, respectively, where the diseases are endemic, but they are not licensed in the United States. In endemic regions, the risk of disease for travelers to urban areas is low. Even in rural areas, the risk is low for travelers whose stay is brief, particularly if not in the summer. Travelers planning prolonged stays in rural areas and whose activities place them at risk of exposure should be advised to consider obtaining these immunizations abroad. Current information on locations of **Japanese B encephalitis** infection and vaccine availability can be obtained from the Division of Vector-Borne Infectious Diseases, Centers for Disease Control (303/221-6400).

Protection Against Vectors. Public health measures to control arthropod vectors are important. Individuals can protect themselves by wearing long-sleeved shirts and trousers, and by using mosquito repellents. Permethrin applied to clothing kills adherent ticks and mosquitoes. Travelers to tropical countries should bring mosquito bed nets and aerosol insecticidal sprays to reduce risk of mosquito bites at night.

The principal vectors of dengue and yellow fever bite during daytime hours but many other vector and pest mosquitoes are most active in twilight hours.

Ascaris lumbricoides Infection

(Ascariasis, Roundworm)

Clinical Manifestations: Asymptomatic infections are common. Nonspecific gastrointestinal symptoms are reported in some patients, but their frequency is not known. During the larval migratory phase, an acute transient pneumonitis (Loeffler's syndrome) associated with fever and marked eosinophilia can occur. Acute intestinal obstruction can develop in patients with heavy infections. The adult worms can be stimulated to migrate by stressful conditions (e.g., fever, illness, or anesthesia) and by some drugs. Worm migration can cause peritonitis secondary to intestinal wall penetration, and common bile duct obstruction with acute obstructive jaundice. *Ascaris* has been found in the appendiceal lumen in acute appendicitis, but an etiologic relationship is uncertain.

Etiology: *Ascaris lumbricoides* is a large roundworm of humans.

Epidemiology: The adult worms live in the small intestine; females produce 200,000 eggs per day. These eggs are excreted in the stool and must incubate in soil for 2 to 3 weeks to embryonate and become infectious. Infection results from ingestion of embryonated eggs. Larvae hatch in the small intestine, penetrate the mucosa, and are passively carried by portal blood to the liver and from there to the lungs. They then ascend through the tracheo-bronchial tree to the pharynx, are swallowed, and mature to adults in the small intestine. The interval between ingestion of the egg and the development of egg-laying adults is approximately 8 weeks. *Ascaris* is cosmopolitan, but is most common in the tropics, in areas of poor sanitation, and wherever human feces are used as fertilizer. If the infection is untreated, adult worms can live for as many as 12 to 18 months, resulting in daily excretion of large numbers of ova.

Diagnostic Tests: Ova can be detected by microscopic stool examination. Occasionally, patients pass adult worms via the rectum or vomit them.

Treatment: Pyrantel pamoate (11 mg/kg, maximum 1 g, in a single dose) is recommended for treatment of asymptomatic and symptomatic infections. Mebendazole (100 mg twice daily for 3 days) is equally effective, but therapy is required for 3 days. Albendazole is an alternative drug. In children younger than 2 years, in whom experience with these drugs is limited, the risks and benefits of therapy should be considered before drug administration. Reexamination of the stools 3 weeks after therapy to determine whether the worms have been eliminated is helpful in assessing therapy, but is not essential. Surgical intervention is occasionally necessary to relieve complete intestinal or biliary obstruction or for volvulus or peritonitis secondary to preformation. If surgery is performed for intestinal obstruction, massaging the worms to eliminate the obstruction is preferable to incision of the intestine.

Isolation of the Hospitalized Patient: No special precautions are recommended.

Control Measures: Sanitary disposal of feces should be undertaken. Children's play areas should be given special attention.

Aspergillosis

Clinical Manifestations: Aspergillosis is manifested by the following types of disease: (1) Aspergillomas are fungus balls that grow in old cavities or bronchogenic cysts and do not invade the lung tissue. (2) Allergic bronchopulmonary aspergillosis manifests as episodic wheezing, expectoration of brown mucous plugs, low-grade fever, eosinophilia, and transient pulmonary infiltrates. (3) Systemic aspergillosis occurs almost exclusively in immunocompromised patients with an underlying disease, usually one that causes neutrophil dysfunction (e.g., chronic granulomatous disease or acute leukemia) or after cytotoxic chemotherapy or immunosuppressive therapy (e.g., in organ transplantation). (4) Sinus infections and eye and brain abscesses frequently occur in patients in certain warm regions of the world such as the Sudan. Otomycosis occurs in the external ear canal. (5) Occasional cases of endocarditis, osteomyelitis, meningitis, vaginitis, skin lesions, keratomycosis, infection of the orbit, and endophthalmitis occur.

Etiology: *Aspergillus fumigatus* and *A flavus* are the most frequent etiologic agents. Other species can also cause aspergillosis.

Epidemiology: *Aspergillus* species are prevalent worldwide and ubiquitous in the environment; they grow on decaying vegetation, in damp hay or straw, and in the soil. Most infected patients other than those who develop otomycosis and allergic bronchopulmonary disease have some impairment in host defenses. Nosocomial outbreaks from nearby construction sites or faulty ventilation systems have occurred. Person-to-person spread does not occur.

The **incubation period** is unknown.

Diagnostic Tests: Dichotomous branching, septate hyphae, identified by direct examination of 10% potassium hydroxide wet preparations or Gomori's methenamine silver nitrate stain of tissue specimens, are suggestive of the diagnosis. Isolation of an *Aspergillus* species in culture is required for definitive diagnosis. The organism is readily recovered from specimens other than blood on Sabouraud or brain-heart infusion media (without cycloheximide). *Aspergillus* species may also be found as laboratory contaminants. Biopsy of a lesion is usually required to confirm the diagnosis. A rise in serum antibody titers occurs in approximately 50% of immunocompromised patients with systemic disease. Serologic tests for antigen currently are experimental but appear promising. In allergic aspergillosis, elevated serum immunoglobulin E, eosinophilia and serum antibody to *Aspergillus* are frequently present.

Treatment: Amphotericin B is the treatment of choice for systemic infection (see Systemic Treatment With Amphotericin B, page 574). Some experts recommend the addition of either flucytosine or rifampin. Surgical excision of a localized lesion is sometimes warranted.

Isolation of the Hospitalized Patient: No special precautions are recommended.

Control Measures: Attempts should be made to eliminate sources of the organism from the environment of immunosuppressed patients. In hospitals, high-efficiency filters have been used to remove *Aspergillus* from the air of operating rooms and laminar flow rooms. Air-conditioner filters can become heavily contaminated with the organism and should be routinely cleaned.

Babesiosis

Clinical Manifestations: Babesiosis is an acute illness with high fever accompanied by chills and drenching sweats; myalgia, arthralgia, nausea, and vomiting can also occur. However, an insufficient number of cases of babesiosis have been recognized to allow accurate characterization of the clinical spectrum of illness. Infection in asplenic patients is usually severe and accompanied by hemolytic anemia. Rare fatalities in splenectomized patients with *Babesia microti* infection have been reported, but infections of asplenic patients in Europe with other species of *Babesia* have frequently caused fatalities.

Etiology: The cause is *B microti* and other *Babesia* species; they are intraerythrocytic protozoa, resembling the plasmodia.

Epidemiology: *B microti* is principally a parasite of rodents and is transmitted to humans through the bite of nymphal ixodes ticks (*Ixodes dammini*). The parasite has been implicated in cases in the northeastern quadrant of the United States, principally on the islands of Nantucket and Martha's Vineyard, several islands in the Long Island complex, and on the Connecticut coastline. Rare human cases and infected rodents have been reported from Wisconsin. Transmission can also occur by blood transfusion. Asymptomatic infections in endemic areas are common, and severe illness appears to be most likely to occur in persons older than 40 years and in those anatomically or functionally asplenic. The disease is not directly transmissible from person to person except through shared blood (e.g., transfusion) or needles.

The **incubation period** can range from weeks to months.

Diagnostic Tests: The parasite can be observed in red blood cells on thick and thin blood smears stained with Giemsa solution. A serologic antibody test is now available at the Centers for Disease Control and some state health departments.

Treatment: Mild and asymptomatic infections frequently do not require treatment. A combination of quinine plus clindamycin has been used successfully in more severe infections. Chloroquine is of no value.

Isolation of the Hospitalized Patient: The routinely recommended blood/body fluid precautions should be scrupulously followed (see Isolation Precautions, page 81).

Control Measures: Specific recommendations concern prevention of tick bites and are similar to those for Lyme Disease and other tick-borne infections (see Control Measures for Prevention of Tick-Borne Infections, page 112).

Bacillus cereus Infections

Clinical Manifestations: Two clinical syndromes of *Bacillus cereus* food poisoning occur. One is a disease with a short incubation period, similar to that of staphylococcal food poisoning, characterized by nausea, vomiting, abdominal cramps, and diarrhea in about one third of patients. The other has a longer incubation period, similar to that of *Clostridium perfringens* food poisoning, and is characterized by abdominal cramps and diarrhea in all patients and vomiting in about one fourth. In both syndromes, illness is mild, not associated with fever, and abates within 24 hours.

B cereus can also cause local skin and wound infections and invasive disease, including bacteremia, meningitis, and pneumonia. Invasive disease occurs most frequently in granulocytopenic, immunocompromised patients. Fulminant *B cereus* endopthalmitis, usually following penetrating trauma, has been described.

Etiology: *B cereus* is an aerobic (facultative anaerobic), spore-forming, Gram-positive bacillus. The short-incubation disease is caused by a preformed, heat-stable toxin. The long-incubation disease is caused by the in vivo production of a heat-labile enterotoxin. This exotoxin also possesses tissue necrosis and cytotoxic properties, and is probably the principal determinant of virulence in nongastrointestinal infections.

Epidemiology: *B cereus* is ubiquitous in the environment and is frequently present in small numbers in raw, dried, and processed foods, but it is an uncommon cause of food poisoning in the United States. Spores of *B cereus* are heat resistant, and the organism can survive brief cooking or boiling. Vegetative forms can grow and produce enterotoxins over a wide range of temperatures (25° to 42°C; 77° to 107.6°F). The disease is acquired by the ingestion of food containing heat-stable toxins or of food contaminated with *B cereus* followed by toxin production in the gastrointestinal tract. The most common sources of contaminated foods are fried rice (causing vomiting), meat, and vegetables (causing diarrhea). The disease is not transmissible from person to person.

The **incubation period** of short-incubation disease is 1 to 6 hours; for long-incubation disease it is 6 to 16 hours.

Diagnostic Tests: Isolation of the organism from the feces (or vomitus) of ill persons who shared the same meal is presumptive etiologic evidence. The recovery of *B cereus* in a concentration of 10^5 or more per gram of epidemiologically incriminated food establishes the diagnosis.

Although frequently dismissed as a contaminant, isolation of *B cereus* from wounds or normally sterile body fluids can be significant, particularly when obtained from immunocompromised patients and confirmed by repeat culture.

Treatment: *B cereus* food poisoning requires only supportive treatment. Oral rehydration or, occasionally, intravenous fluid and electrolyte replacement may be indicated for patients with severe dehydration. Antibiotics are not indicated.

Patients with invasive disease require antibiotic therapy together with prompt removal of potentially infected foreign bodies (catheters or implants). *B cereus* is usually susceptible to aminoglycosides, clindamycin, erythromycin, chloramphenicol, and vancomycin.

Isolation of the Hospitalized Patient: No special precautions are recommended for patients with food poisoning. Drainage and secretion precautions are indicated for patients with draining lesions.

Control Measures: Preventive measures depend on limiting proliferation of *B cereus* in foods by optimum cooking and storage. Prompt refrigeration of boiled rice intended for later use is particularly important.

Bacteroides Infections

Clinical Manifestations: *Bacteroides* species of the oral cavity can cause chronic sinusitis, chronic otitis media, dental infection, peritonsillar abscess, cervical adenitis, retropharyngeal space infection, aspiration pneumonia, lung abscess, empyema, and necrotizing pneumonia. Species from the gastrointestinal flora are recovered in patients with peritonitis, intra-abdominal abscess, pelvic inflammatory disease, postoperative wound infection, and vulvovaginal and perianal infection. Soft-tissue infections involving *Bacteroides* species include synergistic bacterial gangrene and necrotizing fascitis. Invasion of the bloodstream by *Bacteroides* species from the oral cavity or intestinal tract can lead to brain abscess, meningitis, endocarditis, arthritis, or osteomyelitis. Skin involvement includes omphalitis in newborns, cellulitis at the site of fetal monitors, human bite wounds, infection of burns adjacent to the mouth or rectum, and decubitus ulcers. Neonatal infections, such as conjunctivitis, pneumonia, bacteremia, or meningitis, occur rarely. Most *Bacteroides* infections are polymicrobial.

Etiology: Most *Bacteroides* organisms associated with human disease are small, pleomorphic, non-spore-forming, obligately anaerobic Gram-negative bacilli.

Epidemiology: *Bacteroides* infections are caused by endogenous organisms of patients' flora. Members of the *B fragilis* group predominate in the gastrointestinal flora; members of the *B melaninogenicus* and *B oralis* groups are more common in the oral cavity. *Bacteroides* species cause infection as opportunists, usually in conjunction with other endogenous species. Encapsulation of organisms may enhance abscess formation. Endogenous transmission results from aspiration, spillage from the bowel, or damage to mucosal surfaces, such as from trauma or surgery. Peripartum transmission occurs when an infant is exposed during birth to organisms of the vagina or infected tissues. Deficiencies of normal immune mechanisms usually do not predispose to infection but mucosal injury and granulocytopenia do. Except in infections resulting from human bites, no evidence for person-to-person transmission exists.

The **incubation period** is variable and depends on the concentration of organisms and the site of involvement; generally it is 1 to 5 days.

Diagnostic Tests: Anaerobic cultures are necessary for recovery of *Bacteroides* species. Since infections are usually polymicrobial, aerobic cultures of infected clinical specimens are also indicated. A putrid odor of pus or other discharges is suggestive evidence of anaerobic infection; the Gram stain will show leukocytes and bacteria of differing morphology, but the morphologic features of *Bacteroides* species are not sufficiently distinctive to be diagnostic. Use of anaerobic transport tubes or a sealed syringe is recommended for clinical specimens unless specimens can be cultured immediately after collection. Collection of clinical materials, especially from the respiratory tract, must be performed so as to avoid contamination of the specimen with anaerobes normally present on mucosal surfaces.

Treatment: Abscesses should be drained when feasible; those involving brain or liver sometimes will resolve without drainage. Necrotizing lesions should be surgically debrided; the value of hyperbaric oxygenation is controversial.

The choice of antimicrobial agent(s) is based on anticipated (or proven, if available) in vitro susceptibility test results. *Bacteroides* species that cause infections of the mouth and respiratory tract generally are susceptible to penicillin G, ampicillin, broad-spectrum penicillins (such as ticarcillin), and cefuroxime. Some species (e.g., members of the *B melaninogenicus* and *B oralis* groups) produce beta-lactamase and are resistant to those drugs. Other penicillins and first- and second-generation cephalosporins are less active in vitro. Clindamycin is active against virtually all mouth and respiratory tract *Bacteroides* isolates and is advocated by some experts as the drug of choice for anaerobic infections of the oral cavity and lungs. *Bacteroides* species of the gastrointestinal tract usually are resistant to penicillin G, but are predictably susceptible to chloramphenicol, metronidazole, and usually clindamycin. Eighty percent or more of isolates are susceptible to cefoxitin, ceftizoxime, and imipenem. Cefuroxime, cefotaxime, and ceftriaxone are not reliably effective against *Bacteroides* species of the intestinal tract.

Isolation of the Hospitalized Patient: For draining wounds with *Bacteroides* species, drainage/secretion precautions are recommended.

Control Measures: None.

Balantidium coli Infections

(Balantidiasis)

Clinical Manifestations: The most common manifestation is chronic, intermittent episodes of diarrhea. Acute infection is characterized by the rapid onset of nausea, vomiting, abdominal discomfort or pain, and bloody mucoid diarrhea. The organism causes inflammation of the gastrointestinal tract and local lymphatics, causing dilation. Ulceration develops, and secondary bacterial invasion can occur. Fulminant disease can occur in malnourished or otherwise debilitated patients.

Etiology: *Balantidium coli*, a ciliated protozoan, is the largest protozoan known to infect humans.

Epidemiology: Most human infections are asymptomatic. Pigs are believed to be the main reservoir of *B coli*. They excrete cysts in feces; the cysts are infectious when ingested by humans. The excysted trophozoites infect the colon. The patient is infectious as long as the cysts are excreted. The cysts can persist in the environment for months.

The incubation period is unknown; it may be only several days.

Diagnostic Tests: Prompt examination of stools for the parasite is necessary because of the rapid degeneration of trophozoites. Repeated stool examination may be necessary to identify infection as shedding can be intermittent. Materials may also be obtained by scraping lesions during sigmoidoscopy.

Treatment: Tetracycline (which should not be given to children younger than 9 years) is the drug of choice; iodoquinol is the alternative drug. Metronidazole is also effective.

Isolation of the Hospitalized Patient: No special precautions are recommended.

Control Measures: Control measures include sanitary disposal of human feces and avoidance of contamination of food and water with porcine feces.

Blastocystis hominis

Clinical Manifestations: Diarrhea, abdominal pain, malaise, nausea, weight loss, or rectal bleeding can occur. Manifestations can be acute or chronic. Since treatment and even eradication of this protozoan parasite is not always associated with abatement of symptoms, alternative causes should always be sought.

Etiology: *Blastocystis hominis* is a protozoan.

Epidemiology: *B hominis* is recovered from less than 1% to 25% of stools. In most cases, carriage is asymptomatic. The organism is worldwide in distribution. Diarrhea and asymptomatic infection of animals have been reported but the reservoir is largely unknown. Transmission is believed to be fecal-oral, resulting from water contamination. The role of *B hominis* as a pathogen is still unclear. Other potential pathogens or other diseases of the intestinal tract should always be considered in symptomatic patients. Symptoms are not related to the number of organisms visualized microscopically in stool.

The **incubation period** is unknown.

Diagnostic Tests: Stool specimens should be stained with trichrome and examined microscopically. The number of parasites can vary with repeated examinations.

Treatment: Metronidazole for 7 to 10 days has been beneficial in some patients; however, many improve without treatment. A clinical response to metronidazole can also reflect treatment of occult, concurrent giardiasis rather than *B hominis* infection.

Isolation of the Hospitalized Patient: No special precautions are recommended.

Control Measures: None.

Blastomycosis (North American)

Clinical Manifestations: Pulmonary, cutaneous, and disseminated disease occurs. Children most commonly have pulmonary manifestations. Pulmonary lesions resemble tuberculosis; empyema and chest wall sinuses can occur. The cutaneous lesion progresses from a papule to a chronic granulomatous ulcer or elevated mass. Disseminated blastomycosis usually begins with pulmonary infection and can involve the skin, bones, central nervous system, abdominal viscera, and kidneys.

Etiology: The disease is caused by *Blastomyces dermatitidis*, a dimorphic fungus existing in a yeast form at 37°C and in a mycelial form at room temperature. The yeast form is found in infected tissues.

Epidemiology: The source is probably the soil. The major mode of transmission appears to be aerosol inhalation. Person-to-person transmission does not occur. The infection occurs in the United States, Canada, Africa, and India. Outbreaks have been described. Endemic areas in the United States include the southeastern and central states and the Midwestern states bordering the Great Lakes.

The **incubation period** is not known.

Diagnostic Tests: Thick-walled, broad-based, single-budding yeast forms may be seen in 10% potassium hydroxide preparations of sputum, cerebrospinal fluid, urine, or material from lesions. Organisms can be cultured on brain-heart infusion and Sabouraud's dextrose agar at room temperature. Serum antibodies (measured by complement fixation, immunodiffusion, or enzyme immunoassay) develop in some cases but serologic testing is insensitive in diagnosis. A positive immunodiffusion test is a reliable indicator of infection, but a nonreactive test does not exclude the diagnosis. The enzyme immunoassay has greater sensitivity.

Treatment: Ketoconazole and amphotericin B are each effective. Amphotericin B is recommended for life-threatening cases, immunocompromised patients, and infants and children who are at increased risk for adverse hepatic and adrenal effects from ketoconazole. Ketoconazole is the drug of choice for mild and moderately severe pulmonary cases. Mild pulmonary cases with clinical improvement at the time of diagnosis may not require therapy. Therapy is usually continued for 6 months in pulmonary cases and 12 months in patients with bone involvement.

Isolation of the Hospitalized Patient: No special precautions are recommended.

Control Measures: None.

Borrelia

(Relapsing Fever)

Clinical Manifestations: Illness is characterized by the sudden onset of a high fever, chills, headache, and myalgia, followed by splenomegaly and hepatomegaly. Frequently, a fleeting macular rash on the trunk, which can become generalized and/or petechial, occurs. Other possible findings include meningeal irritation, iridocyclitis, epistaxis, and myocarditis. Initial illness of 3 to 6 days is followed by an afebrile period of about 1 week, then a relapse. Relapses become progressively shorter and milder as the afebrile intervals lengthen. Infection during pregnancy is often clinically severe and can result in abortion or, rarely, severe infection in neonates.

Etiology: Relapsing fever is caused by motile spirochetes of the genus *Borrelia. Borrelia recurrentis* is the only species causing louse-borne infection. Among at least 15 species causing tick-borne infections, *B hermsii*, *B turicatae*, and *B parkeri* are the only species found in North America.

Epidemiology: Transmission is vector-borne. Infected lice (*Pediculus humanus*) and soft-bodied ticks (*Ornithodoros* species) are the source of human infections. Louse-borne infections are presently reported in Ethiopia and Sudan; tick-borne infections are widely distributed in many countries. Most human cases in the United States occur in forested western mountain areas, including state and national parks, and result from tick bites. Because soft-bodied ticks have painless bites and feed briefly (10 to 30 minutes), and usually at night, many patients are unaware of having been bitten. Ticks become infected by feeding on rodents and other small mammals and transmit the organisms when they take blood meals. Infection is transmitted vertically in ticks, thereby establishing a reservoir. Lice become infected by feeding on spirochetemic humans and transmit organisms by contaminating the bite wound when they are crushed by the host's scratching. Infected lice and ticks remain contagious throughout their lives. All humans are susceptible. Human-to-human transmission does not occur.

The **incubation period** is 5 to 11 days or more.

Diagnostic Tests: Spirochetes can be observed in darkfield preparations or Wright-stained thin and thick smears of peripheral blood, or Giemsa or acridine orange stains of dehemoglobinized thick smears or buffy-coat preparations. Blood is cultured by intraperitoneal inoculation of immature laboratory mice. Serum agglutinins in convalescent sera against *Proteus* OXK (Weil-Felix reaction) support the diagnosis. Use of more sensitive and specific serologic tests has been limited by species and phase variations in the *Borrelia* antigenic content. Serologic cross reactions with *Borrelia burgdorferi* can occur.

Treatment: Tetracycline chloramphenicol, penicillin, and erythromycin are each effective in producing prompt defervescence and preventing lapses. For children and pregnant women, erythromycin, 40 mg/kg/d for 10 days, is the preferred therapy. Tetracyclines should not be given to children younger than 9 years or to pregnant women. The first dose of the antibiotic should be lower than those subsequently given. For a febrile patient, oral phenoxymethyl penicillin, 7.5 mg/kg, in a single dose (or intravenous penicillin G, 10,000 U/kg, infused over 30 minutes for those unable to take oral medication) is recommended as initial therapy, to be followed by a 10-day course of an effective antibiotic. Because life-threatening Jarisch-Herxheimer reactions can occur, the patient should be monitored closely during the first 8 hours of therapy.

Louse infestation, if present, should be treated.

Isolation of the Hospitalized Patient: The routinely recommended blood/body fluid precautions are indicated for the duration of the illness (see Isolation Precautions, page 81).

Control Measures: Limitation of contact with vectors (lice and ticks) through use of protective clothing, insecticides, insect repellents, and good personal hygiene is indicated. Persons in tick-infested areas should check frequently for attached ticks after possible exposure and remove them promptly (see Control Measures for Prevention of Tick-Borne Infections, page 112). Case reporting is important for public health control.

Brucellosis

Clinical Manifestations: In children, brucellosis is frequently a mild, self-limited disease, especially if caused by *Brucella abortus*. However, in areas where cases associated with goat milk or cheese occur, brucellosis (i.e., caused by *B melitensis*) can be severe in children. The onset of disease can be insidious or acute, with fever, chills, weakness, malaise, weight loss, anorexia, arthralgia, and myalgia. Some patients have abdominal pain, hepatomegaly, or splenomegaly. Endocarditis, pneumonia, meningitis, or meningoencephalitis, osteomyelitis, and abscesses are occasionally reported.

Etiology: *Brucella* species are small, nonmotile, nonencapsulated, non-spore-forming, Gram-negative coccobacilli. The *Brucella* species that infect humans are *B melitensis*, *B suis*, *B abortus*, and *B canis*.

Epidemiology: Brucellosis is an infectious disease of nonhuman mammals, particularly cattle, swine, sheep, goats, and dogs. The disease is transmitted to humans by several modes. In the United States, transmission of brucellosis from animals to humans occurs most commonly by occupational exposure or air-borne spread, rather than by ingestion of infected milk, milk products, or meat. Air-borne spread occurs in heavily contaminated areas (e.g., slaughterhouses or laboratories). In children, however, most disease occurs from ingestion of infected dairy products. Brucellosis is unusual in children in the United States; less than 10% of reported cases in the United States occur in those younger than 19 years. Brucellosis occurs throughout the year, but the prevalence is increased in summer months. Organisms invade through the gastrointestinal tract, eyes, nasopharynx, genital tract, or breaks in the skin. Person-to-person transmission has not been documented.

The **incubation period** varies from a few days to several months. In well-documented, common-source outbreaks, incubation periods have exceeded 30 days.

Diagnostic Tests: *Brucella* species can be recovered by culture from blood, bone marrow, urine, or local sites of involvement in acute disease. The laboratory should be informed that brucellosis is suspected so that care will be taken to minimize the risk in handling these cultures and to maximize the yield of *Brucella* organisms. Cultures should be incubated on special media in the presence of 5% to 10% CO_2 for 3 to 4 weeks. The standard tube (STA) or microagglutination test will detect serum antibodies primarily to the lipopolysaccharide antigens of *B abortus*, *B suis*, or *B melitensis*, but not of *B canis*. Most experts consider a single titer of 1:160 or higher indicative of past or present exposure to *Brucella* organisms or cross-reacting antigens. Alternatively, a fourfold or greater rise in titer in paired serum samples is indicative of recent exposure to *Brucella* or *Brucella*-like organisms. Antibody to *Yersinia enterocolitica*, *Francisella tularensis*, or *Vibrio cholerae* (in either infected or immunized individuals) can result in false-positive tests because of cross-antigenicity with *Brucella* species. False-negative tests may be caused by a prozone phenomenon due to blocking IgG or IgA antibodies. This effect may be eliminated by testing dilutions (at least through 1:1,280) of serum suspected of harboring *Brucella* organisms. IgG antibodies decline rapidly after treatment; the 2-mercaptoethanol (2-ME) test, an agglutination test for IgG antibody, may be used to clarify the diagnostic significance of agglutination titers. A 2-ME titer of 1:160 or greater correlates better than the STA titer with active, recurrent, or persistent infection. No important advantages result for the complement fixation or the antihuman globulin serologic tests, although both detect IgG antibodies and have no prozone effect. Investigational ELISA assays look promising for detecting IgM, IgA, and IgG antibodies. Serologic tests for the diagnosis of *B canis* infections can be obtained through many veterinary diagnostic laboratories. Skin tests are not useful in the diagnosis of brucellosis. In Brucella meningitis, elevated agglutination and ELISA titers in CSF can be helpful in confirming the diagnosis.

Treatment:

- Tetracycline, 30 to 40 mg/kg/d (maximum, 2 g/d), orally, in four doses or doxycycline 5 mg/kg/d (maximum, 200 mg/d), orally, in two doses should be administered for 3 to 6 weeks. A combination of rifampin and a tetracycline, usually doxycycline, is now commonly recommended for refractory cases. If oral therapy cannot be given, the intravenous dosage of tetracycline is 15 to 20 mg/kg (maximum, 1 g/d).
- When the disease is severe, streptomycin, 20 mg/kg/d (maximum, 1 g/d for 2 weeks), or gentamicin 5 to 7.5 mg/kg/d for 5 days, and tetracycline should be given.
- Because tetracyclines can cause staining of developing teeth, trimethoprim-sulfamethoxazole (trimethoprim, 10 mg/kg/d, maximum, 480 mg/d; sulfamethoxazole, 50 mg/kg/d, maximum, 2.4 g/d), given intravenously or orally for 3 to 6 weeks, may be used as an alternative for children younger than 9 years. Recurrent

bacteremia after discontinuation of trimethoprim-sulfamethoxazole treatment has been documented in as many as 30% of patients. Use of streptomycin for 2 weeks or gentamicin for 5 days or rifampin for 3 to 6 weeks with trimethoprim-sulfamethoxazole will reduce the incidence of recurrent bacteremia. Folinic acid can be given to prevent hematologic toxicity from trimethoprim-sulfamethoxazole.

- Patients with relapses after treatment with a tetracycline drug alone should receive combined therapy with a tetracycline or trimethoprim-sulfamethoxazole combined with streptomycin, gentamicin, or rifampin (20 mg/kg/d in two divided doses).
- Prednisone can prevent the Jarisch-Herxheimer reaction, which can occur if the disease is severe or the diagnosis was delayed.

Isolation of the Hospitalized Patient: Drainage/secretion precautions are indicated for patients with draining lesions.

Control Measures: The control of human brucellosis depends on eradication of brucellosis in cattle, swine, and other animals. Pasteurization of all milk and milk products is especially important to prevent disease in children. The certification of raw milk does not eliminate the risk of *Brucella* transmission.

Caliciviruses

Clinical Manifestations: Diarrhea and vomiting are common, often with abdominal pain. Illness is generally self limited, lasting an average of 4 days.

Etiology: Caliciviruses are RNA viruses, with characteristic cup-like depressions on the virus surface. Multiple serotypes have been detected in human infections. Biochemical similarities and antigenic relatedness to the Norwalk agents have been described.

Epidemiology: Outbreaks have been reported primarily in Japan and the United Kingdom in young children in institutional settings. Limited studies suggest that seroprevalence of antibody to calicivirus is widespread, and that infection occurs in early childhood. The mode of transmission has not been established but person-to-person transmission is presumed, and contaminated shellfish, cold foods, and drinking water have been implicated as vehicles. Approximately 3% of children hospitalized for diarrhea excrete calicivirus.

The **incubation period** is 1 to 3 days.

Diagnostic Tests: No tests are generally available. Caliciviruses except for a single strain have not been cultivated in vitro. They are detected by immune electron microscopy, radioimmunoassay, and enzyme immunoassay. Seroconversion may be detected by a blocking ELISA test.

Treatment: Supportive.

Isolation of the Hospitalized Patient: Enteric precautions are advised.

Control Measures: None.

Campylobacter Infections*

Clinical Manifestations: Predominant symptoms are diarrhea, abdominal pain, malaise, and fever. Stools frequently contain frank blood. In neonates, bloody diarrhea can be the only manifestation of infection. Abdominal pain can mimic that of an appendicitis. Mild infection can last only 1 or 2 days and resemble viral gastroenteritis. Most patients recover in less than 1 week, but 20% have a relapse or a prolonged or severe illness. Persistent infection can mimic acute inflammatory bowel disease. Convulsions develop in some young children in association with high fever. Bacteremia is uncommon, but neonatal sepsis occasionally occurs. Reactive arthritis occasionally develops during convalescence.

Etiology: *Campylobacter jejuni* (formerly *C fetus* subspecies *jejuni* or *Vibrio fetus*) is a motile, comma-shaped, Gram-negative rod that causes gastroenteritis. *C fetus* (formerly *C fetus* subspecies *intestinalis*), a related organism, is an infrequent cause of systemic illness in debilitated hosts.

Epidemiology: The gastrointestinal tract of domestic and wild birds and animals is the reservoir of infection. *C jejuni* has been isolated from the feces of 30% to 100% of chickens, turkeys, and water fowl. Poultry carcasses are usually contaminated with the organism. Most farm animals and meat sources can harbor the organism. Pets such as dogs and cats (especially young animals) and hamsters are potential sources. Transmission of *C jejuni* occurs by ingestion of contaminated food, including unpasteurized milk and water, or by direct contact with fecal material from infected animals or persons.

---

*For discussion of *Campylobacter pylori* (now called *Helicobacter pylori* infection), see *Helicobacter pylori*, page 230.

Improperly cooked poultry, untreated water, and unpasteurized milk have been the main vehicles. Person-to-person spread appears to occur, particularly among young children with fecal incontinence and in families. It has also occurred in neonates of infected mothers. Outbreaks of *Campylobacter* diarrhea have been reported in children in day care. In perinatal infection, *C jejuni* usually results in neonatal gastroenteritis, and *C fetus* usually results in neonatal sepsis or meningitis. Enteritis occurs in persons of all ages. Communicability is greatest during the acute phase of the illness. Convalescent excretion is usually brief, typically 2 to 3 weeks, and is shortened by treatment to 2 to 3 days. Asymptomatic carriage is uncommon.

The **incubation period** is usually 1 to 7 days, but can be longer.

Diagnostic Tests: Rapid, presumptive diagnosis is possible in laboratories experienced in examining stool smears by special microscopic or staining techniques. *C jejuni* can be cultured from the feces and occasionally from the bloodstream. Because laboratory identification of the organism requires special techniques, the physician should be aware of whether the laboratory routinely attempts *Campylobacter* isolation or whether it requires special notification.

Treatment:

- Erythromycin shortens excretion of *C jejuni* and, thus, may be beneficial, regardless of the severity of the illness or duration of diarrhea before diagnosis. Treatment with erythromycin usually eradicates the organism from stool within 2 or 3 days.
- Alternative agents for resistant strains should be selected on the basis of susceptibility tests.

Isolation of the Hospitalized Patient: Enteric precautions should be used during the acute illness and until *Campylobacter* can no longer be isolated from stools.

Control Measures:

- Hand washing after handling raw poultry and washing cutting boards and utensils with soap after contact with raw poultry and thorough cooking of poultry are critical. Pasteurization of milk and chlorination of water supplies are also important.
- Infected food handlers and hospital employees who are asymptomatic pose no known hazard for disease transmission and need not be excluded from work if proper personal hygiene measures are carefully maintained.

- Outbreaks of campylobacteriosis are uncommon in day care centers, and specific strategies for controlling infection in these settings have not been evaluated. General measures for interrupting enteric transmissions in day care centers are recommended (see Children in Day Care, page 72). Infants and children in diapers with symptomatic *Campylobacter* infection should be excluded from day care or cared for in a separate protected area until the diarrhea has subsided and preferably should have received at least 2 or 3 days of erythromycin treatment.
- Stool cultures of asymptomatic exposed children ordinarily are not recommended.

Candidiasis

(Moniliasis, Thrush)

Clinical Manifestations: Mucocutaneous infection results in thrush; intertriginous lesions of the gluteal folds, neck, groin, and axilla; paronychia; and onychia. Chronic mucocutaneous candidiasis can be associated with endocrinologic diseases or progressive immunodeficiency, particularly T-cell deficiency. Granulomas of the scalp and face are rare. Respiratory infection is rare and is manifested by a nonspecific pneumonia. Disseminated candidiasis occurs in premature newborn infants and immunocompromised hosts; it may involve the lungs, kidneys, spleen, heart, liver, brain, eye, esophagus, meninges, skin, and mucous membranes. Transient candidemia can occur with or without systemic disease in patients with indwelling catheters or endotracheal intubation, or those receiving prolonged intravenous infusions. Other types of *Candida* infection include vaginitis, cystitis, endocarditis, and enteritis.

Etiology: *Candida albicans* causes most of the infections. Other species, such as *C tropicalis*, can also cause serious infections in compromised hosts. Yeast forms and pseudohyphae can be found in infected tissues.

Epidemiology: *C albicans*, as well as other *Candida* species, can be present in the intestinal tract, vagina, and mucous membranes of healthy individuals. *C albicans* is ubiquitous. Newborns can acquire the organism in utero, during passage through the vagina, or postnatally. Person-to-person transmission occurs. Invasive disease occurs almost exclusively in individuals whose resistance to infection has been impaired. Individuals with AIDS or who are immunodeficient for other reasons, such as diabetes mellitus, or treatment with corticosteroids or antimetabolites, are unusually susceptible. Patients receiving prolonged intravenous hyperalimentation or broad-spectrum antimicrobials also have increased susceptibility.

The **incubation period** is unknown. Most infections are of endogenous origin.

Diagnostic Tests: Typical yeast and pseudohyphal forms are identified by microscopic examination of scrapings suspended in 10% potassium hydroxide. Gram stains of smears from skin and mucous membrane lesions can identify the fungus, although the diagnosis of chronic mucocutaneous candidiasis or thrush of the mucous membranes usually can be made by physical examination. Barium studies and endoscopy are useful in the diagnosis of esophagitis. Cultures of the blood, cerebrospinal fluid, bone marrow, urine, or other material from lesions in compatible clinical circumstances, if positive for *Candida* species, are helpful in the diagnosis. A variety of serologic tests for antibody and experimental tests for antigen detection are available, but these tests have limited use and none has been accepted as a dependable diagnostic aid. A definitive diagnosis requires the isolation of the organism from an otherwise sterile body fluid or tissue (e.g., blood, cerebrospinal fluid, bone marrow, or biopsy specimen) or the demonstration of organisms in a tissue biopsy specimen.

Treatment:

Mucous Membrane or Skin Infections. Oral candidiasis is treated with oral nystatin suspension or clotrimazole troches. However, the safety and effectiveness of clotrimazole have not been established in children younger than 3 years. In immunocompromised patients with oropharyngeal candidiasis, ketoconazole has therapeutic benefit but may not eradicate the organism.

Mild *Candida* esophagitis may be treated with high-dose oral nystatin; more severe disease is treated with ketoconazole for 14 days or with intravenous amphotericin B for at least 5 to 7 days. Fluconazole has recently been approved for the treatment of oropharyngeal and esophageal candidiasis. Although the safety profile of the drug is generally excellent, the number of children younger than 14 years treated with fluconazole is insufficient to establish pediatric safety.

Skin infections are treated with topical nystatin, miconazole, clotrimazole, amphotericin B, econazole, or ciclopirox (see Topical Drugs for Superficial Fungal Infections, page 576). Nystatin is usually effective and is the least expensive of these drugs.

Vaginal candidiasis is effectively treated with clotrimazole or nystatin suppositories.

For chronic mucocutaneous candidiasis, ketoconazole and clotrimazole are effective drugs. Amphotericin B given intravenously and oral flucytosine are also effective. Relapses are common when therapy with any of these agents is terminated, but systemic infection is rare. Keratomycosis is treated with corneal baths of amphotericin B, 1 mg/mL. Some patients with *Candida* cystitis may be successfully treated with bladder irrigations with amphotericin B, 50 µg/mL in distilled water.

Systemic Infections. Amphotericin B is the drug of choice in systemic candidiasis (see Systemic Treatment with Amphotericin B, page 574). Usually a 4- to 6-week course of treatment is necessary, but the length will vary with the clinical response. A shorter course of therapy may be successful for catheter-associated infection, provided the catheter is removed.

Flucytosine (150 mg/kg/d) should supplement amphotericin B if the infection is severe and in patients with central nervous system involvement, as in vitro and clinical studies suggest synergism of flucytosine and amphotericin B against *C albicans*. Susceptibility testing should be performed because some strains of *C albicans* and other *Candida* species are resistant to flucytosine. The dose of flucytosine must be decreased in patients with renal insufficiency. If possible, serum flucytosine concentration should be determined, and the dose should be adjusted to maintain concentrations below 100 µg/mL to avoid toxicity. Adverse side effects include thrombocytopenia, leukopenia, hepatic dysfunction, rash, and diarrhea, especially in azotemic patients. The imidazole derivatives, miconazole, ketoconazole, and fluconazole, administered systemically, can be beneficial in the treatment of systemic candidiasis, but data on their use, especially in children, are limited.

Isolation of the Hospitalized Patient: No special precautions are recommended.

Control Measures: Prolonged broad-spectrum antimicrobial therapy in susceptible patients predisposes to *Candida* colonization and infection and should be avoided whenever possible. Meticulous care of the venous catheter site is recommended in any patient requiring long-term intravenous alimentation; such care should include gauze dressing changes every 48 hours, and the application of a povidone-iodine solution, which is fungistatic as well as bacteriostatic. Transparent dressings are associated with an increased incidence of catheter-related infections.

Oral nystatin or clotrimazole may be effective in preventing oropharyngeal candidiasis in neutropenic patients with leukemia.

Cat Scratch Disease

Clinical Manifestations: The predominant sign is regional lymphadenopathy in a healthy child, adolescent, or adult. Fever and mild systemic symptoms occur in only 30% of patients. Regional or multiple-site lymphadenopathy can occur a few weeks after the appearance of a papule at the inoculation site. Occasionally, infection can produce Parinaud's oculoglandular syndrome involving the conjunctiva and a unilateral preauricular lymph node. Rare complications include encephalitis, osteolytic lesions, hepatitis, thrombocytopenia purpura, erythema nodosum, and chronic, systemic disease.

Etiology: Pleomorphic Gram-negative bacilli have been cultured in brain-heart infusion media from a few patients with cat scratch disease. Using a modified Warthin-Starry silver impregnation stain, bacilli have been visualized primarily in the capillary endothelial cells and in macrophages lining the sinuses close to the germinal centers of affected nodes in about 60% of patients with cat scratch disease.

Epidemiology: Infection is believed to be transmitted to humans by the scratch of infected (but asymptomatic) kittens. Evidence of a cat scratch is present in about two thirds of patients, and history of contact with a cat is present in more than 90% of patients. Occasionally, other animals such as dogs (in 5% of cases) are thought to be the source of infection. No evidence for person-to-person spread exists. However, multiple cases have been observed in families, presumably resulting from contact with the same animal. No age or geographic predilection exists. Infection occurs more frequently in the fall and winter.

The **incubation period** is variable, averaging 3 to 10 days from scratch to the appearance of the primary cutaneous lesion, and 12 days (range, 5 to 50 days) from appearance of the primary lesion to appearance of the adenopathy.

Diagnostic Tests: A cat scratch antigen skin test has been used by some investigators to establish the diagnosis. However, this skin test antigen, which is prepared from suppurative lymph nodes of patients with apparent cat scratch disease, is not a licensed product, is not of proven safety, and is not available commercially. Positive tests in persons without active disease occur in family members of the patient and in those who handle cats frequently. False negative tests occur in 1% to 5% of patients.

If lymph node, skin, or conjunctival tissue is available, the putative agent of the disease, a Gram-negative bacillus, may be identified by the Warthin-Starry silver impregnation stain. Pathologic and microbiologic examinations are also useful to exclude other diseases.

Treatment: The disease is usually self limited, resolving spontaneously in 2 to 4 months. Tender, fluctuant nodes may be aspirated or occasionally excised for relief of symptoms. Incision and drainage and trauma to the node should be avoided.

Anecdotal experience suggests that gentamicin given intramuscularly for 5 to 7 days may be effective in some severely ill patients. Also oral trimethoprim-sulfamethoxazole has been beneficial in some patients.

Isolation of the Hospitalized Patient: No special precautions are recommended.

Control Measures: None are known. Disposing of cats believed to have transmitted infection does not appear to be indicated.

Chlamydial Infections

Chlamydia pneumoniae (TWAR)

Clinical Manifestations: Severe pharyngitis, hoarseness, fever, productive cough, and cervical adenopathy are frequent symptoms. Illness is prolonged and can have a biphasic course. In some patients, sore throat precedes the onset of cough by a week or more. Pharyngitis without exudate and rales are present on physical examination. Most patients are mildly to moderately ill. Usually the white blood cell count is normal and the sedimentation rate is elevated. The chest roentgenogram usually shows a single infiltrate that can involve any part of the lung.

Etiology: *Chlamydia pneumoniae* (formerly termed the TWAR strain) is a new species of *Chlamydia* which is antigenically, genetically, and morphologically distinct from other *Chlamydia* species.

Epidemiology: *C pneumoniae* infection is assumed to be transmitted from person to person. No animal or bird reservoir is known. The disease occurs worldwide. *C pneumoniae* specific serum antibody is present in as many as 45% of adults but is uncommon in children younger than 8 years. The peak age of initial infection is between 5 and 20 years. Recurrent disease is common.

The **incubation period** is unknown.

Diagnostic Tests: The organism can be isolated from posterior oropharyngeal swabs inoculated into the yolk sac of embryonated chicken eggs or HeLa 229 cells. A fluorescent antibody test using monoclonal antibody specific for *C pneumoniae* is available as a research tool. Complement fixation in two thirds of cases and microimmunofluorescent tests in almost all cases demonstrate a serum antibody titer rise during acute infection. A specific IgM titer of 1:16 or greater or an IgG titer of 1:512 or greater is presumptive evidence of recent infection.

Treatment: Erythromycin or tetracycline is recommended. Adolescents and older patients have been treated with erythromycin, 1 g/d for 5 to 10 days, but prolonged or recurrent symptoms have been common, and longer courses of therapy may be needed. For adolescents and adults, tetracycline (2 g/d for 7 to 10 days, or 1 g/d for 21 days, in four divided doses) or doxycycline (200 mg/d for 7 to 10 days in two divided doses) is also appropriate. Tetracycline should not be given to children younger than 9 years. In vitro data suggest that *C pneumoniae* is not susceptible to the sulfonamides.

Isolation of the Hospitalized Patient: No special precautions are recommended.

Control Measures: None.

Chlamydia psittaci (Psittacosis, Ornithosis)

Clinical Manifestations: Psittacosis (ornithosis) is an acute febrile respiratory tract infection with systemic symptoms. Extensive interstitial pneumonia can occur. Myocarditis, pericarditis, endocarditis, thrombophlebitis, hepatitis, thyroiditis, and central nervous system involvement are rare complications.

Etiology: *Chlamydia psittaci* is antigenically and genetically distinct from *C trachomatis*.

Epidemiology: Birds are the major reservoir of *C psittaci*. In the United States, imported birds, especially those smuggled into the country, are an important source. Both healthy and sick birds harbor and transmit the organism, usually via the air-borne route. Excretion of *C psittaci* can be intermittent or continuous for weeks or months. Those in the environment of the infected bird (such as workers at poultry slaughter plants, poultry farms, and pet shops, or pet owners) are at special risk. In addition, laboratory workers are at high risk. The disease is worldwide in distribution and tends to occur sporadically in any season. Infections are rare in children. Patients are potentially infectious during the acute illness, particularly when coughing, but person-to-person transmission has occurred rarely and only from severely ill persons with productive cough.

The **incubation period** is 7 to 14 days.

Diagnostic Tests: Isolation of the agent should be attempted only by experienced laboratories where strict measures to prevent spread of the organism are used in the collection and handling of specimens. The usual method of diagnosis is serologic, by demonstration of a significant increase in complement fixation (CF) antibody titer between acute and convalescent specimens. The CF test does not distinguish between *C psittaci* and *C pneumoniae* infections.

Treatment: A tetracycline is the preferred therapy, except in children younger than 9 years, and should be administered for at least 10 to 14 days after defervescence. Erythromycin is an alternative drug, and is recommended for younger children.

Isolation of the Hospitalized Patient: Drainage/secretion precautions are indicated for the duration of the illness.

Control Measures: Epidemiologic investigation to determine the source of infection is indicated. Suspect birds should be killed and immersed in 2% phenol or a similar disinfectant to prevent spread of the organism from feathers. The specimen should be sealed in an impermeable container and transported on dry ice to the appropriate laboratory. All potentially contaminated caging and housing areas should be thoroughly disinfected and aired before reuse because these areas contain infectious organisms. When cleaning cages and other bird housing areas, care should be taken to avoid scattering the contents. Individuals exposed to common sources of infection should be observed for development of fever or respiratory symptoms; early diagnostic tests should be performed and therapy started if these manifestations develop.

Chlamydia trachomatis

Clinical Manifestations: In neonatal chlamydial conjunctivitis, congestion, edema, and discharge develops a few days to several weeks after birth and lasts for 1 to 2 weeks, occasionally much longer. In contrast to trachoma, scars and pannus formation are rare. Chlamydial pneumonia is usually an afebrile illness and typically presents between 3 and 19 weeks after birth. A repetitive, staccato cough and tachypnea are characteristic but not always present. Rales can be present; wheezing is rare. Conjunctivitis can be present or have occurred previously. Hyperinflation on a chest roentgenogram is prominent. Untreated disease can linger or recur. Severe chlamydial pneumonia has occurred in infants and some immunocompromised adults.

Trachoma is a chronic follicular keratoconjunctivitis with neovascularization of the cornea that results from repeated and chronic infection. Blindness secondary to extensive local scarring and inflammation occurs in 1% to 15% of trachoma patients.

Chlamydia trachomatis as a sexually transmitted pathogen can cause urethritis in both sexes, vaginitis in prepubertal females, cervicitis in postpubertal females, and epididymitis in males. Infection, which is frequently asymptomatic, can persist for many months. Reinfection is common. In postpubertal females, chlamydial infection can progress to acute or chronic pelvic inflammatory disease and ultimately to infertility.

Lymphogranuloma venereum (LGV) is an invasive lymphatic infection with an initial local lesion on the genitalia accompanied by regional lymphadenitis. The disease has a chronic, low-grade course.

Etiology: *Chlamydia trachomatis* is a bacterial agent with at least 15 serologic variants (serovars) divided into the following two biologic variants (biovars): oculogenital (subtypes A-K) and LGV (subtypes L-1-L-3). Trachoma usually is caused by subtypes A-C and genital infections are caused by B and D-K.

Epidemiology: *C trachomatis* is currently the most common sexually transmitted infection in the United States. Oculogenital biovars of *C trachomatis* can be transmitted from the genital tract of infected mothers to their newborn infants. Acquisition occurs in about 50% of infants born vaginally of infected mothers and in some infants delivered by cesarian section with intact membranes. Of infants acquiring *C trachomatis*, the risk of conjunctivitis is 25% to 50% and the risk of pneumonia is 5% to 20%. The nasopharynx is the most commonly infected anatomic site. Asymptomatic infection of the rectum or vagina of the infant can persist for up to 2 years. Prevalence in pregnant women varies between 6% and 12% in most populations, but it can be as low as 2% or as high as 37% in adolescents. Infected women tend to be young, of low socioeconomic status, and from groups with high rates of sexually transmitted diseases.

LGV biovars are worldwide in distribution, but are particularly prevalent in tropical and subtropical areas. LGV is often asymptomatic in women. Perinatal transmission is rare.

Genital infection in adolescents and adults is sexually transmitted. In prepubertal children beyond infancy who have vaginal, urethral, or rectal chlamydial infection, possible sexual abuse must be considered. In infants and children, infection is not known to be communicable. The degree of contagiousness of pulmonary disease is unknown but appears to be low. LGV is infective during active clinical disease, which may last from weeks to many years.

The **incubation period** is variable and depends on the type of infection, but is usually at least 1 week.

Diagnostic Tests: Definitive diagnosis can be made by isolating the organism in tissue culture cells. Available rapid antigen detection tests include (1) direct fluorescent staining for elementary bodies in clinical specimens using monoclonal antibody, and (2) enzyme-linked immunoassay. In addition, several genetic probe methods are now available. Current data indicate that these new diagnostic techniques are specific for culture confirmation. They have not been as sensitive for direct testing of specimens. Rapid antigen detection tests are useful for evaluating urethral and cervical specimens from adults and for eye and nasopharyngeal specimens from infants. They should not be used to test rectal, vaginal, or urethral specimens from children, since fecal bacterial flora cross-react with *C trachomatis* antisera. When evaluating a child for possible sexual abuse, culture of the organism is the only acceptable method for diagnosis.

Serum antibody determination is difficult and not generally available. In children with pneumonia, an elevated serum titer of chlamydia-specific IgM is diagnostic of infection, but this test is available in only a few laboratories.

Indirect laboratory evidence of chlamydial pneumonia includes hyperinflation and bilateral diffuse infiltrates on roentgenographs, eosinophilia of 300 to 400/mm^3 or greater in peripheral blood counts, and elevated total serum IgG (500 mg/dL or more) and IgM (110 mg/dL or more) concentrations. However, the absence of these findings does not exclude the diagnosis.

Treatment:

- ***Chlamydial conjunctivitis and pneumonia*** in young infants is treated with oral erythromycin (50 mg/kg/d in four divided doses for 14 days). Topical treatment will not eradicate nasopharyngeal infection. Sulfonamides may be used after the immediate neonatal period for infants who do not tolerate erythromycin.
- Treatment of **trachoma** is more difficult and recommendations for therapy differ. The most widely used therapy is topical treatment with erythromycin, tetracycline, or sulfacetamide ointment twice daily for 2 months or twice daily for the first 5 days of the month

for 6 months. Oral erythromycin (10 mg/kg) or doxycycline (2.5 to 4 mg/kg) once daily for 40 days is also given.

- For uncomplicated ***C trachomatis genital tract infection*** in adolescents and adults, tetracycline or doxycycline for 7 days is recommended. The alternative is erythromycin for 7 days, which is also the recommended therapy for pregnant patients.
- ***LGV*** is treated with a tetracycline, sulfonamide, or erythromycin for 3 to 6 weeks.

Isolation of the Hospitalized Patient: Drainage/secretion precautions for the duration of the illness are recommended for patients with conjunctivitis or genital tract disease. Patients with pneumonia or LGV need not be isolated.

Control Measures:

Neonatal Chlamydial Conjunctivitis. The recommended topical prophylaxis with silver nitrate, erythromycin, or tetracycline for all newborns for the prevention of gonococcal ophthalmia will not reliably prevent neonatal chlamydia conjunctivitis or extraocular infection (see Prevention of Neonatal Ophthalmia, page 546).

Pregnancy. The identification and treatment of women with *C trachomatis* genital tract infection during pregnancy can prevent disease in the infant. Pregnant women at high risk for *C trachomatis* infection should be screened. Some experts advocate universal testing of pregnant women.

Management of Sexual Partners. Sexual contacts of patients with *C trachomatis* infection or nongonococcal urethritis, mucopurulent cervicitis, epididymitis, or pelvic inflammatory disease should be examined and treated for exposure to *C trachomatis*.

Contacts of Infants With* C trachomatis *Conjunctivitis and/or Pneumonia. Mothers (and their sexual partners) of infected infants should also be treated for *C trachomatis*.

LGV. Nonspecific, preventive measures for LGV are those for sexually transmitted diseases in general, such as education, case reporting, and avoidance of contact with infected patients.

Cholera

Clinical Manifestations: Cholera is characterized by painless, watery diarrhea that is frequently followed by dehydration, hypokalemia, and occasionally hypovolemic shock. Coma, convulsions, and hypoglycemia can occur, particularly in children. Typical cholera stools are colorless with small flecks of mucus ("rice-water"). Mild and asymptomatic infections occur.

Etiology: The disease is caused by a heat-labile enterotoxin elaborated by *Vibrio cholerae*, a Gram-negative, comma-shaped, motile rod that has two biotypes. The E1 Tor biotype is currently the more frequent cause, whereas the classic biotype is unusual, even in the Indian Subcontinent where it can still be found. Serotyping (Ogawa and Inaba serotypes) is based on O (or somatic) antigenic determinants.

Epidemiology: In the last three decades, *V cholerae* biotype El Tor has spread from India and Southeast Asia to Africa, the Middle East, Southern Europe, and the Western Pacific islands (Oceania). In the United States, the Gulf Coast of Louisiana and Texas is now an endemic focus. Humans are the only documented natural host, but free-living organisms can exist in the environment. Ingestion of contaminated water or food, particularly crabs and other shellfish, is the usual mode of acquisition. Adequate cooking of food eradicates the organism. Person-to-person spread is rarely documented. The period of communicability is unknown but presumably is related to the duration of carriage.

The **incubation period** is usually 2 to 3 days, with a range of a few hours to 5 days.

Diagnostic Tests: *V cholerae* can be cultured on selective media and typed by agglutination with specific antisera. A rapid presumptive diagnosis may be made by darkfield microscopy of fresh feces. A rise in vibrio-specific serum agglutinins or vibriocidal antibodies can confirm the diagnosis.

Treatment: Oral or parenteral rehydration therapy to correct dehydration and electrolyte imbalance is the most important modality of therapy. Tetracycline (50 mg/kg/d, maximum, 2 g/d, given orally for 3 to 5 days) results in prompt eradication of vibrios and reduces the duration of the diarrhea. Because tetracyclines cause staining of developing teeth, trimethoprim-sulfamethoxazole (8 mg/kg/d of trimethoprim and 40 mg/kg/d of sulfamethoxazole) or furazolidone (5 to 8 mg/kg/d) is recommended in children younger than 9 years.

Isolation of the Hospitalized Patient: Enteric precautions are indicated for the duration of the illness.

Control Measures:

Hygiene. Because cholera spreads by contaminated food or water and infection frequently requires ingestion of large numbers of organisms, purification or boiling of water can prevent transmission. Cooking crabs, shellfish, and oysters from the Gulf Coast is also recommended.

Antimicrobials. Treatment with tetracycline or trimethoprim-sulfamethoxazole may be effective in preventing coprimary and secondary cases of cholera among household contacts.

Vaccine. The currently available vaccine is of limited prophylactic value. It protects about 50% of those immunized and for only 3 to 6 months. Furthermore, travelers using standard tourist accommodations are at virtually no risk of infection in countries with cholera. Cholera vaccination is not required for travelers entering the United States and the World Health Organization no longer recommends vaccination for travel to or from cholera-infected areas. At present, vaccination is used in the United States primarily to facilitate foreign travel, since a valid International Certificate of Vaccination indicating cholera immunization within 6 months is required by some countries in Asia, the Middle East, and Africa. Some other countries require evidence of recent cholera immunization if, within the previous 5 days, the traveler has been in a country reporting cholera. Travelers to countries requiring evidence of cholera vaccination need only a single primary or booster dose to satisfy International Health Regulations.

A full primary series is two doses administered at least 1 week or more apart. Booster doses are given every 6 months when required. Dose by age is as follows: 6 months to 4 years, 0.2 mL; 5 to 10 years, 0.3 mL; more than 10 years, 0.5 mL, administered subcutaneously or intramuscularly. Vaccine in a dose of 0.2 mL may be administered intradermally to children 5 years or older. Vaccine is not recommended for infants younger than 6 months.

Yellow fever vaccine should not be given concurrently with cholera vaccine, if possible; ideally, these vaccinations should be separated by at least 3 weeks.

Preliminary studies suggest that an investigational vaccine, consisting of purified components of *V cholerae* enterotoxin and combined with killed whole cells, is effective and well tolerated when administered orally.

Clostridial Infections

Botulism and Infant Botulism

Clinical Manifestations: Botulism is a neurologic disorder with onset of symptoms either occurring abruptly within a few hours or evolving gradually over several days. A flaccid paralysis of the bulbar musculature occurs initially and descends symmetrically. Somatic musculature is affected next; hence, patients with rapidly evolving illness may have generalized weakness and hypotonia when first seen. Signs and symptoms in older children or adults can consist of diplopia, blurred vision, dry mouth, dysphagia, dysphonia, and dysarthria. Infant botulism, which occurs predominantly in infants younger than 6 months, is characterized by constipation, listlessness, poor feeding, weak cry, diminished gag reflex, subtle ocular palsies, and generalized weakness and hypotonia ("floppy infant").

Etiology: Human botulism is caused by the neurotoxins A, B, E, F, and G of *Clostridium botulinum* (and occasionally by those of other clostridia).

Epidemiology: Food-borne botulism results when a food contaminated with spores of *C botulinum* is improperly preserved and stored under anaerobic conditions that permit germination, multiplication, and toxin production. Today, almost all food-borne botulism results from improperly home-processed foods. Illness occurs when the unheated food is eaten and botulinal toxin is ingested. Food-borne botulism rarely occurs in infants or children because they usually are not exposed to foods that might contain preformed botulinal toxin.

Infant botulism results when *C botulinum* spores colonize and produce botulinal toxin in the intestine. Infant botulism is not transmitted from person to person. In most cases of infant botulism, the source of spores remains unknown; however, honey is one identified source. Light and dark corn syrups have also been reported to contain botulinal spores, but at lower frequencies than honey.

Wound botulism, although rarely reported, results when *C botulinum* grows in traumatized tissue and produces its toxin. Of the almost 50 cases of documented wound botulism, about half have occurred in children and teenagers.

The usual **incubation period** for food-borne botulism is 12 to 26 hours (range, 6 hours to 8 days); for wound botulism, it is 4 to 14 days between the time of injury and the onset of symptoms. In infant botulism, the incubation period is unknown.

Diagnostic Tests: A toxin neutralization bioassay in mice is used to identify botulinal toxin in serum, stool, or suspect foods. Enriched and selective media are used to isolate *C botulinum* from stool and foods. In infant botulism, the diagnosis is made by demonstrating *C botulinum* organisms or toxin in the feces. Serum has demonstrable toxin in only about 10% of infants with botulism; in comparison in food-borne or wound botulism, toxin is usually present in serum. When constipation makes obtaining a stool specimen difficult, an enema using sterile, nonbacteriostatic water can be given. Electromyography can be helpful in diagnosis; an incremental response of evoked muscle potentials at high-frequency nerve stimulation (more than 20 cycles per second) can be seen, and in infant botulism a characteristic pattern of brief, small, abundant, motor action potentials (BSAP) is often found.

Treatment:

Meticulous Supportive Care. The cornerstone of therapy in all forms of botulism is meticulous supportive care, particularly nutritional and respiratory.

Antitoxin. For food-borne and wound botulism, antitoxin should be administered to symptomatic persons as soon as possible after testing for hypersensitivity to equine sera. Only antitoxin of equine origin is available. Approximately 20% of treated persons experience some degree of hypersensitivity reaction. Trivalent (ABE) Antitoxin* can be obtained by contacting the state health department. If antitoxin is not available through this source, the physician should call the Centers for Disease Control. Antitoxin rarely has been used in infant botulism because of the risk of hypersensitivity, and because experience has shown that it is not needed for full recovery.

Antimicrobials. In infant botulism, antibiotics are used only to treat secondary infections. Aminoglycosides may potentiate the effects of the toxin. Some physicians give penicillin to eradicate bowel carriage of *C botulinum*, but the resulting benefit is uncertain.

Isolation of the Hospitalized Patient: No special precautions are recommended.

Control Measures:

- Prophylactic antitoxin for asymptomatic persons who have ingested a food known to contain botulinal toxin is not recommended. Because of the danger of hypersensitivity reactions, the decision to administer antitoxin requires careful consideration. Consultation in this regard may be obtained from the state health department or the Centers for Disease Control (see Treatment, page 174).
- Elimination of ingested toxin may be facilitated by inducing vomiting and/or by gastric lavage, rapid purgation (e.g., with magnesium sulfate, 15 to 30 g in children and 30 to 45 g in adults), and high enemas. The value of these measures in infant botulism is not clear.
- Exposed persons should have close medical supervision.
- Contacts of wound or infant botulism cases are not at an increased risk of acquiring botulism. Botulinal toxoid (types A, B, C, D, and

---

*Prepared by Connaught Laboratories, Limited, and distributed in the United States through the Centers for Disease Control, Atlanta, Georgia (see Services of the Centers for Disease Control, page 622).

E) is available from the Centers for Disease Control for immunization of laboratory workers whose regular exposure predisposes to high risk.
- Education to improve home canning methods should be promoted. Use of a pressure cooker (116°C; 240.8°F) is necessary to kill spores of *C botulinum.* Boiling for 10 minutes will destroy the toxin. Time-temperature-pressure requirements vary with the product being heated.
- Most sources of spores for infant botulism are unavoidable; however, honey (and perhaps corn syrup) is a source and should not be given to infants younger than 6 months.

Clostridial Myonecrosis (Gas Gangrene)

Clinical Manifestations: The onset is heralded by acute pain at the site of the wound, followed by edema, tenderness, exudate, and progression of the pain. Systemic findings, which occur in conjunction with severe local toxicity, initially include tachycardia disproportionate to the degree of fever, pallor, diaphoresis, hypotension, renal failure, and, later, alterations in mental status. Crepitus, which is not always present, is not pathognomic of *Clostridia* infection. Diagnosis is based on clinical manifestations, including the characteristic appearance of the necrotic muscle at surgery. Untreated gas gangrene can lead to death within hours.

Etiology: Gas gangrene is caused by *Clostridium* species, most commonly *C perfringens* (formerly *C welchii*), that are large Gram-positive anaerobic rods with blunt ends. Other Gram-positive and Gram-negative bacteria are frequently also present.

Epidemiology: Gas gangrene usually results from contamination of traumatic wounds involving muscle injury. The sources of *Clostridia* are soil, contaminated objects, and human and animal feces. Contamination of wounds can occur as long as open lesions are present. Dirty surgical or traumatic wounds with significant devitalized tissue and foreign bodies predispose to disease. Nontraumatic gas gangrene occurs occasionally from *Clostridia* from the patient's intestinal tract.

The **incubation period** is 6 hours to 3 weeks; usually it is 2 to 4 days.

Diagnostic Tests: Anaerobic cultures of wound exudate, affected soft-tissue and muscle, and blood should be performed. Because clostridia are ubiquitous, their recovery from a wound is not diagnostic unless the appropriate clinical manifestations are present. A Gram-stained smear of wound discharge demonstrating characteristic Gram-positive rods and absent or sparse polymorphonuclear cells is indicative of clostridial infection. A roentgenogram of the affected site may demonstrate gas in the tissue.

Treatment:

- Early and complete surgical excision of necrotic infected tissue and removal of foreign material is the most important therapeutic measure.
- High-dose penicillin G (250,000 to 400,000 U/kg/d) should be given intravenously. Chloramphenicol, clindamycin, and metronidazole are alternative drugs for penicillin-allergic patients.
- Hyperbaric oxygen may be beneficial.
- Supportive management of shock, fluid and electrolyte imbalance, hemolytic anemia, and other complications is essential.
- Treatment with antitoxin is of no value. Equine gas gangrene polyvalent antitoxin is no longer available commercially in the United States.

Isolation of the Hospitalized Patient: Drainage/secretion precautions are indicated for the duration of lesion drainage.

Control Measures: Prompt and careful debridement and flushing of contaminated wounds and the removal of foreign material with standard aseptic surgical techniques should be done.

Penicillin G (50,000 U/kg/d) or clindamycin (20 to 30 mg/kg/d) may be of prophylactic value in patients with grossly contaminated wounds.

Clostridium perfringens Food Poisoning

Clinical Manifestations: *Clostridium perfringens* food poisoning is characterized by moderate to severe, crampy, midepigastric pain and watery diarrhea that occur 8 to 24 hours after ingestion of contaminated food. Vomiting is uncommon. Symptoms usually resolve within 24 hours. The absence of fever differentiates *C perfringens* food-borne disease from shigellosis and salmonellosis, and the infrequency of vomiting and the longer incubation period contrast with the clinical features of staphylococcal and chemical food-borne disease. Illness caused by *Bacillus cereus* may be clinically indistinguishable from that caused by *C perfringens.*

Etiology: Disease is caused by a heat-labile cytotoxic enterotoxin produced in vivo by type A *Clostridium perfringens.*

Epidemiology: *C perfringens* is ubiquitous in the environment and frequently is present in raw meat and poultry. Disease follows the ingestion of vegetative bacterial forms which produce and release enterotoxin during the process of spore formation in the lower bowel. Beef, poultry, gravies, and Mexican food are the most common sources. Infection is usually acquired at banquets or institutions (school, camps), or from food caterers or restaurants where food is prepared in large quantities and kept warm for prolonged periods. Illness is not transmissible from person to person.

The **incubation period** is 6 to 24 hours, usually 8 to 12 hours.

Diagnostic Tests: Because the fecal flora of healthy persons frequently includes *C perfringens*, counts of at least 10^6 *C perfringens* spores per gram of feces obtained within 48 hours of onset of disease are required to support the diagnosis in ill persons. To implicate a particular food, the concentration of vegetative bacterial forms should be at least 10^5 per gram in the suspected food. Since *C perfringens* is an anaerobe, special methods of specimen transport, such as anaerobic transport tubes, and laboratory processing are necessary.

Treatment: Usually no treatment is required. Oral rehydration or occasionally intravenous fluid and electrolyte replacement may be indicated for patients with unusually severe dehydration. Antibiotics are not indicated.

Isolation of the Hospitalized Patient: No special precautions are recommended.

Control Measures: Preventive measures depend on limiting proliferation of *C perfringens* in foods by maintaining food warmer than 60°C (140°F) or cooler than 7°C (45°F). Meat dishes should be served hot soon after cooking, or they should be cooled only to core temperatures of 74°C (165.2°F) or higher before serving. Roasts, stews, and similar dishes prepared in bulk should be divided into small quantities for cooking and refrigerated to limit the time such foods are at temperatures at which *C perfringens* grows. Using small quantities of foods will also help decrease leftovers that require storage and reheating.

Pseudomembranous Colitis Due to *Clostridium difficile*

Clinical Manifestations: Initial symptoms of pseudomembranous colitis are diarrhea and abdominal cramps, which progress to spiking fever, systemic toxicity, abdominal tenderness, and passage of stool with blood, mucous, and pus. Characteristically, the disease begins while the patient is in a hospital receiving antimicrobial therapy; but the disease can occur weeks after discharge from the hospital, after discontinuation of therapy, or unassociated with hospitalization or antimicrobial therapy. Severe and fatal disease has been described in severely neutropenic children with leukemia and in infants with Hirschsprung's disease.

Etiology: *Clostridium difficile* is a spore-forming, obligately anaerobic, Gram-positive bacillus. Disease is related to the action of toxin(s) produced by vegetative organisms. At present, two toxins (A and B) have been characterized.

Epidemiology: *C difficile* is widely distributed in soils and the intestinal tract of various animals, including humans. Spores of *C difficile* are acquired from the environment or by fecal-oral transmission from colonized individuals. Intestinal colonization rates in healthy neonates and young infants can be as high as 55% but are usually less than 4% in children older than 2 years and in adults. Hospital and day care facilities are major reservoirs for *C difficile*. Risk factors for the disease are those that increase exposure to organisms and those that diminish the barrier effect of the normal intestinal flora, allowing *C difficile* to proliferate and elaborate toxin(s) in vivo. Penicillins, clindamycin, and cephalosporins are the agents most frequently received by patients who subsequently develop pseudomembranous colitis, but colitis can be associated with almost any antimicrobial agent. Although *C difficile* toxin is rarely recovered from stools of asymptomatic adults, it frequently is recovered from stools of neonates who have no gastrointestinal illness. This finding confounds interpretation of positive toxin assays in patients younger than 6 months.

The **incubation period** is unknown.

Diagnostic Tests: Endoscopic findings of pseudomembranes and hyperemic, friable rectal mucosa suggest pseudomembranous colitis. Tissue-culture assays with toxin neutralization tests are required for confirmation of toxin production. A rapid latex agglutination test for *C difficile* antigen (which does not detect toxin) may be useful for screening patient specimens directly but is not highly specific.

Treatment:

- Antimicrobial therapy should be discontinued in patients who develop significant diarrhea or colitis.
- Orally administered vancomycin (40 mg/kg/d in four divided doses) is the drug of choice for those who require specific therapy. Vancomycin is poorly absorbed from the gastrointestinal tract but

can accumulate in the serum of patients with renal failure. Orally administered metronidazole (35 mg/kg/d in four divided doses)* appears to be effective and is less expensive. However, its safety has not been established in children, and the drug has not been approved for treatment of children with diarrhea. The efficacy of intravenously administered metronidazole or vancomycin is uncertain.

- Antimicrobials are usually given for 10 days.
- As many as 10% to 20% of patients relapse after discontinuing therapy, but they usually respond to a second course of treatment.
- Cholestyramine, which binds toxin, can relieve symptoms.* However, its effect has not been evaluated in children with disease caused by *C difficile*. Because cholestyramine also binds vancomycin, the two drugs should not be administered concurrently.
- Drugs that decrease intestinal motility should not be given.

Isolation of the Hospitalized Patient: Enteric precautions are recommended until diarrhea subsides.

Control Measures:

- Infants and children with *C difficile* colitis should be cared for in a separate, protected area or excluded from day care for the duration of diarrhea.
- Meticulous hand washing techniques, proper handling of contaminated waste (including diapers) and fomites, and limiting the use of antibiotics are the best currently available methods for the control of *C difficile* disease.
- Cleaning procedures that kill *C difficile* spores are currently under study.

Coccidioidomycosis

Clinical Manifestations: The primary pulmonary infection is usually asymptomatic and inapparent. Symptomatic disease may resemble influenza, with cough, fever, and chest pain. Chronic pulmonary lesions are rare in children. A diffuse erythematous maculopapular rash, erythema multiforme, erythema nodosum, and/or arthralgias frequently occur.

Primary extrapulmonary lesions include cutaneous lesions, which usually follow trauma or can occur with dissemination. The progressive disease is similar to tuberculosis; lungs, lymph nodes, bones, joints, abdominal organs, the central nervous system, and the skin are frequently affected sites. Meningitis is more common in children

*Use for this indication is not currently approved by the Food and Drug Administration.

than adults, and is fatal if untreated. Hydrocephalus is a common complication of central nervous system infections. Limited dissemination to one or more sites is common in children.

Etiology: *Coccidioides immitis* is a dimorphic fungus. In soil, it exists in the mycelial phase, the mature hyphal forms of which are termed arthroconidia. From these structures, spores and, later in the infected host, spherules develop.

Epidemiology: *C immitis* is found extensively in the soil of southwestern United States and California, northern Mexico, and certain areas of Central and South America. Climatic conditions (hot summers, little winter frost) combine with soil conditions (alkaline, dry) and local characteristics (rodent burrows, the creosote bush) to produce ideal circumstances for preservation of arthroconidia and their dissemination by aerosols. Individuals are infected by dust-borne arthroconidia or by contact with infected soil, such as occurs when students excavate in endemic regions. The spherule is noninfectious. Person-to-person transmission of coccidioidomycosis does not occur. One episode of multiple infections from a plaster cast that was contaminated with arthroconidia has been reported. In immunocompromised patients, such as those with AIDS, the likelihood of disseminated coccidioidomycosis is increased.

The **incubation period** is 10 to 16 days; the range is from less than 1 week to approximately 1 month, depending on the quantity of arthroconidia inhaled.

Diagnostic Tests: Spherules up to 80 microns in diameter may be visualized in appropriate clinical specimens in selected instances, such as tracheal aspirates, biopsies of skin lesions or organs, urine, or cerebrospinal fluid. Culture of the organism is possible but is a potential infectious hazard to laboratory personnel since conversion of spherules to arthroconidial-bearing mycelium can take place. Suspect cultures should be sealed at the outset and handled cautiously by trained persons thereafter.

Skin tests can be useful in diagnosis. A reactive coccidioidin skin test is characteristic of a hypersensitivity reaction of the delayed type. Conversion of a skin test with coccidioidin (mycelial form) or spherulin (spherule form) from negative to positive in a patient with a clinically compatible syndrome strongly suggests coccidioidomycosis. A positive skin test usually appears 10 to 21 days after infection, but is characteristically absent in progressive disease. Therefore, overreliance on skin test results can lead to incorrect diagnostic conclusions, particularly since dissemination can occur in patients whose skin tests are nonreactive.

Serologic tests are not routinely used in patients with mild illnesses, but they are extremely useful in those with moderate or severe illnesses. Precipitins of both IgG and IgM classes can be detected by immunodiffusion. IgM precipitins are detectable 1 to 3 weeks after symptoms appear and last 3 to 4 months in most cases. Complement fixation antibodies in serum usually are of low titer and transient if the disease is asymptomatic or mild. Higher and persistent complement fixation titers are observed when the disease is severe, and almost always in disseminated infections. In central nervous system coccidioidomycosis, cerebrospinal fluid antibodies are detectable by complement fixation. The concentration and persistence of complement fixation antibody titers in serum in patients with disseminated, severe disease and in cerebrospinal fluid in those with meningitis are useful prognostically and in guiding treatment.

Treatment: Most cases of coccidioidomycosis do not require treatment. Amphotericin B is the recommended therapy in severe progressive pulmonary disease, disseminated infection, central nervous system infections, and in immunocompromised patients, such as those with AIDS. Amphotericin B is administered intravenously.

Experience with agents other than amphotericin B is limited. Ketoconazole has effectively suppressed symptoms and arrested progression of infection in most patients with pulmonary or disseminated coccidioidomycosis. The relapse rate after treatment is high. Efficacy in comparison to that of amphotericin B has not been evaluated. Ketaconazole should not be used in place of amphotericin B in patients with severe disease or who are immunocompromised.

In central nervous system infections, intravenous amphotericin B therapy is augmented by repetitive instillation of this drug into the lumbar, cisternal, or ventricular spaces, frequently by the use of a subcutaneous reservoir (see Systemic Treatment with Amphotericin B, page 574). High doses of ketoconazole given orally along with intraventricular miconazole have also been used successfully.

In some localized forms of the disease (e.g., mandibular, bone), local instillation of amphotericin B has been used with occasional success.

The duration of systemic amphotericin B therapy is variable and depends on the site(s) of involvement, clinical response, and mycologic and immunologic tests. In general, therapy is continued until clinical and laboratory evidence indicates that the active infection has subsided. Minimum treatment for invasive coccidioidomycosis is 1 month, and treatment for 1 year or longer is frequently necessary for central nervous system disease.

Surgical debridement or excision of the lesions in bone and the lung has been advocated for localized, symptomatic, persistent, resistant, or progressive lesions. Surgical treatment (by shunt procedures) of hydrocephalus in central nervous system infections is frequently necessary.

Isolation of the Hospitalized Patient: No special precautions are recommended. Care should be exercised in handling, changing, and discarding dressings, casts, and similar materials in which arthroconidial contamination could occur.

Control Measures: None.

Coronaviruses

Clinical Manifestations: Coronaviruses are a common cause of upper respiratory tract infection in adults and children and have occasionally been implicated in lower respiratory tract disease. Enteric coronaviruses have been identified in the feces of infants and children with gastroenteritis, but their etiologic significance is unproven. Coronavirus-like agents have also been associated with several outbreaks of diarrhea in nurseries and, rarely, with infants with neonatal necrotizing enterocolitis.

Etiology: Coronaviruses are RNA viruses that are large (80 to 160 nm), pleomorphic, enveloped, spherical or elliptical, and have lipid-soluble coats. At least four antigenic groups of respiratory coronaviruses are recognized.

Epidemiology: Human coronaviruses are most likely transmitted by the respiratory route, possibly by aerosols and large droplets, and facilitated by close contact. Because of prolonged carriage of enteric coronaviruses in the stool, fecal-oral transmission can also occur. Although several animal coronaviruses have antigens in common with human strains, no evidence implicates animals as reservoirs or vectors for human disease. Coronaviruses are worldwide in distribution. In temperate climates, outbreaks occur in the winter. Young children have the highest infection rate in outbreaks. The period of communicability is unknown but probably persists for the duration of respiratory symptoms.

The **incubation period** is usually 2 to 4 days.

Diagnostic Tests: Diagnostic tests for human coronaviruses are generally not available. Most strains cannot be isolated by the methods commonly used in diagnostic virology laboratories. Viral particles have been visualized by immune electron microscopy and viral antigens detected by immunoassay techniques. Antibody to coronaviruses can be determined by several assay methods, such as neutralization, complement fixation, indirect hemagglutination, fluorescent antibody, and enzyme immunoassay, but these tests are not routinely available.

Treatment: Supportive.

Isolation of the Hospitalized Patient: For infants and young children, contact isolation is recommended for the duration of symptoms.

Control Measures: None.

Cryptococcus neoformans Infections

(Cryptococcosis, Torulosis)

Clinical Manifestations: Signs and symptoms vary with the organ(s) involved. Infection can involve primarily the central nervous system (meningoencephalitis), lungs (pneumonia), lymph nodes (adenopathy), heart (endocarditis), skin (ulcers), bones and joints, and mucous membranes. Usually, several sites are infected, but manifestations of the involvement of one site predominate.

Etiology: *Cryptococcus neoformans* is an encapsulated yeast.

Epidemiology: The organism is worldwide in distribution. Weathered pigeon droppings frequently contain the fungus. Acquisition is by inhalation of particles containing the organism. The fungus is not transmitted from person to person. It is a frequent cause of infection in adults with AIDS but is rare in pediatric AIDS patients.

The **incubation period**, although not well defined, is probably a few weeks from the time of exposure.

Diagnostic Tests: Encapsulated yeast cells can be demonstrated in wet mounts of sputum or pus or in India ink preparations of cerebrospinal fluid sediment. Precise diagnosis depends on the isolation and identification of the organism by culture at 37°C on Sabouraud's dextrose agar. Media containing cycloheximide, which inhibits growth of *C neoformans*, should not be used. Few organisms may be present in the cerebrospinal fluid, and large quantities of fluid may need to be cultured to recover the organism. The latex particle agglutination test for detection of cryptococcal antigen is a useful and rapid diagnostic tool, particularly with central nervous system disease. Skin testing with the antigen cryptococcin is of no value.

Treatment: Amphotericin B in combination with flucytosine is indicated for meningeal and other serious cryptococcol infections in healthy hosts. In these patients, combination antifungal therapy is superior to amphotericin B alone. In patients with AIDS, therapy with amphotericin B is as effective as combined therapy. Flucytosine often induces cytopenias which complicate management and necessitate discontinuation of the medication. Amphotericin B is administered intravenously and flucytosine is given orally. Meningitis in most patients is treated for at least 6 weeks. Patients with AIDS require maintenance therapy.

Fluconazole has been used successfully in adults with meningitis and is an alternative drug for the treatment of cryptococcosis. Data on its use in children are limited.

Treatment is not indicated for all patients with pulmonary disease because some cases that occur in otherwise healthy hosts can resolve spontaneously.

Isolation of the Hospitalized Patient: No special precautions are recommended.

Control Measures: None.

Cryptosporidiosis

Clinical Manifestations: Frequent, watery diarrhea and low grade fever are the most common presenting symptoms. Other symptoms include abdominal pain, anorexia, and weight loss. In infected immunocompetent individuals, including children, the diarrheal illness is self limited, usually lasting 1 to 20 days (average, 10 days). Immunocompromised patients, especially those with AIDS, can develop chronic, severe diarrhea with malnutrition and dehydration. Although infection is usually limited to the gastrointestinal tract, pulmonary or disseminated infection has occurred in rare instances in immunocompromised patients.

Etiology: *Cryptosporidium* is a coccidian protozoan.

Epidemiology: Cryptosporidia have been found in a variety of biologic hosts, including mammals, birds, and reptiles. Animal handlers become infected in the course of their work. In experimental studies, *Cryptosporidium* has been successfully transmitted from humans to various species of animals. Person-to-person transmission occurs and can cause outbreaks in day care centers, with high attack rates (30% to 40%) of infection. Water-borne outbreaks have occurred. The parasite is not affected by chlorine and is not always removed by water filters.

The estimated **incubation period** is 2 to 14 days.

Diagnostic Tests: Diagnosis can be made by finding oocysts on microscopic examination of the stools, with either the sucrose flotation method or formalin-ethylacetate used to concentrate the oocysts, followed by staining with a modified Kinyoun acid-fast stain. Since shedding can be intermittent, at least two stool specimens should be examined before considering the test to be negative. Oocysts are small (4 to 6 microns in diameter) and can be missed in a rapid survey of the slide. The organism can also be seen on intestinal biopsy. A monoclonal antibody test for detecting oocysts by dual immunofluorescence in stool is also available.

Treatment: Treatment of infection in normal hosts is generally symptomatic and entails rehydration and correction of electrolyte abnormalities. For immunosuppressed patients with severe or chronic infections, no definitive treatment has been established. Spiramycin (a macrolide antibiotic), 4 g/d orally in four divided doses for 3 to 4 weeks, is under study as a treatment regimen for adults and is available for investigational use.* Clindamycin plus quinine have also been given, but the effectiveness of this regimen has not been determined.

Isolation of the Hospitalized Patient: Enteric precautions are recommended.

Control Measures: None.

Cutaneous Larva Migrans

(Creeping Eruption)

Clinical Manifestations: Nematode larvae produce itching, reddish papules at the site of skin entry. As the larvae migrate through the skin and advance several millimeters to a few centimeters a day, they leave intensely pruritic, serpiginous tracks. Larval activity can con-

*For further information, contact the Food and Drug Administration, Washington, D.C. (301/295-8012).

tinue for several weeks or months but eventually is self limiting. The clinical picture of an advancing serpiginous tunnel in the skin with an associated intense pruritus is virtually pathognomonic.

Etiology: Infective larvae of cat and dog hookworms (*Ancylostoma brasiliensis* and *A caninum*) are the usual causes. Other skin-penetrating nematodes are occasional causes.

Epidemiology: Cutaneous larva migrans is a disease of children, utility workers, gardeners, sunbathers, and others who come in contact with sandy soil contaminated with cat and dog feces. In the United States, the disease is most prevalent in the Southeast.

Diagnostic Tests: Since the diagnosis is usually made clinically, biopsies are not usually indicated. Biopsy specimens usually demonstrate an eosinophilic inflammatory infiltrate but the migrating parasite is not visualized. Eosinophilia occurs in some cases.

Treatment: The disease is usually self limited, with spontaneous cure after several weeks or months. Individual larvae can be killed by freezing the area with ethyl chloride spray. Thiabendazole given orally and/or topically is also effective.

Isolation of the Hospitalized Patient: No special precautions are recommended.

Control Measures: Skin contact with moist soil contaminated with animal feces should be avoided.

Cytomegalovirus Infections

Clinical Manifestations: The manifestations of acquired cytomegalovirus (CMV) infections vary with the age and immunocompetence of the host. Asymptomatic infections are the most common, particularly in children. Hepatosplenomegaly can occasionally be a manifestation of acquired disease in childhood. An infectious mononucleosis-like syndrome with prolonged fever and mild hepatitis, occurring in the absence of heterophile antibody, has been described in adults. Pneumonia and retinitis are common manifestations in immunocompromised hosts, particularly those who are under treatment for malignancies, who are infected with the human immunodeficiency virus, or who are receiving immunosuppressive therapy for organ transplantation.

Congenital infections also have a spectrum of manifestations. Usually, infection is asymptomatic, but some congenitally infected infants who appear to be asymptomatic at birth are found in infancy or childhood to have a hearing loss or learning disability. Profound involvement, with intrauterine growth retardation, neonatal jaundice, purpura, hepatosplenomegaly, microcephaly, brain damage, intracerebral calcifications, and chorioretinitis, occurs infrequently.

Infection acquired at birth from maternal cervical excretion is usually not associated with clinical illness. Infection resulting from transfusion from CMV seropositive donors to preterm infants has been associated with lower respiratory tract disease.

Etiology: Human CMV, a DNA virus, is a member of the herpesvirus group.

Epidemiology: Numerous mammalian species harbor their own type of CMV, each of which is relatively species specific. Infection in humans is caused only by human CMV and, very rarely, by simian CMV. Human CMV are ubiquitous and are transmitted both horizontally (by direct person-to-person contact with virus-containing secretions) and vertically. Infections have no seasonal predilection. CMV persists in latent form after a primary infection, and reactivation can occur years later, particularly under conditions of immunosuppression.

Horizontal transmission probably occurs most commonly as a result of salivary contamination, but contact with infected urine can also play a role. Although the virus is not highly contagious, spread of CMV in households and day care centers is well documented. Excretion rates in day care centers may reach 70% in 1- to 3-year-old children. Young children can transmit CMV to their parents and other caregivers, such as day care staff (see also Children in Child Care, page 76). In adolescents and adults, sexual transmission also occurs, as evidenced by seminal and cervical excretion of virus.

Seropositive normal persons carry latent CMV in white blood cells and tissues; hence, blood transfusions and organ transplantation can result in viral transmission. Severe CMV disease is more likely to occur if the recipient is seronegative or is a premature infant. Latent CMV will frequently reactivate in immunosuppressed individuals, and can result in disease if the immunosuppression is severe (e.g., AIDS patients, solid organ transplant and bone marrow transplant recipients).

The **incubation period** for horizontally transmitted CMV infections is unknown for person-to-person spread in households. Infection usually manifests within 3 to 12 weeks after blood transfusions, and between 4 weeks and 4 months after tissue transplantation.

Vertical transmission of CMV to the infant occurs in utero by transplacental passage of maternal blood-borne virus, at birth by passage through an infected maternal genital tract, or postnatally by ingestion of CMV-positive human milk. Approximately 1% of all infants are infected in utero and excrete CMV at birth. In utero fetal infection can occur regardless of whether the mother had primary infection or reactivation during pregnancy. However, infants infected in utero during maternal reactivation are much less frequently affected than those born after maternal primary infection presumably because of prior immunity in the mother. Of infants whose infection resulted from maternal primary infection, 10% to 20% will have mental retardation or sensorineural deafness. Severe disease with manifestations at birth occurs in about 5% of infants infected in utero.

Maternal cervical infection is common and many infants are exposed to CMV at birth. Excretion is higher among young mothers in lower socioeconomic groups. Perinatal acquisition in these infants is thought to be a route of infection. Most infants will remain asymptomatic, but interstitial pneumonia due to CMV can develop in the early months of life.

Virus-positive breast milk can transmit CMV. However, breastfeeding does not cause apparent illness, most likely because of the presence of passively transmitted maternal antibody. However, if seronegative infants are fed CMV-infected milk from milk banks, symptomatic disease can occur.

Diagnostic Tests: The diagnosis of CMV is frequently confounded by the ubiquity of the virus, the high rate of asymptomatic excretion, the frequency of reactivated infections, the development of IgM CMV antibody in some episodes of reactivation, and the simultaneous presence of other pathogens.

Virus can be isolated in tissue culture from urine, pharynx, peripheral blood leukocytes, human milk, semen, cervical secretions, and other tissues and body fluids. Virus present in large quantity can also be identified by electron microscopic examination of urine or tissue. Examination of cells shed in the urine for intranuclear inclusions is an insensitive test.

Complement fixation, the most commonly available serologic test, is the least sensitive method for the diagnosis of CMV infection and should not be used to establish prior infection or passively acquired maternal antibody. Various fluorescence assays, indirect hemagglutination, latex agglutination, and ELISA tests are preferred for this purpose.

Only recovery of virus from a target organ provides unequivocal evidence that the disease is caused by acquired CMV infection. However, a presumptive diagnosis can be made on the basis of a fourfold antibody titer rise in paired sera or by virus excretion.

Proof of congenital infection requires obtaining specimens within 3 weeks of birth. In that period, viral recovery or a strongly positive test for serum IgM anti-CMV antibody is considered diagnostic. Later in infancy, differentiation between intrauterine and perinatal infection is difficult unless clinical signs of the former, such as chorioretinitis or ventriculitis, are present. Special serologic tests that are available only in reference laboratories may help to differentiate between these two possibilities in the first 2 or 3 months of life.

Treatment: The drug ganciclovir (see Antiviral Drugs, page 578) is beneficial in the treatment of retinitis caused by acquired CMV infection in patients with AIDS. This drug has recently been licensed in the United States for the treatment of severe retinitis in immunocompromised adults. Limited data in children suggest that efficacy is similar to that in adults; available data are insufficient to establish safety in children. The drug is useful in other types of CMV organ involvement. The combination of CMV immune globulin* given intravenously and ganciclovir has been reported to be synergistic in the treatment of CMV infections in bone marrow transplant recipients.

Isolation of the Hospitalized Patient: No special precautions are recommended. Hospitalized patients do not need separate rooms. However, since CMV is spread by intimate contact with infectious secretions, hand washing after exposure to secretions is particularly important for pregnant personnel.

Control Measures:

Care of Exposed Persons.

- Exclusion from schools or institutions of children with congenital infection who are excreting CMV is not justified, since asymptomatic infection is common in newborn infants and during infancy and early childhood. Similarly, institution-sponsored screening programs for CMV-excreting children are of questionable value. The intermittent and prolonged shedding of CMV in the urine makes screening programs impractical and prohibitively costly. The child with congenital CMV infection should not be singled out for exclusion or special handling. Hand washing, particularly after changing diapers, is advised in caring for all children.
- Concern arises when a pregnant or immunocompromised patient is exposed to patients with clinically recognizable CMV infection.

*Available through regional offices of the American Red Cross Blood Services.

Many exposed adults and children are already immune, but because most infections are asymptomatic, the history is of no value in assessing susceptibility. Serologic testing can be used to identify nonimmune individuals, although as yet no prophylactic agent can be offered. Follow-up serologic testing will establish if infection has occurred. However, routine serologic screening of personnel is not currently recommended.

- Prevention of exposure of severely immunocompromised patients to recognized cases of CMV infection is prudent.
- Pregnant personnel who may be in contact with CMV-infected patients should be counseled about the potential risks of acquisition and urged to practice good hygiene, particularly hand washing. Approximately 1% of infants in most newborn nurseries, and a higher percentage of older children, may excrete CMV without clinical manifestations. Fetal risks are greatest in the first half of gestation. Amniocentesis has been used in several cases to establish the presence of intrauterine infection, but the sensitivity of this technique is unknown.

Day Care. Educational programs about the epidemiology of CMV, its potential risks, and appropriate hygienic measures to minimize occupationally acquired infection should be provided for women day care workers. The prevalence of CMV in urine or saliva of healthy children can be high, and spread to their mothers and child care workers has been documented. Risk appears to be greater for child care personnel who care for children younger than 2 years. Pregnant personnel should be counseled about these risks. Routine serologic screening for antibody to CMV in day care center workers is not currently recommended.

Immunization. CMV immune globulin* has been developed for prophylaxis of disease in seronegative transplant patients and appears to be moderately effective in kidney transplant recipients. Its use in prevention of CMV transmission to newborn infants has also been studied but the results, to date, are inconclusive. A live CMV vaccine is being tested in normal volunteers and renal transplant patients.

Prevention of Transmission by Blood Transfusion. Transmission of CMV by blood transfusion to preterm infants or others can be virtually eliminated by the use of CMV antibody-negative donors, by freezing blood in glycerol before administration, by removal of the buffy coat, or by filtration to remove the white blood cells.

*Available through regional offices of the American Red Cross Blood Services.

Diphtheria

Clinical Manifestations: Diphtheria usually occurs as membranous nasopharyngitis and/or obstructive laryngotracheitis; these local infections are associated with a low-grade fever and the gradual onset of manifestations during 1 to 2 days. Less commonly, the disease presents as cutaneous, vaginal, conjunctival, or otic infections. Cutaneous diphtheria is more common in tropical areas and among the homeless. Life-threatening complications of diphtheria include thrombocytopenia, myocarditis, and neurologic problems such as vocal cord paralysis and ascending paralysis similar to that of Guillain-Barré syndrome.

Etiology: *Corynebacterium diphtheriae* is an irregularly staining, Gram-positive, nonmotile, pleomorphic rod with three colony types (mitis, gravis, and intermedius). *C diphtheriae* strains may be either toxigenic or nontoxigenic; the ability to produce toxin is not related to colony type.

Epidemiology: Humans are the only known reservoir of *C diphtheriae*. Sources of infection include discharges from the nose, throat, eye, and skin lesions of infected persons. Transmission results primarily from intimate contact with a patient or carrier. Rarely, fomites can serve as vehicles of transmission, and food-borne outbreaks have occurred. Illness is most common in low socioeconomic groups living in crowded conditions. Infection can occur in immunized and partially immunized persons as well as in the unimmunized; disease is most common and most severe in unimmunized or inadequately immunized individuals. The incidence of disease is greatest in the fall and winter, but summer epidemics can occur in warmer climates in which skin infections are prevalent. Communicability in untreated persons usually lasts for 2 weeks or less, but occasionally it can persist for several months. In patients treated with appropriate antibiotics, communicability usually lasts less than 4 days. Occasionally, chronic carriage occurs, even after antimicrobial therapy.

The **incubation period** is usually 2 to 5 days but occasionally longer.

Diagnostic Tests: Specimens for culture should be obtained from the nose and throat and from any lesions. Material should be obtained from beneath the membrane, or a portion of the membrane should be submitted for culture. Because special media are required, the laboratory should be notified that *C diphtheriae* is suspected. In remote areas, throat swabs can be placed in silica gel packs and sent to reference laboratories for culture, as *C diphtheriae* survive drying.

Results of cultures may be available as soon as 8 hours after inoculation. Direct-stained smears and fluorescent antibody-stained smears are unreliable. When *C diphtheriae* is recovered, the strain should be tested for toxigenicity.

Treatment:

Antitoxin.* Because the condition of patients with diphtheria may deteriorate rapidly, a single dose of equine antitoxin should be administered on the basis of clinical diagnosis, even before culture results are available. The site and size of the diphtheritic membrane, the degree of toxicity, and the duration of the illness are guides for estimating the dose of antitoxin; the presence of soft, diffuse cervical lymphadenitis suggests moderate to severe toxin absorption. Suggested dose ranges are the following: pharyngeal or laryngeal disease of 48 hours' duration, 20,000 to 40,000 U; nasopharyngeal lesions, 40,000 to 60,000 U; extensive disease of 3 or more days' duration or brawny swelling of the neck, 80,000 to 100,000 U. The preferred route of administration (after tests for sensitivity with 1:10 antitoxin dilution for conjunctival testing or 1:100 dilution for intradermal testing, see Sensitivity Tests for Reactions to Animal Sera, page 40) is intravenous, to neutralize toxin as rapidly as possible. If the patient is sensitive to equine antitoxin, desensitization (see "Desensitization" for Animal Sera, page 41) is necessary. Antitoxin is probably of no value for cutaneous disease, but some authorities use 20,000 to 40,000 U of antitoxin because toxic sequelae have been reported. Although intravenous immunoglobulin preparations contain antibodies to diphtheria toxin, their use for therapy has not been approved and optimal dosages have not been established. Vigorous cleansing of the lesion with soap and water and administration of antimicrobials for 10 days is recommended.

Antimicrobial Therapy. This therapy is required to eradicate the organism and prevent spread; it is not a substitute for antitoxin. Erythromycin given parenterally or orally (40 to 50 mg/kg/d; maximum, 2 g/d) for 14 days, or penicillin G daily, intramuscularly (aqueous crystalline, 100,000 to 150,000 U/kg/d in four divided doses or procaine, 25,000 to 50,000 U/kg/d, in two divided doses) for 14 days comprise acceptable therapy. Elimination of the organism should be documented by three consecutive negative cultures after completion of treatment.

Carriers. Antimicrobial therapy should also be administered to carriers. If unimmunized, carriers should receive active immunization promptly, and steps should be taken to ensure completion. If previously immunized, carriers should be given a booster dose of a

*To obtain diphtheria antitoxin, see Services of the Centers for Disease Control, page 622.

preparation containing diphtheria toxoid (DTP, DT, or Td). Antimicrobial therapy should be given as (1) oral erythromycin or penicillin G for 7 days, or (2) a single, intramuscular dose of benzathine penicillin G (600,000 U for those weighing less than 30 kg and 1,200,000 U for larger children and adults). Follow-up cultures should be obtained; if they are positive, an additional 10-day course of oral erythromycin should be given. Erythromycin-resistant strains have been identified but their epidemiologic significance has not been determined.

Isolation of the Hospitalized Patient: For pharyngeal diphtheria, patients and carriers of toxigenic strains should be placed in strict isolation until two cultures from both the nose and the throat are negative for *C diphtheriae*. Patients with cutaneous diphtheria should be placed in contact isolation until two cultures of skin lesions are negative. Material for these cultures should be taken at least 24 hours apart after cessation of antimicrobial therapy.

Control Measures:

Care of Exposed Persons. Management is based on individual circumstances, including immunization status and the likelihood of surveillance and adherence to prophylaxis.

- Identification of close contacts of a suspected patient should be promptly initiated. Contact tracing should begin in the household and can usually be limited to household members and other persons with history of habitual, close contact with the suspected case.
- Close contacts, irrespective of their immunization status, should be cultured, given antimicrobial prophylaxis with oral erythromycin or intramuscular penicillin G, and kept under surveillance for 7 days for evidence of disease. The efficacy of antimicrobial prophylaxis is presumed but not proven.
- Asymptomatic, previously immunized close contacts should receive a booster dose of a preparation containing diphtheria toxoid (DTP, DT, or Td) if they have not received a booster dose of diphtheria toxoid within 5 years.
- For asymptomatic close contacts who are unimmunized or whose immunization status is not known, the following should be undertaken: (1) immediate prophylaxis instituted with oral erythromycin (40 to 50 mg/kg/d for 7 days, maximum 2 g/d) or benzathine penicillin G (600,000 to 1,200,000 U given intramuscularly; the lower dose is for patients weighing less than 30 kg); (2) cultures done before and after prophylaxis; and (3) active immunization initiated with DTP, DT, or Td, depending on age.
- Contacts who cannot be kept under surveillance should receive (1) benzathine penicillin G, but not erythromycin for reasons of

compliance; and (2) an initial dose of DTP, DT, or Td, depending on age and the person's immunization history. The use of equine diphtheria antitoxin in unimmunized close contacts who cannot be closely observed is not generally recommended because of the risk of allergic reactions to horse serum, and efficacy of passive immunization has not been established. If antitoxin is used, the usual recommended dose is 5,000 to 10,000 U, injected intramuscularly at a site separate from the site of the toxoid injection, after appropriate testing for sensitivity.

Immunization.

Universal immunization with diphtheria toxoid* is the only effective control measure. Its value is proven by the rarity of the disease in countries in which high rates of immunization with diphtheria toxoid have been achieved. Fewer than five cases have been reported annually in the United States in recent years. As a result of high immunization rates, exposure to persons with diphtheria or to carriers is less frequent now than in the past. However, the decreased frequency of exposure to the organism implies decreased maintenance of immunity secondary to community contact. Therefore, assurance of continuing immunity requires **regular booster injections of diphtheria toxoid every 10 years** after completion of the initial immunization series.

- Immunization for children from age 2 months to the seventh birthday (see Tables 2 and 3) should consist of three doses of DTP vaccine given intramuscularly at 2-month intervals commencing at 2 months of age; a fourth dose at 18 months of age; and a fifth dose given before school entry (kindergarten or elementary school) at 4 to 6 years of age, unless the fourth dose was given after the fourth birthday. The fourth dose can be given at 15 months and concurrently with MMR, OPV, and *Haemophilus* b conjugate vaccine (HbCV).
- Immunization against diphtheria for children younger than 7 years in whom pertussis immunization is deferred or contraindicated (see Pertussis, page 366) should be implemented with DT vaccine† instead of DTP. For children who are younger than 1 year, three doses of DT are given at 2-month intervals; a fourth dose should be given approximately 1 year after the third dose; and the fifth dose should be given before school entry at 4 to 6 years of age. Children who have not received prior doses of DT or DTP and are 1 year or older should receive two doses of DT approximately 2 months apart, followed by a third dose 6 to 12 months later to complete the initial series. A dose of DT can be

*Diphtheria (and tetanus) toxoid vaccines in use in the United States are adsorbed aluminum salts.

†The Immunization Practices Advisory Committee (ACIP) of the U.S. Public Health Service defines primary immunization as consisting of the first four doses; the fifth dose is considered a booster.

given concurrently with MMR, OPV, and HbCV. An additional dose is necessary before school entry at 4 to 6 years of age, unless the preceding dose was given after the fourth birthday.

- Children who have received one or two doses of DTP (or DT) in the first year of life and for whom further pertussis vaccination is contraindicated should receive additional doses of DT until a total of five doses of diphtheria and tetanus toxoids have been received by the time of school entry. The fourth dose is administered 6 to 12 months after the third dose. The preschool (fifth) dose is omitted if the fourth dose was given after the fourth birthday.
- Immunization of children after their seventh birthday (see Table 3) should consist of Td, i.e., adult-type tetanus and diphtheria toxoids. The Td preparation contains not more than 2 flocculating units (Lf) of diphtheria toxoid per dose, as compared with 7 to 25 Lf in the DTP and DT preparations for use in infants and younger children. Td is less likely than DTP or DT to produce reactions in older children and adults. Two doses are given 1 to 2 months apart; a third dose should be given 6 to 12 months after the second. Complete immunization requires three doses followed by boosters every 10 years.
- When children and adults require tetanus toxoid for wound management, the use of preparations containing diphtheria toxoid (DTP, DT, or Td as appropriate for age or specific contraindications) will help ensure continuing diphtheria immunity.
- Active immunization against diphtheria should be undertaken during convalescence from diphtheria in every patient because this exotoxin-mediated disease does not necessarily confer immunity.

Ehrlichiosis (Human)

Clinical Manifestations: Human ehrlichiosis is an acute, systemic febrile illness clinically similar to Rocky Mountain spotted fever but with more frequent leukopenia and less frequent occurrence of rash. The febrile illness is often accompanied by chills, headache, myalgia, arthralgia, nausea, vomiting, anorexia, and acute weight loss. Rash is variable in appearance and location, develops typically about 1 week after onset of illness, but only occurs in approximately one half of reported cases. Diarrhea, abdominal pain and change in mental status are noted less frequently. Reported complications include pulmonary infiltrates, respiratory failure and renal failure. Leukopenia, anemia, hyponatremia, thrombocytopenia, liver function test abnormalities and cerebrospinal fluid pleocytosis (with a predominance of lymphocytes) are common. The disease typically lasts 1 to 2 weeks and recovery generally occurs without sequelae. Fatal as well as asymptomatic infections have been reported.

Etiology: The presumptive cause is *Ehrlichia canis* (or another closely related rickettsial species). *E canis* is causative agent of canine ehrlichiosis.

Epidemiology: Most human cases have been reported from southeastern and south central United States, but a wider distribution is suspected. The disease appears to be transmitted by ticks; which tick transmits the infection to humans is not known. Patients with ehrlichiosis have been somewhat older but similar regarding gender, race, and recognized tick exposures in comparison to those with Rocky Mountain spotted fever. Most human infections have occurred from May through July. The incidence of reported cases appears to be increasing. Epidemiologic data are limited.

The **incubation period** appears to be 1 to 3 weeks; the median has been 11 to 12 days.

Diagnostic Tests: Isolation of *Ehrlichia* from human patients has not been accomplished. The diagnosis of *E canis* infection can be confirmed by demonstrating a fourfold or greater increase in antibody titer between acute and convalescent sera, preferably obtained 2 to 4 weeks apart, using an indirect fluorescent antibody test with *E canis* as antigen. The test is available only through state health departments and the Centers for Disease Control. Microscopic observation of inclusion bodies in the cytoplasm of peripheral leukocytes has been infrequently described.

Treatment: The decision to initiate antibiotic therapy is based on clinical findings and epidemiologic considerations. Tetracycline, in the same dose and schedule used for treatment of Rocky Mountain spotted fever, appears to be effective therapy for human ehrlichiosis. Limited data also suggest that chloramphenicol is also effective. Tetracycline drugs are usually contraindicated in children younger than 9 years. However, in deciding which antibiotic to give a patient with presumed ehrlichiosis who is younger than 9 years, the benefits and risks of a single course of tetracycline therapy should be compared with those of chloramphenicol.

Isolation of the Hospitalized Patient: No special precautions are recommended.

Control Measures: Specific measures concern prevention of contact with ticks and are similar to those for Rocky Mountain spotted fever and other tick-borne diseases (see Control Measures for Prevention of Tick-Borne Infections, p. 112).

Enterovirus (Nonpolio) Infections

Coxsackieviruses, Group A and Group B; Echoviruses and Enteroviruses

Clinical Manifestations: Nonpolio enteroviruses are responsible for significant and frequent illnesses in infants and children and result in protean clinical manifestations. The most common presentation is nonspecific febrile illness, which in infants frequently leads to suspicion of bacterial sepsis. Other common manifestations include the following: (1) respiratory—common cold, pharyngitis, herpangina, stomatitis, pneumonia, and pleurodynia; (2) gastrointestinal—vomiting, diarrhea, abdominal pain, and hepatitis; (3) eye—acute hemorrhagic conjunctivitis; (4) heart—pericarditis and myocarditis; (5) skin—exanthem; and (6) neurologic—aseptic meningitis, encephalitis, and paralysis. Although each of these findings can be caused by several different enteroviruses, some virus/disease associations are particularly noteworthy. These include coxsackievirus A16 in the hand, foot, and mouth syndrome; coxsackievirus A24 and enterovirus 70 in acute hemorrhagic conjunctivitis; enterovirus 71 in encephalitis and polio-like paralysis; echovirus 9 in petechial exanthem and meningitis; coxsackieviruses B1 to B5 in pericarditis and myocarditis and in fulminating encephalomyocarditis; and echovirus 11 in fulminating neonatal hepatic necrosis.

Etiology: The nonpolio enteroviruses are RNA viruses, which include 23 group A coxsackieviruses (types A1 to A24, except type A23), 6 group B coxsackieviruses (types B1 to B6), 31 echoviruses (types 1 to 33, except types 10 and 28), and 4 enteroviruses (types 68 to 71).

Epidemiology: Enteroviruses are ubiquitous in humans, and humans are their only known natural host. Enteroviruses are spread by fecal-oral and possibly oral-oral (respiratory) routes. Attack rates are highest in young children, and infections occur more frequently in lower socioeconomic groups and in tropical areas where hygiene is poor. In temperate climates, enteroviral infections are most common in the summer and fall. In contrast, no seasonal pattern is evident in the tropics. Fecal viral excretion and transmission can continue for several weeks after the onset of infection.

The **incubation period** is usually 3 to 6 days.

Diagnostic Tests: Specimens for viral isolation should be obtained from the throat and rectum and any sites of clinical involvement, such as the cerebrospinal fluid, blood, and biopsy material. Attempts to recover virus are particularly important in patients with serious illnesses during epidemics. Viral isolation from any specimen except the feces usually can be considered causally related to the patient's illness. Because enteroviruses can be carried in the lower gastrointestinal tract for long periods of time, fecal isolates may not be causally related to the patient's illness. Most viral diagnostic laboratories use only tissue culture techniques that are capable of recovering echoviruses, group B coxsackieviruses, and some group A coxsackieviruses. Suckling mouse inoculation, which is not a routine procedure, is required for the recovery of many group A coxsackieviruses. Sera for antibody testing should be collected and stored frozen at the onset of illness and 4 weeks later. The demonstration of a rise in titer of an antibody to a virus recovered from the feces suggests a causal role for the isolated virus. Because no common enterovirus antigen is available for laboratory use, serologic screening without viral isolation is generally not performed.

Treatment: No specific therapy for enteroviral infections exists. Intravenous immune globulin with a high antibody titer to the infecting virus may be of benefit in immunocompromised patients and has been used in life-threatening neonatal infections.

Isolation of the Hospitalized Patient: Enteric precautions are indicated for 7 days after the onset of illness.

Control Measures: Particular attention should be paid to hand washing and personal hygiene.

Escherichia coli and Other Gram-Negative Bacilli

Septicemia and Meningitis in Neonates

Clinical Manifestations: Neonatal septicemia or meningitis caused by *Escherichia coli* and other Gram-negative bacilli cannot be differentiated clinically from serious infections caused by other infectious agents. Moreover, the first signs of sepsis may be minimal and similar to those observed in noninfectious processes. Clinical signs of sepsis include fever, temperature instability, apnea, cyanosis, jaundice, hepatomegaly, lethargy, irritability, anorexia, vomiting, abdominal distention, and diarrhea. Meningitis may be concomitant with sepsis without overt signs attributable to the central nervous system.

Etiology: *E coli* strains with the K1 capsular polysaccharide antigen cause about 40% of cases of septicemia and 75% of cases of meningitis caused by *E coli.* Other important Gram-negative bacilli responsible for neonatal sepsis include non-K1 strains of *E coli, Klebsiella, Enterobacter, Proteus, Citrobacter*, and *Salmonella* species. Anaerobic Gram-negative bacilli are infrequent causes. *Haemophilus influenzae* infection can occur in the newborn period. In contrast to invasive *H influenzae* infections occurring after the new- born period, invasive infections in neonates can be caused by nonencapsulated strains.

Epidemiology: The source of *E coli* and other Gram-negative pathogens in early-onset neonatal infections is usually maternal. In addition, nosocomial acquisition of Gram-negative flora through person-to-person transmission among nursery personnel and from nursery environmental sites, such as fluid reservoirs of incubators, has been documented, especially in preterm infants requiring intensive care management. Predisposing host factors in neonatal Gram-negative infection include maternal perinatal infection, low birth weight, prolonged rupture of membranes, and septic or traumatic delivery. Metabolic abnormalities such as galactosemia, fetal hypoxia, and acidosis have been implicated as predisposing factors. Neonates with immunologic defects, defects in the integrity of the skin or mucosa (e.g., meningomyelocele), or asplenia can also be at an increased risk for Gram-negative infection. In intensive care nurseries, the sophisticated systems for respiratory and metabolic support, invasive procedures (e.g., umbilical catheters), and the frequent use of antimicrobials enable proliferation and selection for multiply antimicrobial-resistant strains of Gram-negative pathogens, and, thus, predispose infants to colonization and infection.

The **incubation period** is highly variable; time of onset of the infection ranges from birth to several weeks of age.

Diagnostic Tests: Blood, urine, cerebrospinal fluid, and other fluids or tissues that might be infected should be stained and examined for bacteria and cultured in any neonate who is to be treated for septicemia. Techniques for detection of bacterial antigens, such as latex particle agglutination, are not commercially available for Gram-negative pathogens implicated in neonatal sepsis, with the exception of *H influenzae* type b and *E coli* K1 (whose capsular antigen cross-reacts with that of group B *Neisseria meningitidis*, thus affecting the interpretation of a positive test).

Treatment:

- Initial empirical treatment for the neonate with suspected septicemia and/or meningitis entails a combination of either a penicillin (usually ampicillin) and an aminoglycoside. An alternative regimen of a penicillin (usually ampicillin) and a cephalosporin that is active against most etiologic Gram-negative bacilli (such as cefotaxime or ceftazidime) can be used, but rapid emergence of cephalosporin-resistant strains, especially *Enterobacter cloacae* and *Serratia species*, can occur. Hence, routine use of cephalosporins in newborn units for empiric treatment of infections is not recommended.
- Once the etiologic agent has been identified and the susceptibilities defined, cefotaxime, an aminoglycoside, or both may be used. Definitive therapy should be based on in vitro susceptibility studies performed on the pathogen.
- Duration of therapy is based on the patient's response; the usual duration of therapy in uncomplicated septicemia is 10 to 14 days, and in meningitis the minimum is 21 days.
- Data on the efficacy of granulocyte transfusions in septic, neutrophil-depleted neonates are limited and remain controversial; some experts recommend this therapy in neonates with bacteriologically proven Gram-negative sepsis and severe neutropenia.
- A therapeutic role for immunoglobulin therapy in meningitis caused by *E coli* or other Gram-negative organisms has not been established.

Isolation of the Hospitalized Patient: The infant with sepsis or meningitis caused by *E coli* or other enteric Gram-negative organisms usually does not require isolation or special precautions. Exceptions include infants with *Salmonella* meningitis (enteric precautions are indicated), infection caused by a multiply resistant organism (contact isolation is indicated), and nursery outbreaks (ill and colonized infants should be cohorted, gowns used if soiling is likely, and gloves used if caretakers are handling feces). Consideration should also be given to contact isolation for infants with infection caused by multiresistant Gram-negative bacilli, such as those resistant to the aminoglycosides (including amikacin) or to cefotaxime and ceftazidime.

Control Measures:

- The physician in charge of the nursery should be aware of all sick infants and the nature of infections in personnel so that clusters of infections are recognized and appropriately investigated. This individual should be notified by other physicians in the community of serious infections in very young infants recently discharged from the nursery, as nursery-acquired infections can become apparent only several weeks to months after discharge.

- Several cases of infection caused by the same genus and species of bacteria occurring in infants in close physical proximity or caused by an unusual pathogen may indicate an epidemic, in which case an epidemiologic investigation should be initiated. Culture surveys of personnel or the environment to identify the source should be based on epidemiologic data.
- The routine performance of ongoing surveillance cultures of the environment or personnel, infants, or families is not recommended.
- An ongoing, in-service educational program for nursery personnel to review and reinforce concepts of infection control, especially hand-washing between all patient contacts, is recommended.
- Periodic review of antimicrobial susceptibility patterns of clinically important bacterial isolates can provide useful epidemiologic and therapeutic information.

Escherichia coli Diarrhea

Clinical Manifestations: At least four different classes of diarrhea-producing *Escherichia coli* have been identified. Features of each are listed in Table 26 and summarized as follows:

- Diarrhea caused by enteropathogenic *E coli* (EPEC) is frequently severe and protracted; it occurs typically in neonates and young infants in developing countries, either sporadically or in epidemics. Neonatal illness is characterized by watery diarrhea and rapidly developing dehydration. Chronic infection can cause failure to thrive.
- Diarrhea caused by enterotoxigenic *E coli* (ETEC) is a self-limited illness of moderate severity with watery stools and abdominal cramps. It occurs in persons of all ages; outbreaks have occurred in adults, usually from ingestion of contaminated food or water, and in newborn nurseries. ETEC is the major cause of traveler's diarrhea.
- Enteroinvasive *E coli* (EIEC) strains that are similar to *Shigella* cause dysentery accompanied by fever, severe diarrhea, vomiting, crampy abdominal pain, and tenesmus. Bloody diarrhea occurs occasionally.
- Enterohemorrhagic *E coli* (EHEC) strains that produce cytotoxins (verotoxins or Shiga-like toxins) cause diarrhea, hemorrhagic colitis, and hemolytic-uremic syndrome. Cases may occur sporadically or in outbreaks. EHEC strains are the only diarrhea-producing *E coli* that are common in the United States.

Etiology: (1) EPEC strains include the following *E coli* serotypes: 026:B6, 055:B5, 086:B7, 0111:B4, 0125:B15, 0126:B16, 0127:B8, and 0128:B12. Most EPEC strains have been shown to adhere abnormally to intestinal mucosa, and some strains may damage epithelial cells by elaborating a Shiga-like cytotoxin. (2) Enteroadherent *E coli*. This term refers to strains for which abnormal adherence, similar to EPEC strains, has been demonstrated in diarrheagenic isolates not belonging to EPEC serotypes. (3) ETEC strains are *E coli* of specific serotypes generally different from EPEC types, which produce either or both heat-labile and heat-stable enterotoxins. (4) EIEC strains include specific serotypes of *E coli* that are different from EPEC types. EIEC strains are closely related to *Shigella*; they have the capacity to invade intestinal epithelial cells. (5) Hemorrhagic colitis is caused by *E coli* 0157:H7 and possibly by other serotypes that produce cytotoxins resembling those found in *Shigella dysenteriae* (Shiga-like toxins).

Epidemiology: The source of most *E coli* diarrhea is infected symptomatic persons or carriers and food or water contaminated with human feces. In contrast, *E coli* 0157:H7 has a bovine reservoir and is transmitted by undercooked meat and unpasteurized milk. Nursery epidemics with EPEC or ETEC result from fecal-oral, attendant-to-infant, or infant-to-infant transmission via the hands of personnel. Mother-to-infant transmission can occur during delivery. During an epidemic, all ill infants usually harbor a single type. Sporadic and epidemic disease (including traveler's diarrhea) in older children and adults caused by ETEC, EIEC, or hemorrhagic colitis-associated strains results from ingestion of contaminated food or water or, rarely, from direct fecal-oral, interpersonal transmission. Diarrhea caused by *E coli* is more common in areas of the world where water supplies are contaminated and sanitation facilities are suboptimal. Two decades ago, nursery epidemics caused by EPEC strains were common; currently, epidemic diseases in newborn infants from these strains are uncommon. The reason for the ecologic change is unknown. EPEC has not been associated with outbreaks in day care settings, but spread in centers caring for young children could occur. Direct person-to-person spread has occurred in day care and institutional outbreaks of *E coli* 0157:H7 diarrhea and from patients with hemolytic-uremic syndrome. Asymptomatic carriage of EPEC is common. The period of communicability is for the duration of excretion of the specific pathogen.

The **incubation period** is from 2 hours to 6 days except in food-borne outbreaks, which usually have incubation periods of less than 24 hours.

Table 26. Classification of *E coli* Strains Associated With Gastrointestinal Symptoms, and Characteristics of Illness They Cause*

	Enteropathogenic *E coli* (EPEC)†	Enterohemorrhagic *E coli* (EHEC)	Enterotoxigenic *E coli* (ETEC)	Enteroinvasive *E coli* (EIEC)
Age groups affected; geographic occurrence	Infants younger than 2 y; worldwide	All ages; worldwide	Infants, children, and travelers; primarily in developing countries	All ages; worldwide
Frequency in U.S.	Uncertain	Probably common	Rare, except in travelers	Rare, except in travelers
Mechanism of action	Probably toxin, enteroadhesion	Cytotoxin	Enterotoxin, adhesion	Epithelial cell invasion and destruction
Onset	Gradual	Abrupt	Abrupt	Abrupt
Stool				
Volume	Moderate	Moderate to large	Large	Small
Consistency	Slimy	Watery to viscous	Watery	Viscous
Color	Clear to bloody	Bloody; may be clear initially	Colorless	Bloody/green
Blood	Late in illness or absent	Present	Absent	Present
PMNs‡	Present	Present	Absent	Present

*Modified from Infectious Disease and Immunization Committee, Canadian Paediatric Society: *Escherichia coli* gastroenteritis. Making sense of new acronyms. *Can Med Assoc J* 1987;136:241-244

†Referred to as enteroadherent if the strain is not among EPEC serotypes but exhibits similar abnormal adherence.

‡PMNs = polymorphonuclear leukocytes on microscopic examination of stained fetal smears

Table 26. Classification of *E coli* Strains Associated With Gastrointestinal Symptoms, and Characteristics of Illness They Cause* *(continued)*

	Enteropathogenic *E coli* (EPEC)†	Enterohemorrhagic *E coli* (EHEC)	Enterotoxigenic *E coli* (ETEC)	Enteroinvasive *E coli* (EIEC)
Bacterial diagnosis	Serotyping	Lack of sorbitol fermentation; confirmation with 0157:H7 antiserum	Toxin detection	Demonstration of invasion in tissue culture or animals
Similar illness	—	Shigellosis	Cholera	Shigellosis
Associated illness	—	Hemolytic-uremic syndrome		

*Modified from Infectious Disease and Immunization Committee, Canadian Paediatric Society: *Escherichia coli* gastroenteritis. Making sense of new acronyms. *Can Med Assoc J* 1987;136:241-244

†Referred to as enteroadherent if the strain is not among EPEC serotypes but exhibits similar abnormal adherence.

Diagnostic Tests: In individual patients with diarrhea, attempts to identify EPEC strains are not recommended because the frequency of sporadic disease caused by EPEC is uncertain, and complete sets of typing sera are not commercially available. EPEC strains can be identified by serotyping with type-specific antisera or by demonstrating abnormal adherence to HEP-2 cells or the gene for adherence factor in specialized laboratories. In nursery outbreaks, fecal specimens should be obtained from both sick and well infants for investigation in a suitably equipped hospital or reference laboratory after other bacterial and viral causes have been excluded. ETEC strains are identified presumptively by serotyping and definitely by the demonstration of enterotoxin production. EIEC strains are identified presumptively by serotyping and definitively by demonstrating invasion of tissue culture cells or the presence of DNA segments associated with invasiveness; these tests are not routinely available. Serotype identification is considered presumptive evidence, as some isolates of ETEC and EIEC serotypes lack the ability to cause diarrhea. EHEC can be confirmed by isolating *E coli* 0157:H7 on sorbitol-MacConkey agar and serotyping with commercially available antisera or by isolation of Shiga-like toxins in specialized laboratories. Inability to ferment sorbitol or delayed sorbitol fermentation is presumptive evidence of *E coli* 0157:H7. Suggested indications for EHEC confirmation include the following: hemorrhagic colitis, hemolytic uremic syndrome, diarrhea in contacts of patients with the hemolytic-uremic syndrome, outbreaks and occasional individual cases of unusually severe diarrheal illness, especially after recent travel.

Treatment: Fluid and electrolyte balance should be corrected and maintained as indicated. Antimotility agents should be avoided.

***Antimicrobial Therapy*.** In EPEC diarrhea in infants, nonabsorbable antibiotics such as neomycin (100 mg/kg/d) or colistin (10 to 15 mg/kg/d) given orally in three to four divided doses for 5 days can be administered.

Trimethoprim-sulfamethoxazole may be considered if diarrhea is intractable. Antimicrobial selection should be based on the susceptibility of the isolates.

For dysentery caused by EIEC strains and for chronic diarrhea caused by EPEC strains, oral, absorbable, or parenterally administered antimicrobials such as ampicillin (50 mg/kg/d) or trimethoprim-sulfamethoxazole (6 to 10 mg/kg/d) can be given.

The role of antimicrobial therapy in hemorrhagic colitis caused by EHEC is uncertain. *E coli* 0157:H7 is cleared rapidly from the stool without antibiotic therapy, usually within 7 days of the onset of diarrhea. Antibiotic therapy does not prevent progression to hemolytic-uremic syndrome.

Late Sequelae. Hemolytic-uremic syndrome (HUS) is a sequela of enteric infection with shiga-like toxins producing *E coli* strains, such as *E coli* 0157:H7. This syndrome includes acute, acquired Coombs-negative hemolytic anemia, thrombocytopenia, and acute renal failure or nephropathy. Most children with hemorrhagic colitis caused by *E coli* 0157:H7 develop mild, self-limited microangiopathic hematologic changes and/or nephropathy in the week after the onset of diarrhea. Close follow-up of patients with hemorrhagic colitis is recommended during this period to detect pallor, edema, or oliguria. Patients with HUS should be cultured for enteric pathogens, including *E coli* 0157:H7, and enteric isolation should be instituted to avoid nosocomial spread. The absence of EHEC in feces does not preclude the diagnosis of HUS.

Isolation of the Hospitalized Patient: Enteric precautions are indicated for patients with all types of *E coli* diarrhea for the duration of the illness. During outbreaks, infants with diarrhea caused by EPEC strains should remain on enteric precautions until cultures of stool taken from the patient after cessation of antimicrobial therapy are negative for the infecting strain. For patients with hemolytic-uremic syndrome, precautions should be continued until stool cultures are negative for *E coli* 0157:H7, or, if these tests are not available, for at least 10 days.

Control Measures:

Nursery and Other Institutional Outbreaks. Strict attention to hand washing techniques is essential in limiting spread. Exposed patients should be observed closely and their stools cultured for the causative organism. Unexposed patients should be kept separate from infants who have been exposed.

In a newborn nursery, management of EPEC infection is based on the number of cases. If only a single case occurs, the infant should be isolated in a unit away from the nursery area. If multiple cases occur, the nursery room should be closed to admissions and not reopened until all infants in the room have been discharged and the room has been cleaned. Infants should be discharged home and not transferred to other infant wards. Personnel caring for infants in the closed nursery cohort should not have duties in other open nursery rooms. If epidemic disease involves more than one room in a nursery, the entire nursery should be closed and not reopened until a strict cohort system can be used in each room of the nursery for the duration of the epidemic. Admissions to a room should be limited to infants born in a 1- to 2-day period. The room should then be closed to admissions until all infants have been discharged and the room has been cleaned. Personnel should be cohorted with the infants.

During an outbreak, the prophylactic administration of neomycin or colistin to all infants in a cohort should be considered, and all infants excreting the causative strain should be treated regardless of symptoms.

Traveler's Diarrhea. This condition is a significant problem for persons traveling in developing countries. Travelers should drink only boiled or carbonated water or other processed beverages; they should avoid ice, salads, and unpeeled fruit. Antimicrobial drugs are not recommended for prevention of traveler's diarrhea in children. The disease has no reported mortality. Although several antimicrobials, such as trimethoprim-sulfamethoxazole, are prophylactically effective in reducing the incidence of traveler's diarrhea, the benefit is usually outweighed by potential risks, including allergic drug reactions, infections induced by antimicrobial therapy (e.g., antibiotic-associated colitis), and the selective pressure of widespread use of antimicrobials leading to antimicrobial resistance. Instead of prophylaxis, empirical treatment at the onset of symptoms is recommended; this approach is effective and can shorten the disease duration to 30 hours or less in most patients.

Hemolytic-Uremic Syndrome (HUS). In a day care outbreak of *E coli* 0157:H7 diarrhea and HUS, cohorting of ill children is recommended. Strict attention to hand washing and hygiene is important, but may not be sufficient to prevent continued transmission. The center should be closed to new admissions and particular care should be exercised to prevent transfer of children to other day care centers in order not to spread the infection further.

Filariasis

(Bancroftian, Malayan, and Timorian)

Clinical Manifestations: Most filarial infections cause no symptoms. Symptoms are caused either by acute inflammation or, most commonly, by inflammation and obstruction of the lymphatic channels where the adult worms develop. In the former, patients develop fever, headache, myalgia, and lymphadenitis. In lymphatic disease, manifestations usually appear 3 months to 1 year after acquisition. Occasionally, moderate lymphadenopathy, particularly involving the inguinal lymph nodes, occurs. Inflammation of the lymphatics of the extremities and genitalia leads to retrograde lymphangitis, epididymitis, orchitis, and funiculitis. Fever, chills, and other nonspecific systemic symptoms also occur. Death of adult worms can result in localized abscesses. Obstructive lymphatic disease with resulting chronically progressive edema of the limbs and genitalia is relatively infrequent. In a few individuals, elephantiasis can result from fibrosis caused by chronic obstruction of the lymphatic channels. Chyluria can occur as a manifestation of Bancroftian filariasis.

Patients with the tropical pulmonary eosinophilia syndrome present with cough, fever, hepatosplenomegaly, marked eosinophilia and high serum IgE concentrations.

Etiology: Filariasis is caused by the following three filarial nematodes: *Wuchereria bancrofti*, *Brugia malayi*, and *B timori*.

Epidemiology: The disease is transmitted by the bite of infected species of various genera of mosquitoes, including *Culex*, *Aedes*, *Anopheles*, and *Mansonia*. *W bancrofti* is found in many scattered areas of the Caribbean, Venezuela, the Guianas, Brazil, sub-Saharan Africa, and Asia, extending into a broad zone from Saudi Arabia through the Indonesian archipelago into Southern China and Oceania. The disease also occurs in small foci in Central America, Colombia, North Africa, and Turkey. *B malayi* is found mostly in India, Southeast Asia, and the Far East. *B timori* is restricted to certain islands at the eastern end of the Indonesian archipelago. Microfilariae infective for mosquitoes are in the patient's blood as long as 1.5 years after the death of the adult worms and several years after the original infection. The infection is not transmissible from person to person or by blood transfusion.

The **incubation period** is not well established; the period from acquisition to the appearance of microfilariae in blood can be 2 to 12 months, depending on the nematode.

Diagnostic Tests: Microfilariae can be detected microscopically, either on routine blood smears obtained at night (10 to 12 PM) or after concentration of blood preserved in formalin. Filtration can be useful, particularly for specimens of chylous fluids. Adult worms can be identified in tissue specimens obtained at biopsy. Serologic tests (indirect hemagglutination and bentonite flocculation) are available, but interpretation of results is affected by cross-reactions of filarial antibodies with those against other helminths. Skin tests are not routinely available. Lymphatic filariasis often must be diagnosed clinically because dependable serologic assays are not available and in elephantiasis the microfilariae may no longer be present. Eosinophilia of 25% frequently occurs in the early, inflammatory phase of the disease.

Treatment: Diethylcarbamazine citrate (Hetrazan)* is the drug of choice. Because allergic reactions caused by disintegrating worms occur in heavy infections, some experts advise pretreatment with antihistamines or corticosteroids. The late obstructive phase of the disease is not affected by chemotherapy. Ivermectin,† an investigational drug in the United States, is effective against the microfilariae and may become the drug of choice for most filarial infections. Resection of the severely enlarged tissues, particularly plastic surgical repair of the genitalia, gives variable results. Chyluria originating in the bladder responds to fulguration; chyluria originating in the kidney cannot be corrected. Prompt identification and treatment of superinfections, particularly streptococcal and staphylococcal infections, are important aspects of therapy.

Isolation of the Hospitalized Patient: No special precautions are recommended.

Control Measures: The mosquito population should be controlled. Treatment of those with asymptomatic infection, i.e., carriers, or an entire community if a substantial percentage are infected, should be considered.

Giardia lamblia

Giardiasis

Clinical Manifestations: Infections are frequently asymptomatic. Patients who develop clinical illness usually have a protracted, intermittent, often debilitating disease, characterized by passage of foul-smelling diarrheal or soft stool associated with flatulence, abdominal distention, and anorexia. Anorexia combined with demonstrable malabsorption can lead to significant weight loss, failure to thrive, and anemia.

Etiology: *Giardia lamblia* is a flagellate protozoan. The infective form is the cyst. Infection is limited to the small intestine and/or biliary tract.

Epidemiology: Giardiasis has a worldwide distribution. Humans are the principal reservoir of infection, but *Giardia* organisms in dogs, beavers, and possibly other animals are infectious for humans and can fecally contaminate water. People become infected either directly

---

*Available from Lederle Laboratories, Pearl River, NY.

†Available from the Drug Service, Centers for Disease Control (see Services of the Centers for Disease Control, page 622).

by hand-to-mouth transfer of cysts from feces of an infected individual or indirectly by ingestion of fecally contaminated water or food. Most community-wide epidemics result from contaminated water supplies. Epidemics resulting from person-to-person transmission occur in day care centers, especially those that care for children who are not toilet trained, and in institutions for the mentally retarded. Staff and family members in contact with these children occasionally become infected. *Giardia* transmission has also been documented among male homosexuals. Those deficient in secretory IgA are very susceptible to giardiasis. Patients with cystic fibrosis also have an increased frequency of giardiasis. Surveys conducted in the United States have demonstrated prevalence rates of *Giardia* in stool that range from 1% to 20%, depending on the geographic location and the age of the patient. Duration of cyst excretion is variable. In about 50% of adults the infection clears spontaneously in 1 to 3 months. The disease is communicable as long as the infected person excretes cysts.

The **incubation period** is usually 1 to 4 weeks.

Diagnostic Tests: The parasite can be detected by microscopic examination of stool or duodenal contents. Because *Giardia* is excreted intermittently, multiple stool specimens obtained on different days should be examined. A single stool examination detects 50% to 75% of infections; sensitivity is increased to about 95% with three specimens. Examination of duodenal contents obtained by direct aspiration or by using a commercially available string test (Enterotest*) is a more sensitive procedure than a single stool examination. Rarely, biopsy of the small intestine is used. To enhance detection, stool should be mixed, placed in fixative, concentrated, and examined by both wet mount and permanent stain. Take-home stool collection kits containing a vial of 10% formalin and a vial of polyvinyl alcohol fixative in childproof containers are convenient for collecting multiple specimens. ELISA and counterimmune electrophoresis (CIE) assays have been developed for the detection of *G lamblia* in stool specimens; ELISA tests are commercially available.

Treatment: Quinacrine hydrochloride is the most effective drug for treatment of symptomatic infections; cure rates are 85% to 95%. However, compliance and consequently cure rates may be lower in children because of quinacrine's bitter taste. Furazolidone is 70% to 80% effective, but since it is the only drug available in liquid suspension, it is more acceptable to children. Metronidazole is an alternative drug; the safety and effectiveness of this drug for children with giar-

---

*Hedeco, Inc., Palo Alto, CA.

diasis have not been established. Paromomycin, a nonabsorbable aminoglycoside that is 50% to 70% effective, has been recommended for the treatment of symptomatic infection in pregnant women. If therapy fails, a course of any of these drugs can be repeated after 2 weeks. Relapse is common in immunocompromised patients and may require continuous therapy for long periods of time.

Treatment of asymptomatic carriers is not recommended because the resulting benefits and risks have not been established.

Isolation of the Hospitalized Patient: Enteric precautions for the duration of the illness are recommended.

Control Measures:

- In day care centers improved sanitation and personal hygiene should be emphasized (see also Children in Day Care, page 68). Hand washing by staff and children should be stressed, especially after using the toilet or handling soiled diapers. When an outbreak is suspected, an epidemiologic investigation should be undertaken to identify and treat all symptomatic children, day care workers, and family members infected with *Giardia*. Persons with diarrhea should be excluded from the day care center until they become asymptomatic. Treatment of asymptomatic carriers has not been demonstrated to be effective in outbreak control. Exclusion of carriers from day care is not recommended.
- Prevention of water-borne outbreaks requires adequate filtration of municipal water obtained from surface water sources because concentrations of chlorine used to disinfect drinking water are not effective against the cysts.
- Backpackers, campers, and persons likely to be exposed to contaminated water should avoid drinking directly from streams. Boiling of water will eliminate the infective cysts.

Gonococcal Infections

Clinical Manifestations: Gonococcal infections in children occur in three distinct age groups.

- Infection in the **newborn infant** usually involves the eye. Other sites of involvement include scalp abscess, which can complicate fetal monitoring; vaginitis; and systemic disease with bacteremia, arthritis, meningitis, or endocarditis.
- In **prepubertal children** beyond the newborn period, gonococcal infection usually occurs in the genital tract. Vaginitis is the most common manifestation; pelvic inflammatory disease and perihepatitis can occur but are uncommon, as is gonococcal

urethritis in the prepubertal male. Anorectal and tonsillopharyngeal colonization can also occur in prepubertal children with gonorrhea of the genitourinary tract.

- In **sexually active adolescents**, as in adults, gonococcal infection of the genital tract in females is most frequently manifest by urethritis, endocervicitis, and pelvic inflammatory disease; in adolescent males, the primary site of infection is usually the urethra. Extension from these primary genital mucosal sites results in epididymitis, pelvic inflammatory disease, and bartholinitis. Infection can involve other mucous membranes and produce conjunctivitis, pharyngitis, or proctitis. Asymptomatic infection of the urethra, endocervix, rectum, and pharynx can occur. Hematogenous spread can involve skin and joints (arthritis-dermatitis syndrome); perihepatitis, meningitis, and endocarditis occur rarely.

Etiology: *Neisseria gonorrhoeae* organisms are Gram-negative diplococci.

Epidemiology: *N gonorrhoeae* infections occur only in humans. The source of the organism is exudate and secretions of infected mucous surfaces. Transmission results from intimate contact, such as sexual acts, parturition, and, very rarely, household exposure in prepubertal children. Sexual abuse should be strongly considered when genital, rectal, or oral infections are diagnosed in children beyond the newborn period and before puberty, and in non-sexually-active adolescents. Approximately 900,000 new cases of gonococcal infection are reported annually in the United States. An unknown number of additional cases are not recognized or reported, and infection of the urethra, cervix, pharynx, or rectum may be asymptomatic. Young men 20 to 24 years of age have the highest reported incidence of infection, followed by those 15 to 19 years of age. For females the highest rates are in adolescents between 15 and 19 years old. Concurrent infection with *Chlamydia trachomatis* is very common. *N gonorrhoeae* is communicable as long as an individual harbors the organism.

The **incubation period** is usually 2 to 7 days.

Diagnostic Tests: Gram-stained smears of exudative material from the eyes, the endocervix of postpubertal females, the vagina of prepubertal girls, male urethra, skin lesions, synovial fluid, and cerebrospinal fluid are useful in the initial evaluation. These smears occasionally contain Gram-negative intracellular diplococci; this finding is particularly helpful when the organism is not recovered in culture. Gram stains of material obtained from the endocervix of pubertal and postpubertal females are less sensitive than culture in the detection of infection but can be of immediate help in the differential diagnosis of a patient with an acute abdomen, or when immediate therapy is indicated. Other *Neisseria* species and Gram-negative cocci may be present in the female genital tract; but these organisms are seldom observed on smear within polymorphonuclear leukocytes. In prepubertal girls, vaginal specimens are adequate and endocervical specimens are unnecessary.

Recovery of the organisms by culture from normally sterile sites, such as blood, cerebrospinal fluid, or synovial fluid, can be accomplished on nonselective chocolate agar with incubation in 5% to 10% CO_2. Selective *N gonorrhoeae* culture media, such as Thayer-Martin (chocolate agar supplemented with antibiotics), inhibit most normal flora and nonpathogenic *Neisseria* found on mucosal surfaces, and rarely obscure the presence of gonococci. These media are used for culture of specimens from the cervix, vagina, rectum, urethra, and pharynx. Specimens for *N gonorrhoeae* culture should be inoculated immediately onto the selective medium prior to transport to the laboratory because *N gonorrhoeae* is extremely sensitive to drying and temperature changes. Transport systems containing selective medium are available commercially; these allow satisfactory shipment of inoculated media if they have been preincubated for 24 hours.

Sexual Abuse. In all prepubertal children beyond the newborn period and in non-sexually-active adolescents who have gonococcal infection, sexual abuse must be considered. Genital, rectal, and pharyngeal cultures should be obtained from all patients before antibiotic treatment. Caution should be exercised in interpreting the significance of *Neisseria* organisms from any site, as *N gonorrhoeae* can be confused with other *Neisseria* species; confirmatory bacteriologic tests should be performed. Isolation of *N gonorrhoeae* from the pharynx of young children poses special problems because of the high carriage rate of nonpathogenic *Neisseria* species. Appropriate cultures should be obtained from persons who have had contact with the abused child. Children in whom sexual abuse is suspected should undergo tests for other sexually transmitted diseases, such as *Chlamydia* and syphilis (for further information, see Sexual Abuse, page 103).

Treatment: Most isolates of *N gonorrhoeae* are relatively susceptible to penicillin. Resistance to penicillin is most frequently mediated by the production of beta-lactamase. The incidence of infections caused by penicillinase-producing *N gonorrhoeae* (PPNG) is increasing in the United States; prevalence varies in different geographic areas. Resistance to penicillin has also been recognized in isolates that do not produce beta-lactamase. These chromosomally mediated resistant

N gonorrhoeae (CMRNG) are less common and can be resistant to multiple antibiotics. High-level resistance to tetracycline has been identified in 30 states. Resistance to spectinomycin is rare. Because of the increased prevalence of penicillin-resistant *N gonorrhoeae*, a third-generation cephalosporin, specifically ceftriaxone or cefotaxime, is now recommended as initial therapy for all ages.

Patients with presumed or proven gonorrhoea should be evaluated for concurrent syphilis. Until universal testing for *Chlamydia* with rapid, inexpensive, and highly accurate tests become available, all patients beyond the neonatal period with gonorrhoea should be treated for presumptive *Chlamydia* infection.

Material for follow-up cultures should be obtained from the infected site 4 to 7 days after completion of treatment to ensure that therapy has been effective.

Specific recommendations for management and antimicrobial therapy are as follows:

Neonatal Disease. Infants with clinical evidence of ophthalmia, scalp abscess, or disseminated infections should be hospitalized. Pretherapy cultures of discharge, blood, and cerebrospinal fluid should be obtained not only to confirm the diagnosis but also to isolate the organism from both mother and infant for antimicrobial susceptibility testing. Susceptibility data are particularly important in the management of infants whose initial response to therapy is poor. Tests for concomitant infection with *Chlamydia trachomatis* should also be considered in patients who do not satisfactorily respond to conventional therapy.

Recommended antimicrobial therapy for nondisseminated infections consists of ceftriaxone, 25 to 50 mg/kg/d, intravenously or intramuscularly, given once daily; or cefotaxime, 25 mg/kg/d, intravenously or intramuscularly, given in 2 or 3 daily doses depending on age. Ceftriaxone should be given cautiously to hyperbilirubinemic infants, especially premature infants. Duration of therapy is 7 days. Regimens suitable for ophthalmic prophylaxis are not adequate treatment for neonatal ophthalmia.

Limited data suggest that uncomplicated gonococcal ophthalmia can be cured with a single dose of ceftriaxone, 50 mg/kg, maximum 125 mg, given intramuscularly or intravenously.

If the gonococcal isolate is proven susceptible to penicillin, aqueous crystalline penicillin G, 100,000 U/kg/d given in divided doses intravenously every 12 hours in the first week of life and every 6 hours thereafter for 7 days, is recommended.

Infants with gonococcal ophthalmia should have their eyes irrigated immediately with saline, then at least at hourly intervals until the discharge is eliminated, and less frequently thereafter.

For newborn infants with disseminated gonococcal infection without meningitis, ceftriaxone 25 to 50 mg/kg/d given once daily or cefotaxime 25 to 50 mg/kg/d given two or three times daily, depending on age, for 7 days, is recommended. For meningitis, ceftriaxone 50 mg/kg/d, given in 1 or 2 daily doses, or cefotaxime 50 mg/kg/d, given two or three times daily, is recommended for 10 to 14 days. Drugs can be given intravenously or intramuscularly. If the isolate is proved susceptible to penicillin, for patients with disseminated disease without meningitis, aqueous crystalline penicillin G 25,000 to 50,000 U/kg/d, intravenously, two to four times daily, depending on age, for 7 days, is recommended; for those with meningitis, 50,000 U/kg/d two to four times daily, depending on age, is given for 10 to 14 days.

Since most neonates with gonorrhoea acquire the organism from their mothers, both the mother and her sexual partner(s) should be investigated and treated appropriately.

Gonococcal Infections in Children Beyond the Neonatal Period and in Adolescents. Recommendations for treatment of gonococcal infections, by age and weight, are given in Table 27.

Children 9 years or older with uncomplicated gonococcal endocervical, urethral, or rectal infection also should be treated for presumtive Chlamydia infection with doxycycline, 100 mg twice daily for 7 days. Tetracycline can be substituted for doxycycline; the dose is 500 mg four times daily and should be given between meals. Compliance, however, may be poorer because the 500-mg dose must be given four times daily and between meals. Children younger than 9 years and pregnant women should not be given tetracycline drugs; erythromycin is recommended. Patients should also be evaluated for coinfection with syphilis.

If infection was acquired from a person proven to have infection caused by a penicillin-susceptible isolate, a single dose of oral amoxicillin, 50 mg/kg (maximum dose, 3 g), or aqueous crystalline penicillin G 100,000 U/kg (maximum dose, 4.8 million units), intramuscularly, plus probenecid, 25 mg/kg (maximum dose, 1 g) followed by doxycycline for 7 days for patients 9 years and older, or erythromycin for younger patients, can be given.

Approximately one half of recurrent infections after treatment with the recommended schedules are caused by reinfection and indicate the need for improved contact tracing and patient education.

Special Problems in Treatment of Children (Beyond the Neonatal Period) and Adolescents.

- Patients with uncomplicated endocervical infection, urethritis, or proctitis who are allergic to penicillins and cephalosporins should be treated with spectinomycin, 40 mg/kg (maximum, 2 g), given intramuscularly. In patients in whom doxycycline or tetracycline is contraindicated or not tolerated, erythromycin base or stearate (adult dose is 2 g/d orally in four divided doses) or erythromycin ethyl succinate (adult dose is 2.4 g/d orally in three divided doses) can be substituted.

- Patients with uncomplicated pharyngeal gonococcal infection should be treated with ceftriaxone 250 mg, intramuscularly, in a single dose.
- Patients who are incubating syphilis (seronegative, without clinical signs) can be cured by regimens that include penicillin, ampicillin, amoxicillin, or ceftriaxone, but not by those that include spectinomycin and possibly not by erythromycin or tetracycline. Data on the effectiveness of the cephalosporins other than ceftriaxone in this circumstance are insufficient. All patients who are treated for gonorrhea should undergo serologic testing for syphilis at the initial visit and 6 to 8 weeks later.
- For disseminated gonococcal infections caused by laboratory-proved, penicillin-susceptible strains of *N gonorrhoeae*, aqueous crystalline penicillin G can be used in a dose of 100,000 to 250,000 U/kg (maximum 10 million units) per day in four to six divided doses daily for 7 to 14 days, depending on the condition (see Table 27). Patients who weigh more than 100 lb (45 kg) should receive a daily dose of 10 million units.

  Long-acting forms of penicillin, such as benzathine penicillin G, have no role in the treatment of gonorrhea.

Acute Pelvic Inflammatory Disease (PID). *N gonorrhoeae* and *C trachomatis* are implicated in most cases, and many cases have a polymicrobial etiology. No reliable clinical criteria distinguish gonococcal from nongonococcal PID. Hence, broad spectrum treatment regimens are recommended (see Pelvic Inflammatory Disease, page 355, including Table 45, page 357).

Acute Epididymitis. Sexually transmitted organisms, such as *N gonorrhoeae* or *C trachomatis*, can cause acute epididymitis, especially in sexually active adolescents and young adults. (Its pathogenesis can also be related to infection in the urinary tract usually caused by Enterobacteriaceae or *Pseudomonas. Haemophilus influenzae* type b is a rare cause in infants and young children.)

The recommended regimen is a single dose of ceftriaxone 250 mg, intramuscularly, plus doxycycline 200 mg/d, given orally, in two divided doses for 10 days (or tetracycline 2 g/d, given orally, in four divided doses for 10 days). Children younger than 9 years should receive a single dose of ceftriaxone 250 mg, intramuscularly, plus erythromycin 50 mg/kg/d (maximum 2 g) given orally in four divided doses.

Table 27. Treatment of Gonococcal Infection in Children Beyond the Newborn Period and Adolescents

Disease	Prepubertal Children Who Weigh < 100 lb (45 kg)	Disease	Patients Who Weigh ≥ 100 lb (45 kg) and Are 9 Years or Older
Uncomplicated vulvovaginitis, urethritis, proctitis, pharyngitis[*,†]	Ceftriaxone, 125 mg, IM, in a single dose	Uncomplicated endocervicitis or urethritis	Ceftriaxone, 250 mg, IM, in a single dose **or** Spectinomycin, 2 g, IM, in a single dose **plus** Doxycycline, 100 mg orally twice daily for 7 d[†]
Ophthalmia, peritonitis, bacteremia, arthritis[†,‡]	Ceftriaxone, 50 mg/kg/d (max. 1 g/d), IV or IM, once daily for 7 d		
Meningitis, endocarditis[‡]	Ceftriaxone, 50 mg/kg/d (max. 2 g), IV or IM, given once or twice daily for 10-14 d for meningitis and for endocarditis	Gonococcal pharyngitis	Ceftriaxone 250 mg, IM, in a single dose
		Disseminated gonococcal infections[*,§]	Ceftriaxone, 1 g/d, IV or IM, given once daily for 7 d **or** Cefotaxime, 1 g, IV, given three times daily for 7 d
		Meningitis, endocarditis[‡]	Ceftriaxone, 1-2 g, IV, given twice daily for 10-14 d (meningitis) or for 28 d (endocarditis)

*Hospitalization should be considered, especially for patients with an uncertain diagnosis, those who may not comply with treatment regimens, those who have purulent joint effusion, and those who have been treated as outpatients and failed to respond.

†Doxycycline (or tetracycline, 500 mg four times daily for 7 days) is recommended on the presumption that the patient has concomitant infection with *Chlamydia trachomatis.* Drug and dosage recommendations are for children 9 years or older. For younger children and women who are pregnant, erythromycin is recommended.

‡Hospitalization is required.

§Such as the arthritis-dermatitis syndrome.

Isolation of the Hospitalized Patient: All newborn infants (including those with ophthalmia) and prepubertal children with gonococcal infections should be placed in contact isolation until effective parenteral antimicrobial therapy has been administered for 24 hours. Special precautions are not indicated for other patients with gonococcal infection.

Control Measures:

Neonatal Ophthalmia. For routine prophylaxis of infants immediately after birth, a 1% solution of silver nitrate, 1% tetracycline, or 0.5% erythromycin ophthalmic ointment is instilled into each eye; subsequent irrigation should not be performed (see Prevention of Neonatal Ophthalmia, page 546). Prophylaxis may be delayed for as long as 1 hour after birth to facilitate maternal-infant bonding.

These prophylactic regimens are ineffective for prevention of chlamydial eye disease.

Infants Born to Mothers With Gonococcal Infections. When prophylaxis is correctly administered, most infants born to mothers with gonococcal infection do not develop gonococcal ophthalmia. However, an occasional case of gonococcal ophthalmia or disseminated gonococcal infection can occur in infants born to mothers with recognized gonococcal disease at parturition. Hence, infants born to mothers with active gonorrhea should receive a single dose of ceftriaxone, 125 mg intravenously or intramuscularly; for low-birth-weight infants, the dose is 25 to 50 mg/kg.

Children and Adolescents With Sexual Exposure to a Patient Known to Have Gonorrhea. Such children should be examined, cultured, and treated the same as those known to have gonorrhea.

Education. Continuing educational efforts to control sexually transmitted diseases are needed, especially for adolescents (see Sexually Transmitted Diseases, page 94).

Other Infections. Patients with gonococcal infection should be evaluated for other sexually transmitted diseases, specifically Chlamydia and syphilis. Hepatitis B vaccination is indicated (see Hepatitis B, Indications for Preexposure Vaccination, page 246).

Pregnancy. All pregnant females should have an endocervical culture for gonococci as an integral part of the prenatal care at the first visit. A second culture late in the third trimester should be done for women at high risk of exposure to gonococcal infection. Recommended therapeutic regimens for patients found to be infected are those previously described for uncomplicated gonorrhea, except that tetracycline should not be used because of the potential toxic effects on the fetus. Women who are allergic to penicillin or probenecid should be treated with spectinomycin.

Case Reporting. All known cases of gonorrhea must be reported. Investigation of the source of infection in the prepubertal child is indicated. Ensuring that sexual contacts are counseled and treated is essential for community control, prevention of reinfection, and prevention of complications in the contact.

Granuloma Inguinale

(Donovanosis)

Clinical Manifestations: Initial lesions are single or multiple, subcutaneous nodules that progress to cutaneous ulceration and granuloma(s). Lesions usually involve the genitalia; anal lesions occur in 10% of the patients, and lesions at distant sites are rare. Extension into the inguinal area results in subcutaneous induration that mimics inguinal adenopathy—the pseudobubo of granuloma inguinale. Fibrosis manifests as sinus tracts, adhesions, and lymphedema.

Etiology: The reputed cause is *Calymmatobacterium granulomatis*, a Gram-negative bacillus. Koch's postulates have not been fulfilled: granuloma inguinale has not been produced by inoculating pure cultures of *C granulomatis* into human volunteers.

Epidemiology: Granuloma inguinale is extremely rare in the United States and most developed countries, but is common in New Guinea and parts of India, Africa, and the Caribbean. The source of infection is persons with active infection, and possibly those with asymptomatic rectal infection. Transmission is usually by sexual intercourse. Infection is only mildly contagious and repeated exposure may be necessary for the development of disease in most cases. Young children can acquire infection by contact with infected secretions. The highest incidence of disease occurs in tropical and subtropical environments. The period of communicability exists throughout the duration of active lesions or rectal colonization.

The **incubation period** is 8 to 80 days.

Diagnostic Tests: The demonstration of Donovan bodies on Wright's or Giemsa's stain of a crush preparation from a lesion is diagnostic. The microorganism can also be detected by histologic procedures on biopsy specimens. Lesions should be cultured for *H ducreyi* to exclude pseudogranuloma inguinale chancroid. Granuloma inguinale is frequently misdiagnosed as carcinoma. The diagnosis can be excluded by histologic examination of the tissue or by the response of the lesion to antibiotics.

Treatment: Tetracycline (which should not be given to children younger than 9 years) and trimethoprim-sulfamethoxazole have been reported to be effective. Gentamicin and chloramphenicol are reserved for resistant cases. Erythromycin has been used in pregnancy. Antimicrobial therapy is continued for at least 3 weeks or until the lesion(s) have resolved. If an antibiotic is effective, some healing is usually noted within 7 days.

Isolation of the Hospitalized Patient: No special precautions are recommended.

Control Measures: Sexual partners should be examined and probably given prophylactic antimicrobial therapy.

Haemophilus influenzae Infections

Clinical Manifestations: In infants and young children, *Haemophilus influenzae* is a major cause of meningitis, otitis media, sinusitis, epiglottitis, septic arthritis, occult febrile bacteremia, cellulitis, pneumonia, and empyema; occasionally it causes neonatal meningitis and sepsis. Other *H influenzae* infections include purulent pericarditis, endocarditis, conjunctivitis, osteomyelitis, peritonitis, epididymo-orchitis, glossitis, uvulitis, septic thrombophlebitis, and possibly chronic bronchitis in adults with chronic lung disease.

Etiology: *H influenzae* organisms are small, pleomorphic, Gram-negative coccobacilli, with six antigenically distinct capsular types (types a to f) as well as nonencapsulated, nontypable strains. Invasive diseases in infants and children are caused by encapsulated strains, nearly always type b. An exception is neonatal sepsis, which can be caused by nonencapsulated organisms. Local respiratory tract disease, including otitis media, sinusitis, and bronchitis, is usually caused by nontypable strains, which are frequent constituents of the normal upper respiratory tract flora.

Epidemiology: The source of the organism is the upper respiratory tract of humans. Asymptomatic colonization is frequent: nonencapsulated strains can be recovered from the throat of 60% to 90% of children, and type b organisms can be recovered from 2% to 5%. The mode of transmission is presumably person to person, by direct contact, or through inhalation of droplets of respiratory tract secretions containing the organism.

Invasive disease caused by *H influenzae* type b is most common in children 3 months to 3 years of age. The age of peak occurrence for epiglottitis, 2 to 4 years of age, is somewhat higher than that for other invasive *H influenzae* type b diseases, such as meningitis. Invasive disease can also occur in older children, and occasionally in adolescents and adults. In temperate climates, invasive disease tends to occur in a biphasic seasonal distribution, with the greatest number of cases in October and November, and from February to April. Meningitis caused by *H influenzae* type b is more frequent in boys, urban dwellers, blacks, Alaskan Eskimos, Apache and Navajo Indians, and day care center attendees. Children, particularly those younger than 4 years, in prolonged, close contact (such as in a household) with a child who has developed invasive disease caused by *H influenzae* type b are at increased risk for serious infection from this organism. In this circumstance, asymptomatic *H influenzae* colonization is more frequent in household contacts of all ages than in the general population. Other predisposing factors to infection include sickle-cell disease, asplenia, certain immunodeficiency syndromes, and malignancies. Children, particularly those younger than 1 year, who have had episodes of documented invasive infection (estimated at approximately 1%) are at risk for recurrence. The exact period of communicability is unknown, but it may be for as long as the organism is present in the upper respiratory tract.

The **incubation period** is unknown and probably widely variable.

Diagnostic Tests: Cerebrospinal fluid (CSF), blood, synovial fluid, pleural fluid, and middle ear aspirate should be cultured on a medium enriched with X and V factors, such as chocolate agar. A Gram stain of an infected body fluid can disclose the organism and allow a presumptive diagnosis to be made. Latex particle agglutination, or other rapid methods for capsular antigen detection in CSF, serum, and concentrated urine aid in the rapid diagnosis of *H influenzae* type b infection and can be helpful in patients in whom antimicrobial therapy was initiated before culture. With capsular antigen detection tests, concentrated urine yields the highest percentage of positive results but is the least specific. Urine, however, can contain antigen in noninfected patients who have received a *Haemophilus* vaccine within several days. The occurrence of antigenuria after immunization with conjugate vaccines is incompletely studied and appears to vary with the type of vaccine. Antimicrobial susceptibility testing should be performed on all clinically important isolates.

Treatment:

- Meningitis possibly caused by *H influenzae* type b can be treated with ampicillin and chloramphenicol, cefotaxime, or ceftriaxone; all are equally acceptable for initial therapy. Depending on the locality, 12% to 40% of *H influenzae* isolates (type b and non-typable strains) are beta-lactamase producing and, therefore, resistant to ampicillin. Chloramphenicol resistance has been reported but is rare. Isolates resistant to both ampicillin and chloramphenicol are very rare in the United States. Based on susceptibility test results, initial therapy of ampicillin and chloramphenicol should be changed to ampicillin for beta-lactamase negative strains, and chloramphenicol for beta-lactamase positive strains. Cefotaxime or ceftriaxone is also acceptable for either beta-lactamase positive or negative strains. For infections caused by strains resistant to ampicillin and chloramphenicol, cefotaxime or ceftriaxone is indicated.
- For patients with uncomplicated meningitis, therapy for 7 to 10 days with high-dose antimicrobials administered intravenously is usually satisfactory. In selected cases, oral therapy with chloramphenicol may be used. Therapy for more than 10 days may be indicated in complicated cases of meningitis caused by *H influenzae* type b.
- For treatment of other invasive *H influenzae* infections, recommendations are similar but primarily based on empirical experience.
- Chloramphenicol pharmacokinetics are unpredictable. Moreover, concurrent treatment with certain drugs, such as phenobarbital, phenytoin, carbamazepine, and rifampin, can alter chloramphenicol metabolism. Conversely, chloramphenicol can interfere with the metabolism of drugs such as phenytoin, tolbutamide, and dicumarol. Hence, if available, serum chloramphenicol concentrations should be monitored in patients receiving either oral or intravenous chloramphenicol.
- Dexamethasone therapy should be considered in infants and children 2 months and older with bacterial meningitis after the physician has considered the benefits and possible risks (see Dexamethasone Therapy for Bacterial Meningitis in Infants and Children, page 566). The regimen is 0.6 mg/kg/d in four divided doses, given intravenously, for the first 4 days of antibiotic treatment, and should be initiated with the first dose of antibacterial therapy.
- **Epiglottitis is a medical emergency. An airway must be established promptly by endotracheal tube or tracheostomy.**
- Infected synovial, pleural, or pericardial fluid should be drained.

- For otitis media, many experts recommend ampicillin for initial therapy. Effective alternative drugs, especially for ampicillin-resistant strains of *H influenzae* include trimethoprim-sulfamethoxazole, erythromycin-sulfisoxazole, cefaclor, cefixime, cefuroxime axetil, and amoxicillin-clavulanic acid.

Isolation of the Hospitalized Patient: Respiratory isolation for 24 hours after initiation of effective therapy is indicated.

Control Measures (for invasive *H influenzae* type b infections):
Care of Exposed Persons.

- Careful observation of exposed household, day care or nursery contacts is essential. Exposed children who develop a febrile illness should receive prompt medical evaluation. If indicated, antimicrobial therapy appropriate for invasive *H influenzae* type b infection should be administered.
- *Rifampin Chemoprophylaxis.* The risk of invasive *H influenzae* type b disease among household contacts younger than 4 years is increased. Asymptomatic colonization with *H influenzae* type b is also more frequent in household contacts of all ages than in the general population. Rifampin eradicates *H influenzae* type b from the pharynx in approximately 95% of the carriers. Limited data indicate that it also reduces the risk of secondary invasive illness in exposed household contacts. Nursery and day care center contacts may also be at increased risk of secondary disease, but experts disagree regarding the magnitude of the risk. Most believe that the risk for children attending day care centers is probably lower than that observed for age-susceptible household contacts, and that secondary disease in contacts is rare when all day care contacts are older than 2 years. Moreover, the efficacy of rifampin in preventing disease in day care groups is not well established and the difficulties in delivering prophylaxis are considerable. Recommendations for contacts are as follows:
- *Household.* Rifampin prophylaxis is recommended for all household contacts,* irrespective of age, in those households with at least one contact younger than 48 months, regardless of the immunization status of the contacts. Prophylaxis is not recommended for households in which all contacts are 48 months or older. In families receiving prophylaxis, the index patient should also receive rifampin prophylaxis; it should be initiated during hospitalization, usually just before discharge. Family members

*A household contact is defined in these circumstances as an individual residing with the index patient, or a nonresident who spent 4 or more hours with the index patient for at least 5 of the 7 days preceding the day of hospital admission of the index patient.

should receive prophylaxis as soon as possible because 54% of secondary cases occur in the first week after hospitalization of the index patient. The time of occurrence of the remaining 46% of secondary cases after the first week suggests that prophylaxis initiated 7 days or more after hospitalization of the index patient, although not optimal, may still be of benefit.

- *Day Care and Nursery School.* The advisability of rifampin prophylaxis in day groups in which a single case has occurred is controversial and a definitive recommendation regarding administration of rifampin prophylaxis for all types of day care groups cannot be made at this time. The following guidelines may be useful: (1) in day care homes resembling households, such as those with children younger than 2 years in which contact is 25 hours per week or more, rifampin prophylaxis can be employed in the same regimen as recommended for household contacts; and (2) in day care facilities where all contacts are older than 2 years, prophylaxis need not be given.

  When two or more cases of invasive disease have occurred among attendees within 60 days, administering rifampin to all attendees and supervisory personnel is recommended.

  The success of rifampin prophylaxis in day care groups appears to depend on strict, prompt compliance by attendees and supervisory personnel.

  Children and staff should be excluded from the day care group until rifampin has been initiated. Children entering the group during the time prophylaxis is given should also receive prophylaxis.

- *Vaccinated Children.* In a cohort (household or day care) in which prophylaxis is given to limit secondary cases, children who have been vaccinated with any *Haemophilus* b vaccine as well as susceptible, unvaccinated children should receive prophylaxis.
- *Pregnancy.* Prophylaxis is not recommended for pregnant women who are contacts of affected infants because the effect of rifampin on the fetus has not been established.
- *Dosage.* Rifampin should be given orally once daily for 4 days (in a dose of 20 mg/kg; maximum dose, 600 mg). The dose for infants younger than 1 month is not established; some experts recommend reducing the dose to 10 mg/kg. For adults, each dose is 600 mg. Rifampin is available in 150 and 300 mg capsules. Patients unable to swallow capsules may be given aliquots of rifampin powder, preweighed by a trained individual, which can then be mixed with a small amount of applesauce immediately before administration. Although rifampin suspension is not commercially available, a liquid suspension (1% in simple syrup) can be prepared (see rifampin package insert). If used, it must be freshly prepared for

administration to each contact group. Rifampin suspension should be shaken vigorously before each administration. The stability of rifampin in solution after the first week following the preparation of the suspension is unknown.

Immunization. *Haemophilus* type b polysaccharide vaccine, consisting of purified type b capsular polysaccharide (abbreviated as PRP), was licensed in 1985 and recommended for administration to children 24 months or older. Subsequently, conjugate vaccines that are more consistently immunogenic and intended for the prevention of *H influenzae* type b infections in younger children have been licensed and have replaced the purified polysaccharide vaccine. These conjugate vaccines consist of the *H influenzae* type b capsular polysaccharide (PRP) or oligosaccharide covalently linked to a carrier protein directly or via an intervening spacer molecule (see Table 28). Protein carriers include diphtheria toxoid, CRM_{197} (a nontoxic mutant diphtheria toxin), an outer membrane protein complex of *Neisseria meningitidis*, and tetanus toxoid.

Currently licensed *Haemophilus* b conjugate vaccines (HbCV) are the following: a polysaccharide-diphtheria toxoid conjugate vaccine (PRP-D), an oligosaccharide-CRM_{197} conjugate vaccine (HbOC), and an outer membrane *N meningitidis* protein conjugate vaccine (PRP-OMP). These vaccines were originally licensed for use in children 18 months old, based on their enhanced immunogenicity in comparison to that of purified PRP vaccine. Studies indicated that these conjugate vaccines had similar immunogenicity in children 15 months and 18 months and provided the basis for subsequent approval of PRP-D, HbOC, and PRP-OMP vaccines for use in children 15 months and older. Prospective efficacy studies of disease prevention have not been performed with the conjugate vaccines in children 15 months or older, but data from the experience in the United States during the period of their use in children 18 months old indicate that they are highly effective.

In October 1990, one of the currently licensed *Haemophilus* b conjugate vaccines, HbOC, was approved in the United States for administration to infants beginning at 2 months of age in a multidose schedule.* This approval was based on safety, immunogenicity, and efficacy in prevention of invasive *H influenzae* type b infections. An efficacy trial with this vaccine was conducted in approximately 60,000 infants in the continental United States. Efficacy in infants completing the initial 3-dose schedule was 100% (95% confidence interval, 68% to 100%). Based on the information available in October 1990, regarding safety, immuno-

***After the *Red Book* went to press, PRP-OMP was also approved for use in infants beginning at 2 months of age. Since the recommended schedule for PRP-OMP differs from that for HbOC, subsequent AAP recommendations should be reviewed.**

Table 28. *Haemophilus b* Conjugate Vaccines (HbCV)

Vaccine Manufacturer and Distributor	Abbreviation for Vaccine (trade name)	Carrier Protein	Saccharide	Spacer	Licensed by the FDA as of October 1990
Connaught	PRP-D (ProHIBit)	Diphtheria toxoid	Poly	6 carbon	Yes, for use at ≥ 15 mo of age
Lederle-Praxis	HbOC (Hib TITER)	CRM_{197} (a non-toxic mutant diphtheria toxin)	Oligo	None	Yes, for use at ≥ 2 mo of age
Merck, Sharp & Dohme	PRP-OMP (Pedvax HIB)	OMP (an outer membrane protein complex of *Neisseria meningitidis*	Poly	Complex, involving a thioether	Yes, for use at ≥ 15 mo of age*
Merieux-Connaught	PRP-T	Tetanus toxoid	Poly	6 carbon	No

*In December 1990, PRP-OMP was approved for use in infants ≥ 2 months of age, and recommendations were subsequently issued by AAP after the *Red Book* went to press.

genicity, and efficacy of HbOC and other licensed conjugate vaccines, the Committee has issued recommendations and guidelines for *H influenzae* type b immunization with the vaccine. Since approval of labeling for use in young infants for PRP-OMP and perhaps other conjugate vaccines is anticipated, further recommendations are anticipated and could be issued during the time the *Red Book* is in press.

Recommendations (as of October 1990):

- *Dosage and route of administration.* The dose of each *Haemophilus* b conjugate vaccine is 0.5 mL, given intramuscularly.
- *Indications and schedule* (see Table 29 for summary):
  - All children should be immunized with an *H influenzae* type b conjugate vaccine at approximately 2 months of age or as soon as possible thereafter, rather than at 15 months as previously recommended. Currently, only HbOC has been approved by the Food and Drug Administration (FDA) for administration to children younger than 15 months.*
  - For routine immunization beginning at approximately 2 to 3 months of age, HbOC should be administered in a three-dose series with the doses given at approximately 2-month intervals. *H influenzae* type b vaccine may be given at the same time as DTP and OPV (see also Simultaneous Administration of Multiple Vaccines, page 16). HbOC should be given intramuscularly in a separate syringe and at a separate site from other vaccines.
  - For children whose immunization was initiated when they were younger than 6 months, three doses in the primary series are required. In this circumstance, immunity may not develop until three doses have been administered; as in efficacy trials performed with HbOC, cases of invasive *H influenzae* type b disease have been observed after one or two vaccine doses.
  - For children who receive the three-dose series, a fourth dose is recommended at 15 months or as soon as possible thereafter. For this dose, the Committee believes that any licensed conjugate vaccine—PRP-OMP, PRP-D, or HbOC—is acceptable. *H influenzae* type b conjugate vaccine and MMR can be administered simultaneously but should be given at separate sites with separate syringes (see also Simultaneous Administration of Multiple Vaccines, page 16). Because several injections are required to complete the immunizations recommended at this age, some may choose to give these injections in more than one patient visit. In this situation, for patients who have not pre-

***After the *Red Book* went to press, PRP-OMP was also approved for use in infants beginning at 2 months of age. Since the recommended schedule for PRP-OMP differs from that for HbOC, subsequent AAP recommendations should be reviewed.**

Table 29. Summary of Recommendations for *Haemophilus influenzae* type b Immunization With HbOC

Age at Initiation of Immunization (mo)	Number of Doses to be Administered	Currently Recommended *H influenzae* type b Vaccine Regimen*
2-6	4	HbOC for first three doses; HbOC, PRP-OMP, or PRP-D for fourth dose
7-11	3	HbOC for first two doses; HbOC, PRP-OMP, or PRP-D for third dose
12-14	2	HbOC for first dose; HbOC, PRP-OMP, or PRP-D for second dose
15-59	1	HbOC, PRP-OMP, or PRP-D
≥60	1†	HbOC, PRP-OMP, or PRP-D

*Safety and efficacy are likely to be equivalent for PRP-OMP, PRP-D, and HbOC administered to children 15 months and older.

†Only indicated for children with chronic illness known to be associated with an increased risk for *H influenzae* type b disease (see text).

viously been immunized against measles, priority should be given to administration of MMR.

- Immunization of children older than 2 months of age at the time of the first dose should be performed as follows:
  - Unimmunized children between 3 and 6 months should receive a four-dose regimen. Optimally, the first three doses of HbOC should be given at 2-month intervals with a minimum of 1 month between doses. A fourth dose of any licensed conjugate vaccine should be given at 15 months or as soon as possible thereafter.
  - Unimmunized infants 7 to 11 months of age should receive a three-dose regimen. Optimally, the first two doses of HbOC should be given at 2-month intervals (with a minimum of 1 month between doses). A third dose of any licensed conjugate vaccine should be given at 15 months of age or as soon as possible thereafter.
  - Unimmunized children 12 to 14 months of age should receive a two-dose regimen at an optimal interval of 2 months (with a minimum of 1 month between doses). No additional doses are indicated for these children. In this situation, HbOC is given for the first dose. Any licensed conjugate vaccine is appropriate for the second dose.
  - Unimmunized children 15 months or older who have not yet reached their fifth birthday (i.e., until 59 months of age)

should receive one dose of any licensed conjugate vaccine, as previously recommended.

- Unimmunized children 5 years of age or older with a chronic illness known to be associated with increased risk of *H influenzae* type b disease should be given a single dose of any licensed conjugate vaccine. Examples include children with anatomic or functional asplenia or sickle-cell anemia, or those who have undergone a splenectomy. Until further data are available, patients with Hodgkin's disease should be immunized approximately 2 weeks or more before the initiation of chemotherapy, or if this cannot be accomplished, 3 months or more after the cessation of chemotherapy. No known contraindications exist to simultaneous administration of *H influenzae* type b vaccine with pneumococcal or meningococcal vaccine when they are given in separate syringes at different sites.
- Unimmunized children who experience invasive *H influenzae* type b disease when younger than 24 months should be subsequently immunized according to the age-appropriate schedule, beginning 1 to 2 months after the acute illness. Children whose disease occurred at 24 months or older do not need immunization because the disease most likely induced immunity.
- At present, rifampin prophylaxis is recommended for all appropriate individuals exposed to a person with invasive *H influenzae* type b disease regardless of the immunization status, as previously recommended (see Care of Exposed Persons, page 223).
- The Committee anticipates that one or more additional *H influenzae* type b conjugate vaccines will be approved for use in children younger than 15 months. The recommended immunization schedule for at least one of these different vaccines may differ from that recommended for HbOC. Until other vaccines are approved, however, they should not be used in children younger than 15 months.

Safety. Conjugate vaccines have been well tolerated in infants and children. No increased incidence of *H influenzae* type b disease during the first two weeks after immunization with HbOC has been demonstrated to date. However, all cases of invasive *H influenzae* type b disease occurring at any time after immunization should be reported promptly to the manufacturer, the FDA, or the Centers for Disease Control. Major adverse reactions should also be reported (see Reporting of Adverse Reactions, page 27).

Helicobacter pylori

(Campylobacter pylori)

Clinical Manifestations: Infection with *Helicobacter pylori* is associated with antral gastritis and primary duodenal ulcer disease. Acute infection may be manifest by epigastric pain, nausea, vomiting, hematemesis, and guaiac positive stools. Symptoms usually resolve within a few days, but chronic gastritis can develop in susceptible individuals. *H pylori* is not associated with autoimmune or chemical gastritis.

Etiology: *H pylori* (formerly *Campylobacter pylori*) are Gram-negative, spirally curved or U-shaped rods that have a tuft of flagella at one end.

Epidemiology: *H pylori* have been isolated from humans, other primates, swine, and ferrets. The role of other animals in human transmission is unknown. The largest reservoir appears to be infected humans but the routes by which organisms are transmitted are unknown. Infection rates are low in children but rise until age 60 years, at which time serologic studies indicate that more than 50% of the population has been infected. The prevalence of histologic gastritis increases progressively with advancing age. Asymptomatic carriage does occur; those individuals usually have abnormal histologic features.

The **incubation period** is unknown.

Diagnostic Tests: The only means to demonstrate *H pylori* is by culture from gastric biopsy tissue on nonselective medium (such as chocolate agar) or selective medium (e.g., Skorrow's or Campypak) at 37°C under microaerobic conditions for 2 to 5 days. Organisms can be visualized on histologic sections stained with Gram, hematoxylin-eosin, silver, Giemsa, or acridine orange staining. Urease activity in biopsy material can be determined. All of these tests require endoscopy and biopsy to obtain tissue. Noninvasive tests include detection of ^{14}C-urea in expired air and serology, which does not differentiate between acute and chronic infection.

Treatment: *H pylori* is susceptible to a wide variety of antibiotics including ampicillin, tetracycline, metronidazole, clindamycin, erythromycin, and bismuth salts, but few have been proved effective in vivo. Combination therapy such as ampicillin or amoxicillin and bismuth subsalicylate appear to be effective in elimination of the organism and in resolving clinical symptoms, but recurrence is common. No current therapy has been associated with eradication of the organism.

Isolation of the Hospitalized Patient: No special precautions are currently recommended.

Control Measures: Disinfection of gastroscopes will prevent transmission of the organism between patients.

Hemorrhagic Fevers Caused by Arenaviruses

Clinical Manifestations: These diseases range from mild infections to severe acute febrile illnesses in which shock is a prominent feature. Headache, myalgia, conjunctival suffusions, and abdominal pain are common early symptoms in all infections and exudative pharyngitis often occurs in Lassa fever. Mucosal bleeding occurs in severe cases as a consequence of platelet dysfunction. Proteinuria is common, but renal failure is unusual. Elevated aspartate aminotransferase can be an indicator of adverse or fatal outcome. Hypovolemic shock develops 7 to 9 days after onset of the illness in more severely ill patients. Upper and lower respiratory symptoms can develop in Lassa fever. Encephalopathic signs with tremor, alterations in consciousness, and seizures can occur in very severe cases of Lassa and Junin virus infections. Sensorineural hearing loss is a common sequela of Lassa fever.

Etiology: Arenaviruses contain RNA. Argentine hemorrhagic fever (AHF) and Bolivian hemorrhagic fever (BHF), the arenavirus diseases occurring in the Western hemisphere, are caused by Junin and Machupo viruses, respectively. Lassa fever, a disease occurring in West Africa, is caused by Lassa virus.

Epidemiology: Contact with virus in urine from persistently infected rodents is the primary source of infection. In addition, all arenaviruses are infectious as aerosols and should be considered highly hazardous for laboratory workers. The geographic distribution and habitats of the specific rodents that serve as reservoir hosts determine the endemic area and groups of persons at risk. Several hundred cases of AHF occur yearly, primarily from February to May, in agricultural workers in the Buenos Aires province. BHF occurs sporadically because its rodent host rarely comes into contact with man. No cases have been reported since 1975. Lassa fever is highly endemic in most of West Africa, where its rodent host lives commensally with man, causing thousands of infections annually. Lassa fever is transmitted from person to person, and nosocomial transmission of Lassa virus has occurred repeatedly. Although Lassa fever predominantly occurs in West Africa, infected travelers from West Africa may come to medical attention elsewhere.

The **incubation period** is from 6 to 17 days.

Diagnostic Tests: A specific diagnosis is made by demonstrating virus-specific IgM in blood, an increase in virus-specific serum IgG antibody titers in serial serum specimens, virus isolation, or by identifying viral antigen in blood or tissues. The increase in serum antibody occurs earlier in Lassa fever (within 3 to 12 days in most patients) than in the South American diseases (between 1 and 3 weeks). These viruses may be recovered from blood of acutely ill patients as well as from various tissues obtained postmortem.

Treatment: Plasma from convalescent patients has proved effective in reducing the mortality of AHF from 16% in untreated patients to less than 1% in those who received 2 units of plasma in the first 8 days of illness. Intravenous ribavirin reduces mortality tenfold in Lassa fever patients treated in the first 6 days of illness.

Isolation of the Hospitalized Patient: Strict isolation precautions for the duration of the illness are recommended for Lassa fever, which is the only one of these infections that has been implicated in nosocomial outbreaks.

Control Measures:

Care of Exposed Persons. No specific measures are warranted for Lassa fever exposure unless direct contamination with excretions or secretions of patients has occurred, in which case prophylactic treatment with oral ribavirin (2 g/d for 10 days), daily temperature recordings for 21 days, and prevention of intimate contact with other individuals during this interval are recommended. No control measures are indicated for persons exposed to AHF or BHF.

Rodent Control. In the village-based outbreaks of BHF, rodent control has proved successful. Rodent control in selected villages has not been considered practical for AHF because the rodent is not commensal with man. Rodent control has reduced Lassa fever infections but has not eliminated infection in household members because the rodents eventually return to the houses.

Hemorrhagic Fevers Caused by Bunyaviruses

Clinical Manifestations: These infections are severe febrile diseases in which shock and bleeding can be significant. Rift Valley fever (RVF) in most cases is a self-limited, dengue-like illness. Occasionally, patients develop hepatitis, hemorrhagic fever with shock and bleeding encephalitis, or retinitis. Congo-Crimean hemorrhagic fever (CCHF) is characterized by hepatitis and more severe bleeding. Early symptoms and signs of fever, headache, and myalgia are followed by distinctive signs of a diffuse capillary leak syndrome, such as facial suffusion, conjunctivitis, and proteinuria. Bradycardia is common, and petechiae and purpura frequently appear on the upper trunk and membranes of the mouth and palate. A hypotensive crisis frequently follows the appearance of frank hemorrhage from the gastrointestinal tract, nose, mouth, or uterus. Characteristic of hemorrhagic fever with renal syndrome (HFRS) is vascular instability and shock. Severe, acute renal insufficiency due to an acute interstitial nephritis is followed by a period of diuresis. Nephropathia epidemica, the clinical form of HFRS in Europe, is a much milder disease consisting of an influenza-like illness and proteinuria; infrequently, acute renal failure also occurs, requiring hospitalization and dialysis.

Etiology: Bunyaviruses are RNA viruses with different geographic distributions. The causative agents of HFRS are Hantaan and related viruses.

Epidemiology: RVF virus occurs in Africa; CCHF virus occurs in Africa, the Middle East, southern portions of West and Central Asia, and Eastern Europe. Hantaan and related viruses occur throughout much of Asia and in Eastern and Western Europe. RVF and CCHF occur in rural areas. RVF virus is believed to be mosquito-borne and may be transmitted mechanically from domestic animals to humans, or from person to person by mosquitoes. RVF can also be transmitted by aerosol and by direct contact with infected animal carcasses. CCHF is transmitted by ticks. Nosocomial transmission of CCHF virus is a serious hazard. Known sources of Hantaan virus are wild mice and roof rats; disease is believed to be transmitted to humans by aerosolized urine. Cases in urban areas have also been recognized. Numerous infections have been acquired in the laboratory by contact with chronically infected laboratory rodents. Viruses related to Hantaan virus have been isolated from rodents in the United States, but their pathogenicity for humans is not established.

Incubation periods range from 3 to 10 days for RVF and CCHF, and are substantially longer for HFRS (21 to 35 days).

Diagnostic Tests: RVF and CCHF viruses are readily recovered from blood and tissues of infected patients. Virus-specific serum IgM antibodies develop within 5 to 10 days of the onset of illness and, thus, are often present at or shortly after admission to the hospital. All three viruses induce serum neutralizing antibodies.

Treatment: Ribavirin has been shown to be effective in reducing renal dysfunction, vascular instability, and mortality in HFRS.

Isolation of the Hospitalized Patient: Patients with CCHF are potentially contagious; strict isolation precautions are recommended. Patients with HFRS and RVF are not considered infectious and require no special precautions.

Control Measures:

Care of Exposed Persons. Persons having direct contact with blood or other secretions and excretions from patients infected with CCHF virus should be monitored daily for fever for 14 days and precluded from intimate contact with other persons during this time. For those with unequivocal exposure, use of prophylactic, oral ribavirin (2 g/d for 10 days) should be considered.

- For **RVF,** aerial dissemination of malathion to kill adult mosquitoes may be useful in circumscribed areas. Vaccination of domestic animals can prevent or limit RVF outbreaks. An effective experimental killed vaccine has been developed by the U.S. Army.
- For **CCHF**, insecticides for tick control have been of limited benefit.
- For **HFRS**, rodent control measures, especially in urban areas, may be effective, but at present they are untested.

Hepatitis A

Clinical Manifestations: Hepatitis A characteristically is an acute febrile illness with jaundice, anorexia, nausea, and malaise. In infants and preschool-aged children, most infections are either asymptomatic or cause mild nonspecific symptoms without jaundice. Fulminant hepatitis A is rare, and chronic infection does not occur.

Etiology: Hepatitis A virus (HAV) is an RNA virus which is classified as a member of the picornavirus group.

Epidemiology: The most common mode of transmission is person to person, resulting from fecal contamination and oral ingestion (i.e., the fecal-oral route). Infection is endemic in developing countries. Spread occurs readily in households and in day care centers, which in the United States have become an important source for HAV infection in the community and for epidemics. In contrast to most other infectious diseases in day care settings, symptomatic (icteric) illness occurs primarily among adult contacts of day care children, whereas most infections in day care attendees are asymptomatic or have nonspecific manifestations. Hence, spread of HAV infection in and from a day care center frequently occurs before recognition of the index case(s). The risk of spread and of an outbreak occurring in a day care center depends on the number of children enrolled who are younger than 2 years and who wear diapers.

Common source food-borne and water-borne epidemics, including several caused by shellfish contaminated by human sewage, have occurred. Transmission by blood transfusion is rare. Nosocomial outbreaks in newborn infants have been reported. On rare occasions, infection has been contracted from nonhuman primates.

Age of infection varies with socioeconomic status and resulting living conditions. In developing countries, infection in the first decade of life is common; in developed countries, infection occurs at an older age. In the United States, infection is most common in young adults. Cases of hepatitis A among intravenous drug users have been reported with increasing frequency. No appreciable seasonal variation in the incidence of infection has been noted. Viral shedding and probably the period of contagiousness last 1 to 3 weeks. The highest titers of HAV in stool of infected patients occur in the 2 weeks before the onset of illness, during which time patients with icteric infection probably are most likely to spread infection. The risk subsequently diminishes and is minimal in the week after the onset of jaundice. No HAV carrier state exists. The presence of serum anti-HAV antibody (IgM and/or IgG) indicates lifelong immunity to HAV.

The **incubation period** is 15 to 50 days, with an average of 25 to 30 days.

Diagnostic Tests: Serologic tests for anti-HAV and IgM-specific anti-HAV antibodies are commercially available. The presence of IgM anti-HAV antibodies usually indicates recent infection. These antibodies are present at the onset of illness and are replaced by IgG anti-HAV antibodies in 2 to 4 months. IgG-specific anti-HAV antibodies alone indicate past infection.

Treatment: Supportive.

Isolation of the Hospitalized Patient: Enteric precautions should be observed. Patients who are not toilet trained or who have diarrhea, stool incontinence, or poor personal hygiene require private rooms and enteric precautions for 1 week after the onset of jaundice. Others do not require a private room. Patients with acute viral hepatitis of unknown type should be managed with the precautions recommended for both hepatitis A and hepatitis B (see Hepatitis B, page 241).

Control Measures:

Care of Household and Sexual Contacts. All household and sexual contacts should receive 0.02 mL/kg of immune globulin (IG) as soon as possible after exposure. Serologic testing of contacts usually is not recommended because it adds unnecessary cost and may delay the administration of IG. The use of IG more than 2 weeks after the last exposure is not indicated.

Newborn Infants of Infected Mothers. Unless the mother is jaundiced at the time of delivery, no special care of the infant is recommended. Neither IG nor withholding of breast-feeding is recommended. If the mother is jaundiced, the infant may be given IG (0.02 mL/kg), although its efficacy in this setting has not been established. In both situations, the need for proper hygiene should be emphasized to the mother.

Day Care Employees, Children, and Their Household Contacts.

Prevention. Prevention of spread of HAV in a day care facility necessitates education of the employees and families about the importance of hygienic measures in preventing fecal-oral spread of HAV and other enteric pathogens. Careful hand washing is imperative, particularly after changing diapers and before preparing or serving food. Because HAV may survive on objects in the environment for weeks, environmental hygiene is also important (see also Children in Day Care, page 79).

Surveillance. Recognition and reporting of day-care-associated hepatitis A cases to local health authorities should be prompt.

Case Identification. Anti-HAV IgM antibody testing should be used to confirm the infection in suspect cases in employees, enrolled children, and in those who are household contacts of a patient with hepatitis.

Uses of Immune Globulin (IG):

- Day care facilities with all children older than 2 years or who are toilet trained. When a case of hepatitis A is identified in an employee or enrolled child, IG (0.02 mL/kg) is recommended for employees in contact with the index case and children in the same room as the index case.
- Day care facilities with children not yet toilet trained. When one case of HAV infection is identified in a day care employee or

child, or in the household contacts of two of the enrolled children, IG (0.02 mL/kg) is recommended for all employees and enrolled children in the facility. During the 6 weeks after the last case is identified, new employees and children should also receive IG.

- If recognition of the day care outbreak is delayed by 3 or more weeks from the onset of the index case or if illness has occurred in three or more families, the disease is likely to have already spread widely. In this situation, IG should be considered for use in all the day care staff and children and for the household contacts of all enrolled children in diapers.

Exclusion. Children and adults with acute hepatitis A should be excluded from the day care facility until 1 week after the onset of the illness and until jaundice, if present, has disappeared; or until IG has been administered to appropriate children and staff in the program, as directed by the responsible health department.

Schools. School room exposure generally does not pose a significant risk of infection and IG is not indicated. However, IG may be given to those who have close personal contact with infected persons. Children and adults with acute hepatitis A should be excluded for 1 week after the onset of the illness and until jaundice has disappeared.

Institutions and Hospitals. In institutions for custodial care, HAV infection can be transmitted easily. If an outbreak occurs, residents and staff in close personal contact with the patients should receive IG, 0.02 mL/kg. Administration of IG to hospital personnel caring for patients with HAV infection is not indicated routinely, unless an outbreak is occurring. Emphasis should be placed on hand washing and proper hygienic procedures in the management of patients.

Food- or Water-Borne Outbreaks. The source is usually recognized too late for IG to be effective. IG may be effective if it can be administered to exposed individuals within 2 weeks of the last exposure to the HAV-contaminated water or food.

Preexposure Prophylaxis for Foreign Travel. IG prophylaxis is recommended for all susceptible travelers to developing countries. For stays of less than 3 months, travelers should receive IG (0.02 mL/kg). For longer stays, 0.06 mL/kg should be given every 5 months. For persons who require repeated immunoprophylaxis, screening for anti-HAV antibody prior to travel can reduce the need for IG by identifying immune persons. Travelers should be counseled to avoid potentially contaminated food or water.

General Measures. Good sanitation and personal hygiene, particularly careful hand washing and sanitary disposal of feces, are important general measures.

Hepatitis B

Clinical Manifestations: Hepatitis B virus (HBV) causes a spectrum of infections, ranging from asymptomatic seroconversion; subacute illness with jaundice and anorexia, nausea, and malaise; to fulminant fatal hepatitis. Anicteric or asymptomatic infection is common in children. Arthralgias, arthritis, or macular rashes can occur early in the course of the illness. Papular acrodermatitis has been noted in young infants. Chronic carriage of hepatitis B surface antigen, with or without chronic liver disease, can result from infection and occurs in a high percentage of infants with perinatal-acquired infection. Chronic carriers, especially those infected at a young age, are at increased risk of developing cirrhosis or hepatocellular carcinoma in later life.

Etiology: The HBV is a DNA-containing, 42-nm hepadnavirus. It contains hepatitis B surface antigen (HBsAg), hepatitis B core antigen (HBcAg), and hepatitis B e antigen (HBeAg). Serum antibodies to each of these antigens are used in diagnostic tests as markers of HBV infection; detection of serum HBsAg indicates current infection.

Epidemiology: The major modes of HBV transmission are contact with blood and through sexual activity. The HBV chronic carrier (defined as a person who is serum HBsAg-positive for 6 months or more) is central to the epidemiology of HBV infection. HBV is also transmitted by percutaneous or mucous membrane exposure to blood, including blood-containing body secretions or other infected body fluids, or by administration of blood products from persons with acute or chronic HBV infections (as indicated by the presence of serum HBsAg). HBV is also found in wound exudate, semen, cervical secretions, and saliva. Although saliva can contain small quantities of virus, it is not an effective vehicle for transmission. Percutaneous contact with contaminated, inanimate objects may transmit infection as the result of prolonged (1 month or longer) survival of HBV in the dried state. Experimental data indicate that HBV is not transmitted by the fecal-oral route or by water.

In children in the United States, infection is most common in populations of high endemicity of HBV infection (e.g., Alaskan Natives, Pacific Islanders, and immigrants from HBV-endemic areas, particularly eastern Asia and Africa); in persons with Down syndrome and other residents of institutions for the developmentally disabled; in patients with hemophilia and others receiving blood products; in hemodialysis patients; and in household contacts of HBV carriers. In high-risk populations, such as Southeast Asian refugees in the United States, child-to-child transmission within and between households occurs. Transmission apparently occurs by exposure of mucous membranes, abraded skin, or unrecognized wounds to saliva from infected persons. In day care facilities, the risk of transmission appears to be negligible (see Children in Child Care, Blood-Borne Infections, page 76). However, day school contacts of deinstitutionalized mentally retarded HBV carriers may be at increased risk of contracting HBV.

Perinatal transmission can occur when mothers are HBsAg-positive. When they are also HBeAg-positive, 70% to 90% of their offspring not receiving appropriate immunoprophylaxis will acquire HBV infection perinatally and become chronic carriers. Prior to routine screening of blood and donors for blood components for HbsAg, transfusions were a major risk for infection.

Adolescents and adults at highest risk of acquiring HBV infection in the United States are intravenous drug users, those having heterosexual activity with multiple partners, and those engaging in male homosexual activity. Others at increased risk include health care workers exposed to blood or blood products, staff of institutions and nonresidential day care programs for the developmentally disabled, and patients receiving chronic hemodialysis. In 30% to 40% of cases of acute hepatitis B, the risk factor is unknown. Seroprevalence studies of markers of past and current HBV infection indicate that prevalence of infection begins to increase between 12 and 18 years of age and steadily increases with advancing age thereafter, especially in Blacks. The prevalence of HBV serologic markers in various population groups in the United States is given in Table 30.

The frequency of HBV infection and patterns of transmission vary markedly in different parts of the world. In the United States, Western Europe, and Australia, it is a disease of low endemicity, with infection occurring primarily during adulthood and with only 0.2% to 0.9% of the population being chronically infected. In contrast, in China, Southeast Asia, most of Africa, most Pacific Islands, parts of the Middle East, and the Amazon Basin, HBV infection is highly endemic. In these areas, most persons acquire infection at birth or during childhood, and 8% to 15% of the population are chronically infected with HBV. In other parts of the world, HBV infection is moderately endemic, and 2% to 7% of the population are HBV carriers. Worldwide, HBV infection is a major cause of not only acute but also chronic hepatitis, cirrhosis and primary hepatocellular carcinoma caused by chronic infection.

Persons are infectious when they are HBsAg-positive, either because of acute infection or chronic carriage. They are capable of transmitting infection through intimate contact with blood or other HBsAg-positive secretions, such as in sexual intercourse or by blood

Table 30. Prevalence of Hepatitis B Serologic Markers in Various Population Groups in the United States*

Population Group	Prevalence of Serologic Markers of HBV Infection	
	HBsAg (%)	Any Marker (%)
Immigrants/refugees from areas of high-risk HBV endemicity	13	70-85
Alaskan Natives/Pacific Islanders	5-15	40-70
Clients in institutions for the developmentally disabled	10-20	35-80
Users of illicit parenteral drugs	7	60-80
Sexually active homosexual men	6	35-80
Household contacts of HBV carriers	3-6	30-60
Patients of hemodialysis units	3-10	20-80
Health care workers having frequent blood contact	1-2	15-30
Prisoners (men)	1-8	10-80
Staff of institutions for the developmentally disabled	1	10-25
Heterosexuals with multiple partners	0.5	5-20
Health care workers having no or infrequent blood contact	0.3	3-10
General population†		
Blacks	0.9	14
Whites	0.2	3

*From Centers for Disease Control. Protection against viral hepatitis: Recommendations of the Immunization Practices Advisory Committee (ACIP). *MMWR.* 1990;39(No. RR-2):5.

†Second National Health and Nutrition Examination Survey, 1976-1980.

donation. The presence of HBeAg correlates with viral replication and increases the risk of infectivity.

The **incubation period** of acute hepatitis B is 45 to 160 days, with an average of 120 days.

Diagnostic Tests: Commercial serologic tests are available for the HBV antigens, HBsAg and HBeAg, and for antibodies to HBsAg, HBcAg, and HBeAg (see Table 31). Some of these tests are used for routine screening of blood donors and transfusions. In acute infection, the test for HBsAg is most commonly used and will detect 90% to 95%

Table 31. Diagnostic Tests for HBV Infections and Immunity

Abbreviation	Hepatitis B Antigen or Antibody	Use
HBsAg	Surface antigen	Detection of carriers or acutely infected persons
Anti-HBs	Antibody to surface antigen (HBsAg)	Identification of persons who have had infections with HBV; determination of immunity after vaccination
HBeAg	e antigen	Identification of carriers at increased risk of transmitting HBsAg
Anti-HBe	Antibody to e antigen (HBe)	Identification of HBsAg carriers with low risk of infectiousness
Anti-HBc	Antibody to core antigen (HBcAg)*	Identification of persons who have had HBV infection
IgM Anti-HBc	IgM antibody to core antigen	Identification of acute or recent HBV infections (including those in HBsAg-negative persons)

*No test is commercially available to measure core antigen (HBcAg).

of cases. However, HBsAg can also indicate chronic infection. The presence of IgM antibody to the HBV core antigen (IgM anti-HBc) is highly specific for establishing the diagnosis of acute or recent HBV infection. In some cases of acute infection, however, serum HBsAg will have disappeared and antibody to surface antigen (anti-HBs) has not yet appeared; in these cases IgM anti-HBc may be present. Anti-HBc is detectable in many persons with prior hepatitis B infection and indicates past infection.

Treatment: No specific therapy for acute HBV infection is available. A variety of therapeutic medications, including interferon, have been demonstrated in some cases to be effective treatment of chronic hepatitis B.

Isolation of the Hospitalized Patient: The routinely recommended precautions for blood and bodily fluids (see Isolation Precautions, page 81) should be scrupulously followed for patients with HBV infection as long as they are HBsAg-positive. Patients with jaundice believed to be caused by a hepatitis virus yet to be identified should also be managed with enteric precautions in view of possible hepatitis A or enterically transmitted, non-A, non-B hepatitis.

Blood of infants whose mothers are HBsAg-positive should be carefully handled because 1% to 2% of these infants are infected in utero. No special care other than removal of maternal blood at birth by a gloved attendant is necessary.

Control Measures: Current control measures to prevent HBV infections involve prevention of person-to-person transmission from blood and blood products, including percutaneous and permucosal exposure; interruption of maternal-infant transmission by immunoprophylaxis; and active immunization of high-risk groups.

Prenatal Screening for HBsAg. Identification of HBsAg-positive pregnant women is essential to prevent perinatal transmission (see Care of Infants Whose Mothers Are HBsAG Positive). Prenatal questioning designed to identify women in high-risk groups in urban populations detects only about 50% of those who are HBsAg-positive. Accordingly, routine screening is recommended for all women. In special situations of increased risk during pregnancy, such as suspected acute hepatitis, history of HBV exposure, or particularly high-risk behavior (e.g., intravenous drug abuse), an additional HBsAg test can be ordered later in pregnancy.

Prevention of HBV Transmission to Medical Personnel and Patients. Universal precautions for blood and bodily fluids should be carefully followed by individuals working in areas of high risk for HBV exposure (e.g., clinical laboratories, dialysis units, patient care likely to involve blood contact, and institutions for developmentally disabled persons). Education of all medical personnel regarding proper disposal of injection and blood drawing equipment can minimize risk of accidental exposure. Whenever feasible, disposable equipment should be used in circumstances in which blood contamination can occur, and the proper physical cleaning and sterilization by autoclaving of nondisposable equipment should be standard policy. Hepatitis B immunization is indicated for personnel at occupational risk (see Indications for Preexposure Vaccination, page 246).

Day Care. Children who are HBV carriers and who have no behavioral or medical risk factors, such as unusually aggressive behavior (e.g., biting), generalized dermatitis, or bleeding problem, should be admitted to day care without restrictions. The risk of HBV transmission in day care appears to be negligible. Routine screening for HBsAg is not warranted. Admission of HBV carrier children with risk factors (e.g., biting, frequent scratching, generalized dermatitis, or bleeding problems) should be assessed on an individual basis by the child's physician, the program director, and the responsible public health authorities. For further discussion, see Children in Day Care, Blood-Borne Virus Infections, page 76.

Adopted Infants and Children from High-Risk Areas. Adopted infants and children from high-risk populations or those with biological mothers of unknown medical or social backgrounds should be screened for HBsAg. Initial screening should be performed at 3 months of age or at the time of adoption if it occurs at a later age, and testing should be repeated 6 months later. If the child is HBsAg-positive, household members should be vaccinated (see Indications for Preexposure Vaccination, page 246).

Immunoprophylaxis. Immunoprophylaxis with hepatitis B (HB) vaccine and/or hepatitis B immune globulin (HBIG) is indicated for persons at high risk of or after exposure to HBV (see Care of Exposed Persons).

Hepatitis B Vaccines. Two types of hepatitis B vaccine have been developed. The first, plasma-derived vaccine, prepared from the plasma of HbsAg carriers, is no longer produced in the United States and its use is now limited to hemodialysis patients, other immunocompromised hosts, and persons with known allergy to yeast. Plasma-derived vaccines are effective and safe, however, and are widely used in other countries. The second type of vaccine, the recombinant vaccines, is produced from common baker's yeast genetically modified to produce the purified vaccine antigen, HBsAg, by insertion of the plasmid containing the gene for HBsAg. Vaccines contain 10 to 40 μg HBsAg protein per milliliter, are absorbed with aluminum hydroxide, and contain thiomersal (1:20,000) as a preservative. The yeast protein content is 5% or less of the final product.

Two recombinant vaccines are currently licensed in the United States. The concentration of HBsAg antigen differs in the two different products but the vaccines are equally immunogenic when administered in doses recommended in the package inserts (see Table 32). For withdrawal of small volumes from vaccine vials, the use of a syringe to which the needle is permanently attached is accurate.

A series of three doses is required for optimal antibody response; it induces an adequate antibody response in more than 90% of healthy adults, and in more than 95% of infants, children, and adolescents.* Field trials of the vaccines licensed in the United States have shown 80% to 95% efficacy in preventing infection or clinical hepatitis among susceptible persons. Protection against illness is virtually complete for persons who develop an adequate antibody response.

---

*An adequate antibody response is ≥ 10 milliInternational units (mIU)/mL, approximately equivalent to 10 sample ratio units (SRU) by RIA or positive by enzyme immunoassay (EIA), measured 1 to 6 months after completion of the vaccine series.

Table 32. Recommended Doses (Given Intramuscularly) and Schedules of Currently Licensed Hepatitis B Vaccines*

	Vaccine†,‡		
Group	Heptavax-B§ (MSD‖) Dose (μg) (mL)	Recombivax HB (MSD‖) Dose (μg) (mL)	Engerix-B¶ (SK**) Dose (μg) (mL)
Infants of HBV carrier mothers	10 (0.5)	5 (0.5)	10 (0.5)
Other infants and children < 11 y	10 (0.5)	2.5 (0.25)	10 (0.5)
Children and adolescents 11-19 y	20 (1.0)	5 (0.5)	20 (1.0)
Adults > 19 y	20 (1.0)	10 (1.0)	20 (1.0)
Dialysis patients and other immuno-compromised persons	40 (2.0)††	40 (1.0)#	40 (2.0)††,§§

*From Centers for Disease Control. Protection against viral hepatitis: Recommendations of the Immunization Practices Advisory Committee (ACIP). *MMWR.* 1990;39(No. RR-2):11.

†**Vaccines should be stored at 2° to 8° C. Freezing destroys effectiveness.**

‡**Usual schedule for each vaccine is three doses, given at 0, 1, and 6 months.**

§Available in U.S. only for hemodialysis and other immmunocompromised patients and for persons with known allergy to yeast.

‖Merck, Sharp & Dohme

¶Alternative schedule: four doses at 0, 1, 2, and 12 months.

**SmithKline Biologicals

††Given as two 1.0-mL doses at different sites.

#Special formulation for dialysis patients.

§§Four-dose schedule recommended at 0, 1, 2, and 12 months.

The duration of protection and need for booster doses are not yet fully defined. Between 30% and 50% of persons who develop adequate antibody after three doses of vaccine will lose detectable antibody within 7 years, but protection against viremic infection and clinical disease appears to persist. Immunogenicity and efficacy of the licensed vaccines in hemodialysis patients are lower than in healthy adults. Protection in this group may last only as long as adequate antibody concentrations persist.

Schedule and Site of Administration. The three recommended doses are given at 0, 1, and 6 months. An alternate schedule consisting of vaccine administration at 0, 1, 2, and 12 months has been approved for

Engerix-B* for postexposure prophylaxis or for more rapid induction of immunity. However, no clear evidence indicates that this regimen provides greater protection than the standard 3-dose series. In addition, different 3-dose schedules, beginning at 2 months of age and with 2-month intervals, have been demonstrated to be effective in infants in high-risk populations whose mothers are HBsAg-negative.

Vaccine is given intramuscularly. In adults and older children, the deltoid area of the upper arm is the recommended site for vaccination because immunogenicity is diminished when injections are given in the buttocks. The anterolateral thigh is preferred for infants. In patients with bleeding diathesis, vaccine may be given subcutaneously. Passively acquired maternal antibody or concurrent administration of immunoglobulin does not interfere with active hepatitis B immunization.

Immunosuppressed Patients. Patients on renal dialysis programs and other immunosuppressed patients should receive twice the recommended dose of plasma-derived HB vaccine for age at each vaccination because their antibody response is diminished. A specially formulated preparation of the recombinant HB vaccine (40 µg HBsAg protein per milliliter adsorbed with 0.5 mg aluminum hydroxide) is available for these immunosuppressed patients.

Boosters and Serologic Testing. For adults and children with normal immune status and for infants born to HBV carrier mothers, booster doses are not necessary after the primary vaccination if the 3-dose series has been completed. The possible need for booster doses after longer intervals than the current 5 to 7 years of follow-up will be assessed as additional information becomes available. Routine serologic testing for HBV immunity is not indicated for these persons.

Hemodialysis patients, in whom protection from the vaccine may be less complete and may persist only as long as serum antibody concentrations are above 10 mIU/mL, should have their serum antibody concentrations measured annually. A booster dose of vaccine should be given when the antibody concentration falls below 10 mIU/mL.

Testing for immunity after vaccination is advised only for persons whose subsequent management depends on their HBV immune status, such as dialysis patients and exposed health care personnel (see Percutaneous or Permucosal Exposure to HBsAg-Positive Blood, page 252), and for persons who would be expected to have a suboptimal response, such as those who received the vaccine in the buttock or who have known HIV infection.

Adverse Effects. The most common side effect is soreness at the injection site. Hypersensitivity to yeast or thiomersal has been reported. The risk of Guillain-Barré syndrome does not appear to be increased in

---

*SmithKline Biologicals

vaccine recipients. Plasma-derived or recombinant vaccines do not contain HIV. The procedures used to prepare the plasma-derived vaccine inactivate the AIDS virus, if present, and genetically engineered vaccines contain no material from humans.

Indications for Preexposure Vaccination (see summary in Table 33).* Persons at substantial risk of HBV infection who are demonstrated or judged likely to be susceptible should be vaccinated. Such persons include the following:

Hemophiliac Patients and Other Recipients of Certain Blood Products. Vaccination is recommended at the time of diagnosis. Prevaccination testing is recommended for those patients who have already received multiple infusions.

Intravenous Drug Abusers.

Sexually Active Heterosexual Persons. Vaccination is recommended for persons with recently acquired sexually transmitted diseases, for prostitutes, and for persons who have had sexual activity with multiple partners in the previous 6 months.

Sexually Active Homosexual Males.

Household and Sexual Contacts of HBV Chronic Carriers. When HBV carriers are identified through routine screening of donated blood, diagnostic testing in hospitals, prenatal screening, screening of refugees from certain areas, or other screening programs, they should be notified of their status, their household and sexual contacts should be tested, and susceptible persons should be vaccinated.

Household Members of Adopted Infants and Children From Countries of High HBV Endemicity Who Are HBsAg-Positive. Adoptees should be screened for HBsAg. Similarly, adoptees from other high-risk populations, such as children whose biological mothers have unknown medical or social backgrounds, should be screened. If the adoptee is HBsAg-positive, household members should be vaccinated.

Populations With High Endemicity of HBV Infection.

- In certain populations in the United States, such as Alaskan Natives and refugees from HBV-endemic areas in which HBV infection is highly endemic, universal hepatitis B vaccination of infants is recommended to prevent disease transmission during childhood. In addition, more extensive programs of "catch-up" childhood vaccination should be considered if resources are available.
- Vaccination is recommended for all infants born in areas in which infection is highly endemic.

*Also see Centers for Disease Control. Protection against viral hepatitis: recommendations of the Immunization Practices Advisory Committee (ACIP). *MMWR.* 1990;39(No. RR-2): 19-21.

Table 33. Persons Who Should Receive Preexposure Immunization*

Hemophiliac patients and other recipients of certain blood products
Intravenous drug abusers
Heterosexual persons who have had multiple sex partners in the previous 6 months and those with recent sexually transmitted disease
Sexually active homosexual males
Household and sexual contacts of HBV chronic carriers
Household members of adoptees from HBV-endemic, high-risk countries who are HBsAg-positive
Specified infants, children, and other household contacts in populations of high HBV endemicity (see text)
Staff and residents of institutions for the developmentally disabled
Staff of nonresidential day care and school programs for developmentally disabled if attended by known HBV carrier; other attendees in certain circumstances
Hemodialysis patients
Health care workers and others with occupational risk
International travelers who will live for more than 6 months in area of high HBV endemicity and who otherwise will be at risk
Inmates of long-term correctional facilities

*For details, see text, and Centers for Disease Control. Protection against viral hepatitis: Recommendations of the Immunization Practices Advisory Committee (ACIP). *MMWR.* 1990;39(No. RR-2):5-22.

- Immigrants and refugees from areas with highly endemic HBV disease (particularly Africa and eastern Asia) should be screened for HBV markers upon resettlement in the United States. If an HBV carrier is identified, all susceptible household contacts should be vaccinated. Even if no HBV carriers are found within a family, vaccination should be considered for susceptible children younger than 7 years because of the high rate of interfamilial HBV infection that occurs among these children.

Staff and Residents of Institutions for the Developmentally Disabled. Susceptible residents of institutions for the developmentally disabled should be vaccinated. Staff who work closely with these residents should also be vaccinated. The risk in institutional environments not only is associated with blood exposure but also may result from bites and contact with skin lesions and other infective secretions. Susceptible residents and staff who live or work in smaller (group) residential settings with known HBV carriers should also be vaccinated.

Nonresidential Day Care and School Programs. Staff of nonresidential programs for developmentally disabled persons, attended by one or more known HBV carriers, have a risk of HBV infection comparable to that among health care workers and, therefore, should be vaccinated. The risk of HBV infection for attendees appears to be lower than the risk for staff. Vaccination of attendees in these programs may be considered, and is strongly encouraged if a classmate who is an HBV carrier behaves aggressively or has special medical problems that increase the risk of exposure to his/her blood or serous secretions.

For implementation of these recommendations, persons discharged from residential institutions who will be entering day care or school programs should be screened for HBsAg.

Hemodialysis Patients. Identification of patients for vaccination early in the course of their renal disease is encouraged.

Health Care Workers and Others With Occupational Exposure to Blood. The risk of acquiring HBV infection from occupational exposures is dependent on the frequency of percutaneous and permucosal exposures to blood or blood products. The risk of a health care worker for HBV exposure depends on the tasks that he or she performs. If those tasks involve contact with blood or blood-contaminated body fluids, such workers should be vaccinated. Vaccination should be considered for other workers depending on the nature of their tasks.

Risks for health care professionals vary during their training and working careers, but are often highest during their training. For this reason, when possible, vaccination should be completed during training and before contact with blood.

International Travelers. Vaccination should be considered for persons who plan to reside for more than 6 months in areas with highly endemic HBV infection and who will have close contact with the local population. Vaccination should also be considered for short-term travelers who are likely to have contact—either from blood or from sexual relations—with residents of such areas. Ideally, vaccination of travelers should begin at least 6 months before travel to allow for completion of the full vaccine series. Nevertheless, a partial series will offer some protection from HBV infection. The alternative four-dose schedule (at 0, 1, 2, and 12 months) may provide better protection during travel if the first three doses can be delivered before travel.

Inmates of Long-Term Correctional Facilities.

Care of Exposed Persons (see Table 34).*

Care of Infants Whose Mothers Are HBsAg-Positive. Neonates born to mothers who are HBsAg positive should be bathed carefully as soon as possible to remove maternal blood and secretions that contaminated their skin during birth. Universal precautions should be in effect. After bathing, the neonates may be managed without special precautions for the rest of their stay in the nursery. Neonates and mothers may have normal contact or may room in.

HBIG (0.5 mL, intramuscularly) should be given as soon as possible after birth, preferably within 12 hours, as part of the routine care of newborns whose mothers are HBsAg-positive. If a mother is found to be positive after this time, HBIG should still be given to the neonate as it may still be of some value. Efficacy of HBIG given at 12 to 48 hours is presumed but unproven. Screening of all women during pregnancy for the presence of HBsAg in serum is essential so that their status can be identified before delivery (see Prenatal Screening for HBsAg), their infants can be appropriately treated, and proper precautions can be taken by exposed persons.

In addition to HBIG, hepatitis B vaccination should be initiated within 7 days of birth, preferably within 12 hours. The dose is 0.5 mL for each vaccine product, and is given intramuscularly. The first dose can be given at the same time as HBIG if it is given with a separate syringe and at a different site. The second and third doses are given 1 and 6 months after the first. If not given in the first 12 hours after birth, the first dose should be administered prior to discharge from the hospital and within 7 days of birth in order to increase the likelihood that vaccination will be initiated.

An alternate schedule is also approved for Engerix-B† (see Schedule and Site of Administration, page 244).

Data on the effectiveness of HB vaccine are not available for infants with birth weights less than 2,000 g. If vaccine administration is delayed for as long as 3 months, a second dose of HBIG (0.5 mL) should be given.

Subsequent doses of hepatitis B vaccine can be given concurrently with DTP but should be given at a separate site and with a different syringe.

In 1% to 2% of cases, the recommended immunoprophylactic regimen of HBIG and hepatitis B vaccination is not effective; therefore, infants should be tested at 9 months of age or later (at least 1 month after the third vaccine dose) for HBsAg and anti-HBsAg to

*Also see Centers for Disease Control. Protection against viral hepatitis: recommendations of the Immunization Practices Advisory Committee (ACIP). *MMWR.* 1190;39(No. RR-2): 19-21.

†SmithKline Biologicals

Table 34. Hepatitis B Virus Postexposure Recommendations*,†

	HBIG‡		Vaccine‡	
Exposure	Dose	Timing	No. of Doses	Timing§
Perinatal	0.5mL	As soon as possible (within 12 h)	3	Within 7 d (preferably within 12 h); repeat at 1 and 6 mo
Sexual‖	0.06mL/kg (max 5mL)	Within 14 d of contact	3	First dose at time of HBIG; repeat at 1 and 6 mo¶
Acute hepatitis B in mother, father, or caretaker				
• Exposed < 12 mo of age	0.5mL	As soon as possible	3	0,1, and 6 mo
• Exposed ≥ 12 mo of age	—	—	(Observe index case; see text)	
Percutaneous or mucosal (also see Table 35)				
• Previously unvaccinated**	0.06mL/kg (max 5mL)	Within 24 h	3	Within 7 d; repeat at 1 and 6 mo¶
• Previously vaccinated**				
▪ Previously known responder	—	—	1††	—
▪ Known non-responder	0.5mL	Within 24 h	1	—
▪ Unknown	0.5mL#	—	1#	—

*See text for details.

†See Table 32 for appropriate dose.

‡Given intramuscularly. If HBIG and vaccine are given concurrently, they should be given at separate sites.

§See Schedule and Site of Administration, page 244, for alternative schedule.

‖Vaccine is recommended for homosexual males, regular contacts of chronic HBV carriers, and heterosexual persons with multiple sexual partners.

¶Vaccination indicated if exposures are likely to recur.

**Test and administer HBIG and vaccine unless adequate anti-HBs (≥ 10 SRU by RIA or positive by EIA) has been demonstrated within 24 months.

††Vaccinate if anti-HBs < 10 SRU by RIA or negative by EIA.

#Give if anti-HBs test indicates susceptibility.

determine the outcome of immunoprophylaxis. Children who are HBsAg-negative and anti-HBsAg negative should receive a fourth dose of vaccine and be retested 1 month later for anti-HBsAg. Those infants who are HBsAg-positive should have follow-up testing to determine if they are chronic carriers (defined as HBsAg-positive for 6 or more months). Further doses of hepatitis B vaccine in this circumstance are of no benefit.

In certain populations, such as Alaskan Natives and Pacific Islanders, hepatitis B is highly endemic and transmission occurs primarily during early childhood. Prenatal screening in these areas is often not feasible because of limited financial or technical resources. In such areas, universal vaccination of newborns with hepatitis B vaccine is recommended as the best means of preventing HBV infection both in the perinatal period and in childhood (see also Indications for Preexposure Vaccination). Vaccine given without HBIG has been shown to prevent 70% to 75% of perinatal HBV infections and an estimated 95% of early childhood HBV infections.

Breast-feeding poses no risk of HBV infection for infants who have started immunoprophylaxis. Studies in Taiwan and England demonstrated that breast-feeding by mothers who are HBsAg-positive does not significantly increase the risk of HBV infection in their newborn infants (who had not received immunoprophylaxis). Administration of HBIG and initiation of active immunization will diminish any risk of transmission.

Adoptees. For management of household members with adopted infants and children from high-risk populations, see Control Measures, page 242.

Household Contacts of Persons With Acute HBV Infection.

- *Exposed infants (younger than 12 months).* Since the risk of severe or chronic HBV infection is higher in infants, and since little information exists about the risk of an infant acquiring HBV infection from close contact with a household member with acute HBV infection, infants in the first year of life should both receive HBIG and be vaccinated when acute HBV infection is diagnosed in the infant's mother, father, or principal caretaker.
- *Exposed children 12 months or older.* In a home with a case of acute HBV infection, the index patient should be followed serologically to determine if the individual becomes an HBsAg carrier. If the index patient becomes an HBsAg carrier, the household contact(s) should be vaccinated. Some experts advise starting HBV immunization as soon as a case has been diagnosed because the household may be in a high-risk category, in which case contacts will be at increased risk during adolescence. In addition, in cases in which follow-up is likely to be poor or unreliable, and the index case does become a carrier, vaccine administration

may be delayed or not given. HBIG is not recommended in these different circumstances.

Sexual Contacts of Persons With HBV Infection. Sexual partners of persons with acute hepatitis B or who are HBsAg-positive are at increased risk of acquiring HBV infection. HBIG has been shown to be 75% effective in preventing such infection. Prescreening sexual partners for susceptibility before HBIG treatment is advisable if it does not delay treatment beyond 14 days after the last exposure. Testing for anti-HBc antibody is the most efficient prescreening test in this situation.

All susceptible persons whose sexual partners have acute hepatitis B infection or whose sexual partners are discovered to be hepatitis B carriers should receive a single dose of HBIG (0.06 mL/kg), if it can be given within 14 days of the last sexual contact or if sexual contact with the infected person is ongoing. In such cases, the susceptible person should receive hepatitis B vaccine in the recommended three-dose schedule. Giving the vaccine with HBIG may improve the efficacy of postexposure treatment. The vaccine has the added advantage of conferring long-lasting protection.

An alternative treatment for persons who are not in high-risk groups for whom vaccine is routinely recommended and whose regular sexual partners have acute HBV infection is to give one dose of HBIG (without vaccine) and retest the sexual partner for HBsAg 3 months later. No further treatment is necessary if the sexual partner becomes HBsAg-negative. If the sexual partner remains HBsAg-positive, a second dose of HBIG should be given, and the hepatitis B vaccine series should be started.

*Percutaneous or Permucosal Exposure to HBsAg-Positive Blood.** For accidental percutaneous (needle stick, laceration, or bite) or permucosal (ocular or mucous-membrane) exposure to blood, the decision to provide prophylaxis must include consideration of several factors: 1) whether the source of the blood is available, 2) the HBsAg status of the source, and 3) the hepatitis B vaccination and vaccine-response status of the exposed person. For any exposure of a person not previously vaccinated, such as from a bite of a child who is an HBV carrier, HBIG is recommended; and if similar exposures are likely to recur, hepatitis B vaccination is also recommended. For further discussion of the management of young children with bites involving an HBV carrier, such as in day care, see Children in Day Care, Blood-Borne Virus Infections, page 76. Such exposures usually involve health care workers, for whom preexposure hepatitis

*From Centers for Disease Control. Protection against viral hepatitis: Recommendations of the Immunization Practices Advisory Committee (ACIP). *MMWR*. 1990;39(No. RR-2): 19-21.

Table 35. Recommendations for Hepatitis B Prophylaxis After Percutaneous or Permucosal Exposure*,†

Exposed Person	HBsAg-Positive Source	HBsAg-Negative Source	Source Not Tested or Unknown
Unvaccinated	HBIG x 1† and initiate HB vaccine‡	Initiate HB vaccine‡	Initiate HB vaccine‡
Previously vaccinated Known responder	Test exposed for anti-HBs§ • If adequate, no treatment • If inadequate, HB vaccine‡ booster dose	No treatment	No treatment
Known nonresponder	HBIG† x 2 or HBIG x 1 plus 1 dose HB vaccine‡	No treatment	If known high-risk source, **may treat as if source were HBsAg-positive**
Response unknown	Test exposed for anti-HBs§ • If inadequate, HBIG† x 1 plus HB vaccine‡ booster dose • If adequate, no treatment	No treatment	Test exposed for anti-HBs§ • If inadequate, HB vaccine booster dose • If adequate, no treatment

*From Centers for Disease Control. Protection against viral hepatitis: Recommendations of the Immunization Practices Advisory Committee (ACIP). *MMWR.* 1990;39(No. RR-2):19-21.
†HBIG dose 0.06 mL/kg IM.
‡HB vaccine dose: See Table 32.
§Adequate anti-HBs is ≥ 10 SRU by RIA or positive by EIA.

B vaccination is recommended and who should be vaccinated whenever an opportunity arises.

After any such exposure, a blood sample should be obtained from the person who was the source of the exposure and should be tested for HBsAg. The hepatitis B vaccination status and anti-HBs response status (if known of the exposed person) should be reviewed. Table 35 summarizes prophylaxis recommendations, according to the U.S. Public Health Service Immunization Practices Advisory Committee; further details are given in Appendix 1.

Appendix 1. Recommendations for hepatitis B prophylaxis following percutaneous or permucosal exposure (from Centers for Disease Control, Protection against viral hepatitis: recommendations of the Immunization Practices Advisory Committee [ACIP]. *MMWR* 1990;39[No. RR-2]:19-21).

The following summarizes prophylaxis for percutaneous or permucosal exposure to blood according to the HBsAg status of the source of exposure and the vaccination status and vaccine response of the exposed person. For greatest effectiveness, passive prophylaxis with HBIG, when indicated, should be given as soon as possible after exposure (its value beyond 7 days after exposure is unclear).

1. *Source of exposure is HBsAg-positive.*
   A. Exposed person has not been vaccinated or has not completed vaccination. Hepatitis B vaccination should be initiated. A single dose of HBIG (0.06 mL/kg) should be given as soon as possible after exposure and within 24 hours, if possible. The first dose of hepatitis B vaccine (Table 32) should be given intramuscularly at a separate site (deltoid for adults) and can be given simultaneously with HBIG or within 7 days of exposure. Subsequent doses should be given as recommended for the specific vaccine. If the exposed person has begun but not completed vaccination, one dose of HBIG should be given immediately, and vaccination should be completed as scheduled.
   B. Exposed person has already been vaccinated against hepatitis B, and anti-HBs response status is known.
      1) If the exposed person is known to have had adequate response in the past, the anti-HBs level should be tested unless an adequate level has been demonstrated within the last 24 months. Although current data show that vaccine-induced protection does not decrease as antibody level wanes, most experts consider the following approach to be prudent:
         a) If anti-HBs level is adequate, no treatment is necessary.
         b) If anti-HBs level is inadequate,* a booster dose of hepatitis B vaccine should be given.
      2) If the exposed person is known not to have responded to the primary vaccine series, the exposed person should be given either a single dose of HBIG and a dose of hepatitis B vaccine as soon as possible after exposure, or two doses of HBIG (0.06 mL/kg), one given as soon as possible after exposure and the second 1 month later. The latter treatment is preferred for those who have failed to respond to at least four doses of vaccine.

---

*An adequate antibody level is ≥ 10 milliInternational units (mIU)/mL, approximately equivalent to 10 ratio units (SRU) by RIA or positive by EIA.

C. Exposed person has already been vaccinated against hepatitis B, and the anti-HBs response is unknown. The exposed person should be tested for anti-HBs.
   1) If the exposed person has adequate antibody, no additional treatment is necessary.
   2) If the exposed person has inadequate antibody on testing, one dose of HBIG (0.06 mL/kg) should be given immediately, and a standard booster dose of vaccine should be given at a different site.

2. *Source of exposure is known to be HBsAg-negative.*
   A. Exposed person has not been vaccinated or has not completed vaccination. If unvaccinated, the exposed person should be given the first dose of hepatitis B vaccine within 7 days of exposure, and vaccination should be completed as recommended. If the exposed person has not completed vaccination, vaccination should be completed as scheduled.
   B. Exposed person has already been vaccinated against hepatitis B. No treatment is necessary.

3. *Source of exposure is unknown or not available for testing.*
   A. Exposed person has not been vaccinated or has not completed vaccination. If unvaccinated, the exposed person should be given the first dose of hepatitis B vaccine within 7 days of exposure, and vaccination should be completed as recommended. If the exposed person has not completed vaccination, vaccination should be completed as scheduled.
   B. Exposed person has already been vaccinated against hepatitis B, and anti-HBs response status is known.
      1) If the exposed person is known to have had adequate response in the past, no treatment is necessary.
      2) If the exposed person is known not to have responded to the vaccine, prophylaxis as described earlier (in section 1.B.2, under "Source of exposure is HBsAg-positive") may be considered if the source of the exposure is known to be at high risk of HBV infection.
   C. Exposed person has already been vaccinated against hepatitis B, and the anti-HBs response is unknown. The exposed person should be tested for anti-HBs.
      1) If the exposed person has adequate anti-HBs, no treatment is necessary.
      2) If the exposed person has inadequate anti-HBs, a standard booster dose of vaccine should be given.

Hepatitis C

(Parenterally Transmitted Non-A, Non-B Hepatitis)

Clinical Manifestations: Hepatitis C typically is characterized by mild or asymptomatic infection with an insidious onset of jaundice and malaise. In some cases, the course is remittent. As many as 50% of the patients can develop chronic liver disease; cirrhosis and possibly hepatocellular concurrence may be involved in some cases.

Etiology: The hepatitis C virus (HCV) is a flavivirus-like single-stranded RNA virus.

Epidemiology: Transmission of HCV can occur by parenteral administration of blood or blood products, but most hepatitis C cases in the United States are not associated with blood transfusions. Approximately 70% to 90% of cases of parenterally transmitted non-A, non-B hepatitis in the United States are caused by HCV. Some evidence indicates that HCV is also sexually transmitted, but the role of person-to-person contact is not well defined. Groups at high risk include parenteral drug users, persons transfused with blood or blood components, health care workers with frequent blood exposure, and persons with sexual or household contact with an infected person. No source or risk factor can be identified in a substantial number of cases. Perinatal transmission probably occurs but the risks and consequences have not been defined. Disease is most frequently recognized in adults; reported cases are infrequent in children younger than 15 years. HCV, like hepatitis B infection, can result in chronic infection. The period of communicability is not known.

The average **incubation period** is 7 to 9 weeks, with a range of 2 to 12 weeks.

Diagnostic Tests: A serologic test for anti-HCV became commercially available in 1990. This test is positive in most patients infected with HCV. However, by this test, anti-HBC may be absent during the acute illness and may only become detectable 6 months after onset of the illness. A positive anti-HCV serologic test does not necessarily indicate continuing infection.

Treatment: Treatment with interferon is investigational; it may be useful in some cases of chronic hepatitis due to HCV.

Isolation of the Hospitalized Patient: The routinely recommended blood and body fluid precautions (see Isolation Precautions, page 81) are indicated for the duration of the illness. Patients with acute viral hepatitis of unknown type should be managed with the precautions recommended for both hepatitis A (see Hepatitis A, page 236) and hepatitis C.

Control Measures:

- In accidental exposure to blood from a patient with hepatitis C, immune globulin (0.06 mL/kg) may be useful in preventing HCV infection, but results of studies evaluating prophylactic efficacy have been equivocal.
- Screening of blood for transfusion for anti-HCV has recently been instituted in order to prevent transfusion-associated hepatitis.

Hepatitis Delta Virus

(Hepatitis D Virus)

Clinical Manifestations: Hepatitis delta virus (HDV) infection produces hepatitis, but only in conjunction with hepatitis B virus (HBV) infection. Infection in a person with acute or chronic HBV infection can result in acute, possibly fulminant hepatitis, or chronic hepatitis which may progress to cirrhosis.

Etiology: Hepatitis delta virus has been characterized as a 35- to 37-nm particle consisting of an RNA fragment and a delta protein antigen (HDAg), both of which are coated with hepatitis B surface antigen (HBsAg). HDV requires HBV as a "helper virus" and cannot produce infection in the absence of HBV.

Epidemiology: HDV can cause an infection at the same time as the initial hepatitis B infection (coinfection), or it can infect an individual already chronically infected with HBV (superinfection). Transmission is similar to that of HBV, i.e., by parenteral, percutaneous, or mucous membrane inoculation. HDV can be transmitted by blood or blood products, intravenous illicit drug use, or sexual contact, as long as HBsAg is present in the patient's blood. Transmission from mother to newborn infant is uncommon. Intrafamilial spread can occur among HBsAg carriers. Some chronic HBV infections can be accompanied by chronic HDV infection. High prevalence areas include southern Italy and parts of Eastern Europe, South America, Africa, and the Middle East. In contrast to HBV infection, HDV is uncommon in the Far East. In the United States, HDV infection is found most frequently in parenteral drug abusers, hemophiliacs, and persons immigrating from endemic areas.

The **incubation period** for HDV superinfection, estimated from inoculation of animals, is about 4 to 8 weeks. When HBV and HDV coinfect, the incubation period is similar to that of HBV infection (45 to 160 days; average 120 days).

Diagnostic Tests: A test for anti-HDV antibody is commercially available. Tests for IgM-specific anti-HDV antibody and delta antigen (HDAg) are research procedures at present. If markers of HDV infection exist, coinfection with hepatitis B virus can usually be differentiated from superinfection of an established HBsAg carrier by testing for hepatitis B core antibody of the IgM class (IgM anti-HBC). Absence of markers of acute hepatitis B infection in a patient with HDV infection suggests that the person is an HBsAg carrier.

Treatment: Supportive.

Isolation of the Hospitalized Patient: The same precautions as for HBV infection, i.e., the routinely recommended blood and body fluid precautions for all patients, should be followed (see Hepatitis B, page 241).

Control Measures: The same control and preventive measures as for HBV infection are indicated, since HDV cannot be transmitted in the absence of HBV infection. HBsAg carriers should take extreme care in avoiding exposure to HDV because no currently available immunobiologic exists for prevention of HDV superinfection.

Enterically Transmitted Non-A, Non-B Hepatitis

Clinical Manifestations: Enterically transmitted, non-A, non-B (ET-NANB) hepatitis is an acute illness with jaundice, malaise, anorexia, fever, abdominal pain, and arthralgia.

Etiology: The agent is believed to be a small (27 to 30 mm in diameter) RNA virus.

Epidemiology: Transmission of ET-NANB hepatitis is by the fecal-oral route. Disease is more common in adults than in children and has an unusually high mortality in pregnant women. Cases have been reported in epidemics or sporadically in parts of Asia, Africa, and Mexico, and have usually been related to contaminated water. Endemic ET-NANB hepatitis has not been recognized in Western

Europe or the United States, but cases have occurred in travelers to endemic areas. The period of communicability after acute infection is unknown.

The mean **incubation period** is about 40 days, with a range of 15 to 60 days.

Diagnostic Tests: No serologic test has been developed. The diagnosis is established by exclusion of acute hepatitis A, B, C, D, and other viral causes of acute hepatitis.

Treatment: Supportive.

Isolation of the Hospitalized Patient: Enteric precautions should be observed for the duration of the illness. However, until hepatitis B and C are excluded, patients should also be managed with precautions recommended for those diseases—i.e., the routinely recommended blood and body fluid precaution for all patients (see Isolation Precautions, page 81).

Control Measures: Good sanitation and avoiding the ingestion of potentially contaminated food and water are the most effective measures. Passive immunoprophylaxis against ET-NANB hepatitis with immune globulin prepared in the United States has not been demonstrated to be effective.

Herpes Simplex

Clinical Manifestations:

Neonatal. In newborn infants, herpes simplex virus (HSV) infection can manifest as (1) generalized, systemic infection involving the liver and other organs and including, occasionally, the central nervous system (encephalitis); (2) localized central nervous system disease; or (3) localized infection that may involve the skin, eyes, and mouth (SEM). Ocular manifestations include conjunctivitis, keratitis, and chorioretinitis. Typical vesicular skin lesions are helpful diagnostically, if present. In about one third of the patients, SEM involvement is the first indication of the infection. In another third, other evidence of systemic or central nervous system disease can occur before the appearance of SEM lesions; and in one third, infants with systemic or localized encephalitis will not have SEM involvement. In the absence of the more pathognomonic SEM lesions (keratitis), the differential diagnosis of respiratory distress, sepsis, and convulsions in newborn infants must include HSV infection. Although common in older children, asymptomatic HSV infection probably occurs rarely, if at all, in neonates.

Neonatal herpetic infections frequently are severe, with a high mortality rate and significant neurologic and/or ocular impairment of survivors, particularly in the absence of antiviral therapy. Recurrent skin lesions are frequently noted in surviving infants but their significance is unknown.

Initial symptoms can occur shortly after birth or as late as 4 to 6 weeks after birth. Disseminated disease usually occurs during the first 2 weeks of life; disease localized to the central nervous system or to the SEM more often occurs during the second or third week.

Children and Infants Beyond the Neonatal Period. Gingivostomatitis is the most commonly recognized manifestation of primary HSV infection. It is characterized by fever, irritability, and an enanthem involving the gingiva and the mucous membranes of the mouth. Most HSV infections at this age are asymptomatic.

Genital herpes is characterized by vesicular lesions of the male or female genital organs, and it is most common in adolescents and adults. Although autoinoculation of HSV type 1 from the mouth to other parts of the body occasionally occurs, sexual abuse must be considered if the disease is seen in prepubertal children, particularly if the causative virus is HSV type 2.

Patients with eczematoid dermatitis who are infected with HSV can develop eczema herpeticum with vesicular lesions concentrated in the areas of eczematous involvement.

In immunocompromised patients, severe local lesions and disseminated HSV infection with generalized vesicular skin lesions and visceral involvement can occur.

HSV tends to persist in a latent form after primary infection. Reactivation of latent virus most often is manifested by "cold sores" (herpes labialis). These lesions appear as single or grouped vesicles in the perioral region, usually on the vermilion border of the lips. Reactivation of genital HSV in the penis, scrotum, vulva, buttocks, and perianal areas, or on the thighs or back can also occur.

Eye infections can be a primary manifestation of HSV infection or a recurrence; they vary in severity from a superficial conjunctivitis to involvement of the deeper layers of the cornea.

HSV encephalitis can result from primary or recurrent infection and is associated with fever, alterations in the state of consciousness, personality changes, and convulsions. It frequently has an acute onset with a fulminant course, leading to coma and death in untreated patients. Cerebrospinal fluid pleocytosis with both lymphocytes and red blood cells is usual. HSV can also cause meningitis, in which the clinical manifestations are nonspecific, usually mild, and self limited.

An herpetic whitlow consists of single or multiple vesicular lesions, usually on the distal parts of fingers.

Etiology: Herpes simplex viruses are large, enveloped viruses containing DNA. The two types have major genomic and antigenic differences. Type 1 (HSV-1) usually involves the face and skin above the waist; type 2 (HSV-2) involves the genitalia and skin below the waist. However, either type of virus can be found in either site, depending on the type of contact.

Epidemiology:

Neonatal. The incidence of neonatal HSV infection is low; estimates range from 1 per 3,000 to 1 per 20,000 live births. Infants who develop HSV infection are significantly more likely to have been born prematurely and/or to be of low birth weight. HSV is most frequently transmitted to an infant during passage through an infected maternal lower genital tract during birth or by an ascending infection, sometimes through apparently intact membranes. Thus, most neonatal infections are caused by HSV-2 but 15% to 20% are due to HSV-1. Late intrauterine infections that manifest soon after birth are not infrequent. Intrauterine infections causing congenital malformations have been implicated in rare cases. Other less common sources of neonatal infection include the following: (a) postnatal transmission from the mother or father, most often from a nongenital infection (e.g., mouth, hands, or around the nipples); or (b) postnatal transmission in the nursery from another infected infant, probably via the hands of personnel attending the infants. Postnatal transmission from personnel with fever blisters to neonates has been extremely rare.

The risk of HSV infection in an infant born vaginally to a mother with a primary (first occurrence) genital infection is high (at least 40% to 50%). The risk to an infant born to a mother with recurrent HSV infection at delivery is much lower—at most 3% to 5%. **Distinguishing between primary and recurrent HSV infection in women by history or physical examination may not be possible.** Surveys suggest that 0.01% to 0.39% of American women shed HSV at delivery. Either primary or recurrent infection can be present without symptoms or nonspecific findings (e.g., vaginal discharge, genital pain, or shallow ulcers). Most infants who develop HSV infection have been born to women without history or clinical findings suggestive of active infection during pregnancy.

Incubation period: see Clinical Manifestations.

Children and Infants Beyond the Neonatal Period. HSV infections are ubiquitous and are transmitted from person to person throughout the year. HSV-1 infection is believed to result from direct contact with infected secretions primarily oral, or with lesions. HSV-2 infections usually result from direct contact with infected secretions through sexual activity. Type 1 strains can be recovered from the genital tract and type 2 strains can be recovered from the pharynx as a result of oral-genital sexual activity. HSV-1 genital infections in children can also result from autoinoculation of virus from the mouth. Nevertheless, sexual abuse must always be considered in prepubertal children with genital herpes.

HSV-1 is usually contracted during the first few years of life by those infected in lower socioeconomic groups; in higher socioeconomic groups, more than half the infected individuals do not contract HSV-1 until after they reach adulthood. The frequency of HSV-2 infection correlates with sexual activity, and HSV infections can occur in association with other sexually transmitted diseases.

Direct inoculation can cause herpetic whitlows of the fingers, usually from hand contact with HSV-containing oral secretions. Direct inoculation of skin can also occur, particularly among wrestlers (e.g., herpes gladiatorum).

The period of time that patients with primary gingivostomatitis or genital HSV can transmit infection is difficult to define. Virus usually can be isolated for at least 1 week, and occasionally for several months. HSV may be shed intermittently from the mouth in the absence of clinical manifestations years after infection. Most primary infections and recurrences are asymptomatic or are associated with minor intraoral or genital lesions. In recurrent lesions, virus is present in the highest concentrations in the first 24 hours after the appearance of vesicles. The amount of virus decreases rapidly in the next 24 hours and usually cannot be recovered after 5 days. HSV can be transmitted during primary infections or during recurrences, regardless of whether symptoms are present.

Genital HSV-2 and HSV-1 infections are commonly transmitted during sexual intercourse and by oral-genital sexual activity, respectively. Many primary infections are asymptomatic. Some individuals may not have recurrences; in others, recurrences can occur as often as every month. Genital HSV-2 infections are more likely to recur than those due to HSV-1. Viral shedding during recurrences can also occur in the absence of clinical signs.

The **incubation period** of genital infection, although not well defined, has been estimated to be 2 to 14 days.

Diagnostic Tests: HSV can be cultured relatively easily. Special transport media are available for specimens that cannot be inoculated immediately. Viral detection usually requires 1 to 3 days after tissue culture inoculation. Newer diagnostic techniques, such as direct fluorescent antibody staining of vesicle scrapings or ELISA detection of HSV antigens, offer more rapid diagnosis. A variety of techniques are available for distinguishing HSV-1 from HSV-2 isolates.

Positive swab cultures obtained from the conjunctiva, nasopharynx, or mouth of infants more than 24 to 48 hours after birth are more likely to indicate viral replication and infection than colonization. For the diagnosis of neonatal HSV infection, specimens for culture can be obtained from skin vesicles, mouth or nasopharynx, eyes, urine, blood, and cerebrospinal fluid. The most sensitive technique for detecting genital HSV infection in symptomatic pregnant women is culture of labial or cervical lesions or, in the absence of lesions, by culture of the cervix and vulva. Multinucleated giant cells and eosinophilic intranuclear inclusions in Papanicolaou-stained smears of the cervix may be present. This method is probably less sensitive than viral isolation in tissue culture.

Acute and convalescent sera can be tested for rises in antibody to confirm acute primary infection, but serologic diagnosis frequently is less helpful than viral isolation, as "acute" sera are often obtained late in the course of the illness. Rises in antibody titer are not usually demonstrable during recurrences.

In children with suspected HSV encephalitis, a brain biopsy is useful before (or soon after) therapy is initiated, as it may identify other treatable causes of encephalitis or confirm a diagnosis of HSV infection. Cerebrospinal fluid cultures are rarely positive for virus in patients with encephalitis.

Treatment: In children, acyclovir and vidarabine have been used primarily for potentially serious infections, as occur in neonates and immunocompromised children. The use of these drugs in less serious conditions has been limited primarily to adults, and information on children in these conditions is limited. For recommended antiviral dosages and duration of therapy, see Antiviral Drugs, page 578.

Neonatal. Acyclovir and vidarabine are both effective in the treatment of neonatal HSV infection localized to the skin, eyes, and mouth. Antiviral treatment is also beneficial in the treatment of localized central nervous system disease and, to a lesser extent, in the treatment of generalized, systemic infection. For reasons of lower toxicity and ease of administration, acyclovir (30 mg/kg/d in 3 divided doses, given intravenously) is the preferred drug. The optimal duration of therapy has not been established; recommended minimum duration is 14 days. Longer courses of 14 to 21 days may be indicated in some cases. Whether 21 days of therapy improves outcome is being studied in a collaborative, multi-institution trial. Relapse of disease after cessation of treatment can occur and is usually related to host factors, but acyclovir resistance has been reported. The need for retreatment of infants with recurrent skin lesions is undetermined and is being investigated.

Antiviral therapy is generally more effective if started early in the course of the disease. The effectiveness of antiviral drugs for prophylactic treatment of exposed newborns has not yet been adequately studied but some experts believe that anticipatory antiviral therapy is warranted for an infant born vaginally to a mother with active HSV infection, particularly if the infant also has other risk factors (e.g., prematurity, invasive instrumentation, or lacerations).

Infants with ocular involvement due to HSV infection should receive a topical ophthalmic drug (specifically, 1% to 2% trifluridine, 1% iododeoxyuridine, or 3% vidarabine), as well as parenteral antiviral therapy. Ophthalmologic consultation is strongly advised.

Genital Infection.

Primary. In adults, acyclovir diminishes the duration of symptoms and viral shedding in primary genital herpes. Oral acyclovir initiated within 6 days of onset of the disease has been demonstrated to shorten by approximately 3 to 5 days the median duration of the signs and symptoms and viral shedding from primary lesions. Intravenous acyclovir should be used only for primary genital herpes in patients with a severe or complicated course that requires hospitalization. Topical acyclovir (5%) ointment applied to primary genital herpes minimally reduces viral shedding and symptoms. Treatment of primary herpetic lesions does not affect the subsequent risk or severity of recurrences.

Recurrent. Antiviral therapy has minimal effect on recurrent genital herpes. Oral acyclovir initiated within 2 days of onset of symptoms shortens the mean clinical course by 1 day. Viral excretion may be diminished, which may shorten the duration of contagiousness. Topical acyclovir is not beneficial.

Oral acyclovir administered daily to adults for suppressive therapy has been effective in decreasing the frequency of recurrences of active disease in persons with frequent recurrences (six or more episodes per year) of genital HSV infection. After 1 year of continuous daily therapy, acyclovir should be discontinued and the patient's recurrence rate should be assessed. Usually, however, the disease recurs at the same frequency as before the course of suppressive therapy. Acyclovir appears to be safe in adults receiving the drug for 3 years, but the long-term effects are unknown. Acyclovir is not recommended for pregnant women.

Other Mucocutaneous HSV Infections.

In Immunocompromised Hosts. Intravenous acyclovir and vidarabine have been effective in the treatment and prevention of dissemination of mucocutaneous HSV infections. Topical acyclovir also can accelerate the healing of recurrent lesions in immunocompromised patients. For prophylaxis of mucocutaneous infection, both oral and intravenous acyclovir have been beneficial in reducing the rate of recurrences during the course of therapy, but not after the therapy is discontinued.

In Immunocompetent Hosts. Insufficient information is available to know if the effects of acyclovir on primary or recurrent nongenital mucocutaneous herpetic disease are similar to those observed for genital HSV infections. In adults, no therapeutic benefit has been demonstrated from use of acyclovir in individuals with recurrent "cold sores." Children with severe primary gingival stomatitis have been treated with acyclovir but no data on efficacy are available.

Ocular. Treatment of eye lesions usually should be undertaken with the help of an ophthalmologist. A variety of DNA inhibitors, such as 1% to 2% trifluridine, 1% iododeoxyuridine, and 3% vidarabine, have been successful for topical therapy of superficial keratitis. Topical steroids are contraindicated in suspected HSV conjunctivitis. However, ophthalmologists may choose to use steroids in conjunction with antiviral drugs to treat more locally invasive infections.

Encephalitis. Acyclovir is the drug of choice for the treatment of patients with HSV encephalitis; it is more likely to be beneficial if treatment is initiated early in the illness. Therapy is less effective in adults than in children, and less effective in comatose and semi-comatose patients than in those who are not.

Isolation of the Hospitalized Patient:

Neonates With HSV Infection. Neonates with HSV infection, or with positive cultures in the absence of disease, should be hospitalized in a private room, if possible, and managed with contact isolation for the duration of the illness.

Neonates Exposed to HSV During Delivery. Neonates with documented perinatal exposure to HSV may be in the incubation phase of infection and should be carefully observed. One method of infection control is to have the infant room–in continuously with the mother in a private room. Infants born vaginally (or by cesarean delivery if membranes have been ruptured for more than 4 to 6 hours) to a mother with active HSV lesions should be physically separated from other infants and placed in contact isolation if they are hospitalized in the nursery during the incubation period. The risk of HSV infection in possibly exposed infants (e.g., those born to a mother with a history of recurrent genital herpes) is low. Although expert opinion varies, special isolation precautions for these infants are not needed in most instances.

Women in Labor and Postpartum Women With HSV Infection. Women in labor who have active HSV lesions, or whose viral cultures or Papanicolaou smear were positive, should be managed during labor, delivery, and the postpartum period with contact or drainage/secretion precautions, depending on the extent of the mucocutaneous disease. These mothers should be instructed on the importance of careful hand washing before and after caring for their infant. A clean covering gown may be used to help avoid contact of the infant with the lesions or infectious secretions. A mother with herpes labialis ("cold sores") or stomatitis should wear a disposable surgical mask when touching her newborn until the lesions have crusted and dried. She should not kiss or nuzzle her newborn until the lesions have cleared. Herpetic lesions on other skin sites should be covered. Breast feeding is acceptable if no lesions are present on the breast and if active lesions elsewhere on the mother are covered.

Children With Mucocutaneous HSV Infection. For patients with severe mucocutaneous HSV infection, contact isolation is advised. Patients with localized recurrent lesions should be managed with drainage/secretion precautions for the duration of the illness, or until the virus no longer can be recovered from the lesions.

Patients With Central Nervous System HSV Infection. Patients with infection limited to the central nervous system do not require special isolation precautions.

Control Measures:

Prevention of Neonatal Infection. Expert opinion varies widely on the appropriate management of pregnant women to minimize the risk of neonatal HSV infection and has changed considerably in recent years. Women with history of previous genital HSV infection and signs or symptoms of infection during pregnancy, or whose sexual partners have genital HSV infection, are at low but increased risk of transmitting HSV to their infants. As a result, in the early 1980s most experts recommended that all pregnant women with history of HSV infection before or during pregnancy should be monitored weekly during the last several months of pregnancy for evidence of HSV infection; those who were HSV-positive or had clinical lesions and whose membranes were intact had a cesarean delivery. This management plan is unsatisfactory for the following reasons: (1) it does not prevent all neonatal HSV infection because most infected infants are born to women who do not, by history, have evidence of prior HSV genital infection; (2) little correlation exists between antepartum HSV infection and viral shedding at delivery; (3) the incidence of neonatal HSV infection is low compared to the incidence of known HSV infection in pregnant women, especially those with recurrent infection; and (4) the difficulty and expense of screening, and the cost and risk of cesarean deliveries without other indications is high relative to the number of cases of neonatal disease that are potentially averted. Similarly, intrapartum cultures have not had sufficient predictive value to be useful.

Although no single management plan can be recommended for all circumstances, current recommendations for prevention of neonatal infection include the following:

Pregnant Women. All pregnant women should be questioned during a prenatal visit about history of HSV infection in themselves or in their sexual partners, and signs and symptoms of current infection should be sought as part of prenatal care.

Women in Labor. During labor all women should be questioned about recent and current HSV symptoms and carefully examined for evidence of genital HSV infection. Cesarean delivery of women in labor who have clinically apparent HSV infection (particularly primary infection) may reduce the risk of neonatal HSV infection unless the membranes have been ruptured for more than 4 to 6 hours. The risk in situations where the membranes have been ruptured for longer periods is uncertain, and many obstetricians prefer to deliver infants by cesarean section whenever the birth canal is infected, even if the membranes had previously ruptured. A history of genital HSV for a woman in labor is not an indication for cesarean section.

Scalp monitors should be avoided when possible in infants of women suspected of having genital herpes.

Care of Exposed Newborns.

Infants Born to Mothers With Active Genital Lesions.

- *By vaginal delivery.* The infant should be observed carefully for skin or scalp rashes, especially vesicular lesions; and unexplained clinical manifestations, including respiratory distress, seizures and signs of sepsis. If any of these manifestations occurs, the infant should be evaluated for possible HSV as well as for bacterial infection. Skin lesions, conjunctiva, nasopharynx, mouth, and urine should be cultured for HSV. Acyclovir should be initiated if culture(s) from the infant are positive, or if HSV infection is strongly suspected while awaiting culture results, bacterial cultures are negative or pending, and no other causes of the infant's clinical manifestations are found.

Some experts obtain HSV cultures of the conjunctiva, nasopharynx, mouth, and urine from asymptomatic infants at 24 to 48 hours of age, since positive HSV cultures from one or more of these specimens obtained at this time are more likely to indicate infection than transient colonization from intrapartum exposure and, thus, may be justification for therapy. In contrast, a positive maternal or neonatal culture taken at the time of delivery (vaginal or cesarean) does not necessarily indicate infection of the newborn.

For asymptomatic infants exposed to herpetic lesions during delivery, the decision to treat empirically with acyclovir is controversial. The infection rate of infants born to mothers with active recurrent genital herpes infections is 5% or less. However, the risk is increased for those infants born of mothers with active primary infection, those born prematurely or who have history of instrumentation or lacerations during delivery. Some experts, hence, recommend emrical acyclovir treatment at birth for infants exposed during delivery to maternal herpes infection who have one or more of these risk factors. However, differentiation of primary from recurrent HSV infection in the mother is often difficult.

- *By cesarean delivery*. The infant should be observed carefully, and cultures should be obtained, as recommended for the potentially exposed infant born by vaginal delivery. Similarly, antiviral therapy should be initiated if culture(s) from the infant are positive, or if HSV is strongly suspected while awaiting culture results (assuming other causes of the infant's manifestations are not identified).

Data confirming the benefit or need for antiviral therapy in these circumstances of the exposed infant born by vaginal or cesarean delivery are not yet available.

Infants Born to Mothers With History of Genital HSV but No Active Lesions at Delivery. These infants should be carefully evaluated, as previously described. The value of the intrapartum cultures, however, from these women is unclear but some experts recommend that they be obtained from the mother and/or the neonate on the day of delivery. One or more positive cultures, however, indicates only exposure and does not necessarily indicate infection.

Other Recommendations:

- The length of in-hospital observation for infants at increased risk for neonatal HSV is empiric and based on factors specific to the infant and local resources, such as the family's ability to observe the infant at home, availability of follow-up care, and clinical assessment.
- Delay of elective or ritual circumcision for about a month for infants at highest risk of disease is prudent.
- Since neonatal HSV infection can occur as late as 6 weeks after delivery, physicians must be vigilant and not ignore a new rash or symptoms which might be due to HSV.

Care of Persons With Dermatitis. Patients with dermatitis are at risk of developing eczema herpeticum. If these patients are hospitalized, special care should be taken to avoid exposure to HSV. They should not be kissed by persons with "cold sores" or handled by people with herpetic whitlow.

Care of Children With Mucocutaneous Infections Who Are in Day Care or School. Oral HSV infections are common in children who are in day care or school. Most of these infections are asymptomatic. In addition, recurrent shedding of virus in saliva in the absence of clinical disease is common. Only those children with HSV gingivostomatitis who do not have control of oral secretions should be excluded from day care. Exclusion of children with "cold sores" from day care or school is not indicated.

Children with uncovered lesions on exposed surfaces and who were infected with HSV as newborn infants or as a result of sexual abuse pose a small potential risk to contacts. If children are certified by a physician to have recurrent HSV infection, covering the active lesions with clothing, a bandage, or an appropriate dressing when they attend day care or school is prudent. If exposed lesions are not easily covered, exclusion of such a child from day care is preferable.

Infected Hospital Personnel. Transmission of HSV in newborn nurseries from infected personnel to newborn infants has rarely been documented. The risk of transmission to infants by personnel who have labial HSV infection ("cold sores") or who are asymptomatic oral shedders of the virus is not known, but probably is low. Compromising patient care by excluding personnel with "cold sores" who are essential for the operation of the nursery must be weighed against the potential risk of infecting newborn infants. Personnel with cold sores who have indirect contact with infants should cover and not touch their lesions, should carefully observe hand washing policies, and must not kiss or nuzzle newborn infants or children with dermatitis. Transmission of HSV infection from personnel with genital lesions is not likely as long as hand washing policies are carefully observed. Personnel with herpetic whitlow should not have responsibility for direct care of neonates, immunocompromised patients, or patients in an intensive care unit.

Histoplasmosis

Clinical Manifestations: Histoplasmosis encompasses a spectrum of clinical diseases. Asymptomatic infection is most common and is recognized from serologic and skin test conversion. Acute pulmonary histoplasmosis is an influenza-like illness with pulmonary infiltrates and hilar adenopathy. Chronic pulmonary histoplasmosis resembles chronic tuberculosis in adults. Acute disseminated histoplasmosis is most frequent in infants younger than 2 years; symptoms include fever, cough, hepatosplenomegaly, adenopathy, pneumonitis, skin lesions, diarrhea, and pancytopenia resembling acute lymphatic leukemia. Chronic histoplasmosis ranges from a single pulmonary lesion to disseminated disease, and is rare in children. Patients with AIDS are at increased risk for disseminated histoplasmosis.

Etiology: *Histoplasma capsulatum* is a dimorphic fungus. In soil, it exists in the mycelial form but converts to a yeast form at the body temperature (37°) of mammals.

Epidemiology: *H capsulatum* is encountered in many parts of the world; it is endemic in the eastern and central United States. Infection is acquired through inhalation of air-borne spores (conidia). The source of the organism is soil or dust in barnyards and other locations harboring bat and bird droppings. Histoplasmosis is not transmitted from person to person.

The **incubation period** is variable but is usually a few weeks from the time of exposure.

Diagnostic Tests: Direct demonstration of intracellular yeast cells in smears of bone marrow or biopsy material from lymph nodes, liver, or spleen is evidence for a presumptive diagnosis. Wright and Giemsa stains usually are adequate, but the Gomori silver methenamine stain is more likely to detect sparse organisms. Bone marrow, blood, sputum, and material from lesions should be cultured on brain-heart infusion and modified Sabouraud's medium at room temperature. Laboratory workers should be aware of the hazards of mycelial-bearing conidia and resulting potential for transmission.

Two skin test preparations, a mycelium-derived antigen* and a yeast-derived antigen,† are available. The yeast-derived antigen has the advantage of decreased likelihood of stimulating preexisting serum antibody titers. A positive reaction with either test indicates either current or previous *Histoplasma* infection.

Both mycelial-phase (histoplasmin) and yeast-phase antigens are used in serologic testing for complement-fixing antibodies to *H capsulatum.* Low titers are often present in healthy persons living in endemic areas. A fourfold rise in yeast-phase titers or a single high titer (more than 1:128) indicates active infections. Serum titers of mycelial but not the yeast-phase antibodies can increase slightly after skin testing with mycelium-derived histoplasmin. In the immunodiffusion precipitin test, H bands are highly suggestive of active infection. Cross-reacting antibodies can result from *Blastomyces dermatiditis* and *Coccidioides immitis* infections.

Treatment: The uncomplicated, primary pulmonary form of histoplasmosis requires no specific therapy. Amphotericin B is effective in progressive, disseminated disease, and is the drug of choice in such cases and in immunocompromised patients (e.g., those with AIDS) with histoplasmosis.

Ketoconazole, an oral imidazole antifungal agent, has been useful in the treatment of histoplasmosis. Based on a limited number of cases, it appears safe in children younger than 2 years. However, in patients with severe disease or who are immunocompromised, amphotericin B is recommended.

---

*Available from Parke-Davis, Morris Plains, NJ

†Available from Berkeley Biologicals, Berkeley, CA

Duration of treatment is determined from clinical and laboratory evidence that active fungal infection has subsided. The minimum duration of treatment with amphotericin B is 6 weeks. For ketoconazole, 3 to 5 months of therapy is necessary.

Isolation of the Hospitalized Patient: No special precautions are recommended.

Control Measures: Investigation for the common source of infection in outbreaks is indicated.

Hookworm Infections

Ancylostoma duodenale and *Necator americanus*

Clinical Manifestations: Intense pruritus ("ground" or "dew" itch) can occur at the site of larval penetration into skin in contact with contaminated soil, usually skin on the soles of the feet and between the toes. The principal manifestation of the subsequent hookworm infection is anemia secondary to blood loss from the intestinal mucosa where the worms are attached. Blood loss results from ingestion by the worms and subsequent bleeding caused by the anticoagulant they secrete. Hypochromic and microcytic anemia, hypoproteinemia, and malnutrition can result in heavily infected persons; eosinophilia is common. Well-nourished, lightly infected individuals are often asymptomatic but epigastric discomfort and tenderness can occur. Stool can be positive for occult blood but does not have gross blood. Pulmonary infiltration with cough and wheezing can occur in patients heavily infected.

Etiology: Infection is caused by *Ancylostoma duodenale* and *Necator americanus*, two worms with identical life cycles but differing epidemiology.

Epidemiology: *A duodenale* is the predominant species in Europe, the Mediterranean region, northern Asia, and the west coast of South America. *N americanus* predominates in the Western hemisphere and in sub-Saharan Africa, Southeast Asia, and a number of Pacific islands. Untreated infected persons can harbor the worms for as many as 30 years, but most patients who do not become reinfected lose the hookworm infection within 2 years. Larvae can remain infective in the soil for several weeks, particularly in damp, shaded areas, and for far shorter periods in drier environments.

Diagnostic Tests: Hookworm eggs can be identified in the feces by direct microscopic examination. In light infections, concentration techniques may be needed. Adult worms or larvae are rarely seen.

Treatment: Pyrantel pamoate (11 mg/kg, maximum 1 g, daily for 3 days) or mebendazole (100 mg twice daily for 3 days) is the drug of choice. In children younger than 2 years, in whom experience with either drug is limited, the risks and benefits of therapy should be considered before drug administration. Pyrantel pamoate has the advantage of single-dose administration. Either treatment may be repeated if necessary. Nutritional supplementation, including iron, is important when anemia is present; severely affected children may require blood transfusion.

Isolation of the Hospitalized Patient: No special precautions are recommended.

Control Measures: Sanitary disposal of feces to prevent contamination of the soil, particularly in endemic areas, is necessary but rarely accomplished. Treatment of all known infected patients can help reduce environmental contamination. The wearing of shoes is also helpful, but this measure is unrealistic in economically deprived areas.

Infectious Mononucleosis Due to Epstein-Barr Virus

Clinical Manifestations: Infectious mononucleosis is typically manifested by fever, exudative pharyngitis, lymphadenopathy, hepatosplenomegaly, and atypical lymphocytes in the peripheral blood. However, the spectrum of disease is extremely variable, ranging from asymptomatic to fatal infection. Infections frequently go unrecognized in young infants and young children. Infection occasionally can be accompanied by a rash, which is more frequent in patients treated with ampicillin. Central nervous system complications include aseptic meningitis, encephalitis, and the Guillain-Barré syndrome. Rare complications include splenic rupture, thrombocytopenia, agranulocytosis, hemolytic anemia, orchitis, and myocarditis. Epstein-Barr virus (EBV) infects B-lymphocytes, which respond by lymphoproliferation. Ordinarily, the replication of the virus and the proliferation of cells is checked by natural killer and T cell responses, but in patients who have congenital or acquired cellular immune deficiencies, fatal disseminated infection or B-cell lymphomas can occur. The status of "chronic" infectious mononucleosis is still controversial and most, if not all, cases appear not to be related to infection with EBV. However, a small group of patients with recurrent symptoms have markedly abnormal serologic tests for EBV.

Elsewhere in the world, two other syndromes caused by EBV assume much greater importance than infectious mononucleosis. Burkitt B-cell lymphoma, found in Central Africa, and nasopharyngeal carcinoma, found in Southeast Asia, appear to be caused by persistent EBV infection.

Etiology: EBV, a DNA virus, is a herpesvirus.

Epidemiology: Humans are the sole source of EBV. Intimate contact is usually required for transmission. EBV is also occasionally transmitted by blood transfusion. Infection frequently is contracted early in life, particularly among lower socioeconomic groups, in which intrafamilial spread is common. Endemic infectious mononucleosis is common in group settings of adolescents, such as in educational institutions. No seasonal predilection exists. Viral excretion can occur for many months after infection, and asymptomatic carriage is common. The period of communicability is indeterminate.

The **incubation period** is estimated to be 30 to 50 days.

Diagnostic Tests: EBV isolation from oropharyngeal secretions is possible, but techniques for performing this procedure are usually not available in routine diagnostic laboratories, and viral isolation does not necessarily indicate acute infection. Hence, diagnosis depends on serologic testing. Nonspecific tests for heterophil antibody, including the Paul-Bunnell test and slide agglutination reaction, are most commonly available. These tests are often negative in infants and children younger than 4 years with EBV infection, but will identify about 90% of cases (proven by EBV-specific serology) in older children and adults.

Multiple specific serologic antibody tests for EBV are available in diagnostic virology laboratories (Table 36). The most commonly performed test is for antibody against the viral capsid antigen (VCA). IgG antibody against VCA is found in high titers early after onset of infection. Therefore, testing of paired sera for anti-VCA may not be useful in establishing infection. Testing for IgM anti-VCA antibody and for antibodies against early antigen (EA) are useful in identifying recent infections. Antibody against EBV nuclear antigens (EBNA) can be identified only several weeks to months after onset of the infection. The demonstration of anti-EBNA antibody excludes recent infection.

Table 36. Serum EBV Antibodies in EBV Infection

Infection	Anti-VCA-IgG*	Anti-VCA-IgM†	Anti-EA (D)‡	Anti-EBNA§
No previous infection	0	0	0	0
Acute infection	+	+	+/0	0
Recent infection	+	+/0	+/0	+/0
Past infection	+	0	0	+

*Anti-VCA-IgG: IgG class antibody to viral capsid antigen.
†Anti-VCA-IgM: IgM class antibody to viral capsid antigen.
‡EA(D): early antigen diffuse staining.
§EBNA: Epstein-Barr nuclear antigen.
0 = < 1:10 or < 1:2 for EBNA.
+ = ≥ 1:10 or ≥ 1:2 for EBNA.

Virus-specific serology is particularly valuable for studying patients who have heterophil-negative infectious mononucleosis. Testing for other viral agents, especially cytomegalovirus, is indicated in these patients.

Treatment: Steroids have been useful for control of tonsillar swelling and other lymphadenopathy but are not recommended for routine cases. Although acyclovir has good in vitro antiviral activity against EBV, the clinical effects of treatment have not been striking.

Isolation of the Hospitalized Patient: No special precautions are recommended.

Control Measures: Patients with a recent history of EBV infection or an infectious mononucleosis-like illness should not donate blood.

Influenza

Clinical Manifestations: Influenza is characterized by the sudden onset of fever, frequently with chills or rigors, headache, malaise, diffuse myalgia, and a dry cough. Subsequently, the respiratory signs—sore throat, nasal congestion, and cough—become more prominent. Conjunctival infection, abdominal pain, nausea, and vomiting can be present. In some children, influenza may appear as a simple upper respiratory tract infection or as a febrile illness with few respiratory signs. In young infants, influenza can produce a sepsis-like picture and occasionally cause croup or pneumonia. Acute myositis characterized by calf tenderness and refusal to walk may develop after several days of influenza, especially type B. Reye syndrome has been associated primarily with influenza B, but also with influenza A infection.

Etiology: Influenza viruses are orthomyxoviruses of three antigenic types (A, B, and C). Epidemic disease is caused by types A and B. Influenza A strains are subclassified by two antigens, hemagglutinin (H) and neuraminidase (N). Three immunologically distinct hemagglutinin subtypes (H1, H2, and H3) and two neuraminidases (N1 and N2) have been recognized as causing human infection. Specific antibodies to these various antigens are important determinants of immunity. Major changes in either of these antigens, such as H1 to H2, are called antigenic shifts. Minor variations within the same subtypes are called antigenic drifts. Antigenic shift has occurred only with influenza A, usually at intervals of 10 or more years. Antigenic drift, which occurs almost annually in both influenza A and B viruses, can during a period of several years result in susceptibility to infection with a type of influenza with which persons were previously infected or immunized.

Epidemiology: Influenza is spread from person to person by direct contact, large droplet infection, or articles recently contaminated by nasopharyngeal secretions. In some explosive outbreaks, air-borne transmission by small particle aerosols has appeared to be an important mode of transmission. During an outbreak of influenza, the highest attack rates occur in school-aged children. Secondary spread to adults and other children within the family is common. The attack rates depend in part on the immunity developed by previous experience with the circulating strain or a related strain by prior natural disease or immunization. Antigenic shift or major drift in the circulating strain is most likely to produce widespread epidemics. In temperate climates, epidemics almost always occur during the winter months and last 4 to 8 weeks within a community; the peak usually occurs within 2 weeks of the onset. In recent years, activity of two or three types of influenza virus in a community has been common and has been associated with a prolongation of the influenza season to 3 months or more. Influenza is highly contagious, especially among institutionalized populations. Patients are most infectious in the 24 hours before onset of symptoms and during the period of peak symptoms. Viral shedding in the nasal secretions usually ceases within 7 days of the onset of illness, but it can persist longer in young children.

The impact of influenza on children is appreciable during interepidemic as well as epidemic years in both healthy children and those with underlying high-risk conditions. Attack rates in healthy children have recently been estimated at 10% to 40% each year, and approximately 1% of these infections can result in hospitalization. The risk of lower respiratory tract disease complicating influenza infection has ranged from 0.2% to 25%. A wide variety of complications, such as Reye syndrome, myositis, and central nervous system manifestations can occur. Reported mortality has been 1% to 4%. The risk of subsequent Reye syndrome, which occurs primarily in school-aged children, has decreased in recent years. In contrast to patterns of respiratory disease in adults, other respiratory viruses (e.g., respiratory syncytial virus and the parainfluenza viruses) cause yearly outbreaks of infection that can produce life-threatening illness in young children. As a result, morbidity and mortality rates in children for influenza are more difficult to determine and the effect of control measures for influenza can be more difficult to measure in children.

Excess rates of hospitalization have been documented for children with influenza who are neonates or who have sickle-cell disease, bronchopulmonary dysplasia, severe asthma, cystic fibrosis, malignancies, diabetes, or chronic renal disease. Pulmonary complications such as bronchitis and pneumonia appear to be more common in these children. Influenza in neonates has been associated with considerable morbidity, including a sepsis-like syndrome, apnea, and lower respiratory tract disease.

The **incubation period** is usually 1 to 3 days.

Diagnostic Tests: Cultures, when performed, should be obtained during the first 72 hours of illness because the quantity of virus subsequently decreases rapidly. Nasopharyngeal secretions, by swab or aspirate, should be placed in appropriate transport media for culture. After inoculation into eggs or tissue culture, virus can usually be isolated within 2 to 6 days. The sensitivity of rapid diagnostic tests such as immunofluorescence for identification of influenza antigen in nasopharyngeal specimens has been variable. Serologic diagnosis can be made retrospectively by a significant change in antibody titer between acute and convalescent sera, as determined by complement fixation, hemagglutination inhibition, neutralization, or ELISA tests.

Treatment: Amantadine and its closely related analogue rimantadine (investigational in the United States) diminish the severity of the signs and symptoms of influenza A but not influenza B. Antiviral therapy should be considered for patients with severe disease or for those with underlying conditions rendering them at high risk for severe or complicated influenza infection. The dosage is 4.4 mg/kg/d, given orally, in two doses, but not to exceed 150 mg/d for children 9 years or younger or who weigh less than 45 kg. For older children or those who weigh more than 45 kg, it is 200 mg/d in two divided doses. Little information is available on the use of amantadine in children younger than 1 year. Therapy should be started as soon as possible after the onset of symptoms and continued for 2 to 7 days, depending on clinical improvement. Amantadine may cause mild central nervous system symptoms that clear with discontinuation of the drug; it has also been reported to increase EEG abnormalities in children with preexisting major motor disorders.

Control of fever with acetaminophen can be important in young children as the fever of influenza can precipitate febrile convulsions. **Children with influenza should not receive salicylates because of the resulting increased risk of developing Reye syndrome.**

Isolation of the Hospitalized Patient: For children hospitalized with influenza or an influenza-like illness, contact isolation is recommended for the duration of the illness. Respiratory secretions should be considered infectious and strict hand washing procedures should be used.

Control Measures:

Influenza Vaccine. The current influenza vaccines produced in embryonated eggs are immunogenic, safe, and associated with minimal side effects. The vaccines are multivalent and contain different viral subtypes; the composition is periodically changed in anticipation of the expected prevalent influenza strains. The two preparations currently in use are the inactivated whole virus vaccine, prepared from the intact, purified virus particles, and the subvirion (split) vaccine, prepared by the additional step of disrupting the lipid-containing membrane of the virus. Only the split virus vaccine should be used for children younger than 13 years.

Immunogenicity in Children. In children with little previous experience with influenza, two doses of vaccine administered 1 month apart are necessary to produce a satisfactory antibody response. Individuals previously primed with a related strain of influenza by infection or vaccination almost uniformly exhibit a brisk antibody response to one dose of the vaccine.

Vaccine Efficacy. The impact of influenza immunization on acute respiratory illness is less likely to be evident in pediatric than adult populations because of the frequency of colds, upper respiratory tract infections, and influenza-like illness caused by other viral agents in young children. The efficacy of the currently available killed vaccines has also been difficult to assess because of yearly variation in the strains of the circulating viruses, and their resulting variation in similarity to the antigens contained in the available vaccines. The protection in healthy subjects from either the whole virus or split virus vaccines against homologous viral-type challenge is usually 70% to 80%, with a range of 50% to 95%.

In infants in the first 6 months of life, efficacy has not been evaluated.

Special Considerations:

- Influenza immunization of high-risk children between 6 and 24 months is occasionally associated with fever at 6 to 24 hours and could exacerbate underlying disease.
- In immunosuppressed children receiving chemotherapy, influenza immunization with a new vaccine antigen results in a sufficient immune response in only a minority of children. The optimal time to immunize children with malignancies who still must undergo chemotherapy, therefore, is when they have been off chemotherapy for 3 to 4 weeks and have peripheral granulocyte and lymphocyte counts greater than 1,000/mm^3. Children who are no longer receiving chemotherapy generally have a high rate of seroconversion.
- The immune response and safety of influenza vaccine in children with hemodynamically unstable cardiac disease, another large group of children potentially at high risk for complications of influenza, is comparable to that of normal children.
- Infants younger than 6 months with high-risk conditions, especially those with cardiopulmonary compromise, may be at as much or greater risk than older children. However, no information is available about the reactivity, immunogenicity, or efficacy of the influenza vaccines in infants during the first 6 months of life. In addition, the effort of influenza antigens in an inactivated vaccine on the infant's future immune response to influenza is not known. Thus, alternative methods of protection for young infants should be considered (see Alternative Methods of Protecting Children against Influenza, page 281).

Recommendations for Influenza Immunization

Targeted high-risk children. The following groups of children, 6 months or older, are particularly in need of yearly immunization:

- Children with chronic pulmonary diseases, including those with moderate to severe asthma, bronchopulmonary dysplasia, and cystic fibrosis.
- Children with hemodynamically significant cardiac disease.
- Children receiving immunosuppressive therapy (for the optimal time of administration, see Special Considerations).
- Children with sickle-cell and other hemoglobinopathies.

Other high-risk children. Other children who should be considered potentially at increased risk for complicated influenza illness and who may benefit from influenza immunization are those with diabetes, chronic renal and metabolic diseases, symptomatic HIV infection (see AIDS and HIV Infections, page 124), and those receiving long-term aspirin therapy, such as children with rheumatoid arthritis or Kawasaki disease who may be at an increased risk of developing Reye syndrome. In children with any disease who are marginally compensated, even uncomplicated influenza can produce adverse effects on the course of the underlying disease.

Close contacts of high-risk patients. Immunization and chemoprophylaxis of adults who are in close contact with high-risk children may be an important means of protection for these children, especially for infants below the age recommended for vaccination. The immunization of pregnant women may be beneficial to the infant, as infants appear to be protected from infection with influenza A virus by transplacentally acquired antibody. The following is recommended:

- Immunization should be encouraged for hospital personnel in contact with pediatric patients.
- Household contacts, including siblings and primary caretakers of high-risk children, should be immunized.
- Children who are members of households with high-risk adults, including those with symptomatic HIV infection, should be immunized.

Other children. Children who are not currently classified as high risk, but for whom control of influenza may be particularly important and for whom vaccination should be considered, are children who are institutionalized, in college or other institutions of higher learning, in boarding schools, or in day care.

Normal children. Although the morbidity from influenza in normal children can be appreciable, routine immunization of normal children at this time is not feasible. Such immunizations would have to be given yearly; for children younger than 9 years, two doses would have to be administered the initial year. However, because the inactivated influenza vaccines are generally safe and immunogenic in normal children, immunization is not contraindicated and should be given at the discretion of the physician and the parent or guardian.

Vaccine Administration. Influenza vaccine should be administered in the autumn, before the start of the influenza season, which is usually December or later. The recommended vaccine, dose, and schedule for different age groups are given in Table 37. Annual vaccination is recommended because of declining immunity in the year after vaccination.

Influenza vaccine may be administered simultaneously (but at a separate site and with a different syringe) with MMR, *Haemophilus* b, pneumococcal, and oral poliovirus vaccines (see Simultaneous Administration of Multiple Vaccines, page 16). Since both influenza and pertussis vaccines in young children can cause febrile reactions,

Table 37. Schedule for Influenza Immunization*

Age	Recommended Vaccine	Dose†	Number of Doses
6-35 mo	Split virus only	0.25 mL	1-2‡
3-8 y	Split virus only	0.5 mL	1-2‡
9-12 y	Split virus only	0.5 mL	1
≥ 12 y	Whole or split virus	0.5 mL	1

*Vaccine is administered intramuscularly.

†Dose given was for 1990-1991 season. Hence, in subsequent years, consult package insert for dose recommendations of each vaccine.

‡Two doses are recommended if the child is receiving influenza vaccine for the first time. If the hemagglutinin and neuraminidase of vaccine strains have not changed, subsequent immunization may be achieved with one dose yearly.

influenza vaccine usually should not be given within 3 days of vaccination with DTP.

Reactions, Adverse Effects, and Contraindications. Febrile reactions in children younger than 13 years are infrequent, especially after split-virus vaccine administration, and occur primarily in young children. Local reactions are infrequent in children younger than 13 years, and occur in approximately 10% of older children immunized with either whole or split-virus vaccine.

Despite concern about the safety of 1976 swine influenza vaccine and Guillain-Barré syndrome (GBS) in older adults, the incidence of GBS after immunization for swine influenza in children or young adults (e.g., military recruits) was not increased. Subsequent studies of immunization with influenza vaccine have not indicated an increased risk of GBS or of other neurologic diseases.

Immunization of children who have asthma with the currently available influenza vaccines is not associated with a detectable increase in adverse reactions, such as bronchial reactivity or leukocyte histamine release.

Children demonstrating severe, anaphylactic reaction to chickens or eggs rarely experience a similar type of reaction to killed influenza vaccines. If influenza vaccine is considered for children with these allergies, skin testing is indicated (see Hypersensitivity Reactions to Vaccine Constituents, page 29). An immediate-reacting IgE skin test using a dilution of influenza vaccine may be a more reliable indicator of allergy than is the history. If skin testing confirms hypersensitivity, these children should not receive influenza vaccine, and if they are older than 1 year, prophylactic amantadine should be offered if an epidemic occurs.

Alternative Methods of Protecting Children Against Influenza - Chemoprophylaxis.

Most studies demonstrating the efficacy of amantadine as a chemoprophylactic agent against influenza A infection have been performed in adults, but several studies in children have indicated a similar beneficial effect in diminishing the spread of influenza among institutionalized children and family members and on pediatric wards. Amantadine appears to be well tolerated in children, except those with preexisting major motor neurologic disorders, and the pharmacokinetics appear similar to those in older patients. Recent studies have demonstrated that a daily dose of 100 mg/d for prophylaxis in adults and children weighing more than 20 kg is as effective as the previously recommended dose of 200 mg/d. The prophylactic dose for children 20 kg or less remains the same as the therapeutic dose (see Treatment, page 276; and Antiviral Drugs, page 578).

Indications. Persons for whom chemoprophylaxis is or may be indicated are as follows:

- Individuals at high risk who were vaccinated after influenza A activity in the community has begun. Chemoprophylaxis during the interval before a vaccine response (2 weeks after the recommended vaccine schedule of 1 or 2 doses has been completed) can be beneficial.
- Nonimmunized persons providing care to high-risk individuals.
- Immunodeficient persons whose antibody response to vaccine is likely to be poor.
- Persons for whom vaccine is contraindicated, specifically those with anaphylactic hypersensitivity to egg protein (see Reactions, Adverse Effects, and Contraindications, page 280).

Isosporiasis

(Isospora belli)

Clinical Manifestations: Protracted diarrhea is the most common presenting symptom and is similar to that caused by *Cryptosporidium.* It can be life-threatening in immunocompromised patients, particularly those with AIDS.

Etiology: *Isospora belli* is a coccidian protozoan.

Epidemiology: Frequency of this parasite, especially in the asymptomatic individual, is unknown. The organism is often missed in microscopic examination of stool samples. Human infection probably occurs by the oral-fecal route; no intermediate host has been identified.

The **incubation period** is unknown.

Diagnostic Tests: Diagnosis is made by demonstration of oocysts or sporocysts in the feces or in duodenal aspirate. A concentration or flotation technique can be helpful.

Treatment: Trimethoprim-sulfamethoxazole or pyrimethamine and sulfadiazine are effective. In patients with AIDS who are allergic to the sulfonamides, treatment of adults with pyrimethamine (75 mg/d) alone, followed by daily prophylactic administration of pyrimethamine (25 mg) has been effective.

Isolation of the Hospitalized Patient: Enteric precautions are prudent, but risk of nosocomial infection is unknown.

Control Measures: None.

Kawasaki Disease

Clinical Manifestations: Kawasaki disease (formerly termed mucocutaneous lymph node syndrome) is an acute, febrile, self-limited, exanthematous, multisystem illness that occurs predominantly in children younger than 5 years. Within 3 days of the abrupt onset of fever, the other characteristic features of the illness usually appear, as follows: (1) discrete bulbar conjunctival injection without exudate; (2) erythematous mouth and pharynx, strawberry tongue, and red, swollen lips; (3) a polymorphous generalized erythematous rash that can be morbilliform, maculopapular, or scarlatiniform, or may resemble erythema multiforme; (4) changes in the peripheral extremities consisting of firm induration of the hands and feet with erythematous palms and soles; and (5) a usually solitary, frequently unilateral cervical lymph node enlarged to more than 1.5 cm in diameter. These early manifestations progress with drying, cracking, and fissuring of the lips usually apparent by the sixth day of illness, and with periungual desquamation and peeling of the palms and soles (to a lesser extent) during the second to third week. These findings constitute the diagnostic clinical features of the illness. For the diagnosis to be made, patients should have fever and at least four of these five features. However, patients with fever and fewer than four of these manifestations can be diagnosed as having Kawasaki disease when coronary artery disease is detected. Associated features include anterior uveitis (80%) in the first week of illness, sterile pyuria (70%), arthritis or arthralgias (35%), aseptic meningitis (5%), carditis with congestive heart failure (less than 5%), pericardial effusion or arrhythmias (20%), and gallbladder hydrops with or without obstructive jaundice (less than 10%).

Without systemic aspirin or intravenous immunoglobulin therapy, the mean duration of fever is 12 days. After the fever resolves, the patient is better but can remain anorectic or irritable for 2 to 3 weeks. During this subacute phase, the characteristic peripheral desquamation can occur, usually between days 10 and 20 of the illness.

Carditis and arthritis can develop at any time during the acute and subacute phases (the first 3 weeks of illness) and generally resolve by 6 to 8 weeks from the onset of the manifestation. Routine two-dimensional echocardiography or angiography demonstrates coronary aneurysm/s in as many as 20% to 25% of the patients. Increased risk for development of coronary aneurysms occurs in males and infants younger than 1 year. Coronary aneurysms appear early in the illness. Serial echocardiograms indicate that in those children developing coronary aneurysms, the first sign of coronary dilation can be seen rarely as early as the seventh day of the illness and occurs at a mean of 10 days. The peak prevalence of coronary aneurysms and coronary dilation is approximately 2 to 4 weeks after the onset of disease. In some children with mild coronary dilation the coronary artery size returns to baseline by 8 weeks after onset of disease. Prospective studies indicate that coronary aneurysms frequently regress to normal lumen size within 1 year. However, coronary stenosis may accompany aneurysm regression, and aneurysm regression does not restore the vessel to normal, as irregular intimal thickening, evidence of thrombosis and recanalization, and persistence of damaged elastic lamina can be found in "regressed" aneurysms. Aneurysms of other vessels (e.g., iliac, femoral, and axillary vessels) can occur. Mitral and aortic regurgitation have been noted during the acute phase or as a late sequela in fewer than 5% of patients.

The current mortality rate in the United States is less than 0.5%. Death results from coronary occlusion with myocardial infarction due to thrombosis or progressive stenosis. Seventy-five percent of fatalities occur within 6 weeks of the onset of symptoms, but myocardial infarction and sudden death can occur months to years after the acute episode. Long-term prognosis is unknown.

Etiology: The etiology is not known.

Epidemiology: Peak age of occurrence in the United States is between 1 and 5 years. Fifty percent of patients are younger than 2 years and 80% are younger than 5 years; children older than 8 years seldom have the disease. The male/female ratio is 1.6:1. The incidence is highest in Asians. Two to four thousand cases are estimated to occur annually in the United States.

Kawasaki disease was first described in Japan, where a pattern of endemic occurrence with superimposed epidemic outbreaks has emerged. A similar pattern of steady or increasing endemic disease with sharply defined community-wide epidemics has been recognized in diverse locations in North America and Hawaii. Epidemics generally occur during the winter and spring at 2- to 3-year intervals. No evidence indicates person-to-person or common-source spread, although the incidence is higher in siblings of children with Kawasaki disease.

Diagnostic Tests: No specific tests are available. The diagnosis is established by fulfillment of the clinical criteria (see Clinical Manifestations) and exclusion of other possible illnesses, including streptococcal infections, viral and rickettsial exanthems, drug reactions, Lyme disease, scalded skin syndrome, toxic shock syndrome, and leptospirosis. An elevated sedimentation rate during the first 2 weeks and an elevated platelet count (above 450,000/mm^3) after the tenth day of illness are common laboratory features. These values usually return to normal within 6 to 8 weeks.

Treatment: Management consists of supportive care in a setting where significant complications of coronary artery disease, carditis, and arthritis can be detected and managed. Specific recommendations are as follows:

IGIV. High-dose immune globulin intravenous (IGIV) therapy initiated within 10 days of the onset of fever in conjunction with aspirin decreases the prevalence of coronary artery dilation and aneurysms detected 2 and 7 weeks later in comparison to treatment with aspirin alone. The mechanism of action of IVIG has not been identified. Significant and rapid resolution of fever and other indicators of acute inflammation has also been demonstrated. Hence, IGIV in conjunction with aspirin is recommended in the treatment of patients who meet the strict criteria for Kawasaki disease (see Clinical Manifestations). IGIV therapy should be initiated as soon as possible and within 10 days of the onset of illness. The efficacy of such therapy if initiated later than 10 days after onset of illness or after aneurysms have been detected has not been established.

Dosage. In the initial studies demonstrating the therapeutic benefit of IGIV, the dosage schedule of IGIV was 400 mg/kg/d in a 2-hour infusion for 4 consecutive days. In a recent well-controlled study, a dosage schedule of 2 g/kg as a single dose during 10 to 12 hours was at least as effective in decreasing the prevalence of subsequent coronary artery disease and ameliorating resolution of fever and other acute inflammatory indices. Complications from this regimen were few and no more than those associated with the 4-day schedule. Hence, IGIV can be given either as a single dose of 2 g during 10 to 12 hours, or the 4-day schedule of 400 mg/kg daily can be used. Advantages of the single dose regimen are shorter duration of intravenous therapy, earlier defervescence, and possible earlier hospital discharge of the child.

Aspirin. Aspirin is given initially in high dosage for its anti-inflammatory effect, and, subsequently, in low dosage for its antiplatelet aggregation action. An anti-inflammatory dose of 80 to 100 mg/kg/d in four divided doses can reduce the duration of fever if started during the first week. Serum salicylate concentrations should be followed during high-dose therapy because gastrointestinal absorption is highly variable. After fever is controlled, aspirin should be decreased. A suggested dose is 3 to 5 mg/kg (maximum, 40 to 80 mg/d) given in one daily dose; this regimen should be maintained for at least 2 months or until both the platelet count and sedimentation rate are normal to reduce the likelihood of spontaneous coronary thrombosis.

Cardiac Care. Children must be examined repeatedly during the first 2 months to detect arrhythmias, congestive heart failure, valvular insufficiency, and myocarditis. Patients should be evaluated by a cardiologist experienced in echocardiographic studies of coronary arteries in children. An echocardiogram should be obtained early in the acute phase of the illness or at the time of diagnosis, 3 weeks after onset, and 8 weeks after onset. Consideration should be given to referring patients to a center with considerable experience in the care of patients with Kawasaki disease. A cardiologist experienced in the management of patients with the complication of documented coronary artery disease should be involved. Patients should receive prolonged low-dose aspirin therapy to suppress platelet aggregation. Dipyridamole in a dose of 4 mg/kg/d, given in three divided doses, is recommended by some experts for patients with persistent coronary artery abnormalities.

Corticosteroids. These drugs are contraindicated except in extremely unusual circumstances. Corticosteroid use has resulted in increased frequency of coronary aneurysms, according to several studies.

Antibiotics. These drugs are not indicated.

Subsequent Immunization. Children who have received IGIV should not receive MMR vaccine until 3 or more months later (see

Active Immunization of Persons Who Recently Received Immune Globulin, page 21).

Isolation of the Hospitalized Patient: No special precautions are indicated.

Control Measures: None.

Legionella pneumophila Infections

Clinical Manifestations: Infection results in at least two distinct syndromes.

- Pneumonia (Legionnaires' disease) is common in adults and varies in severity from a mild, influenza-like illness to severe multisystem disease with gastrointestinal, central nervous system, renal, and progressive pulmonary manifestations. Respiratory failure and death can ensue.
- Pontiac fever is an abrupt-onset, self-limited, influenza-like illness without pneumonia.

Etiology: *Legionella pneumophila* is a fastidious, weakly staining, Gram-negative bacillus with 13 identified serogroups. Other *Legionella* species, such as *L micdadei*, can also cause pneumonia.

Epidemiology: The major environmental reservoir appears to be water. The only proven mode of spread is air-borne transmission. Person-to-person transmission has not been described. Outbreaks have been ascribed to common-source exposure to contaminated air-conditioning cooling towers, evaporative condensers, and potable water. Outbreaks have occurred in hospitals. The disease occurs most commonly in the elderly and immunocompromised. Infection in children is uncommon and is usually asymptomatic or mild and unrecognized. Severe disease has occurred in children with leukemia, severe immunodeficiency, and chronic granulomatous disease.

The **incubation period** for Legionnaires' disease (pneumonia) is 2 to 10 days; for Pontiac fever it is 1 to 2 days.

Diagnostic Tests: *L pneumophila* can be recovered from respiratory secretions and lung tissue by culture on special media. The bacterium can be demonstrated in these specimens by direct immunofluorescence, but this test is less sensitive than culture. Serologic diagnosis is based on the indirect immunofluorescent antibody assay and necessitates a fourfold or greater rise in titer with a convalescent-phase value of 1:128 or more. A single titer of 1:256 or more in a patient with compatible clinical manifestations has been considered presumptive evidence of infection, but similar titers can also be caused by cross-reacting antibodies, such as those to *Mycoplasma pneumoniae* and *Pseudomonas aeruginosa*, and occasionally they are found in healthy individuals. Cross-reacting antibodies often occur in patients with cystic fibrosis. Antibody titers usually rise within 1 to 6 weeks after onset of symptoms but can be delayed for as many as 12 weeks. Titer rises from cross-reacting antibodies can also occur.

Treatment: Erythromycin (50 mg/kg/d; maximum, 2 to 4 g/d) is the drug of choice. Additionally, rifampin (15 mg/kg/d; maximum, 600 mg/d) is recommended for patients with confirmed disease who do not respond promptly to intravenous erythromycin. Duration of therapy is usually 3 weeks.

Isolation of the Hospitalized Patient: No special precautions are recommended.

Control Measures: Methods for decontaminating water supplies in common-source outbreaks have included hyperchlorination (or other chemical decontaminants) and/or superheating (to above 70°C, 158°F).

Leishmaniasis

Clinical Manifestations: The three major clinical syndromes are as follows:

Cutaneous Leishmaniasis. An initial erythematous macule progresses to a papule and ultimately to a shallow ulcer. Lesions can be single or multiple, typically have well-demarcated and raised ulcer borders, and are painless. Lesions are located at the sites of vector bites, most commonly on the exposed areas of the face and arms. Associated satellite lesions and painless regional lymphadenopathy, resembling sporotrichosis, can also occur. Manifestations of Old World (Oriental sore) and New World (American) cutaneous leishmaniasis are similar. In New World disease in Mexico, lesions are often located in the pinna of the ear (*Chiclero* ulcer). Spontaneous resolution of all forms of cutaneous disease is common, but can take months to years. Leishmaniasis should be suspected in nonhealing skin lesions in individuals living in, or traveling to areas where the disease is endemic.

Mucocutaneous Leishmaniasis (Espundia). An initial cutaneous ulcer progresses, probably by hematogenous spread, to involve the nasopharyngeal mucosa months to years later. The ulcers are often extremely disfiguring and do not resolve spontaneously. Mucocutaneous leishmaniasis is a complication of New World cutaneous leishmaniasis.

Visceral Leishmaniasis (Kala-azar). Onset is insidious, leading to a chronic illness with systemic manifestations, including vague constitutional symptoms and fever, with a characteristic semidaily spike (the so-called Dromedary fever). Splenomegaly, hepatomegaly, lymphadenopathy, anemia, leukopenia, and thrombocytopenia occur. Secondary pyogenic and mycobacterial infections are common. Skin changes consisting of darkly pigmented, erythematous areas and other hyperpigmented areas can be present. Untreated visceral disease is inevitably fatal.

Etiology: Cutaneous leishmaniasis is caused by multiple species of *Leishmania. L tropica*, *L aethiopica*, and *L major* cause Old World disease, and *L mexicana*, *L peruviana*, and several species of *L brasiliensis* cause New World disease. Mucocutaneous and visceral leishmaniasis are caused by *L brasiliensis* and *L donovani*, respectively. *Leishmania* species are obligate intracellular parasites.

Epidemiology: Leishmaniasis is a zoonosis; the organism is transmitted to humans from nonhuman mammalian reservoirs (such as dogs and wild animals, including rodents, depending on the geographical region) by the bites of infected sand flies. Clinical manifestations depend primarily on the *Leishmania* species inoculated into the subcutaneous tissue by the vector. Cutaneous Old World leishmaniasis has occurred in most Asian countries, the Soviet Union, the Middle East, North Africa, and, rarely, in southern Europe. New World leishmaniasis occurs primarily in the area extending from the Yucatan region of Mexico to northern Brazil but has been reported as far north as Texas. Mucocutaneous leishmaniasis occurs primarily in the Amazon basin and the central plains of Brazil but also has been reported in Bolivia, Peru, Venezuela, Colombia, Paraguay, and Argentina. Visceral leishmaniasis has a very wide geographic distribution in the Old World, extending from northeastern China to India, the Middle East, Southern Europe, the Mediterranean basin, and most of Central Africa. Small endemic foci have occurred in both Central and South America, particularly in the Honduras and Brazil. Old World cutaneous leishmaniasis is primarily a disease of children. New World cutaneous leishmaniasis caused by *L mexicana* is an occupational disease of harvesters of the chicle plant and, therefore, occurs primarily in young adults. Visceral leishmaniasis is most common in adolescents and young adults, but can occur in young children.

The **incubation periods** of the different types of leishmaniasis range from several days to months. In cutaneous leishmaniasis, the initial lesions typically appear several weeks after the sand fly bite, but this interval can be as long as several years. In visceral leishmaniasis, the incubation period varies, usually from 6 weeks to 6 months. However, incubation periods of as short as 10 days and as long as 10 years have been reported.

Diagnostic Tests: Diagnosis is frequently established by microscopic identification of the intracellular organisms on impression-stained smears or histologic sections of infected tissues. In cutaneous disease, tissue may be obtained by a 3-mm punch biopsy or a needle aspiration of the raised nonnecrotic edge of the suspected lesion. In visceral leishmaniasis, the organisms can be visualized in biopsy specimens or aspirates of bone marrow, liver, lymph node, or splenic pulp. The diagnosis can be confirmed by recovery of the organism from culture of the tissue specimen on a special blood agar medium or by inoculation of homogenized tissue into hamsters. Neither test is routinely available. Culture media and further information can be provided by the Centers for Disease Control (CDC).

The leishmanin (Montenegro) skin test is usually positive in patients with cutaneous or mucocutaneous disease, but the test reagent is not available in the United States. A positive test is denoted by an area of induration at least 5 mm in diameter that appears 48 to 72 hours after injection and is an indication of delayed hypersensitivity to the leishmanial antigen. In patients with visceral leishmaniasis, the skin test is negative during the active infection but becomes positive during recovery as cell-mediated immunity develops. Thus, a positive skin test in a patient with visceral leishmaniasis is a favorable prognostic sign but is not helpful in establishing the diagnosis.

The diagnosis of visceral leishmaniasis can be aided by a positive serologic antileishmanial test. The CDC uses immunofluorescent and complement fixation assays; other assays include indirect hemagglutination, gel diffusion tests, and ELISA. False-positive tests, however, can occur in patients with American trypanosomiasis (Chagas' disease).

Treatment: Cutaneous lesions can heal without treatment. Because currently available antileishmanial drugs can be toxic, treatment is not routinely indicated. However, treatment is indicated when the ulcers are potentially disabling or disfiguring, when healing is delayed, or when the patient is possibly infected with *L brasiliensis.* Drug therapy is always indicated in mucocutaneous and visceral leishmaniasis.The drug of choice in the United States is stibogluconate sodium (Pentostam).* N-methylglucamine antimonate has also been used, but it is not available in the United States. These drugs are generally well tolerated in young, otherwise healthy adults, but potentially serious cardiac and renal toxicity can occur. Cases resistant to these drugs have responded to therapy with amphotericin B. Pentamidine is an alternative drug for visceral leishmaniasis. Local heat (40° to 41°C) has been used successfully for treatment of *L mexicana* lesions.

Isolation of the Hospitalized Patient: No special precautions are recommended.

Control Measures: The identification and treatment of infected individuals are indicated. The elimination or reduction of the sand fly population and/or infected animal reservoirs is difficult and in some settings impossible. Sleeping in tents under fine mesh netting and using insect repellent whenever exposure to the sand fly vector is likely may limit the risk of infection.

Leprosy

(Hansen's Disease)

Clinical Manifestations: Leprosy is a chronic disease involving mainly skin, peripheral nerves, and the mucosa of the upper airway. The clinical forms of leprosy represent a spectrum that reflects the cellular immune response to *Mycobacterium leprae*. Some features typical of the major forms are the following:

- Tuberculoid—one or a few well-demarcated, hypopigmented, and anesthetic skin lesions, frequently with active, spreading edges, and a clearing center. Cell-mediated immune responses are relatively intact.
- Lepromatous—a larger number of papules and nodules, or infiltration of the face, hands, and feet in a bilateral and symmetric distribution. *M leprae*-specific cell-mediated immunity is greatly diminished.
- Borderline (dimorphous)—skin lesions characteristic of both the tuberculoid and lepromatous forms.

---

*Available from the Drug Service of the Centers for Disease Control (see Services of the Centers for Disease Control, page 622).

- Indeterminate—early lesions, usually hypopigmented macules, without developed tuberculoid or lepromatous features.

Serious consequences of leprosy occur from nerve involvement with resulting anesthesia, which may lead to repeated, unrecognized trauma, ulcerations, fractures, and bone resorption.

Etiology: Leprosy is caused by the bacteria *M leprae*.

Epidemiology: The major mode of transmission is contact with humans who have untreated or drug-resistant multibacillary disease (lepromatous or borderline types). A long duration of exposure, such as to a household contact, is typical. The major source of infectious material is probably nasal secretions from patients with untreated multibacillary forms. Organisms are found in large numbers around the nares in these patients; little shedding of *M leprae* from patients' intact skin occurs. Of cases of leprosy reported in the United States, 90% are imported and occur in immigrants and refugees from areas endemic for leprosy, particularly Mexico and Southeast Asia. Indigenous cases continue to occur in Texas, California, Louisiana, and Hawaii. The infectivity of lepromatous patients probably ceases soon after treatment is instituted, frequently within a few days of initiating rifampin therapy or about 3 months after initiating therapy with dapsone or clofazamine.

The **incubation period** ranges from a few months to many years; it is usually 3 to 5 years.

Diagnostic Tests: Histopathologic examination by an experienced pathologist is the best method for establishing the diagnosis and is the basis for the classification of leprosy. Acid-fast bacilli may be found in smears from skin lesions, except from patients with the tuberculoid and indeterminant forms of disease. Organisms have not been successfully cultured in vitro. Drug resistance is tested by the mouse footpad inoculation test. The demonstration of morphologically normal bacilli despite usually effective therapy should suggest possible drug resistance, indicating a need for a change in therapy based on the results of antimicrobial sensitivity testing in mice.

High titers of predominantly IgM serum antibodies against phenolic glycolipid-1 of *M leprae* have been detected in untreated patients. Titers of these antibodies decrease during therapy. This test is experimental.

Treatment: Therapy of patients with leprosy should be undertaken in consultation with an expert in leprosy. The Gillis W. Long Hansen's Disease Center (GWLHDC), Carville, Louisiana (800/642-2477), provides consultation on clinical and pathologic issues and can provide information about local Hansen's disease clinics.

Dapsone is the primary drug used in the treatment of leprosy. It is administered in a dose of 50 to 100 mg/d for adults and 1 mg/kg/d for children. Individuals in high-risk groups for glucose-6-phosphodehydrogenase deficiency should be tested for this condition before dapsone administration. Because primary dapsone resistance of *M leprae* has been reported, dapsone should not be used as monotherapy. Multidrug therapy is necessary in all patients to reduce the risk of drug resistance, and it may also allow the duration of therapy to be shortened. Rifampin (600 mg/d for adults or 10 mg/kg/d for children) should be given with dapsone for 6 months for paucibacillary (indeterminate, tuberculoid, and borderline tuberculoid) disease, with close follow-up to detect relapses. Clofazimine (50 mg/d for adults or 1 mg/kg/d for children) should be added to dapsone plus rifampin for multibacillary (borderline, borderline lepromatous, and lepromatous) disease and continued for at least 2 years and until skin smears are negative. Corticosteroids are used to treat erythema nodosum leprosum (ENL), which commonly occurs in patients with multibacillary forms after drug therapy is initiated. Thalidomide or clofazimine can also be used to treat ENL. Thalidomide is available from the GWLHCD as an experimental drug for selected patients; it should never be given to a woman of childbearing age. Corticosteroids are also indicated for treatment of reversal reactions occurring in patients with borderline disease.

Most patients can be treated as outpatients. Rehabilitative measures, including surgery and physical therapy, may be necessary in some patients.

Isolation of the Hospitalized Patient: No special precautions are necessary. A private room with no formal isolation procedures should be sufficient for a newly diagnosed patient.

Control Measures: Hand washing is recommended for all individuals in contact with a lepromatous patient. Disinfection of nasal secretions, handkerchiefs, and other fomites should be considered until treatment is established. All close household contacts should be examined initially and thereafter annually for 5 years, particularly contacts of patients with multibacillary disease. Household contacts of patients with borderline or lepromatous leprosy who are younger than 25 years should be treated prophylactically with dapsone for 3 years at the same doses used for treatment. Local public health department regulations for leprosy vary and should be consulted. Newly diagnosed cases of leprosy should be reported to public health authorities.

Leptospirosis

Clinical Manifestations: The onset of leptospirosis is usually abrupt, with nonspecific, influenza-like, constitutional symptoms of fever, chills, headache, severe myalgia, and malaise. Gastrointestinal symptoms can also occur. The clinical course is frequently biphasic and protean, and can result in hepatic (abnormal function tests, hepatomegaly, jaundice, and failure), renal (abnormal urinalysis, azotemia, and failure), and central nervous system (aseptic meningitis and altered sensorium) involvement. Myositis is common. Weil's syndrome is severe leptospirosis with jaundice. Conjunctival suffusion, the most characteristic physical finding, occurs in less than half the patients. The duration of the illness varies from less than 1 week to 3 weeks.

Etiology: The etiologic agent is the spirochete *Leptospira interrogans*. Approximately 250 serotypes (serovars) comprising 19 serogroups have been recognized. Disease in the United States has been caused by more than ten serovars, the most common of which are *icterohaemorrhagiae* and *canicola.*

Epidemiology: Many species of wild and domestic mammals (particularly dogs, rats, and livestock) that excrete *Leptospira* organisms in the urine on an acute or chronic basis are the sources for human infection. Most cases in the United States result from recreational exposure. Disease occurs most commonly in the summer among teenagers and adults, and it is most common in the tropics. Those predisposed by occupation include abattoir and sewer workers, veterinarians, farmers, and field workers. Transmission is zoonotic, either by direct or indirect contact with urine or carcasses of infected animals. Indirect contact occurs from swimming, wading, or splashing in pools, streams, or puddles contaminated by leptospiruric animals; occasionally, indirect exposure results in common-source outbreaks. Asymptomatic and symptomatic human infections occur. Communicability exists during the 1-month to more than 3-month phase of leptospiruria in infected animals. Humans with leptospirosis usually excrete the organism in urine for 4 to 6 weeks and occasionally for as long as 18 weeks. Person-to-person transmission is rare.

The **incubation period** is usually 7 to 13 days, with a range of 2 to 26 days.

Diagnostic Tests: The blood and cerebrospinal fluid, in the first 7 to 10 days of the illness, and the urine, after the first week and during convalescence, should be cultured on special media. Because such media are not routinely available, the laboratory should be consulted in cases of suspected leptospirosis. The organism can also be recovered by inoculation of body fluids into guinea pigs. Serum antibody measured by ELISA or agglutination reactions develop in the second week of the illness, but titer rises can be delayed or absent in some patients. Microscopic agglutination is the confirmatory serologic test and is performed in reference laboratories. Direct darkfield examination of the blood and other body fluids has pitfalls that obviate its usefulness; it is not recommended.

Treatment: Penicillin is the drug of choice in severely ill patients. It had been considered beneficial by some if initiated before the fourth day of illness, but a recent study indicates that intravenous, high-dose penicillin (1.5 million units given every 6 hours to adults) for 7 days is effective even in patients in whom therapy is started after the fourth day. Oral doxycycline therapy in mild illness also appears to shorten the course of illness and reduces the incidence of convalescent leptospiruria. Tetracycline drugs should not be given to children younger than 9 years unless the benefits of therapy justify the risk of dental staining.

Isolation of the Hospitalized Patient: The routinely recommended blood and body fluid precautions for all patients (see Isolation Precautions, page 81) are indicated for the duration of hospitalization. In patients with leptospirosis, these precautions also include urine, as it is potentially infective.

Control Measures:

- Vaccination of dogs and livestock prevents disease but not infection and leptospiruria in animals. Its effect on human disease is unproven.
- Protective clothing, boots, and gloves should be worn to reduce occupational exposure.
- Rodent control is indicated.
- Doxycycline, 200 mg, given orally once weekly, is effective prophylaxis and should be considered for high-risk occupational groups with short-term exposure. However, indications for doxycycline use in children have not been established (and tetracycline drugs generally should not be given to children younger than 9 years).

Listeria monocytogenes

(Listeriosis)

Clinical Manifestations: Perinatal and neonatal *Listeria* infections are relatively uncommon and have early-onset and late-onset syndromes similar to those of group B streptococcal infections. Pneumonia, septicemia, and maternal symptoms are common in early-onset disease. Late-onset infection occurs after the first week of life and often results in meningitis. Maternal infection can be associated with transient fever and malaise or amnionitis during labor, or it may be asymptomatic. Infection other than in the perinatal period is uncommon and usually develops in the immunocompromised host, resulting in meningitis and/or septicemia.

Etiology: *Listeria monocytogenes* is a small, aerobic, non-spore-forming, Gram-positive rod that is beta-hemolytic on blood agar.

Epidemiology: *L monocytogenes* is widely distributed in the environment and in animal species, but the source of infections in humans is poorly understood. Asymptomatic fecal and vaginal carriage occurs in humans and is the likely source of sporadic and epidemic neonatal disease. Clustering of cases suggests that exogenous exposure is as important as impaired host resistance in the development of disease. Early-onset neonatal infections result from transplacental or ascending intrauterine infection. Maternal infection has been associated with prematurity and other obstetric complications. Late-onset neonatal infection can result from acquisition of the organism during passage through the birth canal, or possibly from environmental sources. Nosocomial nursery outbreaks have also occurred. Clusters of perinatal infections traced to maternal ingestion of contaminated coleslaw or unpasteurized cheese demonstrate that listeriosis is a food-borne disease. In other outbreaks, milk and other dairy products have been incriminated. Food-borne transmission has also been documented in sporadic cases. Infection is possibly acquired by inhalation or genital contact.

The **incubation period** is unknown. In food-borne transmission, the median period is 21 days.

Diagnostic Tests: The organism can be recovered on routine culture media from blood, cerebrospinal fluid, meconium, gastric washings, placenta, and other infected tissues. Special techniques (e.g., enrichment and selective media) may be needed to recover *Listeria* from the stool and other sites with mixed flora. Gram stain of a fecal smear from an infected newborn infant may demonstrate the organism. The morphologic similarity of the bacterium to diphtheroids can result in its being discarded as a contaminant or saprophyte when recovered on culture. The value of serologic tests is not established.

Treatment:

- Initial therapy with ampicillin and an aminoglycoside is recommended for severe infections because this combination is more effective than ampicillin alone in animal models of *Listeria* infection. After clinical response has been documented or in less severe infections in normal hosts, ampicillin alone may be given. The optimal therapeutic regimen, however, is uncertain. For the penicillin-allergic patient, trimethoprim-sulfamethoxazole is the alternative drug. Cephalosporins, including the newer derivatives, are not active against *Listeria*.
- For neonatal meningitis caused by *Listeria*, 14 days of treatment is usually satisfactory.
- Some authorities have suggested that the cervix and stools of the mother of an infected infant be cultured and the mother treated if either of the cultures is positive. Reculturing during a subsequent pregnancy has also been suggested. The usefulness of these measures has not been established.

Isolation of the Hospitalized Patient: No special precautions are indicated, although drainage/secretion precautions may be considered for heavily infected infants.

Control Measures:

- Antimicrobial therapy of infection diagnosed during pregnancy may prevent fetal or perinatal infection and its consequences.
- The existence of listeriosis in herds of sheep or cattle should preclude the use of untreated manure on crops destined for human consumption, although the role of raw vegetables as a source of infection needs further study.

Lyme Disease

(Borrelia burgdorferi)

Clinical Manifestations: Early disease usually begins with a distinctive skin rash, erythema chronicum migrans, at the site of a recent tick bite. The lesion begins as a red macule or papule that expands to form a large annular erythema, typically with partial central clearing. Patients can develop multiple secondary annular lesions, evanescent red blotches or circles, malar rash or urticaria, conjunctivitis, periorbital edema, or a diffuse erythema. Fever, malaise, headache, mild neck stiffness and arthralgia can occur. These symptoms are typically intermittent and change during a period of several weeks in untreated patients.

Later manifestations of the disease involve the joints, the eyes, the cardiac and nervous systems weeks to months later. Nervous system findings include seventh cranial nerve (Bell's) palsies, aseptic meningitis, and peripheral radiculoneuropathy. Brief, recurrent attacks of nonsymmetric arthritis in large joints are characteristic and chronic arthritis is uncommon in children. Late manifestations can be present without the typical history of early Lyme disease or erythema chronicum migrans.

Adverse pregnancy outcomes—including congenital heart disease, syndactyly, cortical blindness, intrauterine fetal death, prematurity, and rash in the newborn—have occurred in women infected during pregnancy. However, fetal infection and causation of fetal abnormalities rarely have been proven, and the offspring of most women infected during pregnancy have been normal.

Etiology: The cause is a spirochete, *Borrelia burgdorferi*. The organism has been stained and observed in skin, cardiac, retinal, liver, muscle, bone, and synovial lesions and has been cultured from the skin, blood, and cerebrospinal and joint fluid of patients with Lyme disease.

Epidemiology: Lyme disease is clustered primarily in three distinct geographic regions of the United States. Most cases are reported in the Northeast from Massachusetts to Maryland, in the Midwest especially in Wisconsin and Minnesota, and in California. The occurrence of cases in the United States correlates closely with the known distribution and frequency of infection of known tick vectors (*Ixodes dammini* in the Northeast and Midwest, and *I pacificus* in the West). However, cases of Lyme disease have been reported in at least 43 states, many of which are outside the usual range of these ticks. These observations, as well as the recent isolation of the spirochete from other tick species and flying insects, suggest that other arthropods in the United States can occasionally be vectors for Lyme disease. Disease has also been reported from Canada, Europe, Scandinavia, the Soviet Union, China, and Australia. Onset of the illness is generally between May 1 and November 30; most cases occur in June and July. Patients of all ages and both sexes may be affected.

The **incubation period** is 3 to 32 days.

Diagnostic Tests: Diagnosis is made clinically in the early stages of the disease if erythema chronicum migrans is present. In patients without a rash or who manifest a later disease stage, diagnosis is usually made by serology.

Both an indirect fluorescent antibody (IFA) and an ELISA test are available; the ELISA is more widely used and is more sensitive and specific. However, these tests are not yet standardized and results vary between different laboratories. Western blot analysis is more sensitive and specific and frequently complements results of the ELISA test. Both false-negative and false-positive IFA and ELISA test results occur. The IgM antibody titer usually reaches a peak between the third and sixth week after onset of the disease; specific IgG antibody titers usually rise slowly and are generally highest months later when arthritis is present. Patients with Lyme disease may not have elevated titers during the first several weeks of illness, but thereafter most patients with untreated Lyme disease will have a positive serologic test. Titers to the Lyme spirochete are particularly useful in differentiating Lyme disease from other rheumatic syndromes. Lyme spirochetal antibody cross-reacts with other spirochetes, including *Treponema pallidum.* Patients with Lyme disease, however, do not have positive nontreponemal syphilis tests (e.g., VDRL or RPR).

Definitive diagnosis can be made by culture of the Lyme disease spirochete but culture lacks sensitivity. Similarly, spirochetes are rarely seen by direct examination of blood or skin transudate specimens.

Treatment (see Table 38):

Early Stage Disease. At the time of the appearance of erythema chronicum migrans or shortly thereafter, tetracycline (250 mg four times daily), doxycycline (100 mg twice daily) or amoxicillin (500 mg three times daily) is the drug of choice for children 9 years and older. For children younger than 9 years, penicillin V or amoxicillin (25 to 50 mg/kg/d, maximum 1 to 2 grams daily, in three divided doses for either drug) is recommended. Erythromycin (30 mg/kg/d, maximum 750 mg, in divided doses) is an acceptable alternative for the penicillin-allergic patient, although it may be less effective. Length of therapy is dependent on clinical response and manifestations. A patient with early disease should be seen after a 14-day course of antibiotic therapy. If all symptoms have resolved, no further therapy is indicated. If symptoms persist, continued therapy is necessary until they have resolved. Relapses may occur, requiring retreatment with the same or other antibiotic.

Early treatment of erythema chronicum migrans should prevent development of the later manifestations.

Table 38. Recommended Treatment for Lyme Disease in Children

Disease Category	Drug and Dose*
Early Disease	
≥ 9 y	Tetracycline: 250 mg four times daily OR Doxycycline: 100 mg twice daily
< 9 y	Penicillin V: 25-50 mg/kg/d, divided into 3 daily doses (maximum 1-2 g/d) OR Amoxicillin: 25-50 mg/kg/d, divided into 3 daily doses (maximum 1-2 g/d)
Late Disease	
Isolated Bell's palsy	Same as for early disease (oral regimen)
Arthritis	Same as for early disease (oral regimen)
Mild carditis	Same as for early disease (oral regimen)
Persistent arthritis	Ceftriaxone, 75-100 mg/kg, IV or IM, once daily (maximum 2 g/d), or penicillin, 300,000 U/kg/d, IV, given in divided doses every 4 hours (maximum 20 MU/d)
Severe carditis	Penicillin, 300,000 U/kg/d, IV, given in divided doses every 4 hours (maximum 20 MU/d)
Meningitis or encephalitis	Ceftriaxone, 75-100 mg/kg, IV or IM, once daily (maximum 2 g/d)

***Duration of therapy:** oral regimens should be continued 10 to 30 days; parenteral therapy for 14 to 21 days.

Late-Stage Disease. Isolated seventh nerve palsy with normal cerebrospinal fluid findings, mild carditis or arthritis can be treated with one of the oral regimens recommended for early-stage disease. Severe carditis, persistent arthritis, or neurologic involvement should be treated with parenteral antibiotics. Although data are limited, ceftriaxone 75 to 100 mg/kg/d (maximum 2 g/d) is probably the treatment of choice for central nervous system disease. Penicillin G 300,000 U/kg/d, maximum of 20 million U/d, divided into doses every 4 hours, or ceftriaxone could be used for severe carditis or persistent arthritis.

Pregnancy. The most appropriate therapy for Lyme disease during pregnancy has not been determined.

The Jarisch-Herxheimer reaction, with fever, chills, and malaise, can occur when therapy is initiated.

Isolation of the Hospitalized Patient: No special precautions are recommended.

Control Measures:

Ticks. Avoidance of tick-infested areas is the best preventive measure. If a tick-infested area in entered, clothing should cover as much of the arms and legs as possible. Permethrin can be sprayed on clothing to prevent tick attachment. Tick repellents, to be effective, require repeated application every 1 to 2 hours to exposed skin. If "deet"* is used, it should be applied sparingly because seizures have been reported coincident with its application in young children. Daily inspection of family members and prompt removal of any ticks are strongly recommended. (See Control Measures for Prevention of Tick-Borne Infections, page 112.)

Antimicrobial prophylaxis after a tick bite in an endemic area is not warranted. The rate of transmission of *B burgdorferi* appears to be low. Animal studies indicate that transmission requires a prolonged (more than 24 hours) time of tick attachment; in a small study of prophylaxis, no benefit was documented.

Patients with active disease should not donate blood because spirochetemia occurs early in Lyme disease. Patients who were previously treated for Lyme disease can be considered for blood donation.

Lymphocytic Choriomeningitis

Clinical Manifestations: Lymphocytic choriomeningitis (LCM) infection may result in a mild to severe nonspecific illness, including fever, malaise, myalgia, retro-orbital headache, photophobia, anorexia, and nausea. Fever usually lasts 1 to 3 weeks. A biphasic febrile course is frequent. Neurologic manifestations varying from aseptic meningitis to severe encephalitis can occur. Arthralgia or arthritis, respiratory symptoms, orchitis, and leukopenia occasionally develop.

Etiology: LCM virus is an arenavirus.

Epidemiology: LCM is an infection of rodents. House, laboratory, and field mice, as well as hamsters can be infected. Humans are infected incidentally and by inhalation or ingestion of dust or food contaminated with the virus from the urine, feces, blood, or nasopharyngeal secretions of infected rodents. Pet hamsters have been found to

---

*N,N-diethyl-m-toluamide

be a source of infection. The disease is most prevalent in young adults. Human-to-human spread of the virus has not been reported.

The **incubation period** is usually 6 to 13 days; occasionally it is as long as 3 weeks.

Diagnostic Tests: LCM virus can be isolated from blood, cerebrospinal fluid, urine or nasopharyngeal secretions. Acute and convalescent sera can be tested for increases in antibody titers. Infected rodents trapped in houses may be identified by demonstrating serum antibody or viral antigen in liver impression smears using monoclonal antibodies.

Treatment: Supportive.

Isolation of the Hospitalized Patient: No special precautions are recommended.

Control Measures: Control of LCM infection can be achieved by preventing rodent infection in animal and food storage areas of wholesalers and others dealing in the sale of hamsters or other rodents. Because the virus is excreted by rodent hosts for long periods of time, attempts should be made to monitor animal colonies for infection.

Malaria

Clinical Manifestations: The classic symptoms are high fever with chills, rigor sweats, and headache. Other symptoms include nausea, vomiting, arthralgia, and abdominal and back pain. Pallor and even jaundice caused by hemolysis can be present. In general, symptoms are less pronounced in persons with some degree of immunity as a result of repeated or continual malarial infections. Manifestations of malaria in infants can resemble those of sepsis, including only the subtle signs of poor appetite, restlessness, and lethargy. Severe infections caused by *Plasmodium falciparum* can result in coagulopathy, renal and hepatic failure, shock, encephalopathy, coma, and death.

Etiology: Malaria in humans is caused by one of four species of *Plasmodium*: *P falciparum*, *P vivax*, *P ovale*, and *P malariae*.

Epidemiology: Infections usually are acquired by the bite of an infected female *Anopheles* mosquito. Less common modes of transmission include blood transfusion and the use of contaminated needles. Congenital infections also occur. Malaria transmission remains a major problem in much of the tropics and subtropics. Lack of accurate surveillance data from many parts of the world, varying risks of transmission, and changing patterns of drug resistance preclude precise definition of the areas where the risk of acquiring malaria is high and where drug-resistant species occur. The most accurate, current information on risks and drug resistance for any given area can be obtained by contacting local or state health departments; by contacting the Centers for Disease Control Malaria Hotline (404/639-1610); or by consulting the U.S. Public Health Service's annual publication, *Health Information for International Travel.**

Unless properly treated, *P vivax* and *P ovale* persist in a dormant stage (hypnozoite) that can cause periodic relapses for as long as 4 years after initial infection. Untreated *P malariae* infection can also persist subclinically for more than 30 years with periodic recrudescences.

In persons with no preexisting immunity to malaria, the **incubation period** (the time between the causative mosquito bite and the development of symptoms) varies from 6 to 30 days, depending on the *Plasmodium* species involved.

Diagnostic Tests: Diagnosis of malaria depends on the demonstration of *Plasmodium* species in stained smears of peripheral blood. Although parasites can be stained with Wright's solution, Giemsa stain enhances morphologic detail of the parasites and allows greater accuracy of speciation. Thick smears, which must be rendered free of hemoglobin before staining, permit more efficient screening of larger volumes of blood for parasites than do thin smears, which are most useful for making a species diagnosis. In some instances, examination of smears obtained at intervals during a 24- to 48-hour period can be necessary to establish the diagnosis. Serologic tests for antibodies against individual *Plasmodium* species cannot differentiate current from past infection; therefore, these tests are of limited use in the diagnosis of acute malaria.

Treatment: Selection of appropriate therapy depends on the species involved and the patient's travel history. Drugs of choice for treatment of malaria are given in Table 39.

Isolation of the Hospitalized Patient: The routinely recommended blood precautions (see Isolation Precautions, page 81) are indicated for the duration of the illness.

Control Measures: Control measures are directed toward treatment of infected persons with appropriate antimalarial agents; prevention of acute infection by chemoprophylaxis; reduction of contact with

---

*Available from the Superintendent of Documents, U.S. Government Printing Office, Washington, D.C. 20402.

Table 39. Treatment of Malaria

Drug	Adult Dosage	Pediatric Dosage
All *Plasmodium* species except chloroquine-resistant *P falciparum*		
Oral drug of choice: Chloroquine phosphate*	600 mg base (1 g), then 300 mg base (500 mg) 6 h later, and 300 mg base (500 mg/d) at 24 and 48 h	10 mg base/kg (max 600 mg base), then 5 mg base/kg 6 h later, and 5 mg base/kg/d at 24 and 48 h
Parenteral drug of choice: Quinidine gluconate†	10 mg/kg loading dose IV (max, 600 mg) during 1 h, then 0.02 mg/kg/min continuous infusion until oral therapy can be started	Same as above
	OR	
Quinine dihydrochloride‡	600 mg in 300 mL normal saline IV over 2 to 4 h; repeat every 8 h until oral therapy can be started (max 1800 mg/d)	25 mg/kg/d; give 1/3 of daily dose during 2-4 h; repeat every 8 h until oral therapy can be started (max 1800 mg/d)
Chloroquine-resistant *P falciparum*		
Oral drug of choice:		
Quinine sulfate§	650 mg three times a day for 3 to 7 d	25 mg/kg/d in 3 doses for 3 d
plus		
Pyrimethamine-sulfadoxine (Fansidar)	Single dose of three tablets	< 1 y: single dose of a quarter tablet 1-3 y: single dose of a half tablet 4-8 y: single dose of one tablet 9-14 y: single dose of two tablets > 14 y: single dose of three tablets
or		
Mefloquine hydrochloride‖	Single dose of 1250 mg	25 mg/kg in single dose
or		
Tetracycline¶	250 mg four times a day for 7 d	5 mg/kg four times a day for 7 d

Table 39. Treatment of Malaria *(continued)*

Drug	Adult Dosage	Pediatric Dosage
Parenteral drug of choice:		
Quinidine gluconate†	Same as above	Same as above
Quinine dihydro-chloride‡	Same as above	Same as above
Prevention of Relapses: *P vivax* and *P ovale* only		
Drug of choice:		
Primaquine phosphate**	15 mg base (26.3 mg)/d for 14 d or 45 mg base (79 mg)/wk for 8 wk	0.3 mg/kg/d for 14 d

*If chloroquine phosphate is not available, hydroxychloroquine sulfate is as effective; 400 mg of hydroxychloroquine sulfate is equivalent to 500 mg of chloroquine phosphate.

†Some experts consider quinidine more effective than quinine. ECG monitoring is recommended to detect arrhythmias.

‡Available in the U.S. only from the Centers for Disease Control (404/639-3670; nights, weekends, or holidays: 404/639-2888). *P falciparum* infections from Southeast Asia require a loading dose of 20 mg/kg. This loading dose should be administered with careful cardiac and vascular monitoring and adequate hydration.

§For treatment of *P falciparum* infections acquired in Thailand, quinine should be given for 7 days.

||Mefloquine should not be used in children lighter than 15 kg, pregnant women in the first trimester, patients using beta blockers (or other cardiac drugs which may prolong or alter cardiac conduction), or patients with history of epilepsy or psychiatric disorder. Quinidine or quinine may exacerbate the known side effects of mefloquine; patients not responding to mefloquine therapy or failing mefloquine prophylaxis should be closely monitored if they are treated with quinidine/quinine.

¶Physicians must weigh the benefits of tetracycline therapy against the possibility of dental staining in children younger than 9 years.

**Primaquine phosphate can cause hemolytic anemia in patients with glucose-6-phosphate dehydrogenase erythrocyte deficiency. Primaquine should not be used during pregnancy.

mosquitoes through the use of insect repellents, protective clothes, and screens; and elimination of the insect vector through the use of insecticides and other measures.

Chemoprophylaxis for Travelers to Endemic Areas.* The appropriate chemoprophylactic regimen is determined by the traveler's risk of acquiring malaria in the area(s) to be visited and by the risk of exposure to chloroquine-resistant *P falciparum*. Chemoprophylaxis should begin 1 to 2 weeks before arrival in the endemic area, allowing time for development of adequate blood concentration and evaluation of any adverse reactions.

Chloroquine-resistant *P falciparum* has been reported in all areas in which malaria is endemic except Central America west of the Panama Canal, Haiti, the Dominican Republic, the Middle East, and Egypt. Travelers to areas where species have not been reported should take chloroquine alone, once weekly, for the duration of exposure (see Table 40). In addition, chloroquine should be continued for 4 weeks after departure from the endemic area.

Travelers to areas where chloroquine-resistance *P falciparum* exists should take mefloquine alone, once weekly, starting 1 week before travel, continuing weekly during travel, and for 4 weeks after travel has concluded (see Table 40).

Mefloquine is not recommended for use by children lighter than 15 kg body weight, pregnant women during the first trimester, patients taking beta blockers (or other cardiac drugs that can prolong or alter cardiac conduction), patients with history of epilepsy or severe psychiatric disorders (e.g., psychosis) and travelers involved in tasks requiring fine coordination and spatial discrimination, such as airline crews. Because of the frequency of side effects, mefloquine should not be used for presumptive self-treatment.

In travelers for whom mefloquine is contraindicated, chloroquine alone may be an effective alternative (see Table 40). In addition, travelers should carry pyrimethamine-sulfadoxine (Fansidar) for use as presumptive self-treatment if the traveler experiences a febrile illness while taking chloroquine and professional medical care is not readily available. Self-treatment should not be considered a replacement for seeking prompt medical help. Pyrimethamine-sulfadoxine (Fansidar) should not be taken by patients with known intolerance to either drug, pregnant women at term, or infants younger than 2 months.

---

*For further information on prevention of malaria in travelers, see the following: Centers for Disease Control. Recommendations for Prevention of Malaria Among Travelers, *MMWR*. 1990;39(No. RR-3):1-10, and the U.S. Public Health Service's annual publication, *Health Information for International Travel*, Superintendent of Documents, U.S. Government Printing Office, Washington, D.C.

Table 40. Prevention of Malaria*

Drug	Adult Dosage	Pediatric Dosage
Chloroquine phosphate (Aralen)	300 mg base (500 mg salt) orally, once per wk beginning 1 wk before and continuing 4 wk after last exposure	5 mg/kg base (8.3 mg/kg salt) once per wk, up to maximum adult dose of 300 mg base
	CHLOROQUINE-RESISTANT AREAS	
Mefloquine-hydrochloride† (Lariam)	250 mg orally once per wk, beginning 1 wk before travel, and continuing until 4 wk after last exposure	15-19 kg: 1/4 tab/wk 20-30 kg: 1/2 tab/wk 31-45 kg: 3/4 tab/wk > 45 kg: 1 tab/wk Upon return: continue until 4 weeks after last exposure
Alternatives:		
Chloroquine phosphate	Same as above	
plus		
Pyrimethamine-sulfadoxine‡ (Fansidar)	Carry a single dose (3 tablets) for self-treatment of febrile disease when medical care is not immediately available	Used as for adults in following doses: < 1 y: 1/4 tablet 1-3 y: 1/2 tablet 4-8 y: 1 tablet 9-14 y: 2 tablets > 14 y: 3 tablets
or		
Doxycycline§ alone	100 mg daily, starting 1-2 days before exposure and continuing for 4 wk afterwards	> 8 y: 2 mg/kg of body weight orally per d, up to adult dose of 100 mg/d

*At present, no drug regimen guarantees protection against malaria. Travelers to countries with risk of malaria should be advised to avoid mosquito bites by using personal protective measures (see text).

†Mefloquine should not be used by children lighter than 15 kg, pregnant women in the first trimester, people using beta blockers (or other cardiac drugs which may prolong cardiac condition), travelers involved in tasks requiring fine coordination and spatial discrimination (eg, airline crews), or persons with history of epilepsy or psychiatric disorder. Due to the frequency of side effects, especially dizziness, mefloquine should not be used for presumptive self-treatment.

‡Use of Fansidar, which contains 25 mg pyrimethamine and 500 mg sulfadoxine per tablet, is contraindicated in patients with history of sulfonamide or pyrimethamine intolerance, in pregnant women at term, and in infants younger than 2 months.

§Physicians who prescribe doxycycline as malaria chemoprophylaxis should advise patients to limit exposure to direct sunlight to minimize the possibility of photosensitivity reaction. Use of doxycycline is contraindicated in pregnant women and in children younger than 9 years.

Doxycycline alone is an additional alternative regimen for short-term travelers unable to take mefloquine (see Table 40). Travelers taking doxycycline should be advised of the possible side effects, including diarrhea, photosensitivity, and increased risk of monilial vaginitis. Use of doxycyline is contraindicated in pregnant women and usually in children younger than 9 years because of the risk of dental staining.

Prevention of Relapses. To prevent relapses of *P vivax* or *P ovale* infection after departure from areas where these species are endemic, use of primaquine phosphate (0.3 mg base/kg/d for 14 days) can be considered. Primaquine can cause hemolysis in patients with glucose-6-phosphate dehydrogenase deficiency; thus, all patients should be screened for this condition before primaquine therapy.

Protective Measures. All travelers to areas where malaria is endemic should be advised to use personal protective measures. These include the use of mosquito nets while sleeping, remaining in well-screened areas, wearing protective clothing, and the use of mosquito repellents containing "deet."* To be effective, these repellants require repeated application every 1 to 2 hours. Adverse reactions associated with deet include skin rashes, toxic encephalopathy, and seizures. Hence, it should be used sparingly on exposed skin and, where possible, it should be used on clothing to limit skin exposure. Travelers, particularly children, should be advised against using products containing high concentrations of deet directly on skin.

Malassezia furfur Fungemia

Clinical Manifestations: Fever, lethargy, and other signs of neonatal septicemia can occur.

Etiology: *Malassezia furfur* is a lipid-dependent fungus.

Epidemiology: Illness is seen primarily in premature infants and other neonates who are receiving parenteral nutrition that includes fat emulsions. In one study, 64% of infants in an intensive care unit had skin colonization with M furfur, compared to 3% of healthy infants.

Diagnosis: Routine media may not support growth of this organism since medium- and long-chain fatty acids are required. However, Sabouraud's medium overlaid with sterile olive oil provides an effective culture system.

*N,N-diethyl-m-toluamide

Treatment: Removal of catheters and temporary cessation of lipid infusions is usually adequate therapy. Although the organism is frequently sensitive to antifungal drugs, treatment with these drugs without catheter removal is usually not successful. The need for antifungal therapy in addition to catheter removal in patients with positive cultures from sites other than blood has not been determined.

Isolation of Hospitalized Patient: No special precautions are recommended.

Control Measures: None.

Measles

Clinical Manifestations: Measles is an acute, epidemic disease characterized by cough, coryza, conjunctivitis, and a confluent erythematous maculopapular rash and pathognomonic enanthem (Koplik spots). The disease is frequently complicated by middle ear infection and/or bronchopneumonia. Encephalitis has occurred in approximately 1 of every 1,000 cases recently reported in the United States. Survivors of this complication frequently have permanent brain damage. During the era of measles vaccination, death, predominantly from respiratory and neurologic complications, has occurred in 1 of every 1,000 cases reported in the United States. In 1989, 41 measles-associated deaths were reported in the United States, giving a mortality of less than 1 in 500 cases, and in some epidemics the mortality rate has exceeded 1%.

Subacute sclerosing panencephalitis (SSPE), a rare degenerative central nervous system disease characterized by behavioral and intellectual deterioration and convulsions, is a result of a persistent measles virus infection. With widespread measles vaccination, this complication has virtually disappeared.

Etiology: Measles virus is an RNA virus with one antigenic type, classified as a *morbillivirus* in the paramyxovirus family.

Epidemiology: Measles is a disease of man that is transmitted by direct contact with infectious droplets or, less commonly, by air-borne spread. In temperate areas, the peak incidence of infection in unvaccinated populations occurs during the winter and spring. In the prevaccine era, measles was an epidemic disease with biennial cycles in urban areas. Most cases occurred in preschool-aged and young school-aged children, and few persons were still susceptible at the age of 20 years. The childhood immunization program in the United States has been successful, resulting in a 95% reduction in the reported incidence of measles. During the 1960s and 1970s the number of reported cases fell dramatically in all age groups. The decline was greatest in children younger than 10 years and, as a result, the proportion of cases occurring in different age groups has changed. From 1984 to 1988, 58% of reported cases affected children 10 years and older.

In recent years, the incidence of measles in the United States has increased. Recent outbreaks are of two major types. First, outbreaks involving preschool-aged children (younger than 5 years) have occurred primarily in large urban settings. Although some children were too young (less than 15 months) to be immunized according to routine recommendations, most cases occurred in unvaccinated children who were old enough to have been vaccinated and, thus, were theoretically preventable cases. Second, outbreaks involved children and young adults 5 to 19 years of age, most of whom had been vaccinated; these were not preventable by previous immunization guidelines. These outbreaks occurred primarily in adolescents in junior and senior high schools and on college campuses.

The major reasons for the recent recrudescence of measles are as follows: (1) the immunization rate in preschool-aged children 15 months or older in some areas of the country is low; and (2) primary vaccine failure occurs in as many as 5% of individuals appropriately vaccinated at 15 months or older. Although some evidence indicates possible waning immunity after vaccination as a factor, most measles vaccine failures appear to occur in children who did not respond to the vaccine, i.e., primary vaccine failures. Nonetheless, loss of immunity by only a few percent of vaccinees would add substantial numbers to the pool of susceptible persons and contribute to measles transmission in outbreaks.

Patients are contagious from 1 to 2 days before the onset of symptoms (3 to 5 days before the rash) to 4 days after the appearance of the rash. Patients with SSPE are not contagious.

The **incubation period** is generally 8 to 12 days from exposure to onset of symptoms; the average interval from exposure to appearance of the rash is 14 days. In family studies, the average interval between appearance of rash in the source case and subsequent cases is 14 days, with a range of 7 to 18 days. In SSPE, the mean incubation period of 84 cases reported between 1976 and 1983 was 10.8 years.

Diagnostic Tests: Measles virus infection can be diagnosed specifically by viral isolation in tissue culture. However, virus isolation is technically difficult and usually not available. Many measles cases can be diagnosed by antibody determinations on acute sera taken shortly after appearance of the rash and on convalescent sera collected as early as 1, but preferably 3 to 4 weeks later. Some patients will already have experienced a substantial rise in antibody titer if the initial serum is obtained after the rash subsides. Most laboratories, however, can utilize a single specimen to detect the presence of measles-specific IgM antibody. Correct interpretation of serologic data requires knowledge of the time at which specimens were obtained relative to the onset of the rash. This point is especially important when interpreting negative serum IgM results, since IgM antibody may not be detectable on the first day or two after the onset of the rash and is usually undetectable 30 to 60 days after the onset of the rash. IgM-specific measles antibody testing is not always sensitive.

In SSPE, high titers of measles antibody are found in serum and cerebrospinal fluid.

Treatment: No specific antiviral therapy is available.

Isolation of the Hospitalized Patient: Respiratory isolation is indicated for 4 days after the onset of rash. In immunocompromised patients, isolation should be maintained for the duration of the illness.

Control Measures:

Care of Exposed Persons.

Use of Vaccine. Exposure to measles is not a contraindication to vaccination. Available data suggest that live measles virus vaccine, if given within 72 hours of measles exposure, can provide protection. If the exposure did not result in infection, the vaccine should induce protection against subsequent measles infection.

Use of Immune Globulin (IG). IG can be given to prevent or modify measles in a susceptible person within 6 days of exposure. The usual recommended dose of IG is 0.25 mL/kg of body weight given intramuscularly; immunocompromised children should receive 0.5 mL/kg (maximum dose in either instance is 15 mL). IG may be especially indicated for susceptible household contacts of measles patients, particularly those younger than 1 year and immunocompromised persons for whom the risk of complications is highest.

For patients who regularly receive intravenous immune globulin (IGIV), the dose of IGIV (based on milligrams of protein per kilogram body weight) is equivalent to that recommended for IG, since all preparations have a minimum titer based on the same standard that is used for IG. The usual dose of 100 to 400 mg/kg of IGIV should be more than sufficient for postexposure prophylaxis.

Live measles virus vaccine (if not contraindicated) should be given about 3 months after IG administration, by which time passive measles antibodies should have disappeared, provided that the child is at least 12 months old.

HIV Infection. Children and adolescents with symptomatic HIV infection who are exposed to measles should receive IG prophylaxis (0.5 mL/kg) regardless of vaccination status (see AIDS and HIV Infections, page 124). An exception may be the patient receiving IGIV at regular intervals whose last dose was received within 3 weeks of exposure. IG is also indicated for measles-susceptible household contacts with asymptomatic HIV infection, particularly for those younger than 1 year and susceptible pregnant women.

Children Younger Than 1 Year. The risk of complications resulting from measles is high among infants younger than 1 year. Therefore, considering the benefits and risks, infants as young as 6 months may be vaccinated for postexposure prophylaxis if the vaccine is given within 72 hours of exposure. If exposure occurred within the previous 6 days, IG may be given in an attempt to modify the disease.

Hospital Personnel. To decrease nosocomial infection, measures should be taken to ensure that personnel who will be in contact with patients with measles are immune to the disease.

Measles Virus Vaccine. The only measles vaccine currently licensed in the United States is a live attenuated virus vaccine prepared in chick embryo cell culture. It has been attenuated beyond that of the original Edmonston B strain and is, therefore, known as a further attenuated (Moraten vaccine) strain. Measles vaccine is available in monovalent (measles only) formulation and in combination, i.e., measles-rubella (MR) and measles-mumps-rubella (MMR) vaccines. MMR is the vaccine of choice for use in routine vaccination programs for children. In all situations where measles vaccine is to be used, a combination vaccine should be given if the recipients are also likely to be susceptible to rubella and/or mumps.

After administration of a single dose of live vaccine at 15 months or older, approximately 95% or more of vaccine recipients develop serum measles antibody. Evidence extending through 23 years indicates that the protection conferred by a single dose is durable in most persons. However, a small percentage of vaccinated individuals may lose protection after several years. Vaccination is not harmful for individuals already immune. Measles vaccine in seronegative persons produces a mild or inapparent, noncommunicable infection.

Improperly stored vaccine may fail to protect against measles. Since 1979, a stabilizer has been added to the vaccine that makes it more resistant to heat inactivation. However, during storage before reconstitution, measles vaccine must be kept at 2° to 8°C (35.6° to 46.4°F) or colder. It must also be protected from light, which can inactivate the virus. Vaccine must be shipped at 10°C (50°F) or colder and may be shipped on dry ice. Reconstituted vaccine should be stored in a refrigerator and discarded if not used within 8 hours.

Vaccine Recommendations (see Table 41 for summary).

General. Measles vaccine is indicated for persons susceptible to measles, unless otherwise contraindicated. Persons can be considered immune to measles only if they have had a documented episode of physician-diagnosed measles, have laboratory evidence of measles immunity, or have had documented immunization.

Effective measles control necessitates identification and immunization of all susceptible persons, especially preschool-aged children. Because of the continuing occurrence of cases in older children and young adults, increased emphasis must be placed on identifying and appropriately immunizing adolescents and young adults in high school, college, and health care institutional settings.

By 12 years of age, persons should have received two doses of live measles vaccine, the first of which should be given on or after the first birthday. The interval between doses should be one month or more. The Committee recommends that the second dose be given at entry to junior high school or middle school, i.e., at age 11 to 12 years. Some public health jurisdictions will mandate the second dose at school entry and physicians should comply with local requirements. A third dose is not indicated under these circumstances unless the first dose was given before the child's first birthday. Current recommendations for routine reimmunization allow for flexibility in the age of administration of the second dose.

Adolescents and adults should be considered susceptible unless they have documentation of physician-diagnosed measles, have laboratory evidence of immunity to measles, have documentation of two doses of measles vaccine (as previously described), or were born before 1957. However, since implementation of the two-dose schedule is gradual in most areas, one dose will suffice at present for those beyond middle or junior high school entry and before college entry. In future years, an increasing number of students will have received a second dose, and eventually adequate vaccination for all adolescents and young adults will be defined by receipt of two doses.

A parental report of immunization is not considered adequate documentation. A physician should provide an immunization record for a patient only if he or she has administered the vaccine or has seen a record documenting vaccination.

Dose and Vaccine. Live measles vaccine (as a monovalent or combination product) in a dose of 0.5 mL is given subcutaneously.

Table 41. Indications and Contraindications for Measles Vaccination Schedule*

Group	Remarks
	Indications
Unvaccinated, no history of measles (≥ 15 mo)	A two-dose schedule is recommended if born after 1956. The first dose is recommended at 15 months; the second at entry to middle school or junior high school. In localities where revaccination at school entry is mandated by law, such revaccination substitutes for the preceding recommendation
Children 15 mo	Routine immunization (with MMR)
Children 12-15 mo in areas of recurrent measles transmission	Initiate immunization
Children 6-15 mo in epidemic situations†	Immunize; if vaccinated before the first birthday, revaccination at 15 mo is necessary
Children 11-12 y who have received one dose of measles vaccine at ≥ 12 mo	Reimmunize
Students in college and other post-high-school institutions who have received one dose of measles vaccine at ≥ 12 mo	Reimmunize
History of vaccination before the first birthday	Consider unvaccinated and immunize
Unknown vaccine, 1963-1967	Consider unvaccinated and immunize
Further attenuated or unknown vaccine given with IG	Consider unvaccinated and immunize
Egg allergy, nonanaphylactic	Immunize; no reactions likely
Tuberculosis	Immunize; vaccine does not exacerbate
Measles exposure within 72 h	Immunization may protect (alternatively, IG can be given)
HIV-seropositive	Immunize

*See text for details.
†See Outbreak Control (page 321).

Table 41. Indications and Contraindications for Measles Vaccination Schedule* *(continued)*

Group	Remarks
Contraindications	
Pregnancy	Theoretical risk of fetal damage
Anaphylaxis to egg ingestion	Vaccinate with caution after skin testing
Anaphylactic allergy to neomycin	Vaccine contains neomycin
IG within 3 mo	Interference with immune response
Compromised immunity (except those with symptomatic HIV infection)	Possibility of severe infection with vaccine virus

*See text for details.

IG should not be given with the further attenuated measles virus vaccine.

MMR is given for the initial dose. For reimmunization, MMR is also recommended in order to provide additional immunization against mumps and rubella. Recently, the number of cases of mumps in previously vaccinated persons has increased and revaccination may be particularly important for control of mumps. Monovalent measles vaccine may be substituted for MMR if cost is a factor or for reasons of preference.

No unusual reactions have been associated with measles or MMR revaccination. The anticipated side effects are those of the individual vaccines but are expected to be infrequent, as most vaccinees will be immune.

Age for Routine Vaccination (see Tables 2 and 3, pages 17 and 18). In routine circumstances, the first dose should be given at age 15 months and the second dose at entrance to middle school or junior high school, usually at age 11 or 12 years. Revaccination at this age is recommended because of rapid impact on the prevention of measles, since the risk of measles increases substantially soon after entrance to middle school or junior high school. Thus, revaccination boosts immunity in the population soon before the high-risk period, and in individual patients it reinforces possible waning immunity. Vaccination at this age can easily be accomplished within the existing recommendations for health maintenance visits.* Alternatively, for reasons of

*See American Academy of Pediatrics, Committee on Psychosocial Aspects of Child and Family Health. *Guidelines for Health Supervision II.* Elk Grove Village, IL: American Academy of Pediatrics; 1988.

feasibility or local public health regulations, the second dose may be given at school entry (age 4 to 6 years). In jurisdictions where no law stipulates the age of revaccination, parents should be informed of the reasons for the recommendation for revaccination at 11 or 12 years of age.

Colleges and Other Institutions for Education Beyond High School. Colleges and other institutions should require documentation of measles, proof of immunity, or receipt of two doses of measles-containing vaccines before entry of all students. Students without documentation of any measles vaccination should receive a dose on entry followed by a repeat dose 1 or more months later.

Vaccination of Preschool-Aged Children in Areas of Recurrent Measles Transmission. Initial vaccination at 12 months of age, rather than at 15 months, is recommended for preschool-aged children in high-risk areas. Guidelines for defining such areas are as follows: (1) a county with more than five cases among preschool-aged children during each of the last five years; (2) a county with a recent outbreak among unvaccinated preschool-aged children; and (3) cities with large unvaccinated populations.

During an outbreak, monovalent measles vaccine may be given to infants as young as 6 months (see Outbreak Control, page 321). If monovalent vaccine is not available, MMR is not contraindicated and may be given. However, since seroconversion rates for measles, mumps, and rubella antigens are significantly less in children vaccinated before the first birthday than those in children vaccinated in the second year of life or later, children vaccinated before their first birthday should be vaccinated with MMR at 15 months and again at the time of entry to middle school or junior high school (age 11 or 12 years old).

International Travel. Persons traveling abroad should be immune to measles. Because an increasing number of cases of measles in the United States are attributable to exposure in foreign countries, vaccination against measles is particularly important. Consideration should be given to providing a dose of measles vaccine to persons born after January 1, 1957, who travel abroad, who have not previously received two doses of measles vaccine, and who do not otherwise have evidence of measles immunity.

For children traveling to areas where measles is endemic or epidemic, the age for initial measles vaccination should be lowered. Children 12 to 14 months should be given MMR before their departure. Infants 6 to 11 months should receive a dose of monovalent measles vaccine (or MMR) before their departure; at 12 to 15 months they should receive MMR if they remain in a high-risk area, or at 15 months if they return to the United States. Reimmunization, according to the previously given recommendation, should subsequently be implemented.

Since almost all infants younger than 6 months are protected by maternally derived antibodies, immunization is not needed by these infants until they are 6 to 9 months of age. At this time, if they remain in the high-risk area, they should be vaccinated. Vaccines provided through the Expanded Programme on Immunization (EPI) in developing countries meet World Health Organization standards.

Medical Facilities. Evidence of prior measles or receipt of two measles vaccinations is desirable before beginning employment for nurses, nursing and medical students, residents, and other staff born after January 1, 1957. For recommendations during an outbreak, see Outbreak Control (page 321).

Revaccination of Persons Vaccinated According to Pre-1989 Recommendations.

- *Vaccination before 12 months of age.* These children should be considered unvaccinated and receive their initial dose at 15 months of age.
- *Vaccination at 12 to 14 months of age.* These children should be considered to have received an acceptable first vaccination and should receive a second dose, according to previously described recommendation.
- *Recipients of inactivated (killed) vaccine.* Two doses of live measles vaccine separated by no less than one month are recommended for individuals vaccinated at any age with inactivated vaccine, and for those vaccinated with inactivated vaccine followed by live vaccine within 3 months. Recipients of inactivated measles vaccine (available in the United States from 1963 to 1967), when exposed to natural virus, are at risk of developing the atypical measles syndrome, which can be severe and result in serious complications.

  As many as 50% of recipients of inactivated measles vaccine have reactions after revaccination with live measles vaccine. Most of these reactions are mild and consist of local swelling and erythema, with or without low-grade fever lasting 1 to 2 days. Rarely, more severe reactions, including prolonged high fevers, lymphadenopathy, and extensive local reactions, occur and may necessitate hospitalization of the patient. However, recipients of killed measles vaccine are more likely to have serious illness when exposed to natural measles than when given live measles virus vaccine.
- *Persons immunized with unknown vaccine between 1963 and 1967.* The preceding recommendations for recipients of the inactivated vaccine apply to persons vaccinated between 1963 and 1967 with a vaccine of unknown type, as their only vaccination

may have been with inactivated vaccine. Because killed measles vaccine was not distributed in the United States after 1967, persons vaccinated after 1967 and on or after their first birthday with a vaccine of unknown type need not be revaccinated. In Canada, killed measles vaccine was not distributed after 1970.

- *Persons who received IG with vaccine*. Edmonston B measles vaccine was effective when administered with IG, but the response to further attenuated strains (i.e., Schwartz or Moraten) may be impeded by receipt of an IG within 3 months. A person who received further attenuated vaccine or a vaccine of an unknown type with IG should be considered unvaccinated and given two doses of vaccine, as previously described (also see Precautions and Contraindications, page 318).

Measles vaccine can be given simultaneously with other vaccines (see Simultaneous Administration of Multiple Vaccines, page 16).

Adverse Reactions. About 5% to 15% of vaccinees develop a fever of 39.4°C (103°F) or higher beginning about the sixth day after vaccination; the fever generally lasts 1 to 2 days (and as many as 5 days). Most persons with fever are otherwise asymptomatic. Transient rashes have been reported in approximately 5% of vaccinees. Central nervous system conditions, including encephalitis and encephalopathy, have been reported in an approximate frequency of less than one per million doses administered in the United States. Because the incidence of encephalitis or encephalopathy following measles vaccination in the United States is lower than the observed incidence of encephalitis of unknown etiology, some or most of the reported severe neurologic disorders may be only temporally, rather than causally, related to measles vaccination. Limited data indicate that reactions to vaccination are not age related. After revaccination, reactions are expected to be clinically similar but much less frequent in occurrence since most vaccine recipients are already immune.

Convulsions. As with any condition that induces fever during the second year of life, children predisposed to febrile seizures can experience seizures after measles immunization. Most of these seizures are simple febrile seizures and occur in children without known risk factors. These seizures do not increase the risk of subsequent epilepsy or other neurologic disorders. Recent studies have suggested an increased risk of convulsions after administration of measles-containing vaccines to children who have history of previous seizures or whose first-degree family members have history of seizures. Although the exact risk cannot be determined, it appears to be low. The recommendation to immunize children with personal history of convulsions or those whose first-degree relatives have history of convulsions is based on factors indicating that the benefits greatly outweigh the risks. These include the risk from measles disease, the large number of children with personal or family history of seizures (5% to 7%), the low incidence of seizures following measles vaccination, and the lack of association of these seizures with permanent brain damage.

Subacute Sclerosing Pancephalitis (SSPE). Measles vaccine, by protecting against measles, significantly reduces the possibility of developing SSPE. The recent decline in numbers of SSPE cases is additional strong, presumptive evidence of a protective effect of measles vaccination. However, SSPE has been rarely reported in children with no history of natural measles but with history of receiving measles vaccine. Some of these children may have had unrecognized measles before vaccination. No evidence indicates an enhanced risk of SSPE from live measles vaccine given to individuals who previously received live measles vaccine or had natural measles infection.

Precautions and Contraindications:

- *Pregnancy.* Live measles vaccine, when given as a component of MR or MMR, should not be given to women known to be pregnant or who are considering becoming pregnant within 3 months of vaccination. Women who are given monovalent vaccine should not become pregnant for at least 30 days. This precaution is based on the theoretical risk of fetal infection, which applies to the administration of any live virus vaccine to women who might be pregnant or who might become pregnant shortly after vaccination. No evidence substantiates this theoretical risk.

  In the immunization of adolescents and young adults against measles, asking women if they are pregnant, excluding those who are, and explaining the theoretical risks to the others are recommended precautions.
- *Febrile illness.* Children with minor illnesses with or without fever, such as upper respiratory tract infection, may be vaccinated (see Vaccine Safety and Contraindications, page 22). Fever per se is not a contraindication to immunization. However, if other manifestations suggest a more serious illness, the child should not be vaccinated until recovery.
- *Allergies.* Live measles vaccine is produced in chick embryo cell culture. Hypersensitivity reactions rarely follow the administration of live measles vaccine. Most of these reactions are considered minor and consist of wheal-and-flare reactions or urticaria at the injection site. After distribution of more than 174 million doses of measles vaccine in the United States, only five cases of immediate allergic reactions in children with history of anaphylactic reactions to egg ingestion have been reported. These reactions could have been life-threatening; four children experienced difficulty breathing and one of these had hypotension. Persons with

history of anaphylactic reactions (hives, swelling of the mouth and throat, difficulty breathing, hypotension, and shock) after egg ingestion should be vaccinated only with extreme caution (see Hypersensitivity Reactions to Vaccine Constituents, page 29). Persons are not at increased risk if they have egg allergies that are not anaphylactic in type. Such persons should be vaccinated in the usual manner. Persons with allergies to chickens or feathers are also not at increased risk of reaction to the vaccine.

Because measles vaccine contains trace amounts of neomycin (25 μg), persons who have experienced anaphylactic reactions to topically or systemically administered neomycin should not receive measles vaccine. Most often, neomycin allergy manifests as a contact dermatitis which is a delayed-type (cell-mediated) immune response rather than anaphylaxis. In such persons, any adverse reaction to neomycin in the vaccine would be an erythematous, pruritic nodule or papule 48 to 96 hours after vaccination. A history of contact dermatitis to neomycin is not a contraindication to receiving measles vaccine. Measles vaccine does not contain penicillin.

- *Recent administration of an immune globulin.* Vaccination should be deferred for 3 months after a person has received an IG, whole blood, or other antibody-containing blood products because passively acquired antibodies might interfere with the response to the vaccine. If vaccine is given to a person who has received such a product within the preceding 3 months, the person should be revaccinated approximately 3 months later unless serologic testing indicates that measles-specific antibodies were produced. If IG is to be administered in preparation for international travel, administration of vaccine should precede receipt of IG by at least 2 weeks to preclude interference with replication of the vaccine virus.
- *Tuberculosis.* Tuberculin skin testing is not a prerequisite for measles vaccination. Although tuberculosis may be exacerbated by natural measles infection, live measles virus vaccine does not have a deleterious effect and the value of protection against natural measles far outweighs the theoretical hazard of possible exacerbation of unsuspected tuberculosis. If tuberculin skin testing is otherwise indicated, it can be done on the day of vaccination. Otherwise, it should be postponed for 4 to 6 weeks since measles vaccination may temporarily suppress tuberculin skin test reactivity.
- *Altered immunity.* Significantly immunocompromised patients, with the exception of those with HIV infection, should not be given live measles virus vaccine (see Immunodeficient and Immunosuppressed Children, page 47). Replication of the measles

vaccine virus can be potentiated in patients with immunodeficiency diseases and by the suppressed immune responses associated with leukemia, lymphoma, or generalized malignancy, or resulting from therapy with pharmacologic doses of corticosteroids, alkylating drugs, antimetabolites, or radiation. Patients with such conditions should not be vaccinated with live measles virus vaccine. Their risk of exposure to measles can be reduced by vaccinating their close susceptible contacts. Vaccinated persons do not transmit vaccine virus. Management of patients with immune deficiencies, should they be exposed to measles, can be facilitated by prior knowledge of their immune status. Susceptible patients with immune deficiencies should receive IG after exposure (see Care of Exposed Persons, page 310).

After cessation of immunosuppressive therapy, live measles virus vaccine is generally withheld for an interval of not less than 3 months. This interval is based on the assumption that immunologic responsiveness will have been restored in 3 months and the underlying disease for which immunosuppressive therapy was given is in remission or under control. However, because the interval can vary with the intensity and type of immunosuppressive therapy, radiation therapy, underlying disease, and other factors, a definitive recommendation for an interval after cessation of immunosuppressive therapy when live measles vaccine can be safely and effectively administered is often not possible.

- *HIV infection.* Measles vaccination (given as MMR) is recommended for patients with HIV infection, symptomatic or asymptomatic, at 15 months of age. Older children and adolescents with HIV infection who have not been previously immunized against MMR should also be vaccinated. This recommendation is based on reports of severe measles, including fatalities, in these patients and the lack of complications from live virus vaccine in children with HIV infection (see AIDS and HIV Infections, page 125). Regardless of vaccination status, however, symptomatic HIV-infected patients who are exposed to measles should receive IG prophylaxis (see Care of Exposed Persons, page 310).
- *Personal and/or family history of convulsions.* Children with this history should be vaccinated after discussion of the risks and benefits of immunization with parent or guardian (see Adverse Reactions, page 317). The parents or guardians of children who have either a personal or immediate family history of seizures should be advised that such children have a slightly increased risk of seizures after measles vaccination, and they should be advised about appropriate care in the unlikely event that a seizure does occur.

Since fever induced by measles vaccine usually occurs between 5 and 12 days after immunization, prevention of vaccine-related, febrile seizures is difficult. Prophylaxis with antipyretics may be considered; if given, antipyretic prophylaxis should be given before the expected onset of fever and continued for another 5 to 7 days, and is not effective if given after the onset of fever. Parents should be alert to the occurrence of fever after vaccination and should treat their children appropriately.

Children who are receiving anticonvulsants should continue to take such therapy after measles vaccination. However, prophylactic use of anticonvulsants may not be feasible, as therapeutic concentrations of many of the currently prescribed anticonvulsants (e.g., phenobarbital) are not achieved for some time after the initiation of therapy.

Outbreak Control (see Table 42 for summary). All reports of suspected measles cases should be investigated promptly. A measles outbreak exists in a community whenever one case of measles is confirmed. Once this occurs, preventing the spread of measles depends on the prompt vaccination of susceptible persons. Control activities should not be delayed for laboratory results on suspected cases. Persons who cannot readily provide documentation of measles immunity should be vaccinated or excluded from the setting (e.g., school). Documentation of vaccination is adequate only if the date of vaccination is provided. Almost all persons who are excluded from an outbreak area because they lack documentation of immunity quickly comply with vaccination requirements. Persons who have been exempted from measles vaccination for medical, religious, or other reasons should be excluded from the outbreak area until at least 2 weeks after the onset of rash in the last case of measles.

Schools and Day Care Centers. A program of revaccination with MMR vaccine is recommended during outbreaks in day care centers; elementary, middle, junior, and senior high schools; and colleges and other institutions of higher education. Consideration should be given to revaccination in unaffected schools that may be at risk of measles transmission. Revaccination should include all students and their siblings and personnel born in or after 1957 who cannot provide documentation that they received two doses of measles-containing vaccine on or after their first birthday or other evidence of measles immunity. Persons revaccinated, as well as unvaccinated persons receiving their first dose as part of the outbreak control program, may be immediately readmitted to school. Mass revaccination of entire communities is not necessary.

Imposing quarantine measures for outbreak control is both difficult and disruptive to schools and other organizations. Under special circumstances, restriction of an event might be warranted;

Table 42. Recommendations for Measles Outbreak Control*

Outbreaks in preschool-aged children	Age for vaccination should be lowered to 6 mo in outbreak area if cases are occurring in children < 1 year.†
Outbreaks in institutions: day care centers, K-12th grades, colleges, and other institutions	Revaccination of all students and their siblings and of school personnel born in or after 1957 who do not have documentation of immunity to measles.‡
Outbreaks in medical facilities	Revaccination of all medical workers born in or after 1957 who have direct patient contact and who do not have proof of immunity to measles.‡ Vaccination may also be considered for workers born before 1957.
	Susceptible personnel who have been exposed should be relieved from direct patient contact from the 5th to the 21st day after exposure (regardless of whether they received measles vaccine or IG) or, if they become ill, for 7 days after they develop rash.

*Revaccination should be limited to populations at risk, such as students attending institutions where cases occur. Mass revaccination of entire populations is not necessary.

†Children initially vaccinated before the first birthday should be revaccinated at 15 months of age. A second dose should be administered according to local policy.

‡Proof consists of documentation of physician-diagnosed measles disease, serologic evidence of immunity to measles, or documentation of receipt of two doses of measles vaccine on or after the first birthday.

however, such action is not recommended as a routine measure for outbreak control.

Preschool-Aged Children. The risk of complications from measles is high among infants younger than 1 year. Therefore, considering the benefits and risks, vaccination with monovalent measles vaccine is recommended for infants as young as 6 months when exposure to natural measles is considered likely. MMR may be administered to children before the first birthday if monovalent measles vaccine is not readily available. Children vaccinated before the first birthday should be revaccinated when they are 15 months and again during their school years (see Vaccine Recommendations, page 312).

Medical Settings. If an outbreak occurs in an area served by a hospital or within a hospital, all employees with direct patient contact who were born in or after 1957 who cannot provide documentation that they have received two doses of measles vaccine on or after their first birthday or other evidence of immunity to measles should receive a dose of measles vaccine. Since some medical personnel who have acquired measles in medical facilities were born before 1957, vaccination of older employees who may have occupational exposure to measles should also be considered during outbreaks. Susceptible personnel who have been exposed should be relieved from direct patient contact from the fifth to the 21st day after exposure regardless of whether they received vaccine or IG after the exposure. Personnel who become ill should be relieved from patient contact for 7 days after they develop rash.

Meningococcal Infections

Clinical Manifestations: Invasive meningococcal infections usually result in meningococcemia and/or meningitis. Onset is abrupt in meningococcemia with fever, chills, malaise, prostration, and a rash that initially may be urticarial, maculopapular, or petechial. In fulminant cases, purpura, disseminated intravascular coagulation, shock, coma, and death (Waterhouse-Friderichsen syndrome) can ensue within several hours despite appropriate therapy. The signs of meningitis due to meningococcal organisms are indistinguishable from those of acute meningitis caused by *Haemophilus influenzae* and *Streptococcus pneumoniae*. Invasive meningococcal infections can be complicated by arthritis, myocarditis, pericarditis, endophthalmitis, or pneumonia. Other less common meningococcal diseases include primary pneumonia, occult febrile bacteremia, conjunctivitis, and chronic meningococcemia.

Etiology: *Neisseria meningitidis* is a Gram-negative diplococcus with nine serogroups (A, B, C, D, X, Y, Z, 29-E, and W-135). Groups B, C, Y, and W-135 are currently the most prevalent in the United States. Group A has been associated frequently with epidemics elsewhere in the world.

Epidemiology: Asymptomatic colonization of the upper respiratory tract is frequent and provides the focus from which the organism is spread. Transmission is from person to person through infected droplets of respiratory secretions. Disease occurs most frequently in children younger than 5 years; the peak attack rate occurs in the 6- to 12-month age group. Close contacts of patients with meningococcal disease are at an increased risk of developing infection; outbreaks have occurred in semiclosed communities, including day care centers, nursery schools, colleges, and military recruit camps. Patients with deficiency of a terminal complement component (C5-9) are at particular risk for invasive and recurrent meningococcal disease. Patients are considered capable of transmitting infection for approximately 24 hours after the initiation of effective treatment.

The **incubation period** is from 1 to 10 days, most commonly less than 4 days.

Diagnostic Tests: Cultures of blood and cerebrospinal fluid (CSF) are indicated in all patients with suspected invasive meningococcal disease. Cultures of petechial scraping, synovial fluid, sputum, and other body fluids are positive in some patients. Gram stain of a petechial scraping, CFS and buffy coat of blood can be helpful on occasion. Antigen detection tests (e.g., latex agglutination) of CSF, serum, and urine with group-specific meningococcal antisera can allow rapid diagnosis and be particularly useful if antibiotics were administered before the collection of specimens for culture. In some cases, the value of the test is limited by lack of adequate sensitivity and specificity of the reagents, especially that of group B meningococcal antisera (which also reacts with KI *E coli*).

Treatment:

- Penicillin G administered intravenously in a high dose every 4 to 6 hours is the therapy of choice for patients with invasive disease. In the few areas (Spain and parts of Africa) where penicillin in vitro resistance has been reported, chloramphenicol, cefotaxime, and ceftriaxone are acceptable alternatives. In the patient with penicillin allergy of the anaphylactoid type, chloramphenicol is indicated. Five to 7 days of antibiotic therapy is usually adequate for most cases of invasive meningococcal disease.
- Dexamethasone therapy should be considered in infants and children 2 months of age and older with bacterial meningitis after the physician has considered the benefits and possible risks (see Dexamethasone Therapy for Bacterial Meningitis in Infants and Children, page 566). The regimen is 0.6 mg/kg/d in four divided doses, given intravenously, for the first four days of antibiotic treatment, and should be initiated with the first dose of antibacterial therapy.

Isolation of the Hospitalized Patient: Respiratory isolation is indicated for 24 hours after initiation of effective therapy.

Control Measures:

Care of Exposed Persons.

Careful Observation. Exposed household, school, or day care contacts must be carefully observed. Exposed individuals who develop a febrile illness should receive prompt medical evaluation. If indicated, antimicrobial therapy appropriate for invasive meningococcal infections should be administered.

Household, Day Care Center, and Nursery School Contacts. These persons should receive antibiotic prophylaxis as soon as possible, preferably within 24 hours of the diagnosis of the primary case. Prophylaxis is also warranted for persons who have had contact with the patient's oral secretions through kissing or sharing of food or beverages. Prophylaxis is not routinely recommended for medical personnel, except those with intimate exposure (such as occurs with mouth-to-mouth resuscitation, intubation, or suctioning) before antibiotic therapy was begun. Respiratory tract cultures are not of value in deciding who should receive prophylaxis.

Chemoprophylaxis. The drug of choice in most instances is rifampin; sulfisoxazole is recommended when an isolate is known to be sulfa-susceptible.

The recommended regimen for rifampin prophylaxis is 10 mg/kg (maximum dose, 600 mg) every 12 hours, for a total of four doses during 2 days. Some experts recommend reducing the dose to 5 mg/kg for infants younger than 1 month. A liquid preparation can be formulated or the powder can be mixed with other vehicles such as applesauce. For adults, each dose is 600 mg. The four-day rifampin regimen, given for prophylaxis of *Haemophilus influenzae* type b disease of 20 mg/kg (600 mg maximum) once daily for 4 days, has also been demonstrated to be effective for meningococcal prophylaxis.

For sulfisoxazole chemoprophylaxis, the dose is 500 mg daily for infants younger than 1 year, 500 mg every 12 hours for children 1 to 12 years, and 1 g every 12 hours for children older than 12 years and for adults.

Ceftriaxone given in a single intramuscular dose of 125 mg for children younger than 12 years and 250 mg for adults has been demonstrated in a recent study to be more effective than oral rifampin in eradicating the meningococcal group A carrier state. Ceftriaxone is not routinely recommended for prophylaxis because its efficacy has been confirmed only for group A strains. It has the advantages of possible greater efficacy than rifampin, easier dosage administration and availability, and safety in pregnancy.

Immunoprophylaxis. Because secondary cases can occur several weeks or longer after onset of disease in the index case, meningococcal vaccine can be considered as a possible adjunct to chemoprophylaxis when the outbreak is caused by a vaccine serogroup. The result of one study demonstrated efficacy of the vaccine in reducing the occurrence of secondary cases.

Meningococcal Vaccine. A serogroup-specific quadrivalent meningococcal vaccine* against groups A, C, Y, and W-135 *N meningitidis* is available in the United States. The vaccine consists of 50 µg each of the respective purified bacterial capsular polysaccharides. The vaccine is administered subcutaneously as a single 0.5-mL dose.

The Group A component is immunogenic in children 3 months and older. For children younger than 18 months, two doses 3 months apart have been given in epidemic control. If the quadrivalent vaccine is used in infants, response to the other meningococcal group polysaccharides is usually poor. Group C component is effective in children 2 years and older. The duration of protection is not established but is likely to be less than 3 years against group A infections in children immunized when younger than 4 years.

Infrequent and mild adverse reactions occur, principally localized erythema for 1 to 2 days. The safety of the vaccine in pregnant women has not been established.

Indications. Routine vaccination of children with meningococcal vaccine is not recommended. However, vaccine should be administered routinely to children 2 years and older in high-risk groups, including those with functional or anatomic asplenia (see Asplenic Children, page 52) and those with terminal complement component deficiencies. The vaccine should be used to control outbreaks of disease caused by serogroups represented in the vaccine, can be considered as an adjunct to chemoprophylaxis (see Care of Exposed Persons, page 325), and may be of benefit to travelers to countries recognized to have hyperendemic or epidemic disease.

The vaccine is currently given to all American military recruits.

Molluscum Contagiosum

Clinical Manifestations: Molluscum contagiosum is a benign viral disease of the skin characterized by a relatively small number, usually 2 to 20, of asymptomatic discrete, papular, waxy lesions with central umbilication in a generalized distribution. An eczematous reaction may encircle the lesions in about 10% of patients. It has no systemic manifestations.

Etiology: The cause of molluscum contagiosum is a poxvirus.

---

*Meningococcal Polysaccharide Vaccine, Groups A, C, Y, W-135 Combined (Menomune), is available from Connaught Laboratories, Swiftwater, PA.

Epidemiology: Humans are the only known source of the virus. It is spread by direct contact, including sexual contact, or by fomites. The infectivity is generally low, but occasional outbreaks have been reported. The period of communicability is unknown.

The **incubation period** appears to vary between 2 and 7 weeks, but may extend to 6 months.

Diagnostic Tests: The diagnosis can usually be made from the characteristic clinical appearance of the lesions. However, staining of the material expressed from the central core of the lesions reveals characteristic intracytoplasmic inclusions. Electron microscopic examination will identify the typical poxvirus particles.

Treatment: Mechanical removal of the central core of each lesion usually results in resolution. Although lesions may regress spontaneously, removal is advisable to prevent autoinoculation.

Isolation of the Hospitalized Patient: No special precautions are recommended.

Control Measures: No control measures are known for isolated cases. For outbreaks, such as commonly found in the tropics, restricting direct body contact between affected and unaffected children can reduce the spread.

Moraxella catarrhalis Infections

(Branhamella catarrhalis)

Clinical Manifestations: *Moraxella catarrhalis* is a cause of otitis media and paranasal sinusitis in children. It also has been reported to cause bronchopulmonary infection in patients with chronic lung disease and is a rare cause of bacteremia in children (normal or immunocompromised) and conjunctivitis in neonates.

Etiology: *Moraxella catarrhalis* (formerly called *Branhamella catarrhalis* and earlier *Neisseria catarrhalis*) is a Gram-negative diplococcus. Beta-lactamase production mediating resistance to penicillins has been identified in more than 75% of strains.

Epidemiology: The natural reservoir is the upper respiratory tract of humans. *M catarrhalis* is part of the normal flora. Carriage may be more frequent during the fall and winter than during the spring and summer. The mode of transmission is presumed to be direct contact with contaminated respiratory secretions and/or droplet spread. Infection is most frequent in infants but occurs at all ages. Transmission in families, schools, and day care centers has not been studied. The duration of carriage by infected and colonized children, and the period of communicability are unknown.

The **incubation period** is unknown.

Diagnostic Tests: The organism can be isolated readily on common culture media (blood or chocolate agar) after incubation in air or with increased CO_2 (candle jar). In patients with unusually severe infection, in some who are treatment failures, and in neonates or other highly susceptible children, culture of middle ear or sinus fluid is indicated. Recovery of *M catarrhalis* with other pathogens (*S pneumoniae* or *H influenzae*) can occur, indicating a mixed infection.

Treatment: Appropriate antimicrobials for the treatment of common *M catarrhalis* infections are those recommended in general for the initial treatment of otitis media and sinusitis. If an ampicillin-resistant strain is isolated, appropriate antimicrobial choices include amoxicillin-clavulanate, cefixime, cefaclor, erythromycin-sulfisoxazole, and trimethoprim-sulfamethoxazole. If parenteral drugs are needed to treat *M catarrhalis* infection or other concurrent bacterial infections in a mixed infection, in vitro data indicate that the following drugs will be effective: cefuroxime, cefotaxime, ceftriaxone, chloramphenicol, and trimethoprim-sulfamethoxazole.

Isolation of the Hospitalized Patient: No special precautions are recommended.

Control Measures: None.

Mumps

Clinical Manifestations: Mumps is a systemic disease, characterized by swelling of the salivary glands, that can involve multiple organs and can be moderately debilitating. However, approximately one third of infections do not cause clinically apparent salivary gland swelling. Meningeal signs are reported in as many as 15% of cases. Encephalitis occurs in as many as 0.5% of cases and has an average case fatality rate of 1.4%; permanent sequelae are otherwise rare. Orchitis is a common complication after puberty but sterility rarely occurs. Other rare complications include arthritis, renal involvement, thyroiditis, mastitis, and hearing impairment.

Etiology: Mumps is caused by a paramyxovirus.

Epidemiology: Man is the only known natural host. The virus is spread by direct contact via the respiratory route. Infection occurs throughout childhood. Mumps during adulthood is more likely to produce severe disease, including orchitis. Death from mumps is rare; more than half occur in persons older than 19 years. Mumps infection during the first trimester of pregnancy can increase the rate of spontaneous abortion, which has been reported to be as high as 27%. Although mumps virus can cross the placenta, no evidence indicates that mumps infection in pregnancy causes congenital malformations. The infection is more common during the late winter and spring. The incidence has declined markedly since the introduction of the live mumps virus vaccine but in 1986 to 1987 a mild resurgence occurred. Whereas most mumps cases continue to occur in school-aged children 5 to 14 years of age, the reported peak incidence in 1986 to 1987 shifted from children 5 to 9 years old to middle and high school students 10 to 19 years old. Persons 15 years and older accounted for more than one third of reported cases and outbreaks in high schools, colleges, and occupational settings. Outbreaks can occur in highly vaccinated populations, indicating that mumps transmission can be sustained among the few persons not protected by control vaccination. The period of communicability is usually 1 to 2 days but can be as long as 7 days prior to the onset of parotid swelling, and is usually 5, and occasionally as long as 9 days after onset.

The **incubation period** is usually from 16 to 18 days, but cases may occur from 12 to 25 days after exposure.

Diagnostic Tests: Mumps virus can be isolated in tissue culture inoculated with throat washings, urine, and spinal fluid. The complement fixation (CF), neutralization, or hemagglutination inhibition (HAI) test or an ELISA can be used to serologically confirm infection. Although paired sera are desirable, a single serum specimen containing complement fixing antibody against the soluble component of mumps virus suggests recent infection. An ELISA or neutralization test, although not always readily available, should be used for assessing immunity; CF or HAI tests are unreliable for this purpose. Skin tests are unreliable and should not be used to test immune status.

Treatment: Supportive.

Isolation of the Hospitalized Patient: Respiratory isolation is indicated. Patients should be isolated until the swelling has subsided or other manifestations have cleared. Usually, patients can be considered to be no longer contagious 9 days after the onset of parotid swelling.

Control Measures:

School and Day Care. Children should be excluded until 9 days after the onset of parotid gland swelling. For control measures during an outbreak, see Outbreak Control, page 332.

Care of Exposed Persons. Mumps vaccine has not been demonstrated to be effective in preventing infection after exposure. However, mumps vaccine can be given after exposure, as immunization will provide protection against subsequent exposures. No increased risk of reactions or contraindications exist after vaccination of a person during the incubation period of mumps or from vaccination of a person who is already immune. Because approximately 90% of adults who have no knowledge of past infection are immune on serologic testing, mumps vaccine is not routinely advised for those born before 1957 unless they are proven to be susceptible (i.e., seronegative). Mumps immune globulin is of no value and is no longer manufactured.

Mumps Virus Vaccine. Live mumps virus vaccine is prepared in chick embryo cell cultures. Live virus vaccine is administered by subcutaneous injection of 0.5 mL, either alone or as a combined vaccine containing measles and rubella vaccines (MMR). More than 95% of all persons susceptible to mumps develop antibody after a single dose. Serologic and epidemiologic evidence extending through 20 years indicates that vaccine-induced immunity is long lasting and may be lifelong.

Vaccine Recommendations.

- Mumps vaccine should be given routinely to children after the first birthday. It is usually given at 15 months of age as the combined vaccine MMR (see Tables 2 and 3, pages 17 and 18). A second dose of MMR is now recommended at entry to middle school or junior high school. Alternatively, some states mandate the second dose of MMR at school entry for ease of implementation.

  The combined vaccine is recommended to assure immunity to mumps and rubella as well as measles (see Measles, Vaccine Recommendations, page 312). Mumps revaccination is particularly important because mumps can occur in highly vaccinated populations and substantial numbers of cases have occurred in persons with history of mumps vaccination. Administration of MMR is not harmful if given to an individual already immune to one or more of these viruses (from either infection or vaccination).
- Mumps vaccination is of particular value for children approaching puberty and for adolescents and adults who have not had mumps. At office visits of prepubertal children and adolescents, the status of immunity to mumps should be assessed. Persons should be considered susceptible unless they have documentation of physician-diagnosed mumps, adequate immunization for their age, or serologic evidence of immunity.

- *International travel.* Mumps is still endemic throughout most of the world. Although vaccination against mumps is not a requirement for entry into any country, susceptible children, adolescents, and adults born before 1957 would benefit by mumps vaccination (usually as MMR) before beginning travel. Because of concern about inadequate seroconversion due to persisting maternal antibodies and because the risk of serious disease from mumps infection is relatively low, persons younger than 12 months need not be given mumps vaccine before travel.
- Mumps vaccine is not routinely advised for those born before 1957 unless they are considered susceptible, such as if seronegative. However, vaccination is not contraindicated in these persons.
- Mumps vaccine can be given simultaneously with other vaccines (see Simultaneous Administration of Multiple Vaccine, page 16).

Adverse Reactions. Adverse reactions attributed to live mumps vaccine are extremely rare. Temporally related reactions, including febrile seizures, nerve deafness, encephalitis, rash, pruritus, and purpura, may not be related etiologically. The frequency of central nervous system complications after mumps vaccination is lower than the observed background incidence in the normal population. Orchitis has been reported rarely.

Reimmunization with mumps vaccine (monovalent or MMR) is not associated with an increased incidence of reactions. Reactions would be expected only among those not protected by the first dose.

Precautions and Contraindications:

- *Pregnancy.* Susceptible postpubertal females should not be vaccinated if pregnant and should be counseled before vaccination about the potential hazard of fetal infection with vaccine virus. Live mumps virus vaccine can cross the placenta, but virus has not been isolated from fetal tissues of susceptible females who received vaccine and underwent elective abortions. In view of the theoretical risk, however, conception should be avoided for 3 months after vaccination.
- *Allergies.* Mumps vaccine is virtually devoid of allergenic substances derived from the chick embryo cell cultures used for growth of the live vaccine viruses. However, a remote, potential risk of hypersensitivity reactions in patients allergic to eggs does exist. The large-scale use of the vaccine since 1967 has resulted in only rare, isolated reports of allergic reactions. Persons with anaphylactic reactions to eggs should receive live mumps vaccine only with extreme caution (see Hypersensitivity Reactions to Vaccine Constituents, page 29). Mumps vaccine does not con-tain penicillin.
- *Recent administration of immune globulin (IG).* Live mumps vaccine should be given at least 2 weeks before or at least 3 months after administration of IG or blood transfusion because of the pos-

sibility that antibody will neutralize vaccine virus and prevent a successful immunization.

- *Altered immunity.* Patients with immunodeficiency diseases; those receiving immunosuppressive therapy (e.g., patients with leukemia, lymphoma, or generalized malignancy); those receiving pharmacologic doses of corticosteroids, alkylating agents, antimetabolites, or radiation; and patients who are otherwise immunocompromised should not receive live mumps virus vaccine. The exceptions are patients with symptomatic HIV infection who are to be immunized against measles with MMR (see AIDS and HIV Infections, page 124). The risk of mumps exposure for patients with altered immunity can be reduced by vaccinating their close susceptible contacts. Vaccinated persons do not transmit mumps vaccine virus.

  After cessation of immunosuppressive therapy, live mumps virus vaccine is generally withheld for an interval of not less than 3 months. This interval is based on the assumption that immunologic responsiveness will have been restored in 3 months and the underlying disease for which immunosuppressive therapy was given is in remission or under control. However, because the interval can vary with the intensity and type of immunosuppressive therapy, radiation therapy, underlying disease, and other factors, a definitive recommendation for an interval after cessation of immunosuppressive therapy when live mumps vaccine can be safely and effectively administered is often not possible.
- *Febrile illness.* Children with minor illnesses with or without fever, such as upper respiratory tract infections, may be vaccinated (see Vaccine Safety and Contraindications, page 22). Fever per se is not a contraindication to immunization. However, if other manifestations suggest a more serious illness, the child should not be vaccinated until recovery.

Outbreak Control. In determining means to control outbreaks, exclusion of susceptible students from affected schools and schools judged by local public health authorities to be at risk for transmission should be considered. Such exclusion should be an effective means of terminating school outbreaks and rapidly increasing rates of immunization. Excluded students can be readmitted immediately after vaccination. Pupils who have been exempted from mumps vaccination because of medical, religious, or other reasons should be excluded until at least 26 days after the onset of parotitis in the last person with mumps in the affected school. Experience with outbreak control for other vaccine-preventable diseases indicates that almost all students who are excluded from the outbreak area because they lack evidence of immunity quickly comply with requirements and can be readmitted to school.

Mycoplasma pneumoniae

Clinical Manifestations: The most common clinical syndrome caused by *Mycoplasma pneumoniae* is a subacute tracheobronchitis. Tonsillopharyngitis and, occasionally, otitis media or bullous myringitis can also occur. Infection can result in aseptic meningitis, encephalitis, peripheral neuropathy, myocarditis, mucocutaneous eruptions (Stevens-Johnson syndrome), and hemolytic anemia occur but are much less frequent manifestations of *M pneumoniae* infection. Patients with sickle-cell disease may develop more severe pulmonary disease when infected with *M pneumoniae.*

Etiology: Mycoplasmas are organisms without cell walls. *M pneumoniae* is the cause of mycoplasmal pneumonia. The genital Mycoplasmas, *M hominis* and *Ureaplasma urealyticum*, are implicated in neonatal infections and genitourinary tract diseases.

Epidemiology: Infected humans are the only source of infection. Transmission is most likely from symptomatic patients and is presumed to be by droplet spread. Individuals at any age can be infected, but specific disease syndromes are age related. Mycoplasma pneumonia is uncommon in children younger than 5 years but *M pneumoniae* is the leading cause of pneumonia in school-aged children and young adults. Mycoplasmal infections occur throughout the world, in any season, and in all geographic settings. Familial spread frequently occurs during periods of many months, affecting members of a household, the neighborhood, and social contacts. Within the household, the organisms persist for weeks or months. Members of a given group, especially in families, can experience different forms of infection ranging from tracheobronchitis to pneumonia. Military and college populations also have a high incidence of the disease. Asymptomatic carriage after infection can occur for prolonged intervals, commonly for weeks.

The **incubation period** is 2 to 3 weeks.

Diagnostic Tests: Special media are required for culturing *Mycoplasma* species. Isolation of *M pneumoniae* in a compatible clinical situation suggests causation. Because this organism can be excreted from the respiratory tract for several weeks after an acute infection, however, isolation of the organism could indicate either present or recent infection.

Of the different antibody tests used to demonstrate a fourfold or greater increase in titer between acute and convalescent sera, the complement fixation antibody test is most widely available. Since *M pneumoniae* antibody cross-reacts with some other antigens, particularly with those of other mycoplasmas, results of this test should be interpreted cautiously in evaluation of febrile illnesses of unknown origin. However, no cross-reactivity with other respiratory pathogens causing diseases clinically similar to those caused by *M pneumoniae* exists. False-negative results can occur as the sensitivity of this test is 50% to 80%. Serum cold hemagglutinin titers of 1:64 or more are present in 50% of infected patients; fourfold increases in titer between acute and convalescent sera occur more often in patients with severe *Mycoplasma* pneumonia than in those with less severe disease. Other etiologic agents can cause an illness in infants or children associated with a rise of cold hemagglutinins, including adenoviruses and Epstein-Barr virus and measles. A negative test for cold agglutinins does not exclude the diagnosis of mycoplasmal infection.

Recently two rapid diagnostic tests have become commercially available. One is a radiolabeled DNA probe which detects *M pneumoniae* ribosomal RNA in respiratory secretions. Positive tests correlate well with positive cultures; however, cultures are more sensitive, and the test does not detect many infections indicated by antibody conversions. The second test is a slide agglutination reaction to detect *M pneumoniae* antibodies. Since infections are common and resulting antibodies persist for months or years, measurement of antibody in a single serum sample appears to have no diagnostic value.

Treatment: Erythromycin is the preferred antimicrobial agent in children younger than 9 years. Tetracycline is equally effective and may be used in children 9 years and older. However, most studies with these antimicrobial agents have been conducted in adults, and definitive evidence for their efficacy in children is lacking.

Isolation of the Hospitalized Patient: No special precautions are recommended.

Control Measures: Diagnosis of an infected patient should lead to an increased index of suspicion for *Mycoplasma* infection in household members and close contacts. Case finding should be instituted if *Mycoplasma* organisms have affected many individuals in a group. Appropriate therapy for each contact should be given if a compatible clinical illness occurs. Antibiotic prophylaxis for contacts is not indicated. No licensed vaccine is available.

Nocardiosis

Clinical Manifestations: The most common presentation is cutaneous or lymphocutaneous disease after contamination of an abrasion in children with normal immune competence. Usually in these cases the lesions remain localized. Systemic disease occurs most commonly in immunocompromised patients and frequently involves the lung and spreads to the liver, brain, and other organs. Pulmonary infection resembles tuberculosis. Nocardiosis can be the initial infection in patients with chronic granulomatous disease.

Etiology: *Nocardia* species are fungus-like bacteria. Disease is caused most commonly by *N asteroides*, less frequently by *N brasiliensis*, and occasionally by other *Nocardia* species.

Epidemiology: *Nocardia* species are free living in nature in soil and compost, and are found worldwide. Infectious particles are air-borne, and the lung is the probable portal of entry. Direct skin inoculation occurs. Person-to-person transmission does not occur.

The **incubation period** is unknown; it is probably a few days to a few weeks.

Diagnosis: Stained smears of sputum, cerebrospinal fluid, or pus may demonstrate beaded, branching weakly Gram-positive rods that are variably acid-fast. Typical colonial growth occurs on Sabouraud's dextrose agar without added antibiotics. Blood specimens should be cultured on brain-heart infusion medium.

Treatment: Either trimethoprim-sulfamethoxazole or sulfadiazine is the drug of choice. Blood concentrations of the sulfonamide should be maintained at 15 to 20 mg/dL. Immunocompetent patients with lymphocutaneous disease usually respond in 6 to 12 weeks. Immunocompromised patients or those with systemic disease should be treated for 6 to 12 months. The disease can recur months or years after therapy. Patients with meningitis or brain abscess should be monitored with serial brain scans. If no response with the sulfa drugs occurs, streptomycin, amikacin, minocycline, or tetracycline may be added. Tetracycline drugs should not be given to children younger than 9 years unless the benefits of therapy clearly outweigh the risks of dental staining. Incision and drainage of abscesses is beneficial.

Isolation of the Hospitalized Patient: No special precautions are recommended.

Control Measures: None.

Norwalk and Norwalk-like Viruses

Clinical Manifestations: Nausea and diarrhea, frequently accompanied by vomiting, especially in children, followed by fever, headache, malaise, myalgia, and abdominal cramps, characteristically occur. The disease can occur in all age groups. Most cases are self limited, lasting 1 to 3 days.

Etiology: These viruses are 27 to 32 nm in diameter with a distinct structure on electron microscopy and are called small round structured viruses. The agents have been named after the site of the outbreak from which they were derived (e.g., Norwalk, Snow Mountain, or Hawaii) and encompass at least four distinct serotypes. The Norwalk and Snow Mountain agents have similarities to members of the calicivirus family of RNA viruses. A number of other small round viruses, including morphologically distinct astroviruses and caliciviruses (see Caliciviruses, page 158), have also been associated with cases of gastroenteritis, but their importance as causes of these illnesses is less clear.

Epidemiology: Outbreaks of diarrhea due to these agents have been recognized in many areas of the world. Many have occurred as common-source outbreaks associated with ingestion of contaminated water and food, particularly shellfish and salads. Seroepidemiologic studies of Norwalk and Snow Mountain viruses indicate that many persons in the United States are infected during late childhood and adulthood; individuals in developing countries are more likely to be infected in childhood. Sporadic cases, presumably caused by person-to-person and fecal-oral transmission, have also been documented. Air-borne spread has been implicated in one institutional outbreak. Infectivity can last as long as 2 days after resolution of symptoms.

The **incubation period** is 24 to 48 hours.

Diagnostic Tests: These viruses have not been cultivated in cell culture, and laboratory diagnosis is usually available only in research laboratories. The viruses can be visualized in fecal samples by immune electron microscopy or detected by radioimmunoassays and ELISA. These assays may also be used to detect fourfold rises in serum antibody concentrations, which is usually the most sensitive way to diagnose infection.

Treatment: Supportive.

Isolation of the Hospitalized Patient: Enteric precautions are recommended.

Control Measures: No specific control measures are available. To prevent outbreaks, efforts should be directed at optimizing conditions for sanitation, preventing contamination of foods or water, and cleaning environmental surfaces that may be contaminated, such as in bathrooms.

Onchocerciasis

(River Blindness)

Clinical Manifestations: The disease involves the skin, subcutaneous tissues, and eyes. Subcutaneous nodules of variable size containing adult worms develop 6 to 12 months after the initial infection and can appear anywhere on the body. In patients in Central America, the nodules are usually on the scalp or near the eyes. In patients in Africa, they are usually on the torso or adjacent to joints or the limbs. After the worms mature, microfilariae are produced and migrate in the tissues, where they cause a chronic, generalized, pruritic dermatitis. After a period of years, the skin can become lichenified and thickened. Involvement of the eyes, caused by the presence of microfilariae, living or dead, in the ocular structures, leads to photophobia and inflammation of the cornea, iris, ciliary body, retina, and choroid. Blindness can result if the disease is untreated.

Etiology: *Onchocerca volvulus* is a filarial nematode.

Epidemiology: The larvae are transmitted by the bites of an infected *Simulium* black fly which breeds along fast-flowing streams and rivers (hence the colloquial name of the disease, "river blindness"). Disease occurs in parts of southern Mexico, Central America, northern South America, tropical Africa, and the southern Arabian peninsula. Prevalence is greatest among those who live near vector-breeding areas. Humans are capable of infecting flies for up to a decade as the adult worms produce microfilariae. The infection is not transmissible by person-to-person contact or blood transfusion.

The **incubation period** is months. Subcutaneous nodules develop 6 to 12 months after the initial infection.

Diagnostic Tests: Direct examination of a shave biopsy of the epidermis (taken from scapular or posterior hip area) usually will reveal microfilariae. Specimens should be incubated in saline solution overnight and examined unstained under a microscope. In ocular disease, a slit-lamp examination of the anterior chamber of the eye may reveal motile microfilariae or the presence of lesions typical of onchocerciasis. Significant eosinophilia is common, but microfilariae are rarely found in blood. Specific serologic tests are available only at selected research laboratories.

Treatment: Whenever possible, surgical excision of all the nodules should precede chemotherapy in order to diminish allergic reactions to dead worms. Severe allergic reactions, including pruritus, urticaria, and inflammation of the eyes, are frequent. Antihistamines and corticosteroids may be required to reduce and control allergic reactions.

Ivermectin, an investigational drug available from the Centers for Disease Control,* is excellent for the treatment of onchocerciasis and is the drug of choice. One oral dose may be effective. Complications include temporary urticaria, edema, and hypotension (rarely severe) secondary to killing of microfilariae. Contraindications include pregnancy, breast-feeding in the first 3 months after delivery, central nervous system disorders, and age younger than 5 years.

Isolation of the Hospitalized Patient: No special precautions are recommended.

Control Measures: Control measures are directed toward eradication or avoidance of the black fly. Use of ivermectin may result in gradual interruption of transmission by eradication of microfilariae.

Papillomaviruses

Clinical Manifestations: Papillomavirus produce epithelial tumors (warts) of the skin and mucous membranes. Cutaneous non-genital warts include common skin warts, plantar warts, flat warts, and thread-like filiform warts on the neck and face. Those affecting membranes include anogenital warts, epidermodysplasia verruciformes, and respiratory papillomatosis.

Common skin warts are dome shaped with conical projections that give the surface a rough appearance. They are usually asymptomatic and multiple, occurring on the hands and around or under the nails. When small dermal vessels thrombose, black dots appear in the warts. Plantar warts on the foot can be painful and characterized by marked hyperkeratosis, sometimes with black dots. Flat warts, com-

*Available from the Drug Service, the Centers for Disease Control (see Services of the Centers for Disease Control, page 622).

monly found on the face and extremities, are usually small, multiple, and flat topped; they seldom exhibit papillomatosis; and they rarely cause pain. Thread-like filiform warts occur on the face and neck. Most cutaneous warts are benign.

Anogenital warts are of two common types—condylomata acuminata (skin-colored growths with a cauliflower-like surface) or flat warts. They range in size from a few millimeters to several centimeters in diameter. In males they may be found on the shaft of the penis, penile meatus, and perianal areas. In females, the cervix, introitus, labia, perineum vagina, and perianal areas are the usual sites. Most anogenital warts are asymptomatic but occasionally cause itching, burning, or local pain. Some anogenital warts are associated with malignancies, including carcinoma of the cervix.

Laryngeal papillomas, which appear to be comparable to genital warts, are rare; they occur mostly in children younger than 10 years; and they are manifested by a voice change or abnormal cry.

Epidermodysplasia verruciformis is a rare, lifelong, severe infection, believed to be a consequence of an inherited immunodeficiency. The lesions can resemble flat warts but are often similar to tinea versicolor covering the torso and upper extremities. Most appear in the first decade of life but do not undergo malignant transformation until adulthood.

Etiology: Human papillomaviruses (HPV) are members of the *Papovaviridae* and are DNA viruses. More than 50 types have been identified, but a small number of HPV types account for most warts. Those causing nongenital warts are distinct from those causing anogenital warts. Of the latter, only a small number have been associated with malignancies.

Epidemiology: Papillomaviruses are widely distributed among mammals but are species specific. Cutaneous warts occur frequently among school-aged children; prevalence rates are as high as 50%. HPV are thought to be transmitted from person to person by close contact. Nongenital warts are acquired through minor trauma to the skin. An increase in the incidence of warts has been associated with swimming in public pools.

Anogenital warts are primarily transmitted by sexual contact but can be acquired through direct contact with the mother's lesions at the time of delivery. When found in a child beyond infancy, sexual abuse must be considered.

Laryngeal papillomas are believed to be transmitted through aspiration of infectious secretions during passage through the infected birth canal.

The **incubation period** is unknown but is estimated to range from 3 months to several years. Papillomavirus acquired by a neonate at the time of delivery may not cause clinical manifestations for several years.

Diagnostic Tests: Most warts are diagnosed by clinical inspection. Clinical detection of anogenital warts can be enhanced by soaking the area in 3% to 5% acetic acid (vinegar), which causes the lesion to turn white. When the diagnosis is questionable, histologic examination of a biopsy specimen is diagnostic. No culture for HPV is available.

Treatment: Most nongenital warts regress spontaneously within a few months from onset. The optimal treatment for warts that do not resolve spontaneously has not been identified. Most methods of treatment rely on chemical or physical destruction of the infected epithelium, and care must be taken to avoid a deleterious cosmetic result of therapy.

The treatment of choice for anogenital warts in most cases is cryotherapy. Alternative treatments are podophyllin (which is not recommended for children), 5-fluorouracil or trichloracetic acid treatment electrosurgery, laser surgery, and surgical excision. Relapses can occur after treatment. Some experts recommend treatment of all anogenital warts because of their association with genital tract dysplasias.

Laryngeal papillomas are very difficult to treat. Local recurrence is common, and repeated surgical procedures for removal are usually necessary. Extension or seeding of laryngeal papillomas into the trachea, bronchi, or lung parenchyma results in increased morbidity and mortality. Interferon has been used as an investigational treatment and may be of benefit for the patient with frequent recurrences.

Isolation of the Hospitalized Patient: No special precautions are recommended.

Control Measures: Suspected child abuse should be reported to the appropriate local agency. Sexual transmission of anogenital warts can be decreased by using condoms. Other control measures are those for other sexually transmitted diseases (see Sexually Transmitted Diseases, page 103), such as refraining from intercourse until therapy is completed and lesions have healed.

Paracoccidioidomycosis

(South American Blastomycosis)

Clinical Manifestations: Typical features are chronic granulomatous lesions of the mucous membranes, especially the mouth and rectum, and the skin adjacent to the mouth, lymph nodes, and viscera.

Etiology: *Paracoccidioides brasiliensis* is a dimorphic fungus with a yeast and a mycelial (mold) form.

Epidemiology: The infection occurs predominantly in South America, where it is the predominant systemic fungal disease. A few cases have been found in Central America and Mexico. The habitat is not known, but soil is suspected. The mode of transmission is not known.

The **incubation period** is highly variable, ranging from 1 month to many years.

Diagnostic Tests: Round, multiple-budding cells may be seen in 10% potassium hydroxide preparations of sputum or material from lesions. The organism can be cultured easily on most enriched media, including blood agar at 37°C and Sabouraud's agar (preferably with added cycloheximide) at room temperature. Complement fixation and immunodiffusion serologic antibody tests are useful diagnostic aids. Skin hypersensitivity can develop but is nonspecific, as false positive tests in patients with histoplasmosis can occur as the result of immunologic cross-reactivity.

Treatment: The treatment of choice for paracoccidioidomycosis in children is usually ketoconazole. Limited experience indicates that ketoconazole is safe in children younger than 2 years. Miconazole has also been used. Other imidazoles such as fluconazole are being studied and appear to have fewer adverse effects than ketoconazole and miconazole. For acute and severe paracoccidioidomycosis, some experts recommend amphotericin B. Prolonged therapy is necessary.

Isolation of the Hospitalized Patient: No special precautions are recommended.

Control Measures: None.

Paragonimiasis

Clinical Manifestations: The disease has an insidious onset and a chronic course. The initial symptom is cough which eventually becomes productive of blood-tinged sputum; pleural pain and dyspnea follow. Bacterial pneumonitis and lung abscesses can complicate the course. Pleural effusion and pneumothorax have also been reported. Because of pulmonary fibrosis and bronchiectasis, clubbing of the fingers and toes can develop. Abdominal disease, occurring when the worms invade the intestinal wall, is associated with dull pain and diarrhea. Involvement of the lymph nodes can lead to suppuration and abscesses. Invasion of the brain occurs rarely; it can lead to seizures. Symptoms tend to subside after about 5 years, but patients in whom symptoms persisted for 20 years without reinfection have been reported.

Etiology: The adult *Paragonimus westermani* is a fluke, 10 to 12 mm long and 5 to 7 mm wide. The pathologic lesions are caused by the eggs, not the worms (except for those in the brain); the eggs elicit an eosinophilic inflammatory response.

Epidemiology: Transmission occurs when raw or uncooked freshwater crabs or crayfish containing larvae (metacercariae) are ingested. They excyst in the small intestine and penetrate the abdominal cavity, where they undergo further development. After several days, most of the larvae travel to the lungs through the diaphragm, but some remain in the abdomen and others reach aberrant sites. They burrow into the tissues, become encapsulated, and begin laying eggs after about 4 to 6 weeks. When sputum containing eggs is swallowed, the eggs are passed in the stool. Eggs that reach freshwater embryonate, hatch within 3 weeks, and yield miracidia which penetrate snails. Several weeks later cercariae emerge and encyst on and within the muscles and viscera of freshwater crustaceans, and mature into infective metacercariae.

Areas of the highest prevalence are limited to the Far East, especially Japan, Korea, Taiwan, and the Philippines. The disease is also endemic in some parts of Australasia and in West Africa. The Western hemisphere has endemic foci in Colombia, Venezuela, Ecuador, Peru, Costa Rica, and Mexico. Foxes, civets, tigers, leopards, panthers, mongooses, wolves, pigs, dogs, and cats serve as animal reservoirs. No person-to-person transmission occurs.

The **incubation period** is not known.

Diagnostic Tests: Microscopic examination of stools, sputum, pleural effusion, and other tissue aspirates reveals the eggs. Serologic antibody tests are available at the Centers for Disease Control, but these tests do not distinguish active from past infection. Charcot-Leyden crystals and eosinophils in sputum are characteristic.

Treatment: Praziquantel* is the drug of choice. An alternative drug, bithionol,† is effective but is associated with side effects including gastrointestinal disturbances and allergic rashes.

Isolation of the Hospitalized Patient: No special precautions are recommended.

Control Measures: Complete control is impossible because of the animal reservoirs. Boiling of crabs for several minutes until the meat has congealed and turned opaque kills the metacercariae.

Parainfluenza Virus Infections

Clinical Manifestations: Parainfluenza viral infections are the major cause of croup, but they also frequently result in upper respiratory tract infection, pneumonia, or bronchiolitis. Parainfluenza viral infections can be particularly severe and persistent in immunodeficient children.

Etiology: Parainfluenza viruses are large, enveloped RNA viruses classified as paramyxoviruses. Four antigenically distinct types—1, 2, 3, and 4 (with two subtypes, 4A and 4B)—have been identified.

Epidemiology: Parainfluenza viruses are believed to be transmitted from person to person by direct contact and by spread of contaminated nasopharyngeal secretions. Parainfluenza viral infections are ubiquitous and are both epidemic and sporadic. Type 1 viruses tend to produce outbreaks of respiratory illness in the fall of every other year. A major increase in the number of cases of croup in the autumn is indicative of a parainfluenza type 1 outbreak. Type 2 virus can also cause outbreaks of respiratory illness in the fall, but these tend to be less severe, irregular, and less frequent. Parainfluenza type 3 virus usually produces infections over a somewhat longer period, occurring predominantly during the spring and summer in temperate

*Available from Miles Pharmaceuticals, West Haven, CT.

†Available from the Drug Service, Centers for Disease Control (see Services of the Centers for Disease Control, page 622).

climates. Infections with types 4A and 4B are less commonly recognized, sporadic, and generally clinically mild. Infection with type 3 virus is usually first acquired during infancy and is a major cause of lower respiratory tract disease in children in the first year of life. Illness from primary infection with types 1 and 2 occurs predominantly in 2- to 6-year-old children. Reinfections can occur at any age, but are usually milder, causing primarily upper respiratory tract illness. Immunodeficient individuals can develop severe lower respiratory tract disease, with prolonged shedding of the virus. Normal children with primary infection from type 1 shed the virus for an average of 4 to 7 days, with a range of up to 2 weeks. The average period of shedding for type 3 infections is 8 to 9 days, with a range of up to 3 weeks.

The **incubation period** is from 2 to 6 days.

Diagnostic Tests: Virus may be isolated from nasopharyngeal secretions in tissue culture, usually within 4 to 7 days. More rapid identification of viral antigen in the nasopharyngeal secretions can be accomplished by immunofluorescent and ELISA methods, but the sensitivity of the tests can be variable. Serologic diagnosis, made retrospectively by a significant rise in antibody titer between acute and convalescent sera, is generally less helpful and results of tests can be confusing, as heterotypic antibody rises are common with infections caused by other serotypes of parainfluenza and mumps viruses. Furthermore, infection may not always be accompanied by a significant homotypic antibody response.

Treatment: Supportive.

Isolation of the Hospitalized Patient: Contact isolation is recommended for hospitalized infants and young children with parainfluenza viral infections. Prevention of contamination by respiratory secretions and careful hand washing may diminish the possibility of nosocomial spread.

Control Measures: Efforts should be aimed at reducing nosocomial infection. Hand washing should be emphasized.

Parasitic Diseases

Parasitic diseases have traditionally been considered exotic and, therefore, are frequently not included in differential diagnoses in the United States and Europe. Nevertheless, they are among the most common causes of worldwide morbidity and mortality, and many of these infections can be encountered anywhere in the world. Tourists returning to their own countries, immigrants from endemic areas (e.g., refugees from Indochina, Central America, and the Caribbean), and immunosuppressed patients are potential victims of infections in nonendemic areas. In the United States, a noticeable increase in the number of reports of several parasitic infections has occurred in recent years, and many physicians and clinical laboratories are seeing patients with these infections and their diagnostic specimens for the first time.

Consultation and assistance in the diagnosis and management of parasitic diseases are available from government agencies (e.g., Centers for Disease Control [CDC] and state health departments) and university departments of geographic medicine, tropical medicine, infectious disease, international health, and public health.

The CDC distributes a number of drugs for the treatment of parasitic diseases that are not available commercially in the United States. These drugs are indicated by footnotes in the tables on Drugs for Parasitic Infections, page 587, and chapters on specific parasitic infections. To request these drugs, a physician must contact the CDC Drug Service (see Services of the Centers for Disease Control, page 622), and provide the following information: (1) the physician's name, address, and telephone number; (2) the type of infection to be treated and the method by which it was diagnosed; and (3) the patient's name, age, weight, sex, and, if the patient is a woman, whether she is pregnant. Prior consultation with a medical officer from the CDC may be required.

The most important human parasitic infections are discussed in individual sections in this book. The diseases are arranged alphabetically and the discussions include recommendations for drug treatment. A table reproduced from *The Medical Letter* (see Drugs for Parasitic Infections, page 587) gives specific antiparasitic drug and dosage recommendations. Although the recommendations for administration of these drugs given in the discussion of the diseases and in the Table are similar, they may not be identical in all instances because of differences of opinion among authorities. Both sources should be consulted.

Table 43 gives details on some less commonly encountered parasitic diseases.

Table 43. Additional Parasitic Diseases*

Disease and/or Agent	Where Infection May Be Acquired	Definitive Host	Intermediate Host	Humans Infected by	Directly Communicable Person to Person	Diagnostic Laboratory Test in Humans	Diseases in Man: Causative Form of Parasite	Diseases in Man: Manifestation
Angiostrongylus cantonensis	Pacific islands, Eastern Asia, Puerto Rico, Cuba	Rat	Snails and slugs	Eating uncooked, infected mollusks	No	Eosinophils in CSF	Larval worms	Meningoencephalitis
Angiostrongylus costaricensis	Central America	Rodents	Snails and slugs	Eating uncooked, infected mollusks	No	Gel diffusion	Larval worms	Abdominal pains
Anisakiasis	Cosmopolitan, mainly Japan	Marine mammals	Certain saltwater fish	Eating uncooked, infected fish	No	Identification of recovered larvae in granulomas or vomitus	Larval worms	Acute GI disease
Clonorchis sinensis	Far East	Humans, cats, dogs, other animals	Certain freshwater snails	Eating uncooked, infected fish	No	Eggs in stool or duodenal fluid	Larvae and mature flukes	Hepatibiliary disease

Dracontiasis *Dracunculus medinensis*	Foci in India, Africa, Middle East	Humans	Cyclops crustacea	Drinking infected water	No	Adult worm in skin, sub-cutaneous tissues	Adult female worm	Inflammatory response; systemic and local in skin and subcu-taneous tissue
Fascioliasis *Fasciola hepatica*	Foci through-out tropics and tem-perate areas	Humans and many animals	Certain freshwater snails and vegetation	Eating uncooked, infected plants such as watercress	No	Eggs in feces, duodenal fluid or bile	Larvae and mature worms	Disease of liver and biliary tree
Fasciolop-siasis *Fasciolopsis buski*	Far East	Humans, pigs, dogs	Certain freshwater snails, plants	Eating uncooked, infected plants	No	Eggs or worm in feces or duodenal fluid	Larvae and mature worms	Gastroenteritis
Intestinal capillariasis *Capillaria philippinensis*	Philippines	Humans	Fish	Ingestion of uncooked, infected fish	Uncertain	Eggs and parasite in feces	Larvae and mature worms	Protein-losing enteropathy

*For recommended drug treatment, see Drugs for Parasitic Infections (page 587).

Parvovirus B19

(Erythema Infectiosum, Fifth Disease)

Clinical Manifestations: Parvovirus B19 infection is most often manifested as erythema infectiosum (EI), which is characterized by mild systemic symptoms, fever in 15% to 30% of patients, and, frequently, a distinctive rash. On the face, this rash is intensely red with a "slapped cheek" appearance and circumoral pallor. A symmetric maculopapular, lace-like rash can also be noted on the arms, moving caudally to involve the trunk, buttocks, and thighs. The rash can recur and fluctuate in intensity with environmental changes, such as temperature and exposure to sunlight for weeks and sometimes months. Arthralgia and arthritis occur infrequently in children and commonly in adults, especially women.

Infection with the etiologic agent of EI, human parvovirus B19, can also cause asymptomatic infection, a mild respiratory illness with no rash, a rash atypical for EI that is often rubelliform, arthritis in adults (in the absence of manifestations of EI), chronic anemia in immunodeficient patients, and aplastic crisis lasting 7 to 10 days in patients with chronic hemolytic anemias (e.g., sickle-cell disease). Patients with aplastic crisis can have a prodomal illness with fever, malaise, and myalgia, but rash is usually absent.

Parvovirus B19 infection that occurs during pregnancy can cause fetal hydrops and death. Recent data suggest that the risk of fetal death is less than 10% after proven maternal infection. Congenital anomalies among newborn infants associated with B19 infection has not been reported.

Etiology: Human parvovirus B19, a member of the *Parvoviridae* family, has recently been identified as the cause of EI and associated syndromes.

Epidemiology: Humans are the only known hosts. The mode of spread probably involves respiratory secretions and blood; early in the illness, respiratory secretions have been demonstrated to contain viral DNA, and blood has been found to have viral particles. Parvovirus B19 infections are ubiquitous and cases of EI can occur sporadically or as part of community outbreaks. The outbreaks frequently occur in elementary or junior high schools in spring months. Secondary spread among susceptible household members—adults or children—is common, occurring in about 50% of contacts. Rates of infection in schools are less, but infection can be an occupational risk for school and day care personnel, affecting 19% of susceptible persons in a recent outbreak. However, 50% or more of adults have serologic evidence of past infection and are probably not susceptible to reinfection. In children, only 5% to 10% are immune. The timing of the presence of B19 DNA in serum and respiratory secretions indicates that persons with EI are most infectious before onset of illness and are unlikely to be infectious after onset of the rash and other associated symptoms. In contrast, patients with aplastic crises are highly contagious from the onset or prior to the onset of clinical symptoms through the subsequent week or longer. Transmission to hospital personnel can occur in as many as 35% to 40% of susceptible persons.

Household studies of secondary cases suggest that the **incubation period** is usually between 4 and 14 days but can be as long as 20 days. Data from human volunteer studies suggest that rash and joint symptoms occur 2 to 3 weeks after acquisition.

Diagnostic Tests: Laboratory diagnosis can be made by tests currently available in a limited number of laboratories, primarily the Centers for Disease Control (CDC).* One commercial laboratory currently offers serologic testing. More widespread commercial testing is likely to become available, and state laboratories will also be performing serologic tests. The most feasible method for detecting infection in the healthy host is assaying for serum B19-specific IgM antibody, the presence of which confirms infection within the past several months. Serum IgG antibody indicates prior infection and immunity. The best method for detecting chronic infection in the immunocompromised patient is to demonstrate virus by nucleic acid hybridization assay or the polymerase chain reaction assay but these tests are investigational. Virus can also be detected in serum by electron microscopy. B19 antigens can be detected by radioimmunoassay or ELISA. Parvovirus B19 has not been grown in standard tissue-culture systems but has been grown in bone marrow explant cultures. A genetically engineered cell line has been developed that produces viral capsid proteins which will be useful in diagnostic testing.

Treatment: For most patients, supportive care only is indicated. In treating chronic infection in the immunodeficient patient, commercial intravenous immunoglobulin therapy appears to be effective and should be considered.

Isolation of the Hospitalized Patient: For patients hospitalized with EI, no special precautions are indicated.

Contact isolation, including use of gowns and gloves, is indicated for hospitalized children with aplastic crises or immunosuppressed patients with chronic aplastic anemia for the duration of the illness.

*Testing for B19 parvovirus IgM antibody at the CDC is available for selected patients through state health departments.

Masks should also be worn during close contact. Pregnant health care workers should not care for patients with aplastic crises because they are highly contagious.

Control Measures:

- Women who are exposed to children either at home or at work (such as teachers or day care workers) are at increased risk of infection with parvovirus B19. However, because of widespread inapparent infection in both adults and children, all women are at some degree of risk of exposure, particularly those with school-aged children. In view of the high prevalence of B19, the low incidence of ill effects on the fetus, and the fact that avoidance of child care or teaching can only reduce but not eliminate the risk of exposure, routine exclusion of pregnant women from the workplace where EI is occurring is not recommended. When IgG testing for parvovirus B19 antibody becomes more widely available, women at increased risk may be able to have their susceptibility determined.
- Pregnant women who find that they have been in contact with children who are in the incubation period of EI or who are in aplastic crisis should have the relatively low potential risk explained to them, and the option of having serologic tests performed should be offered, if possible. Fetal ultrasound and α-fetoprotein determinations are useful when assessing damage to the fetus.
- Children with EI may attend day care or school, as they are not contagious.
- Transmission of infection can be lessened by routine hygienic practices for control of respiratory infections, which include hand washing and the disposal of facial tissues containing respiratory secretions.
- Pediatricians, as school medical advisors, should act as consultants in providing greater access to testing facilities, assistance in interpreting test results, and reassurance to pregnant women.
- The preventive effect of immune globulin in exposed persons is unknown.

Pasteurella multocida Infections

Clinical Manifestations: The most common manifestation is infection at the site of a scratch or bite of a cat, dog, or other animal. Manifestations usually occur within 24 to 48 hours of the bite or scratch and include swelling, erythema, tenderness, and serous or sanguinopurulent discharge. Regional lymphadenopathy usually occurs; chills and fever can occur. Infectious manifestations in less common foci include septic arthritis, osteomyelitis, meningitis, respiratory infections (e.g., chronic bronchitis, chronic sinusitis, chronic otitis media, pulmonary abscesses, empyema, and pneumonia), appendicitis, hepatic abscess, spontaneous peritonitis, urinary tract infection, and ocular infections, including conjunctivitis, corneal ulcer, and endophthalmitis.

Etiology: *Pasteurella multocida* organisms are bipolar staining, Gram-negative coccobacilli.

Epidemiology: The source of the organism is the oral flora of 70% to 90% of cats, 50% to 66% of dogs, and the mouths of many other animals. The most common source is the mouth of the cat or dog. Transmission occurs from the bite or scratch of an infected animal. Respiratory spread from animal to man also occurs. Human-to-human spread via lesion drainage or respiratory discharge has not been documented.

The **incubation period** is usually less than 24 hours.

Diagnostic Tests: *P multocida* can be isolated from skin lesion drainage or other sites of infection (e.g., joint fluid, cerebrospinal fluid, sputum, pleural fluid, or middle ear drainage). The organism resembles several other organisms morphologically (such as *Haemophilus influenzae, Neisseria* species, and some enteric organisms), but laboratory differentiation is not difficult.

Treatment: The drug of choice for treatment of infections caused by *P multocida* is penicillin or ampicillin. In patients allergic to penicillin, chloramphenicol, or tetracycline (which should not be given to children younger than 9 years) is effective. Parenterally administered newer cephalosporins, such as cefoxitin or cefotaxime, are active against *P multocida* in vitro, but experience with these drugs in the therapy of *P multocida* infection is limited. Other cephalosporins are unlikely to be effective; these include cefazolin, cefalexin, and those given orally; semisynthetic penicillins such as nafcillin and oxacillin; and erythromycin. The duration of therapy is usually 7 to 10 days for local infections and 10 to 14 days for invasive infections. Wound drainage or debridement may be necessary.

Isolation of the Hospitalized Patient: Drainage/secretion precautions are recommended for cutaneous disease.

Control Measures: Limiting contact with wild and domestic animals can prevent *Pasteurella* infections. Animal bites and scratches should be promptly irrigated, cleansed, and debrided; whenever possible, surgical closure of the wounds should be avoided. Antimicrobial prophylaxis with penicillin or the combination of amoxicillin and clavulanic acid may be given, but efficacy of prophylactic regimens has not been proven.

Pediculosis

Clinical Manifestations: Itching is the most common symptom of head lice infestation, but most children with light infestations (1 to 5 lice) do not complain. Itching is usually intense in persons with body or pubic lice infestations. Excoriation can result in a pyoderma with impetigo or regional lymphadenopathy. A characteristic sign of heavy pubic lice infestation is the bluish or slate-colored maculae caeruleae on the chest, abdomen, and thighs. Pubic lice can also infest eyelashes, eyebrows, and body and facial hair.

Parents may become aware of infestation by finding lice or eggs (nits) in their child's hair usually near the nape of the neck. In temperate climates, head lice deposit their eggs on the hair shaft near the scalp. Thus, the duration of infestation can be estimated by the distance of the nit from the scalp; nits 10 or more millimeters from the scalp have been present for 2 weeks or more and are unlikely to be viable.

Etiology: Three species of lice infest humans: *Pediculus humanus capitis*, the head louse; *P humanus corporis*, the body louse; and *Pthirus pubis*, the pubic or crab louse. Ova hatch in a week. Both nymphs and adult lice feed on human blood.

Epidemiology: Head lice infestation in day care and school-aged children, and pubic lice infestations in adolescents and young adults are common in the United States. Head lice occur in all socioeconomic groups, but in the United States, black persons are less commonly infested than white persons. Hair length does not influence infestation. Head or pubic lice infestation is not a sign of uncleanliness. However, body lice generally are found on persons with poor hygiene.

Transmission of *P capitis* occurs by direct contact with infested individuals or indirectly by contact with their personal belongings such as combs, brushes, and hats. Fomites play a major role in body lice transmission, a minor role in head lice transmission, and practically no role in pubic lice transmission. Lice generally cannot survive away from the host for more than 48 hours. Although body lice lay eggs in clothing, eggs generally do not survive away from the scalp at room temperatures for more than 7 days. Pubic lice usually are transmitted through sexual contact. Only body lice have been implicated as vectors of disease (epidemic typhus, trench fever, and relapsing fever). Head lice are not a major health hazard.

The **incubation period** is not known.

Diagnostic Tests: Identification of eggs, nymphs, and lice with the naked eye is possible; the diagnosis can be confirmed by using a hand lens or microscope.

Treatment: Permethrin, a synthetic pyrethroid (10-minute hair rinse); natural pyrethrin-based products (10-minute shampoos); lindane 1% (4-minute shampoo); and malathion 0.5% (8- to 12-hour lotion) are each effective in treating pediculosis of the scalp (see Table 44 for trade names). Lindane-resistant lice have not been reported in the United States. Pyrethrin products are available without prescription. Permethrin, pyrethrin products, and malathion have lower potential toxicity than lindane, but no serious adverse effects have been associated with any of these products when used according to package instructions. Toxicity with lindane has been reported only with misuse, such as ingestion or prolonged administration. When pyrethrin products or lindane is used, many experts recommend a second treatment 7 to 10 days later to kill newly hatched lice. A single treatment of permethrin or malathion appears adequate because these products persist in the hair for at least 2 weeks. Some experts advise a second application 7 days after the first irrespective of the choice of therapy.

Use of a fine-toothed comb aids in the mechanical removal of nits. Applying a damp towel to the scalp for 30 to 60 minutes, soaking the hair with white vinegar (3% to 5% acetic acid) followed by application of a damp towel soaked in the same solution for 30 to 60 minutes, or using a commercial rinse (Step 2*) containing 8% formic acid can facilitate the removal of nits by combing.

For infestation of eyelashes by the crab lice, petrolatum ointment applied twice daily for 8 to 10 days is effective. Nits should be removed mechanically from the eyelashes.

Isolation of the Hospitalized Patient: Contact isolation until therapy has been started is indicated.

Control Measures (for Pediculosis of the Scalp):

- Contacts should be examined and treated if they are infested. Differentiation of nits from benign hair casts (a layer of follicular cells that easily slide off the hair shaft) can be difficult. Bedmates should be treated prophylactically.

---

*GenDerm Corporation, Northbrook, IL.

Table 44. Medications for Treatment of Pediculosis*

Drug	Trade Names (examples)	Manufacturer
Permethrin (synthetic pyrethroid)	Nix	Burroughs Wellcome Co.
Natural pyrethrin-based products	A-200 RID R & C	Beecham Lieming Reed & Carnick
Lindane, 1%	Kwell	Reed & Carnick
Malathion, 0.5%	Ovide	GenDerm

*Compiled from the *Physicians Desk Reference.* Oradel, NJ: Medical Economics Company, Inc.; 1990

- Children should be allowed to return to school or day care the morning after their first treatment since the risk of transmission is promptly reduced by treatment. Reinfestation of children from an untreated, infested contact is more common than treatment failure after proper application of an effective pesticide.
- "No nit" policies requiring that children be free of nits prior to return to day care or school have not been demonstrated to be effective in controlling head lice. The only value of such policies is to ensure that the child has received treatment.
- Clothing, bedding, or cloth toys can be disinfected by machine washing or drying (using hot cycles), since temperatures exceeding 53.5°C (128.3°F) for 5 minutes are lethal to lice and eggs. Dry cleaning or simply storing clothing in plastic bags for about 10 days is also effective.
- For disinfecting combs and brushes, soaking in hot water for 10 minutes or washing with a pediculicide shampoo is recommended.

Pelvic Inflammatory Disease

Clinical Manifestations: Pelvic inflammatory disease (PID) denotes a spectrum of inflammatory disorders of the female upper genital tract usually presenting with pelvic pain; intermenstrual, postcoital, or prolonged vaginal bleedings; deep dyspareunia; or unexplained vaginal discharge. PID may be asymptomatic and includes salpingitis, oophoritis, parametritis, endometritis, and pelvic peritonitis.

Common findings include fever, lower abdominal pain, adnexal tenderness (which may be unilateral), tenderness on motion of the cervix, palpation of an inflammatory mass on bimanual pelvic examination or its demonstration by ultrasonography. The onset of symptoms often follows menses. Most cases are clinically mild, and many patients are afebrile and can have normal sedimentation rates and leukocyte counts.

Complications of acute PID include perihepatitis (Fitz-Hugh-Curtis syndrome) and tubo-ovarian abscess. Important long-term sequelae are tubal infertility (10% to 30% after a single episode, depending on the severity; 50% to 75% after three or more episodes), chronic pelvic adhesions, and ectopic pregnancy.

Etiology: Sexually transmitted organisms, especially *Neisseria gonorrhoeae* and *Chlamydia trachomatis,* are implicated in most PID cases, but many have a polymicrobial etiology. Other organisms isolated from the upper genital tract of PID patients include mixed anaerobic organisms (*Bacteroides* species and *Peptostreptococcus* species), facultative bacteria (*Gardnerella vaginalis, Streptococcus* species, coliform bacteria), and genital tract mycoplasmas (*Mycoplasma hominis, Ureaplasma urealyticum*, and *M genitalium*). The organisms causing upper tract infection are not reliably predicted by cervical culture or known infection in a partner.

Epidemiology: PID is a frequent complication of common sexually transmitted diseases. Approximately 10% to 20% of females with endocervical *N gonorrhoeae* and 10% to 30% of those with endocervical *C trachomatis* develop overt PID. Asymptomatic upper genital tract infection is common in uncomplicated chlamydial infection. In prepubertal females, ascending infection resulting in PID is uncommon. The incidence of PID is highest among sexually active adolescents. Other risk factors include multiple sexual partners, use of an intrauterine device, douching, and a previous episode of PID.

The **incubation period** varies with the etiology (see *N gonorrhoeae* and *C trachomatis,* above).

Diagnostic Tests: The diagnosis is usually made on the basis of clinical findings. The diagnosis is supported by evidence of *N gonorrhoeae* or *Chlamydia* in the cervical secretions, increased leukocytes, in the cervical smear, leukocytosis, and/or an elevated sedimentation rate. Endocervical and rectal cultures for *N gonorrhoeae* and an endocervical test for *C trachomatis* should be obtained before treatment. Laparoscopy definitively diagnoses salpingitis, but this procedure is not usually indicated or practical. If the patient's menses is late or she is not using reliable contraception, a pregnancy test should be done.

Treatment: Treatment is empiric and is directed against the common etiologic agents. No substantial evidence indicates that any of the current antibiotic regimens decreases the incidence of infertility or ectopic pregnancy. Antibiotic treatment should be promptly instituted, based on clinical diagnosis without awaiting culture results, to minimize the risk of progression of the infection and the risk of transmission of the organisms to other sexual partners.

Some experts recommend that all patients with PID be hospitalized, particularly adolescents, in whom the risk of sequelae is high and whose ability to follow a therapeutic regimen may be unpredictable. Hospitalization is indicated if the patient has a suspected pelvic or tubo-ovarian abscess, has overt peritonitis, is pregnant, has an intrauterine device (IUD) in place, is unable to take oral antibiotics, or has failed to respond to 48 hours of outpatient management, or if the diagnosis is uncertain. If the patient has an IUD in place, it should be promptly removed.

Therapeutic regimens recommended by the Centers for Disease Control for antibiotic treatment of PID are summarized in Table 45. These are empiric regimens which provide broad coverage against the etiologic agents of PID. The specific antibiotics listed are examples only. Initial treatment with a parenteral beta-lactim antibiotic is recommended in all cases.

Ambulatory patients should be monitored closely and reevaluated 3 days after treatment is initiated.

Isolation of the Hospitalized Patient: No special precautions are indicated.

Control Measures:

- Male sexual partners of PID patients should be examined, cultured, and treated for presumptive gonorrhea and chlamydial infection because they are likely to have asymptomatic urethral infection and reinfect the index case or other partners.
- Patients should be advised to abstain from intercourse until all symptoms have resolved and both the patient and her partner(s) have completed treatment.
- Patients should be offered a serologic test for syphilis and HIV counseling and screening.
- Patients and their partners with positive cultures for *N gonorrhoeae* and *Chlamydia* should be recultured 4 to 7 days after completing therapy.
- Because of the high risk of reinfection, patients with PID should be rescreened for *N gonorrhoeae* and *C trachomatis* 4 to 6 weeks after completing treatment.

Table 45. Recommended Treatment of Pelvic Inflammatory Disease (PID)

Inpatient Treatment	Ambulatory Treatment*
Regimen A†	
• Cefoxitin 2 g IV every 6 h (or Cefotetan‡ 2 g every 12 h)	• Cefoxitin 2 g IM with concurrent administration of probenecid 1 g PO
PLUS	**OR**
• Doxycycline§ 100 mg IV or PO every 12 h continued for at least 48 h after clinical improvement and followed by doxycycline§ 100 mg orally 2 times a day to complete a 10- to 14-day total course	• Equivalent cephalosporin‡ PLUS • Doxycycline§ 100 mg orally 2 times a day for 10 to 14 days
OR	
Regimen B‡	
• Clindamycin 900 mg IV every 8 h (15 to 40 mg/kg/d)	
PLUS	
• Gentamicin‖: loading dose 2.0 mg/kg IV followed by maintenance 1.5 mg/kg IV every 8 h	
PLUS	
• Doxycycline§ 100 mg, IV or oral, every 12 h continued for at least 48 h after clinical improvement and followed by doxycycline§ 100 mg, orally 2 times a day to complete a 10- to 14-day total course	

*Patients who do not respond on ambulatory regimen within 48 hours should be hospitalized and treated with parenterally administered antibiotic.

†Regimen A provides optimal coverage for *N gonorrhoeae* and *C trachomatis*, and is preferred by some experts when sexually transmitted PID is likely; regimen B may be preferred when a predominant facultative/anaerobic infection is probable (e.g., IUD related). No data are available on the efficacy of oral regimens after discharge from hospital. These regimens do not offer optimal coverage of pyogenic complications caused by anaerobes or gram negatives. In such cases clindamycin 450 mg orally four times a day may be considered.

‡Other cephalosporins such as ceftizoxime, cefotaxime, and ceftriaxone, which provide adequate gonococcal and Gram-negative coverage, may be used. However, ceftriaxone should be used only in mild cases where *N gonorrhoeae* is thought to be the primary etiologic agent.

§Doxycycline administered orally has bioavailability similar to the IV formulation. Patients who do not tolerate doxycycline should receive erythromycin 50 mg orally 4 times a day (40 mg/kg/d) for 10 to 14 days, although this recommendation is based on limited clinical data. Use of doxycycline is ordinarily limited to patients 9 years or older because of the potential for tooth staining. Doxycycline is preferred over tetracycline because of its greater bioavailability and better patient compliance.

‖Although short courses of aminoglycosides (≤ 3 days) in healthy adolescents with normal renal function do not usually necessitate monitoring of serum concentrations, some practitioners may elect to do so.

Pertussis

Clinical Manifestations: Pertussis begins with mild upper respiratory tract symptoms with cough (catarrhal stage) and can progress to severe paroxysms of cough (paroxysmal stage), often with a characteristic inspiratory whoop, followed by vomiting. Fever is absent or minimal. Symptoms subsequently wane gradually (convalescent stage). Older children and adults can have atypical manifestations, with persistent cough and no inspiratory whoop. In infants younger than 6 months, apnea is a common manifestation and whoop can be absent. Duration of the illness in uncomplicated cases is 6 to 10 weeks. Complications include seizures, pneumonia, encephalopathy, and death. Pertussis is a particularly severe disease in the first year of life; pneumonia, seizures, and encephalopathy occurred in 17%, 2.5%, and 0.9%, respectively, in recently reported cases of infants (i.e., children younger than 12 months) in the United States. In those younger than 6 months, the current case-fatality rate is 0.5%. Disease in vaccinated children and older individuals is often milder.

Etiology: *Bordetella pertussis* is a fastidious, Gram-negative, pleomorphic bacillus. A whooping cough syndrome may also be caused by *B parapertussis, C trachomatis*, and certain adenoviruses.

Epidemiology: Humans are the only known hosts of *B pertussis*. Transmission occurs by close contact via large aerosol droplets from the respiratory tract of symptomatic individuals. As many as 90% of nonimmune household contacts acquire the infection. Infants and young children frequently acquire the disease from older siblings, adolescents, and adults who have a mild or atypical illness. In recent years in the United States, adolescents and adults have been increasingly recognized as major sources of pertussis. Asymptomatic carriage has been infrequently demonstrated; its role in transmission has not been established. Pertussis occurs endemically with periodic outbreaks. Widespread active immunization with pertussis vaccine since the 1940s is considered primarily responsible for the current low morbidity and mortality rates of pertussis in the United States. Pertussis can occur at any age but is most common in young children. Currently, approximately 35% of reported cases in the United States occur in infants younger than 6 months, including a substantial proportion in those younger than 3 months; approximately 45% occur in children younger than 1 year, and 66% occur in children younger than 5 years. Mortality and the hospitalization rate are highest in the first 6 months of life.

Communicability is most likely in the catarrhal stage before the onset of paroxysms; subsequently, the risk diminishes rapidly but may last as long as 3 weeks. Erythromycin therapy decreases infectivity and may limit secondary spread. Nasopharyngeal cultures usually become negative for *B pertussis* within 5 days after initiation of erythromycin therapy.

The **incubation period** is 6 to 20 days, usually 7 to 10 days, and rarely more than 2 weeks.

Diagnostic Tests: Culture of *B pertussis* requires inoculation of nasopharyngeal mucus, obtained by dacron or calcium alginate swab, on special media (such as Regan-Lowe or fresh Bordet-Gengou), with incubation for 7 days. Because these media may not be routinely available, the laboratory should be informed when *B pertussis* is suspected. The organism is most frequently recovered in the catarrhal stage or early in the paroxysmal stage and is rarely found after the fourth week of illness. A positive culture is diagnostic. False-negative cultures are common, particularly in patients late in the course of the disease or who are receiving antibiotics. The direct immunofluorescence test of nasopharyngeal secretions has variable sensitivity and specificity, and requires experienced personnel for interpretation. Since false-positive and false-negative results can occur, culture confirmation of all suspected pertussis cases should be attempted. Although absolute lymphocytosis is often present in patients with classical pertussis, it is a nonspecific finding, especially in infants in whom lymphocytosis often develops from other infections. Since the degree of lymphocytosis usually parallels the severity of the patient's cough, this finding can be absent in partially immunized patients, and those with atypical illness. A serologic fourfold or greater pertussis agglutinin titer rise is diagnostic, but the sensitivity of this test is poor. New serologic tests, such as ELISA antibody tests, are promising diagnostic methods but are currently available only in research laboratories.

Treatment:

- Infants younger than 6 months and other patients with potentially severe disease often require hospitalization for supportive care to manage coughing paroxysms, apnea, cyanosis, feeding difficulties, or other complications. Intensive care facilities can be needed for the management of severe cases.
- Antimicrobials given in the catarrhal stage may ameliorate the disease. After paroxysms are established, however, antimicrobials usually have no discernible effect on the course of illness and are recommended primarily to limit the spread of the organisms to others. The drug of choice is erythromycin (40 to 50 mg/kg/d,

orally, in four divided doses; maximum, 2 g/d); some experts prefer the estolate preparation. The recommended duration of therapy to prevent bacteriologic relapse is 14 days. Trimethoprim-sulfamethoxazole (8 mg/kg and 40 mg/kg/d, orally, in two divided doses) is a possible alternative for patients who do not tolerate erythromycin, but its efficacy is unproven.

- Corticosteroids and albuteral (salbutamol), a beta-2-adrenergic stimulant, have shown promise in reducing paroxysms of coughing, but require further evaluation before they can be recommended.
- Pertussis hyperimmune globulin is not effective and is no longer commercially available in the United States.

Isolation of the Hospitalized Patient: The patient should be placed in respiratory isolation for 5 days after initiation of erythromycin therapy. If appropriate antimicrobial therapy is contraindicated, the patient should be isolated until 3 weeks after the onset of paroxysms.

Control Measures:

Care of Exposed Persons.

Day Care. Exposed children, especially those incompletely immunized, should be observed carefully for respiratory symptoms for 14 days (the usual maximum incubation period) after contact has been terminated. Pertussis immunization and chemoprophylaxis should be given as recommended for household and other close contacts. Symptomatic children with cough should be excluded from day care, pending physician evaluation. Children with pertussis, if their medical condition allows, may return or enter a day care facility 5 days after initiation of erythromycin therapy.

Household and Other Close Contacts.

- *Immunization.* Close contacts younger than 7 years who are unimmunized or who have received fewer than four doses of DTP should have pertussis immunization initiated or continued according to the recommended DTP schedule. Children who received their third dose 6 months or more before exposure should be given a fourth dose at this time. Those who have had at least four doses of pertussis vaccine should receive a booster dose of DTP, unless a dose has been given within the last 3 years or they are more than 6 years old.
- *Chemoprophylaxis.* Erythromycin (40 to 50 mg/kg/d, orally, in four divided doses; maximum, 2 g/d) for 14 days, as tolerated, is recommended for all household contacts and other close contacts, such as those in day care. Some experts recommend the estolate preparation. Prompt use of erythromycin chemoprophylaxis in household contacts is effective in limiting secondary transmission.

Chemoprophylaxis is recommended for all household and other close contacts irrespective of age or immunization status, since pertussis immunity is not absolute and may not prevent infection. Furthermore, older children and adults with mild illness that may not be recognized as pertussis can transmit the infection.

For patients who cannot tolerate erythromycin, trimethoprim-sulfamethoxazole is an alternative. However, its efficacy has not been established.

- Persons who have been in contact with an infected individual should be monitored closely for respiratory symptoms for 14 days after last contact with the infected individual.

Immunization. Universal immunization with pertussis vaccine of children younger than 7 years is critical for the control of pertussis. The current vaccine available in the United States (DTP adsorbed) is a suspension of inactivated *B pertussis* cells combined with diphtheria and tetanus toxoids and adsorbed onto an aluminum salt, and, thus, is administered intramuscularly.

Based on household studies of young children exposed to pertussis, vaccine efficacy for children who have received at least three doses is estimated to be approximately 80%. Vaccine-induced immunity persists for at least 3 years and diminishes thereafter with time. Disease in those previously immunized is usually mild. Acellular pertussis vaccines are under evaluation but are not licensed in the United States (as of October 1990).

Schedule for Routine Childhood Immunization (see Tables 2 and 3, pages 17 and 18). Five doses of DTP, given intramuscularly, are recommended.* The first dose is usually given at about 2 months, followed by two additional doses at intervals of approximately 2 months. A fourth dose is recommended 6 to 12 months after the third dose, usually at 15 to 18 months of age, to complete the initial series; a fifth dose is given before school entry (kindergarten or elementary school) at 4 to 6 years of age to protect these children from pertussis in ensuing years and to decrease transmission of the disease to younger children. The fourth dose can be given at 15 months of age, concurrently with other vaccines (see Simultaneous Administration of Multiple Vaccines, page 16).

If pertussis is prevalent in the community, immunization can be started as early as 4 weeks of age, and doses can be given as frequently as 4 weeks apart.

Pertussis immunization is not routinely indicated in individuals 7 years or older.

---

*The Immunization Practices Advisory Committee (ACIP) of the U.S. Public Health Service defines primary immunization as consisting of the first four doses; the fifth dose is considered a booster.

Dose and Route. The DTP dose is 0.5 mL, given intramuscularly. The use of reduced volume of individual doses of DTP vaccine or multiple doses of reduced volume (fractional doses) is not recommended. The effect of such practices on the frequency of serious adverse events and on protection against disease has not been determined.

Antipyretic Prophylaxis. Administration of acetaminophen (15 mg/kg per dose) or other appropriate antipyretic at the time of immunization and at 4 and 8 hours after immunization reduces the incidence of febrile and local reactions. Since convulsions after DTP are almost always associated with fever, antipyretic prophylaxis may benefit children at increased risk of seizures (see Adverse Events Following Pertussis DTP Vaccination, page 363). For such children, administration of an antipyretic every 4 to 6 hours after DTP vaccination should be considered. Caretakers should be aware that antipyretic therapy could also obscure fever caused by concomitant, unrelated infection.

Recommendations for Scheduling Pertussis Vaccine in Special Circumstances.

- In the child in whom pertussis immunization is resumed after deferral or interruption of the recommended schedule, the next dose in the sequence should be given, irrespective of the interval since the last dose (i.e., the schedule is not reinitiated).
- If the fourth dose of DTP is not given until after the fourth birthday, no further doses of pertussis vaccine are necessary.
- For children who have received fewer than the recommended number of doses of pertussis vaccine but who have received the recommended number of DT doses for their age (i.e., those started on DT, then given DTP), dose(s) of DTP should be given to complete the recommended pertussis immunization schedule. However, the total number of doses of diphtheria and tetanus toxoids (as either DT or DTP) should not exceed six before the fourth birthday. A monovalent pertussis vaccine preparation could be used, but currently is only distributed in Michigan by its Department of Public Health.
- Children who have recovered from culture-proven pertussis need not receive further pertussis immunization.
- During pertussis outbreaks, such as in a hospital, pertussis immunization is not usually recommended for adult contacts because monovalent pertussis vaccine is not available.*

*If available (currently only distributed in Michigan), a booster dose of 0.25 mL of monovalent pertussis vaccine may be considered for health care and day care center personnel and for close contacts who have chronic pulmonary disease in addition to antibiotic prophylaxis. However, the efficacy of immunoprophylaxis and chemoprophylaxis in these circumstances is unproven.

Medical Records. Charts of those children in whom DTP vaccination has been deferred should be flagged, and their immunization status periodically assessed to ensure that they are appropriately immunized.

Adverse Events Following Pertussis (DTP) Vaccination.

- *Local and febrile reactions.* Redness, edema, induration and tenderness at the injection site, drowsiness, fretfulness, anorexia, vomiting, crying, and slight to moderate fever are common reactions to pertussis vaccination (Table 46). These manifestations occur within several hours of immunization and subside spontaneously without sequelae. Children with such reactions should receive subsequent doses of pertussis vaccine as scheduled. They are more likely to have the same reactions after subsequent DTP immunization than those in whom reactions have not previously occurred. The incidence of local and febrile reactions also tends to increase with age.

  Bacterial or sterile abscesses at the site of the injection are infrequent (6 to 10 per million injections of DTP). Bacterial abscesses indicate contamination of the product or nonsterile technique and should be reported (see Reporting of Adverse Reactions, page 27). The causes of sterile abscesses are unknown. Their occurrence usually does not contraindicate further doses of DTP.
- *Allergic reactions.* Severe anaphylactic reactions and resulting deaths, if any, are extremely rare. The transient urticarial rashes that occasionally occur after DTP immunization, unless appearing immediately (i.e., within minutes), are unlikely to be anaphylactic (IgE-mediated) in origin. These rashes probably represent a serum sickness-type reaction due to circulating antigen-antibody complexes resulting from one of the DTP antigens and corresponding antibody either acquired from a prior dose or transplacentally. Because formation of such complexes is dependent on a precise balance between concentrations of circulating antigen and antibody, such reactions are most unlikely to recur after a subsequent dose and are not contraindications to further doses.
- *Seizures.* The incidence of seizures occurring within 48 hours of administration of pertussis vaccine is 1:1750, based on a large prospective study.* Most seizures occurring after DTP immunization are brief, self limited, and generalized, and they occur in febrile children. These characteristics indicate that DTP-associated seizures are usually febrile convulsions. These seizures have not been demonstrated to result in the subsequent development of recurrent afebrile seizures (i.e., epilepsy) or other neuro-

*Cody C.L., Baraff L.J., Cherry J.D., Marcy S.M., and Manclark C.R. Nature and rates of adverse reactions associated with DTP and DT immunizations in infants and children. *Pediatrics*. 1981;68:650-660.

Table 46. Adverse Events Occurring Within 48 Hours of Pertussis Immunization*

Categories	Rate (%) per Dose
Redness at site	37.4
Redness > 2.4 in diameter	7.2
Swelling at site	40.4
Swelling > 2.4 in diameter	8.9
Pain at site	51
Fever ≥ 38°C (100.4°F)	47
Fever ≥ 40.5°C (104.9°F)	0.3
Drowsiness	32
Fretfulness	53
Anorexia	21
Vomiting	6
Persistent crying for 3 to 21 h	1
High-pitched, unusual cry	0.1
Convulsions	0.06
Collapse with shock-like state	0.06

*These data are derived from 15,752 DTP immunizations (modified from Cody C.L., Baraff L.J., Cherry J.D., Marcy S.M., and Manclark C.R. Nature and rates of adverse reactions associated with DTP and DT immunizations in infants and children. *Pediatrics.* 1981;68:650-660).

logic sequelae. Predisposing factors to seizures occurring within 48 hours include underlying convulsive disorder, personal history of convulsions, and family history of convulsions (see Infants and Children With Underlying Neurologic Disorders, page 367; and Children With Personal or Family History of Seizures, page 54).

- *Unusual crying.* Persistent, severe, inconsolable screaming or crying for 3 or more hours (1:100*) or an unusual, distinctive, high-pitched cry (1:1000*) is sometimes observed within 48 hours of pertussis vaccination. Distinction between these features and crying due to pain can be difficult and requires close questioning of the patient's caretaker. The significance of such unusual crying is unknown. It has been noted after receipt of immunizations other than pertussis vaccine and is not known to be associated with sequelae.
- *Collapse.* Collapse or shock-like state (hypotonic-hyporesponsive episode) has been observed after pertussis vaccination (1:1750*). A recent follow-up study of a group of children who had experienced such episodes demonstrated no evidence of serious neurologic damage or intellectual impairment as a result of these episodes.

*Cody C.L., Baraff L.J., Cherry J.D., Marcy S.M., and Manclark C.R. Nature and rates of adverse reactions associated with DTP and DT immunizations in infants and children. *Pediatrics.* 1981;68:650-660.

Alleged Reactions. The temporal relation of immunization and severe adverse events, such as death, encephalopathy, onset of a seizure disorder, developmental delay, or learning or behavioral problems, does not establish causation by the vaccine. Many of the manifestations of alleged vaccine reactions have other causes, such as viral encephalitis, other concurrent infections, preexisting neurologic disorders, and metabolic and other congenital abnormalities. For example, whereas infantile spasms frequently have their onset in the first 6 months of life and, in some cases, have been temporally related to the administration of pertussis vaccine, epidemiologic data demonstrate that the vaccine does not cause infantile spasms. Sudden infant death syndrome (SIDS) has occurred after DTP immunization, but several studies provide evidence that DTP immunization does not cause SIDS. A large case-control study of SIDS in the United States demonstrated that SIDS victims were no more likely to have recently received DTP vaccination than control children who did not have SIDS. Since SIDS occurs most commonly at the age when DTP immunization is recommended, coincidental, temporal associations between the death and immunization by chance alone are expected.

Evaluation. Because of alternative causes and these coincidental associations, appropriate diagnostic studies should be undertaken to establish an etiology of serious adverse events occurring temporally with immunization rather than assuming that they are caused by the vaccine. However, the cause of events temporally related to immunization cannot always be established even after diagnostic studies.

Severe acute neurologic illness and permanent brain damage. Permanent neurologic disability (brain damage) and even death have previously been considered uncommon sequelae of rare severe adverse neurologic events temporally related to pertussis vaccine. Because no specific clinical syndromes or neuropathologic findings have been recognized in these cases, determination of whether pertussis vaccine is the cause of a specific child's deficit is not possible. Such adverse events can occur in both vaccinated and unvaccinated children, particularly in the first year of life. Hence, epidemiologic studies have been necessary to determine the risk of severe sequelae after acute events temporally related to pertussis immunization.

The only case-control study that addresses the issue of whether acute neurologic illness associated with DTP immunization results in permanent brain damage is the National Childhood Encephalopathy Study (NCES) in England, conducted from 1976 to 1979. This study examined the causes and natural history of serious acute neurologic illness in 1,182 children aged 2 to 36 months admitted to a hospital, and provided the basis for statements in recent editions of the *Red Book* concerning pertussis vaccination and temporally related severe neurologic disorders. More than 95% of cases of encephalopathy were unrelated temporally to DTP vaccination. Only 35 of these children had received pertussis vaccine within 7 days, and in many of these the temporal relation between acute neurologic illness and vaccination may have occurred by chance. Six of these children had infantile spasms, which was shown in a separate analysis not to be attributable to DTP vaccine. Analysis of the results indicated that very rarely (1:140,000 DTP doses) pertussis vaccine may be associated with the development of severe acute neurologic illness in children who were previously normal. Whereas later neurologic assessment of these children appeared to indicate that permanent neurologic sequelae could occur in some cases, the conclusion of an expert group that subsequently reviewed the NCES was that because of the small number of cases and limitations of the design and methods, the study could not provide valid information regarding whether acute neurologic illness associated with DTP vaccine results in permanent neurologic sequelae. Additional studies have not provided evidence to support a causal relationship between DTP vaccination and serious acute neurologic illness that results in permanent neurologic injury. Although each of these studies individually is of insufficient size to provide definitive answers, the results are consistent with the reanalysis of the NCES findings.

The Committee concludes, based on currently available data, that pertussis vaccine has not been proven to be a cause of brain damage. Although the data do not prove that pertussis vaccine can never cause brain damage, they do indicate that if it does so, such occurrences must be exceedingly rare. Furthermore, in individual cases the role of pertussis vaccine is impossible to determine on the basis of clinical or laboratory findings.

Before administration of each dose of DTP, the child's parent or guardian should be questioned about possible adverse events following the previous dose.

Contraindications and Precautions to Pertussis Immunization. Adverse events after pertussis immunization that usually (but not necessarily always) contraindicate further administration of pertussis vaccine are as follows:

- Encephalopathy within 7 days, defined as severe acute neurologic illness which may be manifest by prolonged seizures, severe alterations of consciousness, or focal neurologic signs. Studies indicate that such events associated with DTP are evident within 72 hours of immunization; prudence, however, usually justifies considering such an illness occurring within 7 days of DTP as a possible contraindication to further doses of pertussis vaccine.

- A convulsion, with or without fever, occurring within 3 days. Children who have experienced a convulsion at any time should be evaluated to determine if additional doses of pertussis vaccine should be given (see Infants and Children With Underlying Neurologic Disorders).
- Persistent, severe, inconsolable screaming or crying for 3 or more hours, or an unusual, distinctive, high-pitched cry within 48 hours.
- Collapse or shock-like state (hypotonic-hyporesponsive episode) within 48 hours.
- Temperature of 40.5°C (104.9°F) or more, unexplained by another cause, within 48 hours.
- Immediate allergic reaction to vaccine—severe or anaphylactic in type.

Although the risks of giving subsequent doses of pertussis vaccine to a child who has had one of these events are not known, the possibility of another reaction of similar or greater severity often justifies discontinuing pertussis immunization. In each case, the decision to give or withhold immunization should be based on the clinical assessment of the prior reaction, the likelihood of pertussis exposure in the child's community, and the potential benefits and risks of pertussis vaccine.

Infants and Children With Underlying Neurologic Disorders. The decision to give pertussis vaccine to infants and children with underlying neurologic disorders can be difficult and must be made on an individual basis after careful and continuing consideration of the risks and benefits (see also Children with Personal or Family History of Seizures, page 54). In some cases, these disorders may constitute a cause for deferring DTP immunization, and based on the medical history of the child, subsequent administration of pertussis vaccine. The different circumstances and recommendations are categorized as follows:

- *A progressive neurologic disorder characterized by developmental delay or neurologic findings.* These conditions are reason for deferral of pertussis immunization. Administration of DTP may coincide with or hasten the recognition of inevitable manifestations of the disorder, with resulting confusion about causation. Examples include infantile spasms, uncontrolled epilepsy, and progressive encephalopathy. Such disorders should be differentiated from those that are nonprogressive and in which the symptoms may change as the child matures.
- *Infants and children with personal history of convulsions.* These patients have an increased risk of convulsions after receipt of pertussis-containing vaccines. A retrospective review of adverse events after the receipt of DTP vaccine indicated a sevenfold greater likelihood of personal history of seizure in children who

had a seizure after receipt of DTP than in children who had local or other nonneurologic, post-DTP adverse events. No evidence indicates that these vaccine-associated seizures produce permanent brain damage, cause epilepsy, aggravate neurologic disorders, or affect the prognosis in children with underlying disorders. However, because the risk of a postvaccine convulsion is increased, pertussis immunization of children with recent seizures should be deferred until a progressive neurologic disorder is excluded or the child's diagnosis has been established. Because outbreaks of pertussis continue to occur in the United States, the decision to defer immunization should be reassessed at each subsequent medical visit; the decision to give DTP should be based on the adjudged risks and consequences of seizure after DTP vaccination in comparison to the risk of pertussis and its complications. Infants and children with well-controlled seizures or those in whom a seizure is unlikely to recur may be vaccinated. Children with associated neurologic deficits may be at increased risk of complications if they develop pertussis. Children traveling to or residing in areas of endemic or epidemic pertussis are at increased risk of developing pertussis. Efforts should be undertaken to ensure pertussis immunization of children attending day care centers, special clinics, or residential care institutions.

- *Infants and children known to have, or suspected of having, neurologic conditions that predispose either to seizures or neurologic deterioration.* Such conditions are tuberous sclerosis and certain inherited metabolic or degenerative diseases. Deferral of pertussis immunization should be considered for these patients. Convulsions or encephalopathy can occur in the normal course of these disorders and, thus, may occur after any immunization. DTP or DT vaccination may be associated with the occurrence of overt manifestations of the disorders with resulting confusion about causation. Hence, children with unstable or evolving neurologic disorders that may predispose to seizures or neurologic deterioration should be observed for a period of time to ascertain the diagnosis and prognosis of the primary neurologic disorder before immunization. Pertussis immunization should be reconsidered at each visit. Children whose condition is resolved, corrected, or controlled can be vaccinated. No evidence indicates that prematurity in the absence of other factors increases the risk of seizures after immunization and is not a reason to defer vaccination (see Preterm Infants, page 46). Similarly, stable neurologic conditions, such as developmental delay or cerebral palsy, are not contraindications to pertussis immunization. Children in the first year of life with neurologic disorders which necessitate temporary deferment of pertussis immunization should not receive either DT or DTP because the risk of acquiring diphtheria or tetanus in children younger than 1 year in this country is remote. At or before the first birthday, the decision to give either DTP or DT should be made to ensure that the child is immunized at least against diphtheria and tetanus. As children become ambulatory, their risk of tetanus-prone wounds increases. Children with neurologic disorders that are recognized after the first birthday frequently will have received one or more doses of DTP. The physician may temporarily defer additional doses of DTP in anticipation of stabilization of the child's neurologic status. If the physician determines that the child probably should not receive further pertussis immunizations, DT immunization should be completed according to the recommended schedule (see Diphtheria, page 194, and/or Tetanus, page 468).

Children With Family History of Convulsions (see also Children with Personal or Family History of Seizures, page 54). A history of seizure disorders or adverse events after receipt of a pertussis-containing vaccine in a family member is not a contraindication to pertussis immunization. Although the risk of seizures after DTP in children with family history of seizures is increased, these seizures are usually febrile in origin and have a generally benign outcome. In addition, this risk is outweighed by the continuing risk of pertussis in the United States and the substantial number of children with family history of seizures who, if not vaccinated, would remain susceptible to pertussis.

Advice to Parents of Children at Increased Risk of Seizures. Parents of children who may be at increased risk of a seizure after pertussis immunization, such as from personal or family history of convulsions, should be informed of the risks and benefits of pertussis immunization in these circumstances. Advice should be provided about fever, its control (see Antipyretic Prophylaxis, page 362), and appropriate medical care in the unlikely event of a seizure.

Pinworm Infection

(Enterobius vermicularis)

Clinical Manifestations: Pinworm infection (enterobiasis) causes pruritus ani and, rarely, pruritus vulvae. Although pinworms have been found in the lumen of the appendix, no evidence indicates that they are causally related to acute appendicitis. Many symptoms, such as grinding of the teeth at night and enuresis, have been attributed to pinworm infections, but without proof of a relationship. Vaginitis, salpingitis, and pelvic peritonitis can occur because of aberrant migration of the adult worm from the perineum.

Etiology: *Enterobius vermicularis* is a nematode.

Epidemiology: Enterobiasis is distributed worldwide and commonly occurs in family clusters, but it has no sex preference or seasonal variation in incidence. In the past, 5% to 15% of the general population in the United States was estimated to be infected, but recent reports suggest that the incidence has declined. Prevalence rates are higher in preschool-aged and school-aged children, in mothers of infected children, and in institutionalized populations. Adult gravid female nematodes usually die after depositing eggs on the perianal skin. Thus, reinfection by autoinfection or infection acquired from others is necessary to maintain enterobiasis in an individual. The period of communicability is as long as the gravid female nematodes are discharging eggs on perianal skin and eggs remain infective in an indoor environment; this period is usually two to three weeks. Humans are the only hosts.

Diagnostic Tests: Diagnosis is made by application of transparent (not merely translucent) adhesive tape to the perianal skin to pick up any eggs; the tape is then applied to a glass slide and examined under a low-power microscopic lens. These specimens are best collected when the patient first awakens in the morning and before washing.

Treatment: The drug of choice is pyrantel pamoate (11 mg/kg in a single dose, maximum 1 g) or mebendazole (given as a single dose of 100 mg and repeated in 2 weeks). In children younger than 2 years, in whom experience with either drug is limited, the risks and benefits of the drugs should be considered before administration can be made. Alternatives include piperazine and pyrvinium pamoate, but they are less effective and cumbersome to use. No unusual cleansing or hygienic measures should be undertaken. Excessive zeal in this regard can induce guilt feelings in parents and is counterproductive. Because of the high frequency of reinfections, families should be informed that recurrence is common. Repeated infections should be treated the same as the first one. Families may need to be treated as a group. Vaginitis is self limited and does not require separate treatment.

Isolation of the Hospitalized Patient: No special precautions are recommended.

Control Measures: Control is difficult in day care centers and schools because the rate of reinfection is extremely high. In institutions, mass and simultaneous treatment, repeated in two weeks, can be effective. Household cohabitants or institutional cohorts of infected patients should be examined for pinworms and treated if necessary.

Plague

Clinical Manifestations: Plague is usually accompanied by fever and painful lymphadenitis (bubonic plague). Pneumonic, septicemic, meningeal, and pharyngeal forms of plague are uncommon.

Etiology: Plague is caused by *Yersinia pestis*, a pleomorphic, bipolar staining, Gram-negative rod.

Epidemiology: Plague is an enzootic infection of wild rodents in many parts of the world, including the western United States, parts of South America, Africa, and Asia. An epidemic occurs when the domestic rodent populations become infected and their infected ectoparasites (fleas) spread the disease to humans. Bubonic plague is transmitted by infected fleas, particularly the oriental rat flea *(Xenopsylla cheopis)* outside the United States and by other rodent fleas in the United States. Direct contact with infected rodents, rabbits, and domestic animals, especially cats, has also been implicated in transmission. Bubonic plague is not directly communicable, except under rare circumstances by human fleas. Pneumonic plague is directly communicable. It is transmitted by the droplet route during direct contact with an animal or individual who is infected.

The **incubation period** is 2 to 6 days for bubonic plague and 2 to 4 days (occasionally shorter but rarely longer) for pneumonic plague.

Diagnostic Tests: *Y pestis* can be isolated by culture of buboes, cerebrospinal fluid, blood, or, in pneumonic plague, sputum. The characteristic bipolar staining of the organism is best seen with Wayson's stain. A Giemsa stain of blood smears can also demonstrate bipolar staining rods. Gram stain and fluorescent antibody studies of the bubo aspirate, cerebrospinal fluid, occasionally peripheral blood, or sputum may provide presumptive evidence of *Y pestis*. Paired sera from the acute and convalescent phases of the illness, 3 to 4 weeks apart, should be obtained to demonstrate seroconversion or a fourfold antibody titer rise by the passive hemagglutination test.

Treatment: Streptomycin (30 mg/kg/d) is the drug of choice. Tetracycline (20 to 30 mg/kg/d given intravenously in four divided doses) or chloramphenicol (75 to 100 mg/kg/d given intravenously in four divided doses) is also effective. Tetracycline should not be given to children younger than 9 years unless the benefits of therapy clearly are greater than the risks of dental staining. Chloramphenicol, with or without streptomycin, should be used for plague meningitis. The optimum duration of antibiotic therapy in plague is not known. Five to 7 days of streptomycin, 10 to 14 days of tetracycline, or 10 days of chloramphenicol is usually sufficient.

Drainage of buboes and abscesses may be necessary, but should not be attempted until at least 24 hours after initiating antimicrobial therapy, because of the potentially highly infectious nature of the drainage.

Isolation of the Hospitalized Patient: All patients should be in strict isolation until pneumonia is excluded and therapy has been initiated. Drainage/secretion precautions are recommended for patients with bubonic plague; strict isolation is mandatory for patients with pneumonic plague. Isolation should be continued for 3 days after the start of effective antimicrobial therapy.

Control Measures:

Care of Exposed Persons. A person with intimate exposure to **bubonic plague** should be placed under surveillance for 7 to 10 days. If human fleas are known to be present, disinfestation of the clothing and residence of the exposed person with an insecticide effective against local fleas should be considered. The person exposed to **pneumonic plague** should (1) have clothing and quarters disinfested with an insecticide powder, if indicated; (2) be given chemoprophylaxis for 7 days with tetracycline (15 mg/kg/d), the preferred drug except for children younger than 9 years, or a sulfonamide (40 mg/kg/d); and (3) be placed in isolation with close observation (including twice daily recordings of temperature) for 7 to 10 days, if reliable close observation as an outpatient is not possible or practical.

Vaccine. An inactivated whole-cell bacterial vaccine* is useful for persons whose occupation may regularly bring them into contact with potentially infected rodents or their fleas (e.g., biologists, geologists, or laboratory workers). Routine vaccination is not recommended for persons living in plague enzootic areas of the western United States. Vaccination is recommended for those traveling to or residing in areas where plague is occurring and where domestic rats are known

*Miles Inc. Cutter Biological, West Haven, CT.

to be infested. Primary immunization consists of three intramuscular injections of vaccine, the first two at 30-day intervals and the third 4 to 12 weeks after the second.

The package insert should be consulted for specific doses. Booster doses of the same amount given in the third injection are indicated at 6-month intervals until a total of five doses are given, then at 12- to 24-month intervals for as long as the danger of exposure exists.

Other Measures. Periodic surveys in high-risk areas to determine the prevalence of infested rats, wild rodents, and fleas should be performed by public health workers. Health officials must be notified when a presumptive diagnosis of plague is made so that control measures can be instituted.

Suppression of the rodent population is important in epidemic control, but it must not be done without prior or concurrent ectoparasite (flea) control during an active plague epizootic. Ratproofing buildings, reducing breeding areas, and rat control on ships by ratproofing and periodic fumigation are important, as is disinfestation of domestic cats and dogs. If field surveys indicate a need, treatment of premises or other human contact areas with residual insecticides should be performed.

Pneumococcal Infections

Clinical Manifestations: *Streptococcus pneumoniae* (pneumococcus) is the most common cause of acute otitis media and is a frequent cause of pneumonia, meningitis, and sinusitis in children. It is also the most common cause of bacteremia in infants and children 1 to 24 months old, some of whom have no evidence of a primary focus of infection.

Etiology: *S pneumoniae* organisms are lancet-shaped, Gram-positive diplococci. Eighty-three pneumococcal serotypes have been identified. Certain serotypes are prevalent in adults; others are prevalent in children. Serotypes in groups 14, 6, 18, 19, 23, 4, 9, 7, 1, and 3 (in order of decreasing prevalence) cause most childhood pneumococcal infections.

Epidemiology: Pneumococci are ubiquitous; many persons carry organisms in the upper respiratory tract without symptoms. Transmission is from person to person, presumably by respiratory droplet contact. Disease is more likely to occur when predisposing conditions (usually immunoglobulin deficiency, symptomatic HIV infection, or some viral upper respiratory tract infections) exist. Pneumococcal infections are most prevalent when respiratory disease is most common, usually during the winter months. The period of communicability is unknown, perhaps as long as the organism is present in respiratory secretions but probably less than 24 hours after effective antimicrobial therapy is begun.

Mortality from pneumococcal disease is highest in patients who have bacteremia or meningitis. Patients with sickle-cell anemia, Hodgkin's disease, congenital or acquired immunodeficiency (including HIV infection, especially in children), nephrotic syndrome, and splenic dysfunction, and those who have undergone splenectomy or organ transplantation are at increased risk of developing severe pneumococcal disease because of impaired immunologic response to the pneumococcus. Certain other patients may also be at an increased risk of severe pneumococcal infections, such as some patients with diabetes mellitus, congestive heart failure, chronic pulmonary disease, and renal failure. Patients with cerebrospinal fluid (CSF) leakage, complicating skull fracture, or neurosurgical procedure can have recurrent pneumococcal meningitis.

The **incubation period** varies by type of infection and can be as short as 1 to 3 days. Illness usually occurs within 1 month after a new pneumococcal serotype is acquired in the upper respiratory tract. Illness is seldom associated with prolonged carriage.

Diagnostic Tests: Material obtained from a suppurative focus should be Gram stained and cultured by appropriate microbiologic techniques. Blood cultures should be obtained in all patients suspected of having invasive pneumococcal disease; cultures of CSF and other body fluid (e.g., pleural fluid) are also often indicated. The white blood cell (WBC) count may be of assistance in suspected bacteremic disease caused by *S pneumoniae*; febrile young children with WBC counts higher than 20,000/mm^3 have an increased likelihood of bacteremia. Although the predictive value of an elevated WBC count for pneumococcal bacteremia is not high, a normal WBC count is highly predictive of the absence of bacteremia. Recovery of pneumococci from an upper respiratory tract culture is not proof of causation of otitis media, pneumonia, or sinusitis because of the frequent presence of these bacteria in uninfected persons. Rapid methods for pneumococcal capsular antigen detection (e.g., latex agglutination, ELISA, coagglutination) in CSF, pleural fluid, serum, and concentrated urine can be useful for a rapid diagnosis in suspected bacteremia, pneumonia, and meningitis; a negative test result, however, does not exclude pneumococcal disease. These tests are particularly useful in patients who have received antibiotics before the collection of specimens for culture.

Treatment:

- Penicillin G is the drug of choice for the treatment of most pneumococcal infections. Because strains of pneumococcus with decreased susceptibility to penicillin G (in vitro minimal inhibitory concentration [MIC] of 0.1 to 1 µg/mL) have been identified, oxacillin disk susceptibility testing should be performed on isolates from blood, CSF, or other infected body fluids. Strains identified to be resistant by oxacillin disk testing should have the MIC of penicillin determined in the laboratory. In many instances, infections caused by strains with decreased penicillin susceptibility respond clinically to high-dose penicillin therapy. However, treatment of meningitis caused by one of these relatively resistant strains should not be treated with penicillin; selection of an antibiotic must be based on susceptibility testing. If the strain is susceptible in vitro, cefotaxime, chloramphenicol, or vancomycin can be used. The latter two drugs are also appropriate alternative drugs for penicillin-allergic patients.

  Penicillin-resistant strains (MIC greater than 1 µg/mL) frequently are resistant to many other antimicrobials, but are susceptible to vancomycin. Among the new beta-lactam antibiotics, cefotaxime and imipenem-cilastatin have the greatest in vitro activity against these strains; clinical efficacy with high-dose cefotaxime (250 to 300 mg/kg/d) has been demonstrated.
- For children with mild to moderately severe infections who are allergic to penicillins, erythromycin and trimethoprim-sulfamethoxazole are alternative drugs. Clindamycin, chloramphenicol, or cephalosporins are also effective therapeutic agents. For treatment of meningitis, CSF concentrations with the macrolides and older cephalosporins (such as cephalothin and cefazolin) are insufficient for these drugs to be used. New cephalosporins such as cefotaxime and ceftriaxone are effective for treatment of meningitis and new beta-lactam-like antimicrobials may be effective.
- The route and dosage of antimicrobial therapy depend on the severity of the illness (see Antimicrobials, page 527). For meningitis, a minimum of 10 days of therapy is generally required.
- In infants and children 2 months and older with bacterial meningitis, dexamethasone therapy should be considered after the physician has considered the benefits and possible risks (see Dexamethasone Therapy for Bacterial Meningitis in Infants and Children, page 566). The regimen is 0.6 mg/kg/d in four divided doses, given intravenously, for the first four days of antibiotic treatment, and it should be initiated with the first dose of antibacterial therapy.
- Treatment of the carrier state is not indicated.

Isolation of the Hospitalized Patient: No specific precautions are recommended.

Control Measures:

Day Care. No isolation precautions are necessary for children in day care who have pneumococcal disease. Prophylactic antibiotic treatment of day care contacts of a person with pneumococcal disease is not recommended.

Active Immunization. The 23-valent pneumococcal vaccine is composed of purified, capsular polysaccharide antigens of 23 pneumococcal serotypes. Each 0.5-mL dose of the vaccine contains 25 µg of each polysaccharide antigen (575 µg total polysaccharide). The vaccine includes the capsular antigens from the serotypes causing 88% of cases of bacteremia and meningitis in adults, nearly 100% of cases of bacteremia and meningitis in children, and 85% of cases of acute otitis media. Like other polysaccharide antigens, some of the pneumococcal serotypes (e.g., types 6 and 14) in the vaccine have limited immunogenicity in children younger than 2 years. The effectiveness of pneumococcal vaccines in preventing pneumonia has been demonstrated in healthy young adults and children older than 17 months predisposed to a high incidence of pneumococcal disease. In one study, vaccinated children with sickle-cell disease or who had undergone splenectomy experienced significantly less bacteremic pneumococcal disease than nonvaccinated patients.

Recommendations for Pneumococcal Vaccination:

- Children 2 years and older with increased risk of acquiring systemic pneumococcal infections or with increased risk of serious disease if they become infected should be vaccinated with 0.5 mL of the pneumococcal vaccine, given subcutaneously or intramuscularly. Included in this high-risk category are children with (1) sickle-cell disease; (2) functional or anatomic asplenia; (3) nephrotic syndrome or chronic renal failure; (4) conditions associated with immunosuppression, such as organ transplantation or cytoreduction therapy; (5) CSF leaks; and (6) HIV infection (see AIDS and HIV Infections, page 124).
- In addition to administering pneumococcal vaccine to children with functional or anatomic asplenia, parents and patients should be informed that vaccination does not guarantee protection from fulminant pneumococcal disease and death (case fatality rates are 50% to 80%). Asplenic patients with unexplained fever or manifestations of sepsis should receive prompt medical attention including treatment for suspected bacteremia, the initial signs and symptoms of which may be subtle. Antimicrobials

selected for initial empirical treatment should be effective against *S pneumoniae*, *Neisseria meningitidis*, and beta-lactamase-producing *Haemophilus influenzae* type b.

- When elective splenectomy is to be performed, pneumococcal vaccine should be given approximately 2 weeks or more before the operation, if possible, to increase the likelihood of eliciting a protective antibody response. Similarly, in planning cancer chemotherapy or immunosuppressive therapy, as in patients with Hodgkin's disease or who are to undergo organ transplantation, vaccination should precede the initiation of chemotherapy or immunosuppression by approximately 2 weeks or more. Vaccination during chemotherapy or radiation therapy should be avoided because antibody responses are poor, and vaccination is not likely to be effective in preventing pneumococcal infection. These patients, including those who received vaccine during chemotherapy, should be immunized 3 months after discontinuation of chemotherapy.
- Vaccination is not recommended for preventing upper or lower respiratory tract infection in healthy children living in the United States.
- Vaccination is not recommended for preventing otitis media during the first 2 years of life, and data are inadequate to evaluate the effectiveness of pneumococcal vaccine in preventing otitis media in children older than 2 years.
- Routine revaccination of children who previously received the 14-valent vaccine with the 23-valent vaccine is not recommended because the increased serotype coverage is modest, the duration of protection is not well defined, and local reactions after revaccination have been reported to be more severe than after initial vaccination. However, revaccination with the 23-valent vaccine should be strongly considered for persons who received the 14-valent vaccine if they are at high risk of fatal pneumococcal infection, such as asplenic patients.
- Revaccination of recipients of the 23-valent vaccine should be considered after 3 to 5 years for children younger than 10 years (at the time of possible revaccination), children at high risk of fatal pneumococcal infection, such as asplenic patients, and for those who have been demonstrated to have rapid antibody decline after initial vaccination, such as those with sickle-cell anemia, nephrotic syndrome, and renal failure, and transplant recipients. Revaccination should also be considered for high-risk older children and adults who were previously (6 years or before) vaccinated. Adult renal transplant recipients who experience increasing frequency of pneumococcal infections 2 or more years after transplant have fewer such infections after revaccination.

- Vaccination generally should be deferred during pregnancy because the effect of the vaccine on the fetus is unknown. The risk of severe pneumococcal disease during pregnancy must be weighed against the potential hazards of the vaccine.
- No data are available to indicate that concurrent administration of pneumococcal vaccine with DTP, poliovirus, influenza, or other vaccines will increase the severity of reactions or diminish antibody responses.

Passive Immunization. Intramuscular or intravenous immunoglobulin administration is recommended for preventing pneumococcal infection in patients with congenital or acquired immunodeficiency diseases.

Chemoprophylaxis (see also Asplenic Children, page 52). Many experts recommend that children with functional or anatomic asplenia receive daily antimicrobial prophylaxis. For prevention of pneumococcal disease, oral penicillin G or V (125 mg twice daily for children younger than 5 years; 250 mg twice daily for children 5 years and older) is recommended. The age at which prophylaxis can be discontinued is an empirical decision since no studies of this question have been performed. Some experts continue prophylaxis throughout childhood and into adulthood in particularly high-risk patients.

The results of a multicenter study demonstrated that oral penicillin V (125 mg twice daily) given to infants and young children with sickle-cell disease reduces the incidence of severe bacterial infection by 84% compared with the placebo control group. Based on this study, a National Institutes of Health Consensus Development Panel recommended daily penicillin prophylaxis for children with sickle-cell hemoglobinopathy beginning before the age of 4 months.

Antimicrobial prophylaxis against pneumococcal infection may be particularly useful for asplenic children not likely to respond to vaccine, such as children younger than 2 years or children receiving intensive chemotherapy or cytoreduction therapy.

Pneumocystis carinii

Clinical Manifestations: In infants, a subacute, diffuse pneumonitis with dyspnea at rest, tachypnea, oxygen desaturation, cough, and usually fever characteristically occurs. In immunocompromised children and adults, the onset can be more acute and fulminant. The chest roentgenogram often shows bilateral interstitial infiltrates, but without a characteristic pattern. Mortality in immunocompromised patients is high, ranging from 10% to 40%.

Etiology: Based on morphology, *Pneumocystis carinii* organisms formerly were presumed to be sporozoa, but recent DNA sequencing suggests that the organism is a fungus.

Epidemiology: *P carinii* is ubiquitous in animals, particularly rodents. Whether *P carinii* in animals is infectious for humans has not been determined. In developing countries, the disease frequently occurs in epidemics and primarily affects malnourished infants and children. Epidemics have also been described in premature infants. In industrialized countries, *P carinii* infections are a major complication of immunosuppression. In the United States, the disease is restricted almost entirely to immuncompromised patients with deficient cell-mediated immunity, including those with congenital immunodeficiency, organ transplant, malignancy under treatment, and particularly AIDS. *P carinii* pneumonia (PCP) is the most common opportunistic infection in infants and young children with perinatally acquired HIV infection and frequently occurs between 6 and 12 months of age. It can be the initial illness in an HIV-infected infant. These infants are not usually malnourished and can have relatively normal T-helper (CD4) cell counts. The prognosis in infants and young children with AIDS who develop PCP is poor; median subsequent survival has been reported to be 1 month. In patients with lymphoma or leukemia, the disease tends to occur during periods of remission. The mode of transmission is unknown. Two hypotheses have been proposed: (1) person-to-person transmission by the respiratory route, and (2) reactivation of latent infection resulting from immunosuppression. Circumstantial evidence suggests that person-to-person transmission can occur, but it has not been proven. Recurrences in immunocompromised patients, especially those with AIDS, are common. The period of communicability and the **incubation period** are not known.

Diagnostic Tests: The most effective procedures are open-lung biopsy, bronchoscopic biopsy, or bronchoalveolar lavage. Percutaneous transthoracic lung-needle aspiration and bronchial washings and brushings have also been used but are less sensitive. Toluidine blue O and methenamine silver nitrate are the most useful stains for identifying the thick-walled cysts; extracystic trophozoites are easier to identify with Giemsa, Wright, Gram-Weigert, or polychrome methylene blue stain. Serologic tests for detecting *P carinii* infection are still experimental and are not recommended for diagnosis. Most healthy persons have detectable serum *P carinii* antibody by age 4 years. Many children and adults with HIV infection and PCP have elevated serum concentrations of serum lactate dehydrogenase.

Treatment: The drug of choice is trimethoprim-sulfamethoxazole (TMP-SMX), usually given intravenously. Oral therapy should be reserved for patients with mild disease who do not have gastrointestinal dysfunction. The rate of adverse reactions in adult patients with AIDS receiving TMP-SMX can be as high as 60%; but studies in adults indicate that 50% of these patients, nevertheless, can be successfully treated with TMP-SMX. The incidence of adverse effects in HIV-infected children treated with TMP-SMX is not known at this time.

Parenteral pentamidine is an alternative drug. It is also associated with a high incidence of adverse reactions, including renal dysfunction, hypoglycemia, hyperglycemia, hypotension, fever, and neutropenia. Its therapeutic efficacy in adults with PCP is the same as that of TMP-SMX.

A minimum duration of 2 weeks of therapy is recommended. In patients with AIDS, 3 weeks is recommended because of the high incidence of recurrence.

A number of potentially useful drugs have been identified by in vitro studies in animal models and human clinical drug trials. These include dapsone, TMP, dapsone with TMP, trimetrexate with folinic acid with or without SMX, aerosol pentamidine, pyrimethamine with sulfadoxine, and DFMO (difluoromethylornithine).

Based on data in adults, corticosteroids appear to be beneficial in the treatment of HIV-infected patients with severe PCP. Optimal dose, timing, and safety have not been determined.

Prophylaxis. HIV-infection chemoprophylaxis has been recommended for adult HIV-infected patients who have already had an episode of PCP (even if receiving zidovudine); and those with a T-helper (CD4) lymphocyte count of less than 200/mm^3 or if T-helper lymphocytes are less than 20% of the total peripheral blood lymphocytes. Two regimens are considered safe and effective: (1) oral TMP-SMX (160 mg TMP-800 SMX) given twice daily with leucovorin (5 mg) once daily; and (2) aerosol pentamidine (300 mg) given monthly. The U.S. Public Health Service has recently published recommendations of an expert panel, giving the indications and use of these regimens in adults.*

These guidelines for adults are also recommended for HIV-infected adolescents. However, for children younger than 13 years, the indications are less well established. Low T-helper (CD4) lymphocyte counts, based on normal values in adults, do not correlate with the risk of PCP, particularly in infants. Prophylaxis for children younger than 13 years is currently recommended in each of the fol-

*Centers for Disease Control. Guidelines for prophylaxis against *Pneumocystis carinii* pneumonia for persons infected with human immunodeficiency virus. *MMWR*. 1989;38 (no. S-5);1-9.

lowing circumstances: (1) prior PCP; (2) less than 400 T-helper (CD4) lymphocytes/mm^3; and (3) infants (younger than 1 year) with established HIV infection.

The dosage regimen for children younger than 13 years is not standardized. TMP-SMX administered on 3 consecutive days weekly has been effective in immunocompromised children without AIDS and is as effective as daily therapy. The current recommended regimen is TMP-SMX given 3 consecutive days of each week in a dosage of 75 mg/m^2 TMP plus 375 mg/m^2 SMX given orally every 12 hours. No information is available on the effectiveness in children of aerosolized pentamidine for prophylaxis. It is an alternative to TMP-SMX in those children to whom aerosol medications can be effectively administered.

Parenteral pentamidine given monthly or biweekly has also been used on a limited basis. The dosage for monthly administration is 4 mg/kg given intravenously. Breakthrough cases of *P carinii*, however, have been reported in patients receiving parenteral pentamidine. Extrapulmonary *P carinii* infection can also occur. Other drugs for prophylaxis include weekly pyrimethamine-sulfadoxine, daily dapsone, or dapsone-TMP. These drugs have not been tested in children.

In immunosuppressed children with cancer, TMP-SMX prophylaxis to prevent *P carinii* has also been effective. The dosage recommendation is the same as for HIV-infected patients, and can be given on 3 consecutive days of each week.

Isolation of the Hospitalized Patient: Infected patients should not have contact with immunocompromised patients until antimicrobial therapy has been given for 48 hours.

Control Measures: Appropriate therapy of infected patients and prophylaxis in immunocompromised patients are the only available means of control.

Poliovirus Infections

Clinical Manifestations: Most poliovirus infections are asymptomatic. Clinical disease occurs, in decreasing order of frequency, as follows: nonspecific febrile illness (abortive poliomyelitis), aseptic meningitis (nonparalytic poliomyelitis), and paralytic disease involving the lower motor neurons (paralytic poliomyelitis).

Etiology: Polioviruses are enteroviruses and consist of three types: 1, 2, and 3.

Epidemiology: Poliovirus infections occur only in humans. Spread is by fecal-oral and possibly oral-oral (respiratory) routes. Transmission from mother to newborn infant has been reported. Infection is more common in infants and young children and occurs at an earlier age under conditions of poor hygiene. However, paralysis is more severe when infection occurs in older individuals. In temperate climates, poliovirus infections are most common in the summer and fall; in the tropics, no seasonal pattern is evident.

Poliomyelitis is rare in the United States at the present time. The last epidemic occurred in 1979 in a group of persons who had declined immunization. Almost all cases since 1980 have been vaccine associated (an average of nine cases per year). The remainder have been imported cases (an average of one case every 2 years). Poliomyelitis is still prevalent in many underdeveloped areas of the world and therefore is a potential threat for unimmunized travelers to these areas, as well as for importation into the United States.

Live oral poliovirus vaccine (OPV) has been associated with paralysis in vaccinees and their contacts. The approximate risk is one case of paralytic disease in immunologically normal vaccine recipients per 7.8 million doses of OPV distributed, and one case of paralytic disease among household and community contacts of vaccinees per 5.5 million doses distributed. The greatest risk of paralysis occurs with the first dose of OPV. From 1973 through 1984, the reported overall frequency of paralysis was one case in 520,000 first doses and one case per 12.3 million subsequent doses. Immunocompromised persons who are exposed to vaccine virus either by exposure to a vaccinee or by receiving the vaccine are at a particularly high risk of acquiring paralytic disease.

Communicability is greatest shortly before and after onset of clinical illness when virus is present in the throat and excreted in large amounts in the feces. Virus persists in the throat for about 1 week after the onset of illness, and is excreted in the feces for several weeks and occasionally for months. Patients are potentially contagious as long as fecal excretion persists. In recipients of OPV, the virus persists in the throat for 1 to 2 weeks; it is excreted in the feces for several weeks, although in rare cases it has been excreted for more than 2 months. Immunodeficient patients may excrete virus for prolonged periods.

The **incubation period** of abortive poliomyelitis is 3 to 6 days. For the onset of paralysis in paralytic poliomyelitis, the incubation period is usually 7 to 21 days, but occasionally it is as short as 4 days.

Diagnostic Tests: Poliovirus can be recovered from the feces, throat, and, rarely, from cerebrospinal fluid by isolation in tissue culture. Specimens should be obtained from all patients with paralytic disease suspected to be poliomyelitis for isolation of the virus. Fecal material is most likely to yield viruses. Rectal swabs have low sensitivity and are discouraged. If a poliovirus is isolated, it should be sent to the Centers for Disease Control through the state health department for testing to distinguish wild poliovirus from vaccine strains. Since infants who are immunized with poliovirus vaccine can excrete virus in the feces for several weeks, absolute proof that a disease is caused by the poliovirus necessitates positive isolation from a nongastrointestinal, nonpharyngeal source. The incidental isolation of poliovirus from enteric sites in healthy young infants should be assumed to be the result of exposure to vaccine virus, unless a reason to suspect otherwise exists. Serologic testing of acute and convalescent sera should be performed in patients suspected of having paralytic poliomyelitis. However, experience indicates that interpretation of serologic tests can be difficult. Cultures of stool from at least two specimens collected within the first 15 days after onset of symptoms represents the diagnostic test of choice for confirming polio.

Treatment: Supportive.

Isolation of the Hospitalized Patient: For patients suspected of excreting wild poliovirus, enteric precautions are indicated for the duration of hospitalization or until virus can no longer be recovered from the feces.

Control Measures:

Immunization of Infants and Children. Two types of trivalent vaccine are available—live oral poliovirus vaccine (OPV) and inactivated poliovirus vaccine (IPV) given parenterally. OPV contains poliovirus types 1, 2, and 3, which have been produced in monkey kidney cell cultures. IPV is a mixture of the three types of poliovirus inactivated with formalin. Earlier products were grown in monkey kidney cell culture and required four doses for a primary series. An enhanced-potency IPV, (licensed in the United States in 1988), which is produced in human diploid cell culture, is the inactivated poliovirus vaccine currently in use in this country. It is highly immunogenic; after only three doses it induces a seroconversion rate equal to that of OPV. Both IPV and OPV are effective in preventing poliomyelitis.

Based on consideration of the risks and benefits, OPV is currently the vaccine of choice for immunization of children in the United States because it (1) induces intestinal immunity, (2) is simple to administer, (3) is well accepted by patients, (4) results in immunization of some contacts of vaccinated persons, and (5) has essentially eliminated disease caused by wild polioviruses in the United States. Multiple doses of OPV are given to ensure that infection occurs with all three types of poliovirus and induces complete immunity. No evidence exists for waning immunity. Breast-feeding does not affect the success of immunization; hence, no interruption of the feeding schedule is necessary.

To ensure that vaccination is undertaken among fully informed persons, parents of prospective vaccinees should be made aware of the reasons and circumstances for specific vaccine recommendations at particular ages, and of the benefits and risks of poliovirus vaccines for both individuals and the community. Parents who refuse OPV for their children after being informed of the risks and benefits should be offered IPV for their children.

Recommendations for OPV. Ordinarily, the first dose of OPV is administered when the infant is approximately 2 months; a second dose is given when the infant is 4 months (see Table 2, page 17). A minimum interval of 6 weeks, but usually 2 months, is recommended. A third dose of OPV is recommended when the child is 18 months to complete the primary series, but can be given at any time between 12 and 24 months, including at 15 months. MMR, DTP, and the *Haemophilus* conjugate vaccines can be given concurrently (see Simultaneous Administration of Multiple Vaccines, page 16). A supplementary dose of OPV should be given before the child enters school (at 4 to 6 years). Two doses produce an antibody response in excess of 90% to all three serotypes, and in the United States an additional dose at age 6 months is usually not warranted. In geographic areas where polio is endemic, however, a third dose administered 2 months after the second dose is desirable. In these endemic areas, a dose may also be given when the newborn infant is discharged from the hospital. Because successful immunization is less likely in newborn infants, the otherwise recommended series of three doses of OPV should be given subsequently, beginning at 2 months of age.

For children who are not immunized in the first year of life (see Table 3, page 18), two doses of OPV should be given approximately 6 to 8 weeks apart, followed by a third dose 6 to 12 months later. If the risk of exposure to polio is substantial, the third dose should be given 6 to 8 weeks after the second dose. If the third dose is administered before the fourth birthday, a supplementary (fourth) dose should be given before the child enters school (at 4 to 6 years of age).

Children at any age who are partially immunized should receive the number of doses necessary to complete the required series of three doses. If the schedule has been interrupted, the series does not need to be reinitiated; instead, it is continued.

Indications for OPV are summarized in Table 47.

Table 47. Persons for Whom OPV Immunization Is Indicated

Normal infants and children receiving routine immunization.
Unimmunized or partially immunized children who are at imminent risk of exposure to poliovirus.
Adults at future risk of exposure to poliomyelitis who had received one or more doses of OPV or IPV.
Adults at imminent (within 4 weeks) risk of exposure to poliomyelitis who are unimmunized.
Adults at imminent (within 4 weeks) risk of exposure to poliomyelitis who have had a partial or complete series with IPV.

Recommendations for IPV. Persons who have refused OPV or in whom OPV is contraindicated (see Precautions and Contraindications to Immunization, page 388) should be immunized with IPV. OPV should not be used in households with an immunodeficient person, including those known to be HIV-infected, because OPV is excreted in the stool by healthy vaccinees and can infect an immunocompromised household member, which may result in paralytic disease (see Adverse Vaccine Reactions, page 389). Only IPV should be used for all those requiring poliovirus immunization in such households. For adults needing polio immunization, IPV should be given in most cases (see Immunization Recommendations for Adults, page 386).

The primary series of IPV consists of three doses administered subcutaneously and results in antibody responses to the three serotypes in more than 95% of vaccine recipients. The first two doses should be given at 4- to 8-week intervals, and the third dose should be given 6 to 12 months after the second dose. In infancy, the primary schedule of IPV is usually concomitant with the first two doses and the fourth dose of DTP; the two vaccines should be given in separate syringes. When entering school, children should receive another dose of IPV.

Children partially immunized with IPV should receive sufficient doses of IPV or OPV to complete the primary immunization series. For IPV-immunized persons, booster doses of IPV have previously been recommended every 5 years; however, for recipients of enhanced-potency IPV, the need for 5-year boosters has not been established. Incompletely immunized children who are at an increased risk of exposure to poliovirus should be given the remaining recommended doses of IPV or, if time is a limiting factor, at least a single dose of OPV (unless they are immunocompromised or live in a household with an immunocompromised member).

Indications for IPV are summarized in Table 48.

Table 48. Persons for Whom IPV Immunization Is Indicated

Persons with compromised immunity who are unimmunized or partially immunized.
Symptomatic and asymptomatic persons known to be infected with the human immunodeficiency virus (HIV).
Household contacts of an immunodeficient individual, including those known to be HIV infected.
Partially immunized or unimmunized adults in households (or other close contacts) of children to be given OPV, provided that immunization of the child can be assured (see page 387).
Unimmunized adults at future risk of exposure to poliomyelitis.
Adults at future risk of exposure to poliomyelitis who have been partially immunized with IPV or OPV.*
Adults at future risk of exposure to poliomyelitis who have had a primary series of IPV.*
Individuals refusing OPV immunization.

*OPV is also acceptable.

Immunization Recommendations for Adults.

- Routine primary poliovirus vaccination of previously unvaccinated adults (generally those 18 years or older) residing in the United States is **not** indicated.
- *Immunization is recommended for certain adults who are at a greater risk of exposure* to wild polioviruses than the general population, including the following:
  1. Travelers to areas or countries where poliomyelitis is or may be epidemic or endemic.
  2. Members of communities or specific population groups experiencing disease caused by wild polioviruses.
  3. Laboratory workers handling specimens that may contain polioviruses.
  4. Health care workers in close contact with patients who may be excreting polioviruses.

All persons should be fully informed of the two available poliovirus vaccines and of the benefits, risks, and reasons for immunization with one or the other vaccine. Recommendations for immunization of these individuals are as follows:

- *Unvaccinated Adults.* Primary immunization with IPV is recommended, whenever feasible. IPV is preferred because the risk of vaccine-associated paralysis after OPV is slightly higher in adults than in children. Two doses of IPV should be given at intervals of

1 to 2 months; a third dose should be given 6 to 12 months after the second dose.

If time does not allow three doses of IPV to be given according to the recommended schedule before protection is required, the following alternatives are recommended:

1. If 2 months or more are available before protection is needed, three doses of IPV should be given at least 1 month apart.
2. If 1 to 2 months are available before protection is needed, two doses of IPV at least 1 month apart should be given.
3. If less than 1 month is available, a single dose of either OPV or IPV should be given.

In these instances, the remaining doses of vaccine to complete the primary immunization should be subsequently given at the recommended intervals, if the person remains at an increased risk.

- *Incompletely Immunized Adults.* Those who previously received less than a full primary course of OPV or IPV should be given the remaining required doses of vaccine, either OPV or IPV, regardless of the interval since the last dose and the type of vaccine that was previously received.
- *Adults Who Are at an Increased Risk of Exposure to Poliomyelitis and Who Previously Completed a Primary Course of OPV.* Such adults can be given another dose of OPV or IPV. The need for further supplementary doses has not been established. Adults who previously completed a primary course of IPV may be given a dose of either IPV or OPV. If IPV is used exclusively, additional doses may be given every 5 years, but their need in enhanced-potency IPV recipients has not been established.

Management of Unimmunized or Inadequately Immunized Adults in Households in Which Children Are To Be Given OPV (or Other Close Contacts of Such Children). Adults who have not been adequately immunized against poliomyelitis with OPV or IPV are at risk, albeit small, of developing OPV-associated paralytic poliomyelitis when children in the household or day care facility in which they work are given OPV (see Adverse Vaccine Reactions, page 389). The physician should avoid any unnecessary delay in infant immunization with OPV while minimizing the risk to adult contacts, who may include parents, older relatives, baby-sitters, day care center staff, and others with prolonged contact and opportunity for fecal-oral acquisition. The Committee recommends administering OPV to the infant regardless of the history of immunization in the adult contact, after the responsible adult has been informed of the small risk involved and advised to take precautions concerning contact with feces. An acceptable alternative, provided complete immunization of the infant can be ensured, is to immunize the adult household contacts according to the following guidelines:

- For a previous recipient of a partial course of OPV or IPV, a dose of enhanced-potency IPV is given to the susceptible adult and the first dose of OPV is given to the infant.
- For a susceptible adult with no previous immunization or an unknown immunization status, two monthly doses of the IPV are given; at the time of the second monthly visit, the first dose of OPV is administered to the infant. This process can be facilitated by giving the initial IPV dose to the mother and other adult contacts when the infant is discharged from the hospital. The remaining OPV dose or doses can then be administered to the infant at the appropriate (2-month) intervals.

No procedures should be adopted that decrease the likelihood of children being adequately immunized against poliomyelitis.

Precautions and Contraindications to Immunization.

- Although no convincing evidence indicates that adverse effects of either OPV or IPV occur in the **pregnant woman** or developing fetus, immunization during pregnancy should be avoided for reasons of theoretical risk. However, if immediate protection against poliomyelitis is needed, OPV is recommended.
- **Patients with immunodeficiency diseases**, such as AIDS or other manifestations of HIV infection, combined immunodeficiency, hypogammaglobulinemia, and agammaglobulinemia, should not be given OPV because of the risk of vaccine-associated disease. Furthermore, patients with altered immune states because of such diseases as leukemia, lymphoma, or generalized malignancy, or because of immunosuppressive therapy with pharmacologic doses of corticosteroids (see Immunodeficient and Immunosuppressed Children, page 47), alkylating drugs, antimetabolites, or radiation therapy, also should not receive OPV because of the risk of paralytic disease. Although a protective immune response to IPV in the immunodeficient patient cannot be ensured, IPV is safe and some protection may result from its administration.
- Use of IPV rather than OPV to immunize **asymptomatic persons known to be infected with the HIV virus** is indicated, as one or more other household members are likely to be immunodeficient (see AIDS and HIV Infection, page 124).
- OPV should not be used for immunizing **household contacts of persons with immunodeficiency disease, altered immune states, immunosuppression due to therapy for other disease, or known HIV infection**. IPV is recommended for these individuals. However, many immunosuppressed individuals will be immune to polioviruses by virtue of previous immunization or exposure to a wild-type virus when they were immunologically competent, and their risk of paralytic disease is thought to be less than that of congenitally immunodeficient individuals. Nevertheless, their house-

hold contacts should not receive OPV. If OPV is inadvertently administered to a household-type contact of an immunodeficient patient, close contact between the patient and the recipient of OPV should be avoided for approximately 2 months after vaccination (the period of maximum excretion of vaccine virus).

- Because of the possibility of immunodeficiency in other children born to a **family with one or more immunodeficient children,** OPV should not be given to members of a household with this history until the immune status of the recipient and other family members is documented and immunodeficiency has been excluded.

Adverse Vaccine Reactions. In rare instances, administration of OPV has been associated with paralysis in healthy recipients and their contacts. The greatest risk occurs with the first dose of OPV. Immunocompromised persons are at particularly high risk. For previously unvaccinated adults, the risk is slightly higher than that in children (see also Epidemiology, page 382). Other than efforts to identify those with immunodeficiency, no procedures are currently available for identifying persons likely to experience this type of adverse reaction. Vaccinees and their parents should be informed of the extremely small risk of vaccine-associated paralysis for vaccinees and their susceptible, close personal contacts.

No serious side effects of currently available IPV have been documented. Because IPV contains trace amounts of streptomycin and neomycin, hypersensitivity reactions in individuals sensitive to these antibiotics are possible.

Case Investigation and Epidemic Control. Each suspected case of poliomyelitis should be reported promptly to the state health department. Poliomyelitis should be considered in the differential diagnosis of all cases of acute flaccid paralysis. If the course is clinically compatible with polio, specimens should be obtained for viral studies, and an immediate epidemiologic investigation should be undertaken. If evidence implicates vaccine-derived poliovirus, no vaccination plan need be employed, as no outbreaks associated with vaccine virus in the United States have been documented. If evidence implicates wild poliovirus and a possibility of transmission, a vaccination plan designed to contain spread should be employed. Within an epidemic area, OPV should be provided for all persons who have not been completely immunized or whose immunization status is unknown, with the exceptions noted in Precautions and Contraindications to Immunization (page 388).

Q Fever

Clinical Manifestations: Acute Q fever is usually characterized by the abrupt onset of fever, chills, weakness, headache, and anorexia as well as other nonspecific systemic symptoms. Cough and chest pains can occur and can signify pneumonia, which occurs in about half the patients. Weight loss and weakness may be pronounced. Hepatosplenomegaly is frequently noted. The illness lasts 1 to 4 weeks, with a gradual resolution. Rash is unusual. Endocarditis and hepatitis are the major manifestations of the chronic disease. Although the mortality from acute Q fever is less than 1%, mortality among patients with endocarditis is 30% to 60%.

Etiology: *Coxiella burnetii*, the cause of Q fever, is unique among rickettsiae because it undergoes a host-dependent phase variation.

Epidemiology: Animal infection is widespread, usually subclinical, and primarily involves a large variety of domestic farm animals (especially sheep, goats, and cows), but also cats, rodents, marsupials, and other species. Tick vectors may be important in maintaining some animal reservoirs. Infectious spore-like forms can persist in the soil for many years. Human disease is uncommon, but many infections are asymptomatic. The disease occurs endemically throughout the world, typically in areas where cattle are raised and sheep and goats are herded. The disease has been transmitted to humans by inhalation of infected material, tissues, or dust from infected cats or animals on farms, in research facilities, and in other settings. Some animal workers, ranchers, research laboratory workers, and individuals in other occupations or with avocational interests that place them in close contact with infected animals or tissues have a heightened risk of disease. Q fever has occurred among flocks of sheep used as experimental subjects in medical research facilities, and transmission to research investigators and technical personnel has been documented. Handling of animal fetuses and products of conception is a major means of infection. Although seasonal trends are not obvious, in some areas the disease coincides with the lambing season in the early spring. Because the birth of farm animals, such as sheep, goats, and cows, are somewhat controllable events, the disease can be spread throughout the year in areas where planned animal births are permitted. Evidence for human intrauterine infection has been reported.

The **incubation period** is usually between 9 and 20 days.

Diagnostic Tests: Isolation of *C burnetii* from blood is usually not attempted because of the hazard to laboratory workers. Specific antiphase I and antiphase II immunofluorescent, ELISA, complement fixation, and immune adherence hemagglutination antibody tests using paired serum specimens are used diagnostically. Specific IgM, IgG, and IgA tests using immunofluorescence or ELISA methods are available in reference and research laboratories. *C burnetii* infection does not cause a positive serum Weil-Felix test.

Treatment: Tetracycline is the drug of choice. Chloramphenicol is an alternative but its efficacy has not been proven. Tetracyclines should not be given to children younger than 9 years unless the benefits clearly are greater than the risks of dental staining. Therapy should be continued until the patient is afebrile for 2 to 3 days. In chronic Q fever, relapses necessitating repeated courses of antimicrobial therapy can occur. The organism can remain latent in tissues for years; treatment of chronic disease is extremely difficult. Relapses can occur following discontinuation of treatment.

Isolation of the Hospitalized Patient: No special precautions are recommended.

Control Measures: Experimental vaccines for domestic animals and laboratory workers are promising but are not commercially available. Recommendations have been made to reduce the risk of infection in research facilities involving sheep.* Special safety practices are recommended for nonpropagative laboratory procedures involving *C burnetii*; and for all propagative procedures, necropsies of infected animals, and manipulation of infected human and animal tissues. Otherwise, no specific management is recommended for persons who have been exposed. Flash pasteurization of milk at 71.6°C (161.1°F) for 15 seconds or 62.9°C (145.2°F) for 30 minutes destroys the organism, but the epidemiologic role of milk in transmission is uncertain.

Rabies

Clinical Manifestations: Infection with rabies virus characteristically produces an acute febrile illness with rapidly progressive central nervous system manifestations, including anxiety, dysphagia, and convulsions, and almost invariably progresses to death. Some patients may present with paralysis.

Etiology: Rabies virus is an RNA virus classified in the rhabdovirus family.

---

*Bernard AW, Parham GL, Winler WG, Helmick CG. Q fever control measures: Recommendations for research facilities using sheep. *Infect. Control.* 1982;3:461-465.

Epidemiology: A large animal reservoir of sylvatic rabies exists in the United States, including skunks, bats, raccoons, foxes, and other species. In some areas, these wild animals infect domestic dogs and cats. Rabies in small rodents, rabbits, and hares is rare, but in some areas where raccoon rabies is spreading (e.g., the mid-Atlantic states), an increasing number of woodchucks have been found to be rabid. The virus is present in saliva and is transmitted by bites or by licking of mucosa or open wounds. Most rabies cases in humans throughout the world result from dog bites in areas in which canine rabies is enzootic. Although experimental evidence has shown that dogs and cats can harbor the virus in their saliva as long as 12 days before the appearance of recognizable illness, most dogs and cats become ill within 3 days of virus shedding, and no case of rabies in the United States has been attributed to a dog or cat that has remained healthy throughout the standard 10-day period of confinement. Airborne transmission has been reported in the laboratory and in bat-infested caves. Transmission has also occurred by transplantation of corneas from patients dying of undiagnosed rabies. Person-to-person transmission by bite has not been documented, although the virus has been isolated from the saliva of patients.

The **incubation period** in humans ranges from 5 days to more than 1 year, but 2 months is the average.

Diagnostic Tests: Infection in animals can be diagnosed by demonstration of virus-specific fluorescence in brain tissue. Suspected rabid animals should be killed in a manner that does not render brain tissue unfit for examination. Virus can be isolated from brain, saliva, and other tissues in suckling mice or in tissue culture. However, virus isolation takes much longer than fluorescent microscopy of brain. The diagnosis in suspected human cases sometimes can be made premortem or postmortem by fluorescent microscopy of skin biopsies from the nape of the neck, by isolation of the virus from the saliva or cerebrospinal fluid, or by detection of antibody in the serum and cerebrospinal fluid in unvaccinated persons. The laboratory should be consulted before submission of specimens so that appropriate materials can be collected and transport arranged.

Treatment: Only three patients with human rabies have survived with intensive, supportive care; all other patients have succumbed despite treatment. Once symptoms have developed, no drug or vaccine improves the prognosis.

Isolation of the Hospitalized Patient: Strict isolation is recommended for the duration of the illness despite the absence of a proven risk of transmission to human contacts. Those attending the patient should be aware of the possible hazards of contamination with saliva. If the patient has bitten someone, or his saliva has contaminated an open wound or mucous membrane, the involved area should be thoroughly washed and immunization started (see Care of Exposed Persons, page 394).

Control Measures:

Case Reporting. All patients who are suspected of having rabies should be reported promptly to public health authorities.

Exposure Risk and Decision to Give Immunoprophylaxis. Exposure to rabies results from a break in the skin caused by the teeth or claws of a rabid animal or by the contamination of scratches, abrasions, or mucous membranes with saliva from a rabid animal. The decision to immunize an exposed individual ordinarily should be made in consultation with the local health department, which can provide information on the risk of rabies in a particular area for each species of animal, and in accordance with the guidelines in Table 49. In the United States, skunks, raccoons, and bats are more likely to be infected than other animals, but foxes, coyotes, cattle, dogs, and cats occasionally are infected. Bites of rodents (such as squirrels and rats) or lagomorphs (rabbits and hares) rarely require specific antirabies prophylaxis. Additional factors must be considered when deciding if immunization is indicated. An unprovoked attack is more suggestive of a rabid animal than a bite during attempts to feed or handle an animal. Properly immunized dogs and cats have only a minimal chance of developing rabies. However, in rare instances rabies has developed in properly vaccinated animals, or in improperly vaccinated, unusual pets.

Handling of Suspect Animal. A suspect dog or cat that has bitten a human should be captured, confined, and observed by a veterinarian for 10 days. Any illness in the animal should be reported immediately to the local health department. If the animal develops signs of rabies, it should be killed and its head removed and shipped under refrigeration (iced, not frozen) to a qualified laboratory for examination. Because clinical signs of rabies in a wild animal cannot be interpreted reliably, a suspect wild animal should be killed at once and its brain examined for evidence of rabies. The exposed person need not be treated if examination of the brain by fluorescent antibody procedures is negative for rabies.

Care of Hospital Contacts. Immunization of hospital contacts of a patient with rabies should be reserved for individuals who were bitten or whose mucous membranes or open wounds have come in contact with the saliva, cerebrospinal fluid, or brain tissue of a patient with rabies (see Care of Exposed Persons). Other hospital contacts of a patient with rabies do not require immunization.

Care of Exposed Persons.

Local Care. The immediate objective of postexposure treatment is to prevent virus from entering neural tissue. Prompt and thorough local treatment of all bites and scratches is essential, as virus may remain localized to the area of the bite for a variable time. All wounds should be thoroughly flushed and cleaned with soap and water. Quaternary ammonium compounds (such as Zephiran) which were recommended in the past are no longer considered superior to soap. The need for tetanus prophylaxis and measures to control bacterial infection should also be considered. The wound, if possible, should not be sutured.

Immunoprophylaxis. After local care is completed, concurrent use of both passive and active immunoprophylaxis is required for optimal therapy (see Table 49). Wherever possible, human rather than equine products should be used for passive immunization, and human diploid cell or fetal rhesus lung diploid vaccine should be used for active immunization. Physicians can obtain expert counsel from their local or state health departments.

Active Immunization. Human diploid cell vaccine (HDCV), 1 mL, is given intramuscularly in the deltoid area or anterior thigh on the first day of treatment, and repeat doses are given on days 3, 7, 14, and 28. A sixth dose is recommended in some European countries but not in the United States, as five doses appear to be equally protective. Serologic testing after HDCV immunization generally has not been necessary, but it has been advised for recipients who may be immunosuppressed.

Care should be taken to ensure that the vaccine is administered intramuscularly. Intradermal vaccine is not advised for postexposure treatment. Because antibody responses in adults who received vaccine in the gluteal area sometimes have been less than in those who were injected in the deltoid muscle, the latter site should always be used except in infants.

- *Adverse reactions and precautions with HDCV.* Reactions primarily reported in adults after vaccination with HDCV are less common than with previously available vaccines. Reactions are uncommon in children. In a study using five doses of HDCV, local reactions such as pain, erythema, and swelling or itching at the injection site were reported in approximately 25% of the recipients; mild systemic reactions such as headache, nausea, abdominal pain, muscle aches, and dizziness were reported in about 20% of the recipients. Several cases of neurologic illness resembling Guillain-Barré syndrome that resolved without sequelae in 12 weeks and a focal, subacute, central nervous system disorder temporally associated with HDCV have been reported. The rate of neurologic abnormalities after HDCV is approximately 1 in 150,000.

Table 49. Postexposure Antirabies Treatment Guide*

Species of Animal	Condition of Animal at Time of Attack	Treatment of Exposed Human
Wild Skunk Fox Coyote Raccoon Bat Other carnivores	Regard as rabid unless proven negative by laboratory test	RIG† and HDCV‡
Domestic Dog and cat	Healthy, under surveillance	None§
	Unknown (escaped)	Call public health official for advice
	Rabid or suspected rabid	RIG† and HDCV§
Livestock		Consider individually‖
Rodents and lagomorphs (rabbits and hares)		Consider individually‖

*These recommendations are only a guide. They should be applied in conjunction with knowledge of the animal species involved, circumstances of the bite or other exposure, vaccination status of the animal, and presence of rabies in the region.

†RIG = Rabies Immune Globulin (Human).

‡HDCV = Human Diploid Cell Vaccine, given intramuscularly. Discontinue vaccine if fluorescent antibody stains of tissues from the animal killed at the time of attack are negative for rabies antigen.

§Begin RIG + HDCV at the first sign of rabies in a biting dog or cat during a holding period (10 days).

‖**See Exposure Risk and Decision to Give Immunoprophylaxis, page 393.**

Immune-complex-like reactions in persons receiving booster doses of HDCV have been observed. The reaction, characterized by onset 2 to 21 days postinoculation, presents with a generalized urticaria and can include arthralgia, arthritis, angioedema, nausea, vomiting, fever, and malaise. In no instances were these illnesses life-threatening. Current estimates suggest that this immune-complex-like illness can occur in as many as 6% of adults receiving booster doses as part of a preexposure immunization regimen;

it is rare in persons receiving primary immunization, which includes most children receiving vaccine in the United States. All serious, systemic, neuroparalytic or anaphylactic reactions to the rabies vaccine should be reported immediately (see Reporting of Adverse Reactions, page 27).

If the patient has a serious allergic reaction to HDCV, vaccine produced in rhesus diploid cells by the Michigan State Department of Health can be given. This vaccine is designated as Rabies Vaccine Absorbed (RVA).* It is administered on the same schedule as HDCV.

Although the safety of the use of rabies vaccine during pregnancy has not been established, pregnancy should not be considered a contraindication to the use of vaccine after exposure.

- *Nerve tissue vaccines*. Nerve tissue vaccines are not licensed in the United States, but are available in many areas of the world. These preparations induce neuroparalytic reactions in 1:2,000 to 1:8,000 recipients. Immunization should be discontinued if meningeal or neuroparalytic reactions develop. Corticosteroids can be used for treatment of complications, but they should be used only for life-threatening reactions because they definitely increase the risk of rabies in experimentally inoculated animals.

Passive Immunization. Rabies Immune Globulin (Human) (RIG)† should be used concomitantly with the first dose of vaccine for post-exposure prophylaxis to bridge the time between onset of treatment and active antibody production by the vaccinee. The exception to the concomitant use of vaccine and RIG is the patient previously immunized with HDCV (or another rabies vaccine if the patient is known to have developed serum antibody); these patients should be given two doses of vaccine only, one immediately (day 0) and the other on day 3. If vaccine is not immediately available, RIG should be given alone and vaccination started later. If RIG is not immediately available, vaccine should be given followed by RIG when obtained in the first 8 days after the beginning of treatment. If administration of both vaccine and RIG are delayed, both should be used regardless of the interval between exposure and treatment; but every effort should be made to give RIG as soon as possible after exposure.

RIG is virtually free of hypersensitivity reactions. The recommended dose is 20 IU of RIG per kilogram of body weight. Rarely is RIG not available. Antirabies serum of equine origin (ARS)‡ may be used in a dose of 40 IU per kilogram of body weight. Allergic reactions may occur in as many as 40% of persons. A careful history must

*Available from Michigan Department of Public Health (tel. 517/335-8050).

†Available from Miles Inc. Cutter Biological, West Haven, CT, or Merieux Institute, Miami, FL.

‡Available from Sclavo Inc., Wayne, NJ.

be obtained and appropriate tests for hypersensitivity performed before administration of serum of equine origin (see Sensitivity Tests for Reactions to Animal Sera, page 40). Approximately one half of the antibody preparation is used to infiltrate the wound(s); the remainder is given intramuscularly. RIG is supplied in 2-mL (300 IU) and 10-mL (1,500 IU) vials. ARS is supplied in 5-mL vials (1000 IU). Passive antibody can inhibit the response to rabies vaccines; therefore, the recommended dose should not be exceeded. Vaccine should never be administered in the same parts of the body or with the same syringe used to give RIG.

The following persons should receive two 1-mL doses of HDCV (one dose on each of days 0 [exposure] and 3): (1) those who previously received postexposure prophylaxis with HDCV or RVA; (2) those who received a three-dose, intramuscular, preexposure regimen of HDCV or RVA; (3) those who received a three-dose, intradermal, preexposure regimen of HDCV with the Merieux product in the United States; and (4) those who have a documented adequate rabies titer after previous vaccination with any other rabies vaccine. RIG is not recommended in these circumstances.

- *Complete postexposure antirabies treatment*, including RIG or ARS, should be given if an exposed person immunized previously with vaccines other than HDCV has not had prior documentation of a serum antibody response.

Preexposure Control Measures, Including Immunization. The relatively low frequency of reactions to HDCV has made practical preexposure immunization for persons in high-risk groups, such as veterinarians, animal handlers, certain laboratory workers, children living in areas where rabies is a constant threat, and persons traveling to live in areas where rabies is common. Others, such as spelunkers whose vocational or avocational pursuits in exploring caves result in frequent exposures to dogs, cats, foxes, skunks, or bats, should also be considered for preexposure prophylaxis. Both intramuscular (1mL volume) and intradermal (0.1-mL volume) dosage forms of HDCV are available. RVA is licensed for intramuscular administration (1 mL doses only). The latter is cheaper and only slightly less immunogenic. The schedule is the same for both routes of administration: three injections given on days 0, 7, and 28. This series of immunizations has resulted in the development of antibodies in virtually 100% of persons properly vaccinated. For this reason, routine serologic testing for rabies antibody is no longer indicated. The preferred site of administration for intradermal vaccine is the deltoid area. A single case of rabies immunization failure in an individual living in a foreign country who was vaccinated intradermally has been reported, and is probably related to the immunosuppressive effect of the concurrent administration of chloroquine for malaria prophylaxis. Therefore, such individuals should receive HDCV by the intramuscular route.

Serum antibody titers decline by 2 years after the primary series given intramuscularly. Booster vaccination with HDCV (1 mL intramuscularly or 0.1 mL intradermally) or with RVA intramuscularly will produce an effective anamnestic response. However, significant allergic reactions have been associated with booster vaccination in about 6% of individuals; therefore, boosters are not routinely recommended unless the risk of exposure to rabies virus is likely to be continuous or frequent. This group includes veterinarians, animal handlers, and laboratory workers exposed to high concentrations of rabies virus (e.g., in certain research or production laboratories). In these persons, rabies serum antibody titers should be determined at 6-month intervals, and booster doses of vaccine should be administered as appropriate to maintain antibody concentrations. The Centers for Disease Control currently specifies complete virus neutralization at a 1:5 or greater titer by the rapid fluorescent-focus inhibition test as acceptable. The World Health Organization specifies 0.5 IU/mL or greater as acceptable.

Public Health. A variety of approved public health measures (including immunization of dogs and cats and the elimination of stray dogs and selected wildlife) are used to control rabies in animals. Nonvaccinated dogs, cats, or other pets bitten by a known rabid animal should be destroyed immediately. If the owner is unwilling to have this done, the animal should be vaccinated and placed in strict isolation for 6 months. If the animal has a current vaccination (within 1 to 3 years, depending on the vaccine administered and local regulations), it should be revaccinated and restrained by leashing and confinement for 90 days.

Physicians should also urge parents and teachers to caution children against provoking or attempting to capture stray or wild animals as personal or family pets.

Rat-bite Fever

Clinical Manifestations: Rat-bite fever is a zoonotic illness characterized by fever of abrupt onset, a maculopapular or petechial rash predominantly on the extremities, muscle pain, and headache. Usually the patient experienced a rat bite in the preceding 10 days. With *Streptobacillus moniliformis* infection (streptobacillary fever), the bite usually heals promptly, and nonsuppurative migratory polyarthritis or arthralgia occurs in about 50% of the patients. Sore throat is an additional manifestation of *Streptobacillus* infection after ingestion of infected milk (called Haverhill fever). Complications include soft-tissue abscesses and endocarditis. With *Spirillum minus* infection, a period of initial apparent healing is usually followed by ulceration at the site of the bite, regional lymphadenopathy, a distinctive rash of red or purple plaques, and, rarely, arthritic symptoms.

Etiology: Rat-bite fever is caused by either of two organisms: *Streptobacillus moniliformis*, a microaerophilic, Gram-negative, pleomorphic rod; and *Spirillum minus*, a small, Gram-negative, spiral organism with bipolar flagellar tufts.

Epidemiology: *S moniliformis* and *S minus* are found in upper respiratory tract secretions of infected animals. *S moniliformis* is transmitted by the bite of rats, squirrels, mice, cats, and weasels, and by the ingestion of contaminated food or milk products. *S minus* is transmitted by the bite of rats and mice. Rarely, *S moniliformis* and *S minus* infections are indirectly transmitted from person to person, such as by blood transfusion. Streptobacillary disease accounts for most cases of rat-bite fever in the United States; *S minus* infections occur primarily in Asia. Both infections are currently rare.

The **incubation period** for *S moniliformis* is usually 3 to 10 days; for *S minus* it is 7 to 21 days.

Diagnostic Tests: *S moniliformis* can be isolated when blood, joint fluid, or material from the site of the bite is inoculated into appropriate bacteriologic media or laboratory animals. Since it is a fastidious organism, the laboratory should be notified that rat-bite fever is suspected.

S minus has not been recovered on artificial media. Organisms can be seen in blood smears by darkfield microscopy or on Wright-stained smears. *S minus* can be recovered from blood, lymph nodes, or local lesions by intraperitoneal inoculation of mice or guinea pigs.

Treatment: Procaine penicillin (20,000 to 50,000 U/kg/d) should be administered intramuscularly for 7 to 10 days for rat-bite fever caused by either agent. Tetracycline (which should not be given to children younger than 9 years), chloramphenicol, or streptomycin may be substituted in the patient who is allergic to penicillin. Patients with endocarditis should receive intravenous penicillin G (150,000 to 250,000 U/kg/d in four to six divided doses) for at least 4 weeks. The addition of streptomycin initially may be useful.

Isolation of the Hospitalized Patient: No special precautions are recommended.

Control Measures: Exposed persons should be observed for symptoms. Rat control is important.

Respiratory Syncytial Virus

(See also Ribavirin Therapy of Respiratory Syncytial Virus, page 581.)

Clinical Manifestations: Respiratory syncytial virus (RSV) causes acute respiratory illness in patients of any age. In infants and young children, it is the most important cause of bronchiolitis and pneumonia. During the first few weeks of life, particularly in preterm infants, respiratory signs can be minimal; lethargy, irritability, and poor feeding, sometimes accompanied by apneic episodes, may be the major signs. Reinfection throughout life is common. Infection in older children and adults usually manifests as an upper respiratory tract illness, occasionally with bronchitis.

Etiology: Respiratory syncytial virus, a large, enveloped RNA virus, is a paramyxovirus. Strain variation results in two major groups (A and B or 1 and 2). The clinical and epidemiologic importance of this variation is yet to be determined.

Epidemiology: Humans are the only source of infection. Transmission is usually by direct or close contact, which may involve droplets. Virus can persist on environmental surfaces for many hours, and for one half hour or more on the hands. Infection among hospital personnel can occur by self-inoculation with contaminated infant secretions. Nosocomial infections are frequent among both personnel and infants. Initial infection occurs most commonly during the first year of life. Severe illness can develop in infants and young children with underlying cardiopulmonary disease. Immunodeficient children are also at risk for severe disease with prolonged viral shedding.

RSV usually occurs in annual epidemics during the winter and early spring and infects essentially all children during the first 3 years of life. Spread among household and day care contacts, including adults, is common. The period of viral shedding is usually 3 to 8 days, but it may be longer, especially in young infants in whom shedding may continue for as long as 3 to 4 weeks.

The **incubation period** ranges from 2 to 8 days; 4 to 6 days is most common.

Diagnostic Tests: Viral isolation from nasopharyngeal secretions can usually be accomplished within 3 to 8 days. RSV is a relatively labile virus, and infectivity decreases rapidly at room temperature and after freeze-thawing. The laboratory should be consulted for optimal methods of collection and transport of specimens. Rapid diagnostic procedures, including immunofluorescent and ELISA techniques, for the direct detection of viral antigen in clinical specimens are commercially available. The sensitivity of these assays in comparison to culture varies between 53% and 96%, but most are in the range of 80% to 90%. Serologic testing of acute and convalescent sera can be used to confirm infection; however, infection may not always be accompanied by detectable seroconversion, especially in young infants.

Treatment: Ribavirin, administered by small-particle aerosol for 12 to 18 hours each day for 3 to 7 days, is approved for treatment of hospitalized infants. (For indications and details of use, see Ribavirin Therapy of Respiratory Syncytial Virus, page 581.)

Isolation of the Hospitalized Patient: Contact isolation is recommended for young children and infants. Strict adherence to these infection control procedures, such as prevention of contamination by respiratory secretions and careful hand washing, will help control nosocomial spread. In several studies, the use of eye-nose goggles by staff has been shown to further decrease nosocomial transmission of RSV.

Control Measures: Efforts should be made to reduce nosocomial infection, particularly during epidemics of RSV. Hospital personnel with upper respiratory tract illnesses occurring during RSV epidemics are likely to be infected with RSV and can transmit infection. They should therefore not have direct contact with infants, unless their reassignment will compromise nursing or medical care. No vaccine is yet available.

Rhinovirus Infections

Clinical Manifestations: Rhinovirus infections are usually the most frequent cause of the common cold in adults and a major cause in children. Rhinoviruses can also be involved in bronchitis, sinusitis, otitis media, and, perhaps, lower respiratory tract disease in young children. However, their role in the latter has not been proved. Rhinoviruses can precipitate asthmatic attacks.

Etiology: Rhinoviruses are RNA viruses classified as picornaviruses. At least 100 antigenic types have thus far been classified. Infection with one type appears to confer lasting type-specific immunity, but it offers no protection against other types.

Epidemiology: Humans are the only known hosts. Transmission occurs by close person-to-person contact, aerosol, fomites, and self-inoculation after contamination of the hands. Infections occur throughout the year, but peak activity is usually in the fall and spring. Several serotypes usually circulate simultaneously, but the prevalent types in a population tend to change from year to year. By adulthood, antibody to about half the serotypes has usually developed. Household spread is common. The period of communicability is variable, but it tends to correlate with the presence of clinical symptoms and the amount of virus shed. Rhinoviruses may be shed from nasopharyngeal secretions for as long as 3 weeks.

The **incubation period** is approximately 2 to 5 days.

Diagnostic Tests: Inoculation of nasal secretions in appropriate tissue cultures for viral isolation is the best means of making a specific diagnosis. The large number of antigenic types makes serologic testing impractical.

Treatment: Supportive.

Isolation of the Hospitalized Patient: Contact isolation is advisable for hospitalized young children and infants. Respiratory secretions should be considered infectious for the duration of the illness. Careful hand washing should diminish the possibility of nosocomial spread.

Control Measures: Frequent hand washing and hygienic measures in schools, households, and other settings where transmission is common may help reduce rhinovirus spread.

Rickettsial Diseases

The rickettsiae are pleomorphic bacteria, have arthropod vectors, and, with the exception of louse-borne epidemic typhus, are transmitted to humans only incidentally. They are obligate intracellular parasites and, except for *Rickettsia quintana*, cannot be grown in cell-free media. They have typical bacterial cell walls and cytoplasmic membranes, and divide by binary fission. Their natural life cycles involve specific animal species as reservoirs (with the exception of *R prowazekii*, the cause of epidemic typhus), and animal-to-human or vector-to-human transmission occurs as a result of environmental or occupational exposure.

Ticks are the vector for many of these diseases. Thus, control measures concern prevention of tick transmission of rickettsia to humans (see Control Measures for Prevention of Tick-Borne Infections, page 112).

The rickettsial infections have many features in common, including the following:

- Multiplication of the organism in an arthropod host (except Q fever).
- Intracellular replication.
- Limited geographic and seasonal occurrence related to arthropod life cycles, activity, and distribution.
- Humans are incidental hosts (except for louse-borne typhus).
- Local, primary lesions occur with some rickettsial diseases.
- Fever, rash (except in Q fever and in most cases of ehrlichiosis), headache, myalgias, and respiratory symptoms are prominent features.
- Generalized capillary and small-vessel endothelial damage, thrombus formation, and tissue necrosis are common pathologic features (except in Q fever).
- With the exception of Q fever and rickettsialpox, nonspecific serum *Proteus* agglutinins (Weil-Felix reaction) develop during infection. However, their presence is frequently unreliable in diagnosis, since both false-positive and false-negative test results can occur.
- Species-specific serum antibodies are detectable in convalescence.
- Various serologic tests for detecting these antibodies, including indirect immunofluorescence (IFA), complement fixation, microagglutination, indirect hemagglutination, latex fixation, enzyme immunoassay, radioisotope precipitation, and radioimmunoassay, are available or are being developed in reference or research laboratories. The IFA test is recommended because of its relative simplicity, sensitivity, and specificity.
- Immunity after natural infection is usually of long duration against reinfection by the same agent (except in the case of scrub typhus, caused by *R tsutsugamushi*). Among the four different groups of rickettsial diseases, generally partial or complete cross-immunity is conferred by infections with rickettsiae within groups but not between groups.
- Infections usually respond to tetracyclines and to chloramphenicol if given early and in adequate dosage, although these drugs are rickettsiostatic and not rickettsicidal. Tetracycline drugs should not be given to children younger than 9 years unless the benefits of therapy clearly are greater than the risks of dental staining in comparison to the relative benefits and risks of chloramphenicol.
- Treatment early in the course of illness can blunt serologic responses.
- Many rickettsial diseases, especially Rocky Mountain spotted fever and Q fever, are reportable to state and local health departments.

For details, consult chapters on the following rickettsial diseases:

- Ehrlichiosis
- Q Fever

- Rickettsialpox
- Rocky Mountain Spotted Fever
- Endemic Typhus
- Epidemic Typhus

A number of other epidemiologically distinct but clinically similar tick-borne spotted-fever infections caused by rickettsia have been recognized. The etiologic agents of some of these infections share the same group antigen as *R rickettsii*; these include *R conorii*, the etiologic agent of Boutonneuse fever (also known as Kenya tick-bite fever, African tick typhus, Mediterranean spotted fever, India tick typhus, and Marseille fever) endemic in southern Europe, Africa, and the Middle East; *R sibericus*, the etiologic agent of Siberian tick typhus endemic in central Asia; and *R australis*, the etiologic agent of Queensland tick typhus endemic in eastern Australia. Each of these infections has clinical, pathologic, and epidemiologic features similar to those of Rocky Mountain spotted fever and are treated similarly, but they are usually milder and associated with a small indurated lesion that develops at the site of the tick bite ("tache noire") with resultant eschar and regional lymph node enlargement. The specific diagnosis is confirmed serologically. These conditions are of importance among persons traveling to endemic areas.

Rickettsialpox

Clinical Manifestations: Rickettsialpox is characterized by generalized erythematous papulovesicular eruptions that also can be present on the palms, soles, and mucous membranes after the appearance of a primary lesion at the site of the bite of the mouse mite vector. A black scab or eschar develops at the site about the time of fever onset. Systemic disease lasts about 1 week and consists of chills, fever, headache, myalgias, anorexia, photophobia, and regional lymphadenopathy. The disease is self limited, nonfatal, and without complications.

Etiology: Rickettsialpox is caused by *Rickettsia akari*, which is classified with the spotted-fever-group rickettsiae and antigenically is related to *R rickettsii*.

Epidemiology: The natural host for *R akari* in the United States is *Mus musculus*, the common house mouse. The disease is transmitted by the mouse mite *Allodermanyssus sanguineous*. Disease risk is heightened in areas infested with mice. The disease was first recognized in apartment house dwellers in New York City and was found in large urban settings, paralleling the distribution of mice. The disease has also been recognized in the Soviet Union, Korea, and Africa. All age groups are affected. No seasonal pattern of disease occurs. The disease is not communicable between humans. It is currently very rare in the United States.

The **incubation period** is 9 to 14 days.

Diagnostic Tests: *R akari* can be isolated from blood during the acute stage of the disease, but isolation should be attempted only in specialized laboratories. The Weil-Felix test for all *Proteus* OX agglutinins is negative. An indirect fluorescent antibody or complement fixation test for *R rickettsii* (the cause of Rocky Mountain spotted fever) will demonstrate fourfold rises in the species-specific rickettsial antibody titers between acute and convalescent sera, since antibodies to *R akari* have extensive cross-reactivity with those against *R rickettsii*.

Treatment: A tetracycline or chloramphenicol will shorten the course of the disease. Tetracyclines should not be given to children younger than 9 years unless the benefits clearly are greater than the risks of dental staining. Treatment should be given for 6 to 10 days.

Isolation of the Hospitalized Patient: No special precautions are recommended.

Control Measures: Disinfestation with residual insecticides and rodent control measures limit or eliminate the vector. No specific management of exposed persons is necessary.

Rocky Mountain Spotted Fever

Clinical Manifestations: Rocky Mountain spotted fever (RMSF) is a systemic, febrile illness with a characteristic rash usually occurring before the sixth day. Fever, headache, myalgia, toxicity, and nausea or vomiting are major clinical features. Abdominal pain and cough are less frequently noted. The rash is initially erythematous and macular, and later can become maculopapular, frequently petechial. The palms and soles characteristically are involved. Rash first appears on the wrists and ankles, spreading within hours proximally to the trunk. Although the early development of a rash is a useful diagnostic sign, in some cases the rash fails to develop or develops only late in the illness. The disease can last as long as 3 weeks and can be severe with prominent central nervous system, cardiac, pulmonary, gastrointestinal, renal, or other organ involvement; disseminated intravascular coagulation; and shock leading to death.

Etiology: *Rickettsia rickettsii* is an obligate intracellular pathogen and a member of the spotted fever group of rickettsiae.

Epidemiology: The disease is transmitted to humans by the bite of ticks. Many small wild animals and dogs have antibodies to *R rickettsii*, but their exact role as natural hosts is not clear since ticks are both reservoirs and vectors of *R rickettsii*. In ticks, the agent is transmitted transovarially and between stages. Persons with occupational or recreational exposure to the tick vector (e.g., pet owners, animal handlers, and outdoor persons) are at an increased risk of acquiring the disease. Persons of all ages, races, socioeconomic status, and both sexes can be infected, but most cases occur in those younger than 15 years, probably because they are most frequently in tick habitats. Laboratory-acquired infection has occurred by accidental inoculation, aerosol contamination, and tick bite. Transmission has occurred rarely by blood transfusion. Mortality is highest in males, in persons older than 30 years, in nonwhites, and in persons with no known tick bite or attachment as the result of delay in disease recognition and initiation of appropriate antimicrobial therapy.

The disease is widespread in the United States; most cases are reported in the south Atlantic and southeastern and south central states. Focal sites in an affected area can account for much of the morbidity in an area. The dog tick (*Dermacentor variabilis*) is primarily responsible for transmission in these geographic areas, and summer is the season of highest prevalence. In the western United States, the upper Rocky Mountain states have the highest incidence; the vector is usually the wood tick (*D andersoni*). The Lone Star tick (*Amblyomma americanum*) is a vector of *R rickettsii* in south central United States. Transmission parallels the tick season in a given geographic area. Spring and summer are the seasons of highest prevalence. The disease also occurs in Canada, Mexico, and Central and South America.

The **incubation period** is usually about 1 week, but ranges from 1 to 14 days. It appears to be related to the size of the rickettsial inoculum.

Diagnostic Tests: Culture of *R rickettsii* is usually not attempted because it is dangerous to laboratory personnel; only those laboratories with adequate biohazard containment equipment should attempt isolation of rickettsiae. The diagnosis can be established retrospectively by one of the multiple rickettsial group-specific serologic tests by the finding of a fourfold increase in antibody titer between acute and convalescent sera, as determined by indirect fluorescent antibody (IFA), complement fixation, latex agglutination, indirect hemagglutination, or microagglutination tests. Antibodies are detected by

IFA 7 to 10 days after onset of illness. A microtiter ELISA has been developed to characterize the IgM and IgG responses to *R rickettsii*. The complement fixation and microagglutination tests are highly specific for this disease, but lack sensitivity, particularly if the patient has received early antibiotic treatment. Criteria for diagnosis with single convalescent serum specimens have been established. The nonspecific and insensitive Weil-Felix serologic reaction (*Proteus* OX-19 and OX-2 agglutinins) becomes positive 10 to 14 days after the onset of the illness. No microbiologic test is readily available for rapid diagnosis early in the illness. However, *R rickettsii* have been identified by immunofluorescent staining of skin biopsy specimens at the site of the rash. With adequate specimens, this method can be 70% sensitive and 100% specific, but it is not widely available.

Treatment: Early initiation of treatment based on clinical diagnosis and epidemiologic considerations affords the highest likelihood of success in patients with suspected RMSF. Chloramphenicol or a tetracycline is the drug of choice. Tetracycline drugs are contraindicated in children younger than 9 years, especially when a nontoxic alternative antimicrobial is also effective. However, having compared the benefits and risks of tetracycline in children younger than 9 years with those of chloramphenicol, some experts consider a tetracycline drug to be appropriate therapy for children of any age with presumed RMSF. Therapy is continued until the patient is afebrile for at least 2 to 3 days. A usual course is 6 to 10 days.

Isolation of the Hospitalized Patient: No special precautions are recommended.

Control Measures: Control of ticks in their natural habitat is not practical. Avoidance of tick-infested areas is the best preventive measure. If a tick-infested area is entered, persons should wear protective clothing and apply tick/insect repellents to clothes and exposed body parts for added protection. They should be taught to thoroughly inspect themselves, their children (bodies and clothing), and pets for ticks after spending time outdoors during the tick season, and to remove them promptly (see Control Measures for Prevention of Tick-Borne Infections, page 112).

No licensed *R rickettsii* vaccine is currently available in the United States.

Roseola

(Exanthem Subitum, Sixth Disease)

Clinical Manifestations: Roseola infantum is a common, acute, febrile illness of young children characterized by fever for several days and rapid defervescence, followed by an erythematous maculopapular rash for 1 to 2 days. Convulsions may occur during the febrile episode. Encephalitis is a rare complication.

Etiology: The causative agent has recently been identified as a herpes virus, human herpesvirus 6 (HHV-6). A roseola-like illness has occasionally been associated with several viral agents, such as parvovirus B19, echovirus 16, other enteroviruses, and several adenoviruses.

Epidemiology: Humans are the only known hosts. The mode of transmission is unknown. HHV-6 has been isolated from the lymphocytes of peripheral blood and the secretions of some infants with roseola. The attack rate is highest in children between the ages of 6 and 24 months. Infection is rare before 3 months or after 4 years of age. Specific antibody to HHV-6 can be found in most cord bloods, declines in the first few months of life, and then is rapidly acquired, and by age 4 years almost all individuals are seropositive. These findings suggest that infection is ubiquitous, acquired early in life, and asymptomatic or unrecognized in most children. Secondary cases are rarely identified, although occasional outbreaks have been reported. Cases occur sporadically throughout the year, but in temperate climates the greatest number of cases tend to occur in the spring or summer. The period of communicability is unknown but is probably greatest during the febrile phase and before the appearance of the rash.

The **incubation period**, estimated from outbreaks, is 5 to 15 days.

Diagnostic Tests: No diagnostic tests are commercially available.

Treatment: Supportive.

Isolation of the Hospitalized Patient: No special precautions are recommended.

Control Measures: None.

Rotavirus Infections

Clinical Manifestations: Infection can result in diarrhea, usually preceded or accompanied by emesis and low-grade fever. In severe cases, considerable dehydration and acidosis may occur. Infection can also be accompanied by respiratory symptoms, such as cough and coryza.

Etiology: Rotaviruses (RV) are members of the family *Reoviridae* and are RNA viruses, with at least five distinct antigenic groups (A to E). Group A viruses are major causes of infantile diarrhea and consist of two subgroups and at least four serotypes that have been isolated from humans. Group B viruses have caused large outbreaks of gastroenteritis in adults and children in China. Group C viruses have a worldwide distribution.

Epidemiology: Most, if not all, human infections result from contact with infected humans. RV infections in animals occur in many species, but transmission from animals to humans has not been documented. RV is present in high titer in stools of infected patients, which is the only body specimen consistently positive, and it usually persists for a week after the onset of symptoms. Transmission is believed to be by the fecal-oral route. Since RV occurs in all children in developed and developing countries, however, its usual mode of transmission is probably unrelated to contamination of food or water. Respiratory transmission has been suggested because of the low inoculum size, ubiquitous occurrence of infection in all children, and the rapid spread in outbreaks in isolated areas that is inconsistent with contact with a common vehicle of infection. Spread within families, hospitals, and day care centers and other institutions is common.

RV is the most common cause of nosocomially acquired diarrhea in children and is an important cause of acute gastroenteritis in children attending day care. Human RV infections occur throughout the world and are the single most common agent of diarrhea in infants younger than 2 years who require medical attention in developed countries. Death from dehydration, although unusual in developed countries, is a major cause of mortality in developing countries. Disease is most prevalent during the cooler months of the year in temperate climates. Seasonal variation in tropical climates is less pronounced. Although clinically apparent cases of gastroenteritis occur most commonly when the infant is between 6 and 24 months old, other age groups show serologic evidence of infection. Asymptomatic infections are common in newborn infants. Reinfection, frequently without clinical symptoms, is known to occur in adult contacts.

The **incubation period** is usually from 1 to 3 days.

Diagnostic Tests: ELISA and latex agglutination assays for RV detection in stool are commercially available. In research laboratories, virus can also be identified in stool by viral isolation and electron microscopy. Epidemiologic analysis of strains can be performed by determination of the viral RNA migration patterns on polyacrylamide gel electrophoresis. Strains can be further characterized by subgroup and serotype, using an ELISA test with monoclonal antibodies.

Treatment: No specific therapy is available. Parenteral and oral fluids are given to correct dehydration. Orally administered human immunoglobulins have been used to treat immunocompromised patients with prolonged infections.

Isolation of the Hospitalized Patient: Strict adherence to enteric precautions is indicated for the duration of the illness.

Control Measures:

- *Day Care.* General measures for interrupting enteric transmission in day care centers are recommended (see Children in Day Care, page 72). Children with RV diarrhea in whom stool cannot be contained by diapers or toilet use should be excluded until the diarrhea ceases.
- Specific, effective control measures have not been established. Live attenuated, orally administered vaccines prepared from animal strains of RV or from reassortants between human and animal RV are being evaluated for safety and efficacy.

Rubella

Clinical Manifestations:

Postnatal Rubella. Rubella is usually a mild disease characterized by an erythematous maculopapular discrete rash, postauricular and suboccipital lymphadenopathy, and slight fever. Some 25% to 50% of infections are asymptomatic. Transient polyarthralgia and polyarthritis occasionally occur in children and are common in adolescents and adults, especially females. Encephalitis and thrombocytopenia are rare complications.

Congenital Rubella. The most commonly described anomalies associated with congenital rubella are ophthalmologic (cataracts, microphthalmia, glaucoma, chorioretinitis), cardiac (patent ductus arteriosus, peripheral pulmonary artery stenosis, atrial or ventricular septal defects), auditory (sensorineural deafness), and neurologic (microcephaly, meningoencephalitis, mental retardation). In addition, infants with congenital rubella are frequently growth retarded and have radiolucent bone disease, hepatosplenomegaly, thrombocytopenia, jaundice, and purpuric-like skin lesions ("blueberry muffin" appearance).

Etiology: Rubella virus is an RNA virus classified as a rubivirus in the togavirus family.

Epidemiology: Humans are the sole source of infection. Postnatal rubella is transmitted chiefly through direct or droplet contact from nasopharyngeal secretions. The peak incidence of infection is in the late winter and early spring. Asymptomatic infection is common. The period of maximum communicability appears to be the few days before, and 5 to 7 days after, onset of the rash. Volunteer studies indicate the presence of rubella virus in nasopharyngeal secretions from 7 days before to 14 days after the onset of the rash. Infants with congenital rubella can continue to shed virus in nasopharyngeal secretions and urine for 1 year or more and transmit infection to susceptible contacts. In approximately 10% to 20% of these patients, virus can be isolated from the nasopharynx when the infant is 6 months old.

Before the widespread use of rubella vaccine, rubella was an epidemic disease, occurring in 6- to 9-year cycles, and most cases occurred in children. Currently in the United States the incidence of rubella has declined by more than 99% from the prevaccine era. The risk of acquiring rubella has declined sharply in all age groups, including adolescents and young adults. In the vaccine era, more cases have occurred in young, unvaccinated adults and in outbreaks in colleges and occupational settings in which young adults are grouped together. Serologic surveys have indicated that 10% to 20% of young adults are susceptible to rubella; this rate is similar to that in the prevaccine era. This degree of susceptibility in young adults is predominantly due to under use of vaccine in this population and not to waning immunity in immunized persons.

The **incubation period** for postnatal rubella ranges from 14 to 21 days, usually 16 to 18 days.

Diagnostic Tests: Rubella virus most consistently can be isolated from the nose by inoculation of appropriate tissue culture. Throat swabs, blood, urine, and cerebrospinal fluid can also yield virus, particularly in congenitally infected infants. Serologic testing is also useful in confirming the presence of infection, particularly in the absence of typical clinical manifestations. Acute and convalescent sera should be tested; a fourfold or greater rise in titer or seroconversion is indicative of infection. Many virology laboratories can detect specific rubella IgM antibody, the presence of which is indicative of recent postnatal infection or congenital infection in a newborn infant. Every effort should be made to establish a laboratory diagnosis when rubella infection is suspected in pregnant women or in newborn infants. The diagnosis of congenital rubella infection in children older than 1 year is difficult. Serology is usually not diagnostic. Viral isolation is confirmatory but is possible in only a small proportion of congenitally infected children older than 1 year. Until recently, the hemagglutination inhibition antibody test was the most frequently used method of screening for the presence of rubella antibodies. However, this test has generally been supplanted by a number of equally or more sensitive assays for determining rubella immunity, including latex agglutination, fluorescence immunoassay, passive hemagglutination, hemolysis-in-gel, and enzyme immunoassay tests. Some individuals who have not had antibody detected on routine testing by hemagglutination inhibition have been shown to be immune by more sensitive tests.

Treatment: Supportive.

Isolation of the Hospitalized Patient: For postnatal rubella, contact isolation is required for 7 days after the onset of the rash. Contact isolation is also required for congenitally infected infants and infants suspected of having congenital rubella. Infants with congenital rubella should be considered contagious until they are 1 year old, unless nasopharyngeal and urine cultures after 3 months of age are negative for rubella virus. Virus is detectable in the nasopharynx of a small number of these children when they are 1 year or older.

Control Measures:

School and Day Care. Children with postnatal rubella should be excluded from school or day care for 7 days after the onset of the rash. Patients with congenital rubella in day care should be considered contagious until they are 1 year old, unless nasopharyngeal and urine cultures are negative for rubella. Mothers should be made aware of the potential hazard of their infants to susceptible pregnant contacts.

Care of Exposed Persons. When a pregnant woman is exposed to rubella, a blood specimen should be obtained as soon as possible and tested for rubella antibody. The presence of antibody in a properly performed test indicates that the individual is immune and not at risk. Those previously determined to be immune can also be reassured. If antibody is not detectable, a second blood specimen approximately 3 weeks later should be tested. If antibody is present in the second specimen, infection can be assumed to have occurred. If the test is negative, it should be repeated 6 weeks after the exposure to rubella. At this time, a negative test indicates that infection has not occurred; a positive test indicates that infection did occur. The testing should be done by the same laboratory, and each specimen should be tested simultaneously with the previously obtained sera.

To determine if the index patient has rubella, detection of rubella-specific serum IgM antibody or isolation of virus from the nose can also be useful.

The routine use of immune globulin (IG) for postexposure prophylaxis of rubella in early pregnancy is not recommended. Administration of IG should be considered only if termination of the pregnancy is not an option. Limited data indicate that IG in a dose of 0.55 mL/kg may prevent or modify infection in an exposed, susceptible person. In one study, the attack rate of clinically apparent infection was reduced from 87% in control subjects to 18% in recipients of IG. However, the absence of clinical signs in a woman who has received IG does not guarantee that fetal infection has been prevented, since in this study serologic testing indicated that 44% of the IG recipients were infected and since infants with congenital rubella have been born to mothers who were given IG shortly after exposure.

Live rubella virus vaccine given after exposure does not prevent illness. However, immunization of exposed, nonpregnant persons may be indicated because if the current exposure does not result in infection, the immunization will protect the individual in the future. Immunization of a person who is incubating natural rubella or who is already immune is not contraindicated.

Rubella Virus Vaccine. The live rubella virus vaccine currently distributed in the United States is the RA 27/3 strain of rubella virus grown in human diploid cell cultures. It contains no penicillin. Serum antibody is induced in more than 98% of the recipients.

Available data indicate that one dose confers long-term, probably lifelong, immunity. Previously, rubella reimmunization was not recommended. However, in conjunction with the recently recommended two-dose measles immunization schedule (see Measles, Vaccine Recommendations, page 312), two doses of rubella vaccine are now advisable. Although primary rubella vaccine failures have not been a major problem, the potential consequences of rubella vaccine failure are substantial (i.e., congenital rubella), and an additional dose of rubella vaccine should provide an added safeguard against such failures.

Vaccine Recommendations (see Table 50 for a summary). Rubella vaccine is administered in a single subcutaneous dose of 0.5 mL, either alone, as a combined preparation that also contains measles vaccine (MR), or, usually, in combination with measles and mumps vaccines (MMR).

Routine Childhood Immunization. Rubella vaccine is currently recommended to be administered in combination with measles and mumps vaccine (as MMR) when a child is 12 months of age or older (see Tables 2 and 3, pages 17 and 18).

A second dose of rubella vaccine administered as MMR is also now advised. The recommended age for this second dose is determined by the measles vaccination schedule (see Measles, Vaccine Recommendations, page 312).

Susceptible Girls and Boys. Before the onset of puberty, susceptible children should be immunized. Review of the records of both boys and girls during medical visits before puberty for documented evidence of rubella immunization or serologic evidence of naturally acquired immunity is indicated. Clinical diagnosis of infection is usually unreliable and should not be accepted as indicative of immunity.

Special emphasis must continue to be placed on the immunization of postpubertal adolescent and adult males and females, including college students and military recruits. Those who have not been immunized or who have not been proven serologically to be immune to rubella should receive vaccine. Women should be informed of the theoretical risk of injury to the fetus if they are pregnant or become pregnant within 3 months of being immunized (see Precautions and Contraindications, page 416, for further discussion). Specific recommendations are as follows:

- Postpubertal females who are not known to be immune to rubella should be immunized. They should not receive vaccine if they are pregnant. Postpubertal females, after receiving rubella vaccine, should be warned not to become pregnant for 3 months.
- Premarital serology tests for rubella immunity will enhance efforts to identify susceptible women before pregnancy.
- Prenatal or antepartum screening for rubella susceptibility should be routinely undertaken, and vaccine should be administered to susceptible women in the immediate postpartum period before discharge. In this situation, previous administration of Rho (D) Immune Globulin (Human) or blood products is not a contraindication to vaccination, but serologic testing should be done 6 to 8 weeks after vaccination in these cases in order to ascertain that seroconversion has occurred. Testing of other vaccines is usually not necessary. Physicians can help ensure immunization of susceptible women by inquiring about the immune status of the

Table 50. Indications and Contraindications for Rubella Vaccine

Indications	Contraindications
Children ≥ 12 mo (with measles and mumps vaccines [as MMR] in a two-dose schedule*)	Pregnancy
	Immunodeficiency or immunocompromised state†
Susceptible individuals in the following groups:	IG or blood in past 3 mo‡
Prepubertal girls and boys	
Adults, especially premarital or postpartum women	
College students	
Day care personnel	
Health care personnel	
Military personnel	

*See Measles, Vaccine Recommendations, page 312.
†Exception is AIDS (see text).
‡Rubella vaccine may be given postpartum concurrently or after the administration of anti-Rho (D) IG or blood products (see text for indications for subsequent serologic testing for seroconversion).

mothers of their patients during visits for newborn infants and well-child care. Breast-feeding is not a contraindication to postpartum immunization.

- A special effort should be made to be certain that all individuals are protected who plan to attend or work in educational institutions or day care centers, or obtain employment where they may be exposed to or spread rubella.
- Both male and female health care personnel who may be exposed to patients with rubella should be protected for their own benefit as well as for the prevention of transmission of rubella to pregnant patients.

Immunization should be performed unless documented evidence of rubella immunization or serologic evidence of naturally acquired immunity is provided.

Rubella vaccine can be given simultaneously with other vaccines (see Simultaneous Administration of Multiple Vaccines, page 16).

Adverse Reactions. Those associated with rubella vaccine include rash, fever, and lymphadenopathy 5 to 12 days after vaccination in a small percentage of children. In addition, joint pain, usually in small peripheral joints, has been noted in approximately 0.5% of children and 1% to 3% of girls who are more than 12 years of age. Arthralgia and arthritis tend to be more frequent in previously unvaccinated postpubertal females. Joint involvement usually begins 7 to 21 days after vaccination and is generally transient. Persistent or recurrent arthralgic complaints have been reported in vaccinated adult women but are uncommon, and the etiologic relationship to vaccination is unclear. The incidence of joint manifestations after vaccination is lower than that following natural infection at the corresponding age. Furthermore, in those reimmunized, the likelihood of these manifestations can be expected to be considerably less than that in previously immunized individuals (most of whom are already immune). Transient peripheral neuritic complaints, such as paresthesia and pain in the arms and legs, have also been reported, although rarely. Central nervous system manifestations and thrombocytopenia have been reported, but no causal relationship with vaccine has been established.

Precautions and Contraindications:

- *Pregnancy.* Rubella vaccine should not be given to pregnant women. If vaccine is inadvertently given, or if pregnancy occurs within 3 months of immunization, the patient should be counseled on the theoretical risks to the fetus. The maximal theoretical risk for the occurrence of congenital rubella is estimated to be 1.4%, based on data accumulated by the Centers for Disease Control from more than 200 susceptible women who received the current rubella vaccine (the RA27/3 strain) during the first trimester. Of the offspring, 2% had subclinical infection but none had congenital defects. In view of these observations, receipt of rubella vaccine in pregnancy is not ordinarily an indication for interruption of pregnancy. Pregnant women immunized with rubella vaccine who are known to be susceptible should be reported to the Division of Immunization, Centers for Disease Control.

  Routine serologic testing of postpubertal women before immunization is not necessary. Serologic testing is a potential impediment to protection of these women against rubella. However, a sample of blood may be obtained before vaccination and stored for at least 3 months. If a woman becomes pregnant or has become pregnant after vaccination, the prevaccination specimen can be tested. Demonstration of rubella antibody in the prevaccine specimen indicates immunity and eliminates anxiety about fetal injury from rubella vaccine virus.

  Vaccinating susceptible children whose mothers or other household contacts are pregnant does not cause a risk. Susceptible children should receive the vaccine. Most vaccinees intermittently shed small amounts of virus from the pharynx 7 to 28 days after vaccination, but no evidence of transmission of the vaccine virus has been found in studies of more than 1,200 susceptible household contacts.

- *Altered immunity.* The following persons should not receive rubella vaccine: (1) patients with immunodeficiency diseases; (2) patients on immunosuppressive therapy (such as those with leukemia, lymphoma, or generalized malignancy); (3) patients receiving pharmacologic doses of corticosteroids, alkylating agents, antimetabolites, or radiation; and (4) otherwise immunocompromised persons. The exceptions are patients with symptomatic HIV infection who are to be vaccinated against measles with MMR (see AIDS and HIV Infection, page 124).

  After cessation of immunosuppressive therapy, rubella vaccine is generally withheld for an interval of not less than 3 months. This interval is based on the assumption that immunologic responsiveness will have been restored in 3 months and the underlying disease for which immunosuppressive therapy was prescribed is in remission or under control. However, because the interval can vary with the intensity and type of immunosuppressive therapy, radiation therapy, underlying disease, and other factors, a definitive recommendation for an interval after cessation of immunosuppressive therapy when rubella vaccine can be safely and effectively administered is often not possible.
- *Recent administration of immune globulin (IG).* Rubella vaccine should be given at least 2 weeks before or at least 3 months after the administration of IG or blood transfusion because of the possibility that antibody will neutralize vaccine virus and prevent a successful immunization. However, rubella vaccine may be given postpartum at the same time as anti-Rho (D) IG or after blood products are given.
- *Febrile illness.* Children with minor illnesses with or without fever, such as upper respiratory tract infection, may be vaccinated (see Vaccine Safety and Contraindications, page 22). Fever per se is not a contraindication to immunization. However, if other manifestations suggest a more serious illness, the child should not be vaccinated until recovery.

Surveillance of Congenital Infections. Accurate diagnosis and reporting of the congenital rubella syndrome and vaccine complications are extremely important in assessing the control of rubella. All birth defects in which rubella infection is etiologically suspected should be thoroughly investigated and reported to the Centers for Disease Control through the local or state health departments.

Salmonellosis

Clinical Manifestations: *Salmonella* infections are categorized as asymptomatic carriage, gastroenteritis, enteric fever (caused by *S typhi* or other *Salmonella* species), bacteremia without focality, and focal infections (such as meningitis, osteomyelitis, and abscesses). The presence of one infectious focus does not preclude the presence of another. For example, gastroenteritis can be complicated by bacteremia and/or a metastatic focal infection. The most commonly recognized illness is gastroenteritis, in which diarrhea, abdominal cramps and tenderness, and fever are common symptoms. The site of infection is usually the small bowel but colitis can occur.

In enteric fever, the onset is typically gradual and manifestations can include fever, constitutional symptoms (e.g., headache, malaise, anorexia, and lethargy), abdominal pain and tenderness, hepatomegaly, splenomegaly, rose spots, and changes in mental status. Constipation can be an early feature; diarrhea can occur later, usually in the second week of illness. Sustained or intermittent bacteremia can occur in both enteric fever and *Salmonella* bacteremia without focal infection. Patients with the latter syndrome have an illness characterized by fever without manifestations of enterocolitis or enteric fever. Recognizable focal infections ultimately may occur in as many as 10% of patients with *Salmonella* bacteremia.

Etiology: *Salmonella* organisms are Gram-negative rods of the family Enterobacteriaceae. Classification of *Salmonella* has been controversial. Three primary species, *S typhi* (one serotype), *S choleraesuis* (one serotype), and *S enteritidis* (more than 1,700 serotypes) have been identified. Also, on the basis of somatic antigens, some divide *Salmonella* organisms into groups A through E. Organisms from all groups can cause human disease. Current usage refers to each serotype as a species. Frequent isolates in the United States in recent years have been *S typhimurium* (group B), *S heidelberg* (B), *S enteritidis* (D), *S newport* (C2), *S infantis* (C1), *S agona* (B), and *S saint-paul* (B).

Epidemiology: The principal reservoirs for nontyphoidal *Salmonella* serotypes are animals, including poultry, livestock, and pets; other sources include contamination in animal product and meat processing plants, contaminated water, unpasteurized milk, and infected humans. *S typhi* is found only in humans. Modes of transmission include ingestion of contaminated food or water (primary route); contact with infected animals (e.g., pet turtles); person-to-person transmission via the fecal-oral route; and contact with contaminated medications, dyes, and medical instruments. Ingestion of raw milk, which may be contaminated even though certified, can produce severe disease. Nontyphoidal *Salmonella* infections are common.

Age-specific attack rates are highest in those younger than 5 years and older than 70 years, and peak in the first year of life. Invasive infections and mortality are most common in infants, the elderly, and those with underlying disease, particularly hemoglobinopathies, malignancy, and other immunosuppressive conditions. Most reported cases are sporadic in occurrence, but outbreaks in the home and institutions are common. Nosocomial epidemics, including outbreaks of meningitis in newborn nurseries, have been reported. Typhoid fever is uncommon in the United States but is endemic in many less developed areas of the world.

The risk of communicability exists throughout the duration of fecal excretion. This period is extremely variable; frequently it lasts several weeks or more and can be prolonged by antibiotic therapy. Chronic carriage with nontyphoidal serotypes and in children with typhoid fever for more than 1 year is uncommon.

The **incubation period** for gastroenteritis is from 6 to 72 hours, but is usually less than 24 hours. For enteric fevers, the incubation period is from 3 to 60 days, but is usually 7 to 14 days.

Diagnostic Tests: Cultures of stool, rectal swabs, blood, urine, bone marrow aspirates, and foci of infection, as indicated by the suspected *Salmonella* syndrome, should be obtained. Serologic tests for *Salmonella* agglutinins ("febrile agglutinins" or the Widal test) may suggest the diagnosis of *S typhi* infection. However, because of false-positive and false-negative results, these tests are not as reliable as bacterial cultures for a diagnosis of typhoid fever.

Treatment:

- Antimicrobial therapy is usually not administered to patients with uncomplicated gastroenteritis caused by nontyphi *Salmonella* species because it does not shorten the duration of the disease and can prolong the duration of excretion of *Salmonella* organisms. Antimicrobial therapy is warranted in *Salmonella* gastroenteritis occurring in patients with an increased risk of invasive disease and other complications, including infants younger than 3 months, patients with malignancy, hemoglobinopathy, or other immunosuppressive illnesses, recipients of immunosuppressive therapy, or patients with severe colitis.

- Chronic gastrointestinal disease predisposes to *Salmonella* infection and to invasive disease. Ampicillin, amoxicillin, or trimethoprim-sulfamethoxazole is recommended for susceptible strains in these patients. Strains acquired in developing countries are often resistent to these antibiotics but susceptible to new cephalosporins, such as ceftriaxone or cefotaxime, and to fluoroquinolones (e.g., ciprofloxacin). However, the fluoroquinolones are not approved for patients younger than 21 years and in most cases should be used only for *Salmonella* infections in adults.
- In invasive *Salmonella* disease (such as osteomyelitis, typhoid fever, non-*S typhi* bacteremia, or *S choleraesuis* infections), the drugs indicated are chloramphenicol, ampicillin, or amoxicillin. Trimethoprim-sulfamethoxazole is an alternative antimicrobial if the patient has specific drug allergies, or if a resistant organism is isolated or is strongly suggested by epidemiologic factors. Drug choice, route of administration, and duration are based on susceptibility of the organism, disease state, and clinical response. For susceptible *S typhi*, the administration of chloramphenicol for at least 2 weeks is usually recommended. For *Salmonella* meningitis, a third-generation cephalosporin, such as ceftriaxone or cefotaxime, or parenteral trimethoprim-sulfamethoxazole is recommended.
- Chronic (more than 1 year) *S typhi* carriage can be eradicated in some patients by high-dose parenteral ampicillin, large-dose oral amoxicillin, the fluoroquinolones (in adults only), or cholecystectomy.
- Antipyretics can cause precipitous declines in temperature and shock, and should be avoided in patients with enteric fever syndromes.
- Heparin should not be used to treat asymptomatic disseminated intravascular coagulation that occurs in many patients with enteric fever.
- Corticosteroids should be administered to patients with severe typhoid fever, which is characterized by delirium, obtundation, stupor, coma, or shock. Prompt therapy may be lifesaving. The duration of corticosteroid therapy should be brief. Large doses of dexamethasone (an initial dose of 3 mg/kg followed by eight doses of 1 mg/kg every 6 hours) are administered intravenously for 48 hours.

Isolation of the Hospitalized Patient: Enteric precautions should be used for the duration of the illness. In patients with typhoid fever, enteric precautions should be continued until cultures of three consecutive stools taken after cessation of antimicrobial therapy are negative for *S typhi*.

Control Measures:

Important measures include proper sanitation methods for food processing and preparation, sanitary water supplies, education about hand washing and personal hygiene, sanitary sewage disposal, exclusion of infected persons who are food handlers from working, prohibition of the sale of turtles for pets, case reporting to appropriate health authorities, and investigations of outbreaks. Determination of serotype is of primary importance in the detection and investigation of outbreaks.

Day Care. Outbreaks of salmonellosis are very unusual in day care programs, and specific strategies for controlling salmonellosis in day care have not been evaluated. General measures for interrupting enteric transmission in day care centers are recommended (see Children in Day Care, page 72). When *S typhi* disease is identified in a symptomatic day care attendee or staff member, the stools of other attendees and staff members should be cultured, and all infected persons should be excluded until three consecutive stool cultures are negative. When species other than *S typhi* are identified in a symptomatic day care attendee or staff member with enterocolitis, older children and staff do not need to be excluded once asymptomatic. Asymptomatic contacts need not be cultured. If multiple symptomatic infected persons are identified, the decision to exclude these persons or cohort them in the program should be made in consultation with public health authorities. Antimicrobial therapy is not recommended for colonized individuals, persons with uncomplicated enterocolitis, or those simply exposed to a colonized or infected individual.

Typhoid Vaccine. Resistance to infection with *S typhi* is enhanced by typhoid vaccination, but the degree of protection with currently available vaccines is limited and can be overcome by ingestion of a large bacterial inoculum. Two vaccines are now available in the United States for civilian use; a third, an acetone-inactivated parenterally administered vaccine, efficacy of which ranges from 66% to 94%, is available only to the Armed Forces in the United States. The two available to civilians are (1) a parenteral heat-phenol-inactivated vaccine that has been widely used for many years, and (2) a newly licensed oral live-attenuated vaccine prepared from the Ty21a strain of *S typhi* (Vivotif*). Since data are unavailable regarding its efficacy for children younger than 6 years and are limited concerning adverse reactions in this age group, the vaccine manufacturer recommends that the Ty21a vaccine not be given to children younger than 6 years.

In field trials, Ty21a has been demonstrated to have similar efficacy to that of the parenteral vaccine. Vaccine efficacy ranges from 51% to 76%.

---

*Manufactured by the Swiss Serum and Vaccine Institute, Berne, Switzerland.

Indications. In the United States, vaccination is recommended only for the following groups:

- *Travelers to areas where typhoid fever is endemic and a recognized risk of exposure will occur.* Risk is greatest for travelers to developing countries, especially Latin American, Asia, and Africa, who will be exposed to potentially contaminated food and drink. Such travelers need to be cautioned that typhoid vaccine is not a substitute for careful selection of food and drink, since typhoid vaccines are not 100% effective.
- *Persons with intimate exposure to a documented typhoid fever carrier*, such as occurs with continued household contact.
- *Laboratory workers with frequent contact with S typhi.*

The vaccine is not recommended for persons attending summer camps, nor for those in areas of natural disaster, nor for control of common-source outbreaks.

Dosages. For *primary vaccination*, the following is recommended:

- Children 10 years or older and adults:

  Oral Ty21a vaccine. One enteric-coated capsule is taken on alternate days for a total of four capsules. Each capsule should be taken with cool liquid, no warmer than 37°C, approximately one hour before meals. The capsules must be kept refrigerated and all four doses must be taken to achieve maximal efficacy.

  OR

  Parenteral inactivated vaccine. The dose is 0.5 mL subcutaneously, given on two occasions, separated by 4 or more weeks.*

- Children < 10 years of age:

  Oral Ty21a vaccine.† *Recommendations are the same as for older children and adults.*

  OR

  Parenteral inactivated vaccine. The dose is 0.25 mL subcutaneously, given on two occasions, separated by 4 or more weeks.

Booster doses.† There are recommended only in circumstances of continued or repeated exposure to *S typhi.* If parenteral vaccine is used, booster doses should be given every 3 years. Even if more than 3 years have elapsed since the earlier vaccination, a single booster dose of parenteral vaccine is sufficient. Less reaction follows booster vaccination by the intradermal route than by the subcutaneous route. (The acetone-inactivated parenteral vaccine should not be given by

---

*If parenteral vaccine is used and time is insufficient for two doses of vaccine separated by 4 or more weeks to be given, three doses of the parenteral vaccine at weekly intervals are given. However, this schedule may be less effective

†The vaccine manufacturer recommends that Ty21a should not be given to children < 6 years.

the intradermal route because of the potential for severe local reactions.) No experience has been reported using oral live-attenuated vaccine as a booster; however, using the primary series of four doses of Ty21a as a booster for persons previously vaccinated with parenteral vaccine is a reasonable alternative to administration of a parenteral booster dose. The following routes and dosages of parenteral vaccine for booster vaccination are recommended:

- Children 10 years and older and adults: one dose, 0.5 mL subcutaneously or 0.1 mL intradermally.
- Children 6 months to 10 years: one dose, 0.25 mL subcutaneously or 0.1 mL intradermally.

The optimal booster schedule for persons who have received Ty21a vaccine has not yet been determined. However, continued efficacy 5 years after vaccination has been demonstrated in one study. The manufacturer of Ty21a recommends revaccination with the entire four-dose series every 5 years. This recommendation may change as more data become available on the duration of protection produced by the Ty21a vaccine.

Precautions and Contraindications. Reported side effects with oral Ty21a vaccine have been rare and consist of abdominal discomfort, nausea, vomiting, and rash or urticaris. In safety trials, adverse reactions occurred with equal frequency among groups receiving vaccine and placebo.

Parenteral inactivated vaccines produce several systemic and local adverse reactions, including fever (14% to 29%), headache (9% to 30%), and severe local pain and/or swelling (6% to 40%). Because of adverse reactions, 13% to 24% of vaccinees are reported to miss school or work. More severe reactions have been sporadically reported, including hypotension, chest pain, and shock.

The only contraindication to parenteral typhoid vaccination is a history of severe local or systemic reactions following a previous dose. No experience has been reported with parenteral inactivated vaccine or oral Ty21a vaccine in pregnant women. Oral Ty21a, since it is a live-attenuated vaccine, should not be used in immunocompromised persons, including those known to be infected with HIV. Parenteral inactivated vaccine presents a theoretically safer alternative for these patients.

Scabies

Clinical Manifestations: The disease begins with an intensely pruritic, papular eruption. In older children and adults, the sites of predilection are the interdigital folds, flexor aspects of the wrists, extensor surfaces of the elbows, anterior axillary folds, belt line, thighs, navel, penis, areas surrounding the nipples, abdomen, outer borders of the feet, and lower portion of the buttocks. In infants younger than 2 years, the eruption is often vesicular and is likely to occur on the head, neck, palms, and soles, but these areas are usually spared in older children and adults. The distribution of typical scabies lesions does not parallel that of the adult female mite because the eruption is caused by the immature stages of the mite and sensitization to the proteins of the parasite. Itching is more intense at night. The characteristic mite burrow appears as a white, tortuous, thread-like line. Most burrows are obliterated by scratching long before a patient is seen by a physician.

Etiology: The mite *Sarcoptes scabiei* subspecies *hominis* is the cause of the disease.

Epidemiology: Humans are the source of the infection. Transmission occurs most often by close personal contact. Minimum contact with a patient with crusted scabies (Norwegian) can result in transmission because of the large number of mites in the exfoliating scales. Scabies can be transmitted as long as the patient remains infected and untreated, including during the interval before symptoms develop.

Scabies occurs worldwide in cycles thought to be 15 to 30 years long. In the past, epidemics were attributed to poverty, poor sanitation, and crowding because of war and economic crises. The current wave of infection in the United States and Europe has evolved in the absence of major social disturbances and has affected persons from all socioeconomic levels without regard to age, sex, or standards of personal hygiene. Scabies is endemic in many developing countries.

The **incubation period** in persons without previous exposure is usually 4 to 6 weeks. Persons who were previously infected develop symptoms 1 to 4 days after repeat exposure to the mite, but these reinfections are usually milder.

Diagnostic Tests: Diagnosis is confirmed by identification of the mites' eggs or scybaia (feces) from skin scrapings of several unexcoreated lesions. Prior application of water, alcohol, or mineral oil to the skin facilitates collecting the scrapings, which should be placed on the slide under a cover slip and examined microscopically under low power.

Treatment: Infected children and adults should apply lotion or cream containing a scabicide over the entire body below the head. Because scabies can affect the head, scalp, and neck in infants and young toddlers, treatment of the entire head, neck, and body in this age group is required. The drug of choice is 5% permethrin, a synthetic pyrethroid (Elimite*). Alternative drugs are lindane (Kwell, Scabene) and cro-

---

*This recently licensed product differs in its concentration of permethrin from that used for the treatment of pediculosis (1%). It is available from Herbert Laboratories, Irvine, CA.

tamiton (Eurax). Permethrin should be removed by bathing after 8 to 14 hours, lindane after 8 to 12 hours, and crotamiton after 48 hours. Crotamiton can be applied once daily for a period of 2 to 5 days but it is associated with frequent treatment failures.

Lindane applications should not be in excess of those recommended to avoid the possibility of neurotoxicity from absorption through the skin. Lindane should be used cautiously in young infants and pregnant women.

Isolation of the Hospitalized Patient: Contact isolation until after the start of effective therapy is indicated.

Control Measures:

Care of Exposed Persons.

- Prophylactic therapy is recommended for household members. Signs of scabies can appear as late as 1 to 2 months after exposure, and patients can transmit scabies during this interval. All members of the household should be treated at the same time to prevent reinfection. Bedding and clothing worn next to the skin should be laundered in a washer with hot water and a hot drying cycle. The parasites do not survive more than 3 to 4 days without contact with the skin. Clothing that cannot be laundered should be removed from the patient and stored from several days to a week or more to avoid reinfestation.
- Children should be allowed to return to day care or school the day after treatment has been completed.
- Epidemics and localized outbreaks may require stringent and consistent measures to treat contacts. Environmental disinfection is rarely warranted. Caretakers who have had prolonged skin-to-skin contact with infected patients may benefit from prophylactic treatment.

Schistosomiasis

Clinical Manifestations: Initial entry of the infecting larvae (cercariae) through the skin frequently can be accompanied by a transient, pruritic papular rash. After penetration, the organism enters the bloodstream, migrates through the lungs, and ultimately lodges in the venous plexus draining either the intestines or the bladder (depending on the *Schistosoma* species). While the worms are maturing, a syndrome of fever, malaise, cough, rash, abdominal pain, and nausea can develop, usually from 3 to 12 weeks after infection. In acute infections with heavy infestation due to *S mansoni* or *S japonicum*, a mucoid, bloody diarrhea accompanied by tender hepatomegaly occurs. In chronic infection, lightly infected individuals can be asymptomatic; heavily infected individuals can have a range of symptoms caused primarily by inflammation and fibrosis triggered by the eggs produced by adult worms. Portal hypertension can develop and cause hepatosplenomegaly, ascites, and esophageal varices. In *S haematobium* infections the bladder becomes inflamed and fibrotic. Symptoms include dysuria, urgency, terminal microscopic and gross hematuria, and nonspecific pelvic pain.

Etiology: The trematodes (flukes) *S mansoni*, *S japonicum*, *S haematobium*, and, rarely, *S mekongi* and *S intercalatum* cause the disease. All species have similar life cycles.

Epidemiology: Humans are the principal hosts for the major species. Persistence of schistosomiasis depends on the presence of an appropriate snail as an intermediate host. Eggs excreted in stool (*S mansoni* and *S japonicum*) or urine (*S haematobium*) into freshwater hatch into motile miracidia, which infect snails. After development in the snails, cercariae emerge and penetrate the skin of humans encountered in the water.

S mansoni occurs throughout tropical Africa and in Madagascar, several Caribbean islands, Venezuela, Brazil, and the Middle East. *S japonicum* is found in China, Japan, the Philippines, and elsewhere in Southeast Asia. *S haematobium* occurs in Africa, Madagascar, the Middle East, Mauritius, and in small foci in India. Children are frequently involved in transmission and infection because of habits of promiscuous defecation, urination, and frequent wading in infected waters. Communicability lasts as long as live eggs are excreted in the urine and feces. Adults of the *S mansoni* species have been documented to live up to 26 years in the human host. Thus, schistosomiasis can be seen in patients many years after they have left the endemic areas.

Diagnostic Tests: Microscopic examination of concentrated stool specimens or urine is used to detect characteristic eggs. In light infections, several specimens may have to be examined before eggs are found. Biopsy of rectal mucosa may be necessary; the fresh tissue obtained should be compressed between two glass slides and examined unstained for eggs. Serologic tests are available through commercial laboratories and the Centers for Disease Control, which aid in diagnosing patients whose stool or urine examinations are negative.

Treatment: The drug of choice for all species is praziquantel given in 1 to 3 doses during a single day; the alternative drug for *S mansoni* is oxamniquine (for dosages, see Drugs for Parasitic Infections, page 587).* For *S haematobium*, the alternative drug is metrifonate (10 mg/kg every 2 weeks for three doses).† No satisfactory alternative drug for *S japonicum* is available.

Isolation of the Hospitalized Patient: No special precautions are recommended.

Control Measures: These include the elimination of the intermediate snail host, treatment of infected populations, sanitary disposal of human waste, and education about the source of infection. No vaccine is currently available. Travelers to endemic areas should be advised to avoid contact with freshwater streams and lakes.

Shigellosis

Clinical Manifestations: In mild infections, the clinical manifestations consist only of watery or loose stools for several days, with minimal or no constitutional symptoms. Abrupt onset of fever, systemic toxicity, headache, and profuse watery diarrhea occurs in patients with small bowel infection. Convulsions can occur. Abdominal cramps, tenderness, tenesmus, and mucoid stools with or without blood characterize large bowel disease (bacillary dysentery). Rare sequelae include Reiter's syndrome following *S flexneri* infection and hemolytic-uremic syndrome from *S dysenteriae* infection.

Etiology: *Shigella* organisms are Gram-negative rods that belong to the family Enterobacteriaceae; four species including many serovars have been identified. *Shigella sonnei* currently accounts for more than half the cases in the United States. *S flexneri* accounts for a large percentage of the rest. *S dysenteriae*, type 1 (the Shiga bacillus) is rare in the United States (having fewer than 1% of reported isolates) unless it is imported by travelers; but it is widespread in rural Africa and the Indian subcontinent. *S boydii* is uncommon.

Epidemiology: Feces of infected humans are the source. No animal reservoir is known. Predisposing factors include crowded living conditions, low hygienic standards, closed population groups with substandard environmental sanitation (e.g., residential homes for

---

*Available from Pfizer Inc., New York City, NY.

†Available from the Centers for Disease Control (see Services of the Centers for Disease Control, page 622).

retarded children), and travel to countries with low standards of food sanitation. Fecal-oral, person-to-person contact is the common route of transmission by which children are infected. Other modes of transmission include ingestion of contaminated food or water, homosexual transmission, and contact with a contaminated, inanimate object. Houseflies have been suspected as vectors, causing physical transport of infected feces. Infection is most common in children 1 to 4 years old; it is an important problem in day care centers in the United States. The risk of communicability exists until the organism is no longer present in the feces. Even without antimicrobial therapy, convalescent carriage usually ceases within 4 weeks of the onset of illness. Chronic carriage (more than 1 year) is rare.

The **incubation period** varies from 1 to 7 days, but is usually 2 to 4 days.

Diagnostic Tests: Culture of feces or rectal swab specimens should be performed. Blood should be cultured only in severely ill patients because bacteremia is rare. A stool smear stained with methylene blue may reveal polymorphonuclear leukocytes and/or erythrocytes, a finding indicative of enterocolitis, but the finding is not specific for *Shigella* infection.

Treatment:

Antimicrobial Therapy. This therapy is effective in both shortening the duration of diarrhea and eliminating the organism from feces, and it is recommended for most patients with dysentery. The small bowel form of the disease is often self limited (lasting 48 to 72 hours) but may progress to dysentery. In cases of mild illness the primary indication for treatment is to prevent further spread of the organism. Resistance to antimicrobials is common (plasmid-mediated, multiple antibiotic resistance has been identified in all *Shigella* species); and antimicrobial susceptibility testing should be done on clinical isolates. For cases in which susceptibility is unknown or an ampicillin-resistant strain is isolated, the drug of choice is trimethoprim-sulfamethoxazole. Strains acquired in developing countries are often resistant to trimethoprim-sulfamethoxazole but susceptible to nalidixic acid. For susceptible strains, ampicillin is effective. Amoxicillin is ineffective for the treatment of *Shigella* infections. For patients 9 years or older, tetracycline is useful if the strain is susceptible. The oral route is acceptable, except in seriously ill patients.

Antidiarrheal Drugs. Such drugs that inhibit intestinal peristalsis are usually contraindicated because they may prolong the clinical and bacteriologic course of the disease.

Isolation of the Hospitalized Patient: Enteric precautions are indicated until cultures of three consecutive stool specimens taken after cessation of antimicrobial therapy are negative.

Control Measures:

Day Care. General measures for interrupting enteric transmission (especially hand washing) in day care centers are recommended (see Children in Day Care, page 72). When *Shigella* infection is identified in a day care attendee or staff member, the stools of other symptomatic attendees and staff members should be cultured. Stools of household contacts with diarrhea should also be cultured. All symptomatic individuals in whom *Shigella* is isolated from stool should receive antimicrobial therapy (see Treatment) and should no longer have diarrhea before readmission to the program. If several individuals are infected, consideration can be given to using a cohort system until the stool cultures are negative. Efforts should be made to prevent transfer of children to other day care centers in order not to spread the outbreak.

General Control Measures. Strict attention to hand washing is essential to limit spread. Other important control measures include sanitary water supply, food processing, and sewage disposal; exclusion of infected persons as food handlers; prevention of food contamination by flies; and case reporting to appropriate health authorities (e.g., hospital infection control officer and public health department).

Vaccination. Several candidate vaccines have been tested but none is available for general use.

Staphylococcal Infections

Clinical Manifestations: *Staphylococcus aureus* causes a wide variety of suppurative infections, ranging from localized to invasive diseases such as septicemia. Localized diseases include furuncles, impetigo (bullous and nonbullous), and wound infections. Suppurative and/or invasive infections include osteomyelitis, arthritis, endocarditis, and pneumonia. Meningitis is rare. *S aureus* also causes toxin-mediated diseases, such as toxic shock syndrome (see Staphylococcal Toxic Shock Syndrome, page 435), scalded skin syndrome, and food poisoning (see Staphylococcal Food Poisoning, page 434).

Coagulase-negative staphylococci, primarily *S epidermidis*, cause bacteremia in premature infants and immunocompromised patients and are frequently associated with vascular access device, cerebrospinal fluid shunt infections, and endocarditis in patients with prosthetic valves. Coagulase-negative staphylococci can also cause urinary tract infections, especially in adolescents.

Etiology: Staphylococci are Gram-positive cocci which appear microscopically in grape-like clusters. Staphylococci multiply aerobically and anaerobically; they are resistant to heat to 50°C (122°F), high salt concentrations, and drying; and they can survive on clothing and in dust.

Coagulase-negative staphylococci are classified in 11 species. Most infections are caused by *S epidermidis*. Slime production by *S epidermidis* is associated with invasiveness. *S saprophyticus* causes urinary tract infections.

Epidemiology: *S aureus* microbes are ubiquitous and can be part of the normal human flora. *S aureus* colonizes the anterior nares and moist body areas in approximately 30% of humans. Persons who have skin or draining staphylococcal lesions are important disseminators of *S aureus*. Carriers can also transmit staphylococci. Infants who have been colonized while in the nursery can be the source of family dissemination. Person-to-person transmission is the usual mode of spread, occurring via the hands, nasal discharges, and, rarely, by aerosol. Communicability is a constant possibility as long as lesions or the carrier state persist. Open, draining lesions are particularly likely to lead to the spread of the organism. Most staphylococcal abscesses and toxin-related diseases are caused by *S aureus*. Staphylococci on skin and the mucous membranes cause infection when skin or mucous membranes or other host defenses are compromised, either locally or systemically. Infection is usually caused by the patient's endogenous *S aureus* strain. The presence of foreign bodies, such as intravascular catheters and prosthetic heart valves, predispose to infection.

Coagulase-negative staphylococci are ubiquitous on skin and mucosal surfaces. Carriers can transmit infection and person-to-person spread is the common mode of dissemination. When host defenses are compromised, organisms on the skin or mucous membranes can cause disease. Infection is usually the result of invasion by a patient's endogenous strain. The presence of foreign bodies, such as shunts or intravascular catheters, predisposes to infection.

The **incubation period** is usually 1 to 10 days for bullous impetigo and the scalded skin syndrome. For other staphylococcal lesions, it is extremely variable. A long delay can occur between acquisition of the organism and onset of disease.

Diagnostic Tests: Gram-stained smears of material from lesions can provide presumptive evidence of infection. Isolation of the organisms by culture of blood, tissue, pleural fluid, bones, or lesions is definitive. The positive coagulase test or mannitol fermentation differentiates *S aureus* from coagulase-negative staphylococci. Occasionally, when clusters of cases occur, examination of antibiotic susceptibility, plasmid typing, or phage type patterns of the isolated strains can help determine the source of the outbreak.

Treatment:

S aureus.

- Serious infections require intravenous therapy with a penicillinase-resistant penicillin, such as nafcillin or oxacillin, because most *S aureus* strains in the community and in hospitals produce penicillinase and are resistant to penicillin and related antimicrobial agents. First- or second-generation cephalosporins (e.g., cephalothin or cefuroxime) or clindamycin are also useful. The newer third-generation cephalosporins are usually not as active in vitro against staphylococci, and some may be inadequate for effective treatment. Some 5% to 10% of patients allergic to the penicillins will also be hypersensitive to the cephalosporins. Intravenous vancomycin can be used for *S aureus* strain which are resistant to the penicillinase-resistant penicillins, and for patients who are allergic to both penicillin and the cephalosporins. All *S aureus* strains are usually susceptible to vancomycin. The choice of antibiotics for systemic therapy should be based on results of susceptibility tests.
- Drainage of abscesses is desirable and usually required.
- Skin and soft-tissue infection, such as impetigo or cellulitis due to *S aureus*, can usually be treated with oral penicillinase-resistant beta-lactam drugs, such as cloxacillin, dicloxacillin, or a cephalosporin. For superficial skin lesions, topical antibacterial therapy with mupirocin or bacitracin ointment and hot soaks may be sufficient.

Coagulase-Negative Staphylococcal Infections.

- Serious infections require intravenous therapy with antibiotics. Penicillin is active against susceptible strains. However, most strains causing infection are resistant to penicillin, in which case a semisynthetic penicillinase-resistant penicillin, such as methicillin, nafcillin, or oxacillin, can be used. Methicillin-resistant strains can be common, especially in nosocomial infections (in some hospitals 40% or more of isolates may be resistant). Methicillin resistance has been reported in as many as 83% of patients with prosthetic valve endocarditis. Most of these organisms are susceptible to vancomycin, which is the drug of choice for methicillin-resistant organisms. Rifampin and gentamicin are also effective but rapid emergence of resistance limits their use. When either is used in combination with vancomycin, increased antibacterial activity has been reported.

- Intravenous vancomycin should be strongly considered for initial treatment of all severe infections caused by coagulase-negative staphylococci.
- Removal of foreign bodies and drainage of diseases is desirable and often required.

Endocarditis. This infection can be caused by either *S aureus* or, in patients with prosthetic cardiac valves, coagulase-negative staphylococci (usually *S epidermidis*). Recommendations for antimicrobial treatment of endocarditis have been formulated by the American Heart Association's Council on Cardiovascular Disease in the Young and should be consulted (Bisno et al. Antimicrobial treatment of infective endocarditis due to viridans streptococci, enterococci, and staphylococci. *JAMA*. 1989;261:1471-1477).

Isolation of the Hospitalized Patient:

S aureus Infections. Patients with draining lung abscesses or pneumonia should be placed in contact isolation for 48 hours after starting effective therapy. For patients with wound and skin infections, including infected burns, which are draining openly (i.e., not adequately covered by a dressing), contact isolation should be implemented. For patients with small lesions adequately covered by dressings, drainage/secretion precautions are adequate. For patients with the scalded skin syndrome and bullous impetigo, contact isolation is indicated. When prevalence of multiply-resistant staphylococci is low, patients infected or colonized with these strains can be managed by contact isolation to avoid transmission. Precautions should continue for the duration of the illness. No special precautions are necessary for patients with other staphylococcal infections, such as bacteremia.

Coagulase-Negative Staphylococcal Infections. Patients with draining abscesses should be placed in contact isolation for 48 hours after starting therapy. For patients with wound and skin infections, including infected burns, which are draining openly (i.e., not adequately covered by a dressing), contact isolation should be implemented. For patients with small lesions adequately covered by dressings, drainage/secretion precautions are adequate. Precautions should continue for the duration of the illness. No special precautions are necessary for patients with other staphylococcal infections, such as bacteremia.

Control Measures:

- Maximum precautions to avoid transmission of staphylococci via hands and clothing of personnel should be a hospital routine. Careful hand washing before and after every patient contact is mandatory.

- Carriers require no special treatment. Routine culturing of hospital personnel is not recommended. However, identification of carriers who disseminate a strain which has been implicated in epidemic disease in a closed population is necessary. Consideration should be given to removing these personnel from areas of patient contact and treating them with topical intranasal antibiotics and occasionally with appropriate orally administered antibiotics. The goal of therapy in this instance is to eliminate carriage of an epidemiologically virulent strain. The carrier state can be very difficult to eradicate.
- Persons involved in hospital outbreaks of staphylococcal disease should be observed and warned of the possibility of delayed disease and the spread to family members.
- Epidemic *S aureus* disease in newborn nurseries presents special problems. Approaches include the following:
  - Infants with definite or suspected staphylococcal disease should be placed on contact isolation.
  - The cohorting of infants and staff should be instituted in the affected nursery. For example, all infants in a room should be discharged and the room carefully cleaned before new infants are admitted to that room. Staff, especially nursing staff, taking care of one cohort should not take care of another cohort, when more than one patient cohort is present.
  - Meticulous patient care techniques for infection contact should be reemphasized. Careful hand washing by personnel is of paramount importance.
  - Cultures of infants (umbilicus and anterior nares) and personnel (nares and hands) should be obtained to determine prevalence of colonization and to identify staphylococcal strains involved in the outbreak for antimicrobial susceptibility testing, phage typing, or plasmid typing. Occasionally, personnel colonized with the outbreak strain will need to be removed from patient contact until carriage has been eliminated.
  - During epidemics, full-term infants may be bathed with hexachlorophene (3%) as soon after birth as possible and daily until they are discharged. The hexachlorophene should be thoroughly washed off after bathing. Care must be exercised in using hexachlorophene because systemic absorption can result in central nervous system damage. Hexachlorophene should not be used for routine bathing and should be used only for full-term infants.
  - Application of triple dye or bacitracin ointment to the umbilical stump of all infants twice daily throughout the nursery stay can also be helpful.

- In unusual circumstances, treatment with oral antistaphylococcal agents of all infants and personnel who are carriers may be necessary.
- Persons involved in hospital outbreaks should be observed and warned of the possibility of delayed disease and the spread to family members.
- Surveillance in the nursery should be continued for several weeks after the epidemic has apparently terminated.
- Surveillance of recently discharged infants for infections should be performed. Observation for disease in neonates, both in the nursery and at home for several weeks, is the most reliable index of *S aureus* outbreaks.

Staphylococcal Food Poisoning

Clinical Manifestations: Staphylococcal food poisoning is characterized by the abrupt onset of severe cramps, nausea and vomiting, diarrhea, and, occasionally, low-grade fever. Its short incubation period (30 minutes to 7 hours), brevity of illness, and usual lack of fever help distinguish it from other types of food poisoning except that caused by *Bacillus cereus*. Chemical food poisoning usually has a shorter incubation period. *Clostridium perfringens* food poisoning usually has a longer incubation period and infrequently is accompanied by vomiting, which is common in staphylococcal and *B cereus* food poisoning. Patients with food-borne salmonellosis and shigellosis often have fever and the incubation period is longer.

Etiology: The enterotoxins produced by strains of *Staphylococcus aureus* and, rarely, *S epidermidis* are the cause. Of the eight immunologically distinct heat-stable enterotoxins (A,B,$C_{1\text{-}3}$,D,E,F), enterotoxins A and D are the most common in the United States. Enterotoxin F is identical with toxic shock syndrome sssociated toxin (TSST-1) and has not been implicated in outbreaks of food poisoning.

Epidemiology: Illness is caused by preformed toxin present in food containing enterotoxigenic staphylococci. Contamination is usually by food handlers who may be healthy but colonized with this organism. Food products most commonly involved include filled pastries, egg and potato salads, poultry, and ham. The disease is not transmissible from person to person.

The **incubation period** is 30 minutes to 7 hours.

Diagnostic Tests: Isolation of the same phage types of *S aureus* from stools or vomitus of affected persons, the vehicle of transmission, and the food handler responsible for contaminating the food is the method of diagnosis in an epidemic. Lesions on the hands of food handlers may be the source of contamination and should be cultured. Other possible sources that should be cultured include the nose, throat, and rectum. Identification of enterotoxin or staphylococcal organisms in incriminated foods and phage typing of isolates of staphylococci can be performed by the Food and Drug Administration. The vomitus and stools of patients may contain the offending *Staphylococcus* species and should be cultured.

Treatment: Supportive. Antibiotics are not indicated.

Isolation of the Hospitalized Patient: No special precautions are recommended.

Control Measures: Optimum cooking and refrigeration of foods, particularly meat, dairy, and bakery products, will help to prevent the disease. Food handlers with staphylococcal infections should be excluded from food preparation.

Staphylococcal Toxic Shock Syndrome

Clinical Manifestations: Toxic shock syndrome (TSS) is an acute febrile illness with myalgia, vomiting, diarrhea, pharyngitis; a diffuse macular erythroderma which desquamates; and mucous membrane and conjunctival hyperemia. The temperature is usually higher than 38.9°C (102°F). The erythematous, sunburn-like rash is usually present during the acute phase, with desquamation of the skin of the palms and soles occurring 7 to 10 days later. Hypotension and, in severe cases, shock and multiorgan system dysfunction can occur. The organ systems that can be involved include renal (abnormal urinalysis, elevated BUN, or serum creatinine levels), hepatic (elevated serum enzyme and bilirubin levels), hematologic (preponderance of immature and mature neutrophils in peripheral blood, and thrombocytopenia), and central nervous system (disorientation or alterations in consciousness without focal neurologic signs).

The case definition established by the Centers for Disease Control is based on the following six major diagnostic criteria:

1. Fever of 38.9°C (102°F) or higher.
2. Presence of a diffuse macular erythroderma.
3. Desquamation 1 to 2 weeks after onset of illness, particularly of the palms and soles.

4. Hypotension, defined as a systolic blood pressure of 90 mm Hg or less for adults, and below the fifth percentile for children younger than 16 years; or an orthostatic drop in diastolic blood pressure of 15 mm Hg or more with a change from lying to sitting; orthostatic syncope; or dizziness.
5. Involvement of three or more of the following organ systems: gastrointestinal, muscular, mucous membrane, renal, hepatic, hematologic, and central nervous system.
6. Negative results on blood and cerebrospinal fluid cultures (blood culture may be positive for *Staphylococcus aureus*), and, if obtained, negative serologic tests for Rocky Mountain spotted fever, leptospirosis, and measles.

TSS is probable when four or more major criteria, one of which is desquamation, or all five other than desquamation are fulfilled. The syndrome can be confused with Kawasaki disease, scarlet fever, Rocky Mountain spotted fever, measles, and leptospirosis. Telogen effluvium, including hair thinning or patchy hair loss, and nail splitting, ridging, or loss frequently occur 1 to 2 months after onset. Persistent neuropsychologic sequelae have been reported but appear to be infrequent.

Etiology: In most patients the etiologic agent is TSST-1-producing strains of *S aureus*; however, TSST-1-negative strains of *S aureus* have been implicated.

Epidemiology: The disease was first described in 1978, although a review of medical literature suggests that it was recorded as "staphylococcal scarlet fever" as early as 1927. In 1980 the disease became widely recognized, with the documentation of an increased risk of illness among menstruating women who used tampons. Since then, the incidence of menstrually associated cases has decreased. The disease was first reported in children, but 60% of the cases now occur among women between 15 and 30 years old. Approximately 55% of the cases in women occur during their menstrual period. Nonmenstrual TSS cases have been associated with cutaneous or subcutaneous lesions, childbirth or abortion, surgical wound infections, vaginal infections occurring at times other than during menstruation or the postpartum period, and other sources of focal staphylococcal infection, including sinusitis and pneumonia. On occasion, the source of infection may be unknown. Patients currently considered at high risk include (1) menstruating women using tampons or other inserted vaginal devices; (2) persons with focal *S aureus* infection; (3) women using diaphragms or contraceptive sponges; and (4) persons with scarlet fever syndrome. TSS is frequently a life-threatening or fatal disease; with treatment, the case fatality rate is 2% to 4%. No evidence of person-to-person transmission or identified common exposures has been found.

The median **incubation period**, based on postoperative TSS, is 2 days.

Diagnostic Tests: Because *S aureus* may be isolated from the anterior nares and vagina of 10% to 20% of healthy individuals, and approximately 10% of such strains can produce TSST-1, the identification of TSST-1-producing *S aureus* is only presumptive evidence. The diagnosis is made on the basis of clinical criteria (see Clinical Manifestations).

Treatment:

- Management of the hypotensive patient depends on the severity of the illness and its complications. Aggressive intravenous fluid replacement for hypovolemic shock has been necessary, and some patients have required vasopressor agents.
- Although antimicrobial agents do not necessarily affect the outcome of the acute illness, antistaphylococcal antibiotics are recommended to eradicate the focus of TSST-1-producing *S aureus*, reduce the risk of a recurrent episode, and treat the occasional patient with staphylococcal bacteremia or bacteriuria.
- Any vaginal tampons (menstrual) or incision and wound packing (nonmenstrual) should be removed. Infected wounds should be explored and drained, even if the wound does not show prominent signs of inflammation.
- Additional types of therapy have been required in some patients to correct electrolyte and acid-base imbalance and to manage the complications of prolonged shock, acute renal failure, adult respiratory distress syndrome, myocardial failure, and disseminated intravascular coagulation with thrombocytopenia.
- To avoid recurrent episodes, menstruating patients should not use tampons during subsequent menstrual periods. From 18% to 68% of menstrual-onset patients have recurrent episodes of illness during subsequent menstrual periods. Treatment with antistaphylococcal antibiotics during the initial episode and discontinuing the use of tampons reduce this risk.

Isolation of the Hospitalized Patient: Drainage/secretion precautions are recommended for the duration of the illness.

Control Measures: None are known.

Group A Streptococcal Infections

Clinical Manifestations: The most common clinical illness produced by group A streptococcal (GAS) infection is acute tonsillitis or pharyngitis. Some untreated patients develop secondary purulent complications, including otitis media, peritonsillar abscesses, and suppurative cervical adenitis. The significance of streptococcal upper respiratory tract disease is its nonsuppurative sequelae, rheumatic fever and acute glomerulonephritis. Scarlet fever occurs most commonly in association with pharyngitis, and, rarely, with pyoderma, and has a characteristic sandpaper-like rash, which is caused by one or more of the several erythrogenic exotoxins produced by GAS strains. Severe scarlet fever with systemic toxicity is rare today. With this exception, the epidemiology, symptoms, sequelae, and treatment of scarlet fever are no different from those of streptococcal pharyngitis.

The second most common site of GAS infection is the skin. Streptococcal skin infections (i.e., pyoderma and impetigo) can result in glomerulonephritis, which occasionally can be epidemic, but rheumatic fever is not a sequela. Less commonly, GAS infection causes perianal cellulitis, vaginitis, erysipelas, septicemia, myositis, endocarditis, pericarditis, pneumonia, septic arthritis, osteomyelitis, and, in neonates, omphalitis. A toxic-shock-like syndrome caused by GAS has been recently described and is associated with local tissue destruction, shock, renal impairment, acute respiratory distress syndrome, and a 30% case-fatality rate.

Etiology: More than 80 immunologically distinct protein types of Group A beta-hemolytic streptococci (*Streptococcus pyogenes*) have been identified. Most of these serotypes can be divided into groups commonly associated with either skin or respiratory infections. Epidemiologic studies suggest an association between certain serotypes (e.g., types 1, 3, 5, 6, and 18) and recent outbreaks of rheumatic fever, but a "rheumatogenic" factor has not been identified. Several serotypes are clearly associated with pyoderma and acute glomerulonephritis. Pharyngitis-associated nephritis, however, is often associated with other types of nephritogenic strains (e.g., type 12). Groups C and G streptococci have been associated with pharyngitis but not with rheumatic fever.

Epidemiology: Pharyngitis usually results from contact with a person who has active streptococcal pharyngitis. Fomites and household pets such as dogs have not been demonstrated to be vectors of GAS infection. Transmission of GAS infection almost always occurs by contact with respiratory secretions. Outbreaks of pharyngitis, such as occur in schools, are usually spread by this route. Close contact, such as occurs in schools, day care centers, and military installations, increases transmission. Food-borne outbreaks have occurred and are a consequence of human contamination of food in conjunction with improper refrigeration procedures.

Streptococcal pharyngitis can occur at any age, but it is most frequent among school-aged children. The classic clinical presentation of streptococcal pharyngitis is uncommon in children before they are 3 years old, as is rheumatic fever. The young infant with GAS respiratory infection frequently exhibits a low-grade fever with serous or seromucoid rhinitis. Toddlers (1 to 3 years old) may display a protracted, atypical illness consisting of low-grade fever, irritability, anorexia, and cervical adenitis. Streptococcal infections are less frequent in adults than in children except during epidemics. Both sexes and all races are similarly susceptible. Pharyngitis, impetigo, and their nonsuppurative complications are associated with crowding, which is often present in socioeconomically disadvantaged populations.

Geographically, both streptococcal pharyngitis and impetigo are ubiquitous. Impetigo is more common in tropical climates and in warm seasons, presumably in part because of the presence of insect bites and other minor skin trauma. Streptococcal pharyngitis occurs more frequently in the late fall, winter, and spring in the United States, presumably because of close person-to-person contact indoors and in schools.

Throat culture surveys of asymptomatic children during school outbreaks of pharyngitis have yielded streptococcal prevalence rates usually between 15% and 30% but as high as 50%. Serologic studies indicate that these asymptomatic persons are most commonly carriers with a previously undetected streptococcal infection. Continued convalescent carriage can persist for several months. The carrier state is not associated with an appreciable risk of rheumatic fever.

Communicability of streptococcal pharyngitis is maximum during acute infection and gradually diminishes during a period of weeks in untreated individuals. Transmission by a carrier is unlikely, perhaps because of a decreased production of M protein (the organism's major virulence factor), diminished numbers of organisms, and the disappearance of bacteria from nasal secretions. The occurrence of transmission during the incubation period is uncertain.

Rates of rheumatic fever in the United States have decreased for several decades. The recent outbreaks of rheumatic fever, in different geographic areas of the United States, occurring in both schoolchildren and in military populations, demonstrate that acute rheumatic fever can still occur. The reasons for the local outbreaks of rheumatic fever are not clear, but the introduction of specific streptococcal strains may be a factor.

The acquisition of GAS on normal skin precedes the development of impetigo. The organism can be acquired from others with impetigo, possibly by physical contact. Less commonly, individuals with streptococcal pharyngitis or upper respiratory tract carriage can infect their open skin lesions (e.g., insect bites or burns) or those of others. Infections of surgical wounds, puerperal sepsis, and neonatal infections (which most often begin with omphalitis) usually result from contact transmission via the hands. At times, anal or vaginal carriers and persons with local suppurative infections can transmit infection, particularly to surgical or obstetrical patients and newborn infants in nosocomial outbreaks.

The **incubation period** of streptococcal pharyngitis is 2 to 5 days. In impetigo, a 7- to 10-day period between the acquisition of GAS on normal skin and the development of lesions has been demonstrated.

Diagnostic Tests: The **throat culture** remains the basis of the management of children with pharyngitis because most cases of acute pharyngitis are not caused by streptococcal infection, and the clinical differentiation of viral and streptococcal pharyngitis is often impossible. A swab specimen from the tonsils and posterior pharynx should be obtained and cultured on sheep blood agar medium, to confirm streptococcal infection. Bacitracin-sensitivity disks (containing 0.04 units of bacitracin) on the culture plate or use of latex, coagglutination, or precipitation techniques will usually differentiate group A from other beta-hemolytic streptococci. False-negative cultures may occur, and recovery of GAS from the pharynx does not distinguish patients with true streptococcal infection, as evidenced by an antibody response, from streptococcal carriers who have pharyngitis resulting from other causes (i.e., viral infection). Moreover, the degree of positivity of the culture does not reliably distinguish infection from carriage.

Most rapid antigen diagnostic tests are based on direct extraction of group A carbohydrate antigen from throat swabs. Because these tests vary in methodology, sensitivity, and specificity, the value and reliability of specific tests should be individually considered. Their accuracy is also dependent on the experience of the person performing the test. Therefore, when a patient suspected of having streptococcal pharyngitis has a negative rapid antigen test, a duplicate swab should be processed for culture. Although the specificity of these tests is generally high, sensitivity can be as low as 60% to 70% and can vary with the number of organisms present (i.e., the amount of antigen). Although weakly positive cultures may be more common in carriers, at least one third of such patients will have streptococcal disease.

Tests for antibody in acute and convalescent sera, such as the antistreptolysin O (ASO) and antideoxyribonuclease B (anti-DNase B), are useful in confirming a recent GAS infection. These tests can be helpful in diagnosing patients with nonsuppurative complications of streptococcal infection (acute rheumatic fever or acute glomerulonephritis). However, they are of no immediate value in the diagnosis or management of acute streptococcal infection. As with any serologic test, a rise in titer in sera obtained 3 to 6 weeks apart (4 to 6 weeks for anti-DNase B) is much more reliable than a single high titer. The upper limits of normal titers vary with age, population, and season of the year.

Indications for Throat Culture. Factors to be considered in the decision to obtain a throat culture are the child's clinical signs and symptoms, the season, the child's age, and the family and community epidemiology. Children with typical findings of pharyngitis should be cultured. An important reason for culturing even those with classic findings is to establish the presence or absence of streptococcal disease and to help in the management of contacts who subsequently may become ill. Additionally, the best way to diagnose streptococcal infection in individuals with suggestive but not classic findings is by culture. In children younger than 3 years, GAS is a less frequent cause of pharyngitis, and rheumatic fever in this age group is extremely rare in the United States. However, streptococcal pharyngitis has been reported in out-of-home child care groups.

Indications for culturing contacts vary according to circumstances. Siblings and other household contacts of a child who has developed acute rheumatic fever or glomerulonephritis should be cultured and, if positive, treated regardless of whether the contact is currently or recently symptomatic. Household contacts of an index patient with streptococcal pharyngitis who have recent or current symptoms suggestive of streptococcal infection should be cultured. Culturing asymptomatic household contacts is not recommended except during outbreaks or in other specific epidemiologic situations (e.g., the presence of a person in the family with rheumatic heart disease).

Posttreatment throat cultures are indicated only in patients who are at high risk for rheumatic fever or who are symptomatic. The recent outbreaks of acute rheumatic fever do not provide sufficient evidence to alter this general recommendation. Repeated courses of antibiotic therapy are usually not indicated in asymptomatic patients who continue to harbor GAS after appropriate therapy, except for those who have or have had, or whose family members have or have had, rheumatic fever or rheumatic heart disease, or in other special epidemiologic circumstances (e.g., outbreaks of rheumatic fever).

Children and families in whom recurrent or relapsing GAS pharyngitis occurs at close intervals during a particular streptococcal season present a special problem. These illnesses may be caused by the same strain (i.e., a true relapse) or by heterologous strains. In assessing such a situation, confirming that the cultured bacteria is GAS and not beta-hemolytic streptococci of other serogroups is important. Poor compliance with oral treatment and bacteriologic resistance to the therapeutic agent (e.g., erythromycin resistance, which occurs in 4% to 5% of strains in the United States) should be excluded as causes. An alternative course of therapy (such as benzathine penicillin) should be considered. Culturing asymptomatic household members is usually not helpful. However, if multiple members have symptomatic pharyngitis or other forms of GAS infection, simultaneous cultures of all household members and treatment of all persons with positive cultures may be of value.

In schools or other environments where large numbers of individuals are in close contact, GAS upper respiratory tract carriage in healthy children can be as high as 5% to 15%, in the absence of an outbreak of streptococcal disease. Therefore, classroom or school culture surveys are not routinely indicated and should be undertaken only if an outbreak of streptococcal disease, rheumatic fever, or glomerulonephritis is occurring.

Treatment:

Pharyngitis.

- Penicillin V remains a very effective antimicrobial for the treatment of GAS pharyngitis and should be used unless the patient is allergic to penicillin. Penicillin prevents rheumatic fever, even when therapy is started as long as 9 days after the onset of the acute illness. Thus, for patients seen early, a brief delay for processing of the throat culture does not increase the risk of rheumatic fever. In patients with acute rheumatic fever, a full therapeutic course of penicillin should be given to eradicate GAS, which may or may not be recoverable on initial throat culture.

  The dose of orally administered penicillin V is 200,000 U (125 mg) in those less than 60 lb to 400,000 U in others (250 mg), three or four times daily for 10 days. With good compliance, two divided doses of oral penicillin totaling 800,000 U (500 mg) daily are effective. To prevent rheumatic fever, treatment should be given for at least 10 days, regardless of the promptness of clinical recovery. Although different preparations of oral penicillin vary in absorption, their clinical efficacy is similar. Relapses may occur more frequently with oral penicillin than with intramuscularly administered benzathine penicillin G.

- Benzathine penicillin G, 600,000 U, is administered intramuscularly to children less than 60 lb (27.3 kg); for larger children and adults, the dose is 1,200,000 U, intramuscularly. Intramuscular therapy ensures treatment for an adequate time and avoids the problem of compliance. Mixtures containing shorter-acting penicillins in addition to benzathine penicillin G have not been shown to be superior to benzathine penicillin G alone, except in reducing discomfort from the injection. If a mixture is used, it must contain benzathine penicillin G in the recommended doses. Although data are limited, the combination of 900,000 U of benzathine penicillin G and 300,000 U of procaine penicillin G may be satisfactory for children less than 60 lb. Less discomfort is associated with an injection of benzathine penicillin if the preparation is brought to room temperature before administration.
- Orally administered erythromycin is indicated for patients allergic to penicillin, and treatment should also be given for 10 days. Erythromycin estolate (20 to 30 mg/kg/d in two to four divided doses) or erythromycin ethyl succinate (40 to 50 mg/kg/d in three to four divided doses) is effective in treating streptococcal pharyngitis; the maximal dose is 1 g/d. Although GAS strains resistant to erythromycin are prevalent in some areas of the world (e.g., Asia), they remain uncommon (approximately 4% to 5%) in the United States.
- An oral cephalosporin (e.g., cefalexin, cephradine, cefadroxil, cefaclor, cefixime, and cefuroxime axetil) for 10 days is an acceptable alternative for the patient allergic to penicillin, although 5% to 15% of patients truly allergic to penicillin can also be allergic to the cephalosporins. A cephalosporin should not be used in patients with an immediate (anaphylactic) type hypersensitivity to penicillin. Cephalosporins are also more expensive. Tetracyclines and sulfonamides should *not* be used for treating GAS infection; many strains are resistant to tetracycline, and sulfonamides will not eradicate the organism, although sulfonamides are effective for continuous prophylaxis in preventing recurrent rheumatic fever (see Secondary Prophylaxis of Rheumatic Fever, page 445). Although data suggest that beta-lactamase production by upper respiratory tract flora may interfere with penicillin effectiveness in the treatment of GAS pharyngitis in some patients, directing treatment against these organisms is controversial and is usually not necessary in patients with acute pharyngitis. Successful retreatment using beta-lactamase-resistant antibiotics, however, has been reported for patients who have failed penicillin treatment.
- Pharyngeal carriers of GAS appear to be at little risk of developing nonsuppurative sequelae of streptococcal infection or of spreading infection to those who live and work around them; they usually

do not warrant antibiotic treatment. However, carriers present a difficult diagnostic problem when they develop symptomatic upper respiratory tract infection because differentiation between acute streptococcal infection or chronic carriage is frequently not possible. In these circumstances, a single course of therapy is reasonable.

- Children and families with recurrent, documented, symptomatic GAS pharyngitis for many weeks pose special treatment considerations. The entire family should be cultured simultaneously (see Indications for Throat Culture, page 441). Those harboring GAS should be treated (preferably with intramuscularly administered benzathine penicillin G) and recultured after treatment. If they are still harboring GAS, a second course of treatment (benzathine penicillin G or erythromycin) should be given. These persons should be recultured after this second treatment; if one or more persons still harbor GAS but are asymptomatic, no further treatment is necessary (except in persons with present or past rheumatic fever or family history of rheumatic heart disease, or in outbreaks, circumstances in which an expert should be consulted). Several antibiotic regimens have been evaluated and appear effective in preventing GAS relapses; these include penicillin prophylaxis, 10 days of penicillin therapy with rifampin given concurrently during the last 4 days of therapy, clindamycin, dicloxacillin, and amoxicillin/clavulanate. However, the efficacy of these regimens has not been established sufficiently to recommend their routine use.

Impetigo.

- Local antibacterial preparations, such as bacitracin or mupirocin ointment may be useful in limiting person-to-person spread of streptococcal impetigo. With multiple spreading lesions or impetigo in multiple family members, day care groups, or athletic teams, GAS impetigo should be treated systemically with antibiotic regimens, as recommended for pharyngitis.
- More intensive, parenteral treatment is required for infections such as endocarditis, pneumonia, septicemia, meningitis, arthritis, and osteomyelitis.

Late Sequelae. Acute rheumatic fever and acute glomerulonephritis are serious late sequelae of GAS infections. During epidemics, as many as 3% of untreated patients with acute streptococcal pharyngitis/tonsillitis may develop rheumatic fever. In endemically occurring infection, the attack rates are much lower but still constitute a serious risk, particularly in developing countries. The risk of rheumatic fever can be virtually eliminated by adequate treatment of the antecedent GAS infection, but the prevention of acute nephritis by antimicrobial treatment is less certain. Suppurative complications, such as peritonsillar abscess and cervical adenitis, are prevented by prompt therapy.

Isolation of the Hospitalized Patient: Drainage/secretion precautions should be used in patients with pharyngitis until 24 hours after the initiation of effective therapy. With pneumonia, contact isolation is indicated until 24 hours after the initiation of effective therapy. The presence of empyema may necessitate a longer period of isolation. For burns with secondary GAS infections, contact isolation or drainage/secretion precautions, depending on the extent of the infection, should be observed for 24 hours after the start of effective therapy.

Control Measures: The most important means of controlling GAS disease and its sequelae is prompt identification and treatment of infections.

School and Day Care. Children with streptococcal pharyngitis or skin infections should not return to school or day care until at least 24 hours after beginning antimicrobial therapy, and until they are afebrile. Close contact with other children during this time should be avoided.

Care of Exposed Persons. Contacts who have recent or current clinical evidence of a streptococcal infection should be cultured and treated if the culture is positive to reduce the risks of a delayed, nonsuppurative complication or further transmission. Rates of GAS acquisition are higher among sibling contacts (25%) than among parent contacts in nonepidemic settings; rates as high as 50% for sibling contacts and 20% for parent contacts have been reported during epidemics. Approximately 50% to 80% of contacts who acquire the organism will become ill. Asymptomatic persons may be at some risk of nonsuppurative complications, as studies indicate that as many as one third of patients with rheumatic fever had no history of recent streptococcal infection and another third of the patients had minor respiratory infections that were not brought to medical attention. However, asymptomatic family contacts need not be cultured except in unusual epidemiologic circumstances or when the contacts are at risk of developing complications of infection (see Indications for Throat Culture, page 441). Short courses of antibiotics for contacts are inappropriate. Under specific conditions (e.g., a large family with documented, repeated intrafamily transmission during a prolonged period), physicians may elect to treat all family members (see Indications for Throat Culture). These circumstances arise infrequently.

Secondary Prophylaxis of Rheumatic Fever. Patients who have a well-documented history of rheumatic fever (including cases manifested solely by Sydenham's chorea) and those who show definite evidence of rheumatic heart disease should be given continuous antibiotic prophylaxis (secondary prophylaxis) because asymptomatic, as well as optimally treated symptomatic GAS infections, can trigger a rheumatic recurrence. Prophylaxis should be initiated as soon as the diagnosis of active rheumatic fever or rheumatic heart disease is made. Secondary prophylaxis should be long term and perhaps for life in patients with rheumatic heart disease. The risk of recurrence declines with the interval from the most recent attack, and patients without rheumatic heart disease are at a lower risk of recurrence than those with cardiac involvement. These considerations influence the duration of secondary prophylaxis in adults but should not alter the practice of secondary prophylaxis in children, adolescents, and young adults. Secondary prophylaxis should be continued in patients with rheumatic heart disease, even after prosthetic valve replacement, because these patients remain at risk for recurrence of rheumatic fever. When streptococcal infections occur in family members of rheumatic fever patients, they should be treated vigorously (see Indications for Throat Culture, page 441, and Treatment, page 442).

The following three regimens for secondary prophylaxis are effective:

1. benzathine penicillin G, 1,200,000 U, intramuscularly, once every 3 or 4 weeks;
2. penicillin V, orally, 200,000 U (125 mg) for those less than 60 lb to 400,000 U (250 mg) for others twice a day;
3. sulfadiazine, orally, 1 g once a day for patients more than 60 lb (27.3 kg), and 0.5 g once a day for patients less than 60 lb (sulfisoxazole in similar doses is probably equally satisfactory).

The first regimen is the most reliable because the success of oral prophylaxis depends primarily on patient compliance, although inconvenience and the pain of injection may cause some patients to discontinue intramuscular prophylaxis. In some countries, and in situations where the risk of GAS recurrence is great, benzathine penicillin G is given every 3 weeks because of greater effectiveness; in the United States every 4 weeks appears adequate in most patients. Sulfadiazine is as effective as oral penicillin.

Allergic reactions to oral penicillin are similar to those with intramuscular penicillin, but they usually are less severe and occur less frequently. These reactions also occur less often in children than in adults. Anaphylaxis is extremely rare in patients receiving oral penicillin. Allergic reactions to penicillin include a serum sickness-like reaction, characterized by fever and joint pains, which may be mistaken for an acute rheumatic fever recurrence. Sulfadiazine reactions are infrequent and usually minor; blood counts may be advisable after 2 weeks of prophylaxis, as leukopenia has been reported. Sulfadiazine prophylaxis in late pregnancy is contraindicated because of interference with fetal bilirubin metabolism. Febrile mucocutaneous syndromes (erythema multiforme, Stevens-Johnson syndrome, or epidermal necrolysis) have been associated with penicillin as well as sulfonamides. When an adverse event occurs with any of these therapeutic regimens, the drug should be stopped immediately and an alternative drug considered. For the exceptional patient allergic to both penicillin and sulfonamides, erythromycin (250 mg twice daily) may be used.

Bacterial Endocarditis Prophylaxis. Patients with rheumatic valvular heart disease also require additional short-term antibiotic prophylaxis at the time of certain procedures (including dental and surgical procedures) to prevent the possible development of bacterial endocarditis (see Prevention of Bacterial Endocarditis, page 536). Patients who have had rheumatic fever without evidence of valvular heart disease do not need prophylaxis for endocarditis. Penicillin should not be used for endocarditis prophylaxis in patients who are receiving oral penicillin for secondary rheumatic fever prophylaxis because of relative penicillin resistance of viridans streptococci in the oral cavity in such patients. Erythromycin is the alternative antibiotic recommended in such patients.

Group B Streptococcal Infections

Clinical Manifestations: Group B streptococci are a major cause of perinatal bacterial infections, including endometritis, amnionitis, and urinary tract infections in parturient women and systemic and focal infections in infants from birth until 4 or more months of age. Two distinct forms of bacteremic disease occur in neonates. Early-onset disease is characterized by respiratory distress, apnea, shock, pneumonia, and, occasionally, meningitis, and it usually occurs in the first 3 days of life. Late-onset disease, which typically occurs after the fifth to seventh day, is frequently accompanied by meningitis; osteomyelitis, septic arthritis, or other focal infections can also occur. Group B streptococci less commonly cause infections in older persons, particularly those with diabetes and immunocompromised hosts.

Etiology: Group B streptococci (*Streptococcus agalactiae*) are divided into the five following serotypes: Ia, Ib, Ia/c, II, and III. All serotypes are associated with infections in newborn infants, children, and adults. Serotype III is the predominant cause of early- and late-onset neonatal meningitis.

Epidemiology: Group B streptococci (GBS) are common inhabitants of the gastrointestinal tract and the female genitourinary tract. Less commonly, they colonize the pharynx and skin. The colonization rate in pregnant women and newborn infants ranges from 5% to 35%. Colonization during pregnancy can be intermittent. Neonatal GBS disease has an incidence of 1 to 5 cases per 1,000 live births; the incidence varies considerably among hospitals. Early-onset disease occurs in approximately one infant per 100 to 200 colonized women. Transmission from mother to infant occurs during delivery and in utero shortly before delivery. After delivery, person-to-person transmission can occur, and GBS can be acquired in the nursery from colonized infants or hospital personnel (probably via hand contamination), or in the community after hospital discharge. The risk of early-onset disease is increased in low-birth-weight infants; in those born after prolonged labor and/or prolonged rupture of amniotic membranes; and in infants born of women with perinatal infection. Low or absent concentration of type-specific serum antibody also appears to be a predisposing factor. The period of communicability is unknown, but it may extend throughout the duration of colonization or active disease. Infants can remain colonized for several weeks after birth and after treatment of symptomatic infections.

The **incubation period** of early-onset disease is less than 3 days. In late-onset disease the incubation period from GBS acquisition to disease is unknown; onset of infection usually occurs from 7 days to 3 months of age with a mean of 3 to 4 weeks.

Diagnostic Tests: Gram-positive cocci in fluids that are ordinarily sterile (cerebrospinal, pleural, joint fluid, or urine) provide presumptive evidence of infection. Cultures of blood and body fluids are necessary to establish the diagnosis. Serotype identification by type-specific antisera is available in a few laboratories. GBS antigen may be rapidly detected in biologic fluids (serum, cerebrospinal fluid, and urine) by latex particle agglutination or other immunologic tests, and it constitutes evidence of infection. The sensitivity and specificity of rapid diagnostic tests are variable, and false positive results occur in 5% to 8% of urine samples, especially bagged urine specimens that become contaminated during collection.

Treatment:

- Penicillin or ampicillin plus an aminoglycoside is the initial treatment of choice for a newborn infant with presumptive, invasive, life-threatening infection.

- Penicillin G or ampicillin alone can be given when GBS is identified in a focus of infection and clinical response has been documented. Before so doing, however, some experts advise determination of the susceptibility of the organism to penicillin and/or ampicillin.
- The recommended dosage of penicillin G for meningitis for infants 7 days or younger is 100,000 to 150,000 U/kg/d, intravenously in two or three divided doses; for infants more than 7 days old, 200,000 to 250,000 U/kg/d, in four divided doses, intravenously, is recommended. For ampicillin, the recommended dosage for infants 7 days or younger is 100 mg/kg/d in two or three divided doses, intravenously; for infants more than 7 days old, 150 to 200 mg/kg/d in four divided doses, is recommended. The optimal dose, however, is unknown. Some experts recommend higher doses of penicillin (300,000 to 400,000 U/kg/d) and of ampicillin (200 to 300 mg/kg/d).
- For meningitis, a second lumbar puncture at approximately 24 hours after initiation of therapy to document bacteriologic cure has prognostic importance. Cerebrospinal fluid cultures should be repeated if response to therapy is in doubt after 36 to 72 hours of treatment.
- For infants with bacteremia without a defined focus, treatment should be continued for 10 to 14 days. For infants with uncomplicated meningitis, 14 days of treatment is usually satisfactory, but longer periods of treatment may be necessary. Musculoskeletal infections may require longer treatment, depending on the severity of infection, response to treatment, and complications. Treatment duration should be guided by the patient's clinical and bacteriologic responses.

Isolation of the Hospitalized Patient: No special precautions are recommended except during a nursery outbreak of GBS disease (see Control Measures).

Control Measures:

Chemoprophylaxis. Parenteral administration of ampicillin to high-risk, colonized, pregnant women (e.g., those with premature onset of labor, premature rupture of membranes, or fever) throughout labor has been demonstrated to decrease transmission of GBS to the infant and rates of disease in infants. Studies of the use of a penicillin administered to infants in the delivery room indicate varying effectiveness in prevention of disease. At present, no generic recommendations for the prevention of neonatal GBS disease have been made. Chemoprophylaxis should be considered for individual patients or for hospital policy.

Intrapartum treatment with ampicillin is recommended by some experts for a woman with a previously infected infant to prevent a subsequent neonatal infection. Treatment of the twin of an index case is indicated because of the high frequency of coinfection in both infants.

Neonatal Infection Control. Routine cultures of infants to determine GBS colonization are not recommended. Epidemiologic evaluation of late-onset cases in a special care nursery may exclude a nosocomial source.

Nursery Outbreak. Cohorting of ill and colonized infants and the use of a gown and gloves during an outbreak are recommended. Other methods of control (e.g., treatment of asymptomatic carriers with penicillin or treatment of the umbilical cord with triple dye or hexachlorophene) are impractical or unreliable.

- Routine hand washing by personnel caring for infants colonized or infected with GBS is recommended to prevent spread to other infants.

Non-Group A or B Streptococcal Infections

Clinical Manifestations: Streptococci of groups other than A or B may be associated with invasive disease in newborn infants, older children, and adults. Urinary tract infection, endocarditis, upper and lower respiratory tract infections, and meningitis are the principal clinical syndromes.

Etiology: Streptococcal groups D (enterococcal species, such as *Enterococcus faecalis*, and nonenterococcal species, such as *Streptococcus bovis* and *S equinus*), C and G are common pathogens. Streptococcal groups F, H (*S sanguis*), and K (*S salivarius*) are also potential pathogens. The association of streptococci of other groups with human infection is less clear. Nongroupable streptococci, such as *S viridans* and anaerobic streptococci (peptostreptococci), can be pathogenic in a variety of infections.

Epidemiology: The common habitats in humans of these streptococcal groups are skin (C, F, G), oropharynx (C, F, G, H, K), gastrointestinal tract (D, F, G), and vagina (C, D, F, G). The normal habitants of different species of *S viridans* include the oropharynx, teeth surfaces, skin, and the intestinal and genitourinary tracts. Intrapartum transmission probably causes early-onset neonatal infections.

The **incubation period** and the period of communicability are unknown.

Diagnostic Tests: Microscopic examination of fluids that are ordinarily sterile can yield presumptive evidence of Gram-positive coccal infections. The diagnosis is established by culture and serogrouping of the isolate, using group-specific antisera.

Treatment: Enterococcal group D streptococci and occasional strains from other groups (e.g., C and G) are less susceptible to penicillin and cephalosporins than are most other streptococcal isolates. In invasive enterococcal infections, including endocarditis, ampicillin or vancomycin in combination with an aminoglycoside should be used. A similar combination may be required for optimum treatment of serious groups C and G infections. In other situations, ampicillin or penicillin G alone is given.

Endocarditis. Guidelines for antimicrobial therapy have been formulated by the American Heart Association's Council on Cardiovascular Disease in the Young and should be consulted for appropriate regimens and details of therapy (Bisno et al. Antimicrobial treatment of infective endocarditis due to viridans steptococci, enterococci, and staphylococci. *JAMA*. 1989;261:1471-1477).

Isolation of the Hospitalized Patient: No special precautions are recommended.

Control Measures: Patients with valvular or congenital heart disease should receive antibiotic prophylaxis to prevent streptococcal endocarditis at the time of dental and selected other surgical procedures (see Prevention of Bacterial Endocarditis, page 536).

Strongyloidiasis

(Strongyloides stercoralis)

Clinical Manifestations: Asymptomatic infection is common. Infective larvae first entering the body can produce transient pruritic papules at the site of penetration of the skin, usually on the feet. Larval migration through the lungs can cause pneumonitis, with coughing productive of blood-streaked sputum. The intestinal phase of infection can be accompanied by vague abdominal pain, distention, vomiting, and diarrhea that consists of mucoid, voluminous stools. Malabsorption has been reported. In immunocompromised patients, complications include disseminated strongyloidiasis (due to hyperinfection), diffuse pulmonary infiltrates, and sepsis from Gram-negative bacilli.

Etiology: *Strongyloides stercoralis* is a nematode (roundworm).

Epidemiology: Strongyloidiasis is endemic in the tropics and subtropics, including the southern and southwestern United States, wherever suitable moist soil and improper disposal of human waste coexist. Humans are the principal hosts. Dogs, cats, and other animals may also be reservoirs. Transmission involves penetration of the skin by infective larvae, either from autoinfection or contact with infected soil. Because some larvae mature into the infective forms in the colon, autoinfection is a common, low-grade phenomenon with this parasite. In immunocompromised patients, autoinfection becomes more frequent and causes hyperinfection with resulting disseminated strongyloidiasis, in which the patient's organs and tissues become suffused with the larvae, and the number of adult worms in the small intestine becomes extraordinarily high. In addition, because these larvae penetrate the wall of the colon, bacteremia and meningitis with enteric flora can occur. Even mild immunosuppression associated with treatment with corticosteroids can precipitate hyperinfection. The period of communicability lasts as long as the patient is infected, which can be several decades.

The **incubation period** is not known.

Diagnostic Tests: Stool examination reveals the characteristic larvae, but several specimens may have to be examined before a positive one is found. The string test (Enterotest) or duodenal aspirate is more likely to show larvae. Serodiagnosis can be helpful but is only available in a few reference laboratories, and false negatives do occur. The ELISA test is positive in approximately 85% of cases. Cross-reaction with the antigens of filarial worms also occurs and limits the specificity of serodiagnosis. Eosinophilia (greater than 30%) is common. In disseminated strongyloidiasis, larvae can be found in the sputum.

Treatment: Thiabendazole (50 mg/kg/d, maximum 3 g, given in two divided doses for 2 days) is curative in most patients. Side effects of nausea, vomiting, and malaise are common. Treatment may have to be repeated or prolonged in the hyperinfection syndrome. Relapses occur and should be treated. Ivermectin given in a single dose has been reported to be effective in this infection.

Isolation of the Hospitalized Patient: No special precautions are recommended.

Control Measures: Sanitary disposal measures for human waste should be followed. Education about the risk of infection through bare skin is important. For the individual who has an immunologic defect or who requires immunosuppressive therapy, examination of the stool, and possibly duodenal fluid and respiratory secretions for *S ster-*

coralis, should be considered before immunosuppressive therapy is started. Serologic tests are perhaps the most sensitive for indicating infection but they do not distinguish between past and current infection. Persons with positive tests should have several stool examinations to demonstrate larvae; a string test may be necessary.

Syphilis

Clinical Manifestations:

Congenital Syphilis. This disease may have multisystem manifestations. It can result in stillbirth, liver failure, pneumonitis, or hemorrhage. Late manifestations of congenital syphilis can involve the central nervous system, bones, teeth, eighth nerve, eye, skin, and cartilage. Congenital syphilis can be asymptomatic, especially in the first weeks of life.

Acquired Syphilis. This disease can be divided into three stages. The primary stage appears as one or more painless, indurated ulcers of the skin and mucous membranes, most commonly on the genitalia but potentially involving any area of the body. The secondary stage is characterized by a rash, which can appear in many forms, but is most frequently maculopapular and classically involves the palms and soles. The mucous membranes can be involved (condyloma lata, mucous patches). Generalized lymphadenopathy, fever, malaise, splenomegaly, sore throat, headache, and arthralgia can be present. A variable latent period follows, which can be interrupted by recurrences of secondary syphilis symptoms. The tertiary stage is marked by aortitis, various neurologic abnormalities (neurosyphilis), and/or gummatous changes of the skin, bone, and/or viscera. These commonly occur 15 years or more after the primary infection, and, thus, have not been reported in children, except for meningovascular syphilis, which occurs earlier.

Etiology: *Treponema pallidum* is a thin, motile spirochete.

Epidemiology: Syphilis occurs throughout the world but is most frequent in large urban areas. In HIV-infected adults, syphilis is common and may be increased in severity. In adults in the United States infection in males is two times more common than in females, but the ratio is decreasing. In the pediatric age group, the disease is most common in adolescents. Congenital syphilis is acquired from an infected mother via transplacental or perinatal transmission of *T pallidum*. Transmission can occur at any time during pregnancy. In untreated early syphilis, 40% of pregnancies result in stillbirths or perinatal deaths. Infection also commonly occurs during or just before delivery.

Acquired syphilis is contracted from direct contact with ulcerative, denuded lesions of the skin or mucous membranes of infected persons. Acquired syphilis is almost always transmitted by sexual contact. The possibility of sexual abuse must be considered in any young child with acquired syphilis. Open, moist lesions of the primary or secondary stages teem with spirochetes. Infectious lesions usually do not occur more than 1 year after infection, although rare relapses with infectious secondary lesions have occurred as long as 4 years later. In untreated women, syphilis may be transmitted to the fetus, regardless of the duration of the disease; the rate is almost 100% during the secondary stage and slowly decreases with increasing duration of disease. The moist secretions of early congenital syphilis are also highly contagious. Organisms are rarely found in lesions more than 24 hours after treatment has begun.

The **incubation period** for acquired primary syphilis is typically about 3 weeks, but ranges from 10 to 90 days after exposure.

Diagnostic Tests: Spirochetes can be identified by microscopic darkfield examination. Specimens should be scraped from moist, mucocutaneous lesions or aspirated from a regional lymph node. Since false-negative results are common and the procedure may not be reliable in inexperienced hands, serologic testing, follow-up, and often repeated darkfield testing are necessary. Darkfield examinations of specimens from mouth lesions are difficult to interpret unless direct fluorescent antibody techniques are used because of the difficulty of distinguishing *T pallidum* from nonpathogenic treponemes by simple darkfield examination.

Serologic tests for syphilis provide only indirect evidence of infection. Serologic tests can be divided into two categories: (1) nontreponemal tests and (2) treponemal tests.

The nontreponemal tests for syphilis are flocculation tests using cardiolipin, lecithin, and cholesterol as antigen and include the Venereal Disease Reference Laboratory (VDRL) slide test, rapid plasma reagin card test (RPR), and the automated reagin test (ART). These tests measure antibody directed against lipoidal antigen that results from interaction of host tissues with *T pallidum* and/or from *T pallidum* itself. These tests are inexpensive, rapidly performed, and convenient for screening large numbers of sera. They provide quantitative results, which are helpful as indicators of disease activity and useful for follow-up after treatment. Nontreponemal tests may be falsely negative—i.e., nonreactive—in early primary, late acquired, and late congenital syphilis.

A reactive nontreponemal test from a patient with typical lesions usually indicates the need for treatment. However, any reactive nontreponemal test should be confirmed by one of the specific treponemal tests to exclude a false-positive test, which can be caused by conditions such as infectious mononucleosis, connective tissue disease, tuberculosis, and endocarditis. Treatment should not be delayed pending the treponemal test results in symptomatic patients or patients at high risk of infection. A sustained fourfold decrease in titer of the nontreponemal test with treatment demonstrates adequate therapy; a similar titer increase after treatment suggests reinfection or relapse. The quantitative nontreponemal test usually becomes nonreactive after successful therapy within 1 year in primary syphilis, and within 2 years in secondary syphilis.

Specific treponemal antibody serologic tests include the fluorescent treponemal antibody absorption (FTA-ABS) test, the microhemagglutination test for *T pallidum* (MHA-TP), and the *T pallidum* immobilization test (TPI). The latter has been the standard against which all subsequent tests have been compared, but it is rarely used today and is only available in a few laboratories. Positive FTA-ABS and MHA-TP tests usually remain reactive for life, even with successful therapy.

Treponemal specific serologic tests are also not 100% specific in the diagnosis of syphilis, particularly in subjects with other spirochetal diseases such as yaws, pinta, leptospirosis, rat-bite fever, and Lyme disease. However, nontreponemal serology can be used to differentiate Lyme disease from syphilis, as the VDRL is uniformly nonreactive in Lyme disease.

The usual sequence in performing these tests is initially a nontreponemal test followed by the more expensive and specific treponemal test on sera reactive in the nontreponemal test. The probability of syphilis is high in a sexually active patient whose serum is reactive on both a nontreponemal and a treponemal test. Western blot analysis and ELISA using *T pallidum* surface proteins have been successfully used to demonstrate specific IgG antibodies in sera from infected mothers and IgM antibodies in sera from their newborn infants. These tests as well as a new IgM fluorescent antibody test are currently investigational.

Testing During Pregnancy. All women should be screened serologically for syphilis early in pregnancy with a nontreponemal test (e.g., VDRL or RPR). In areas of high syphilis prevalence and in patients considered at high risk for syphilis, an additional nontreponemal test should be done at the beginning of the third trimester (28 weeks) and again at delivery. For those treated during pregnancy, follow-up serology is necessary to assess the efficacy of therapy.

Evaluation for Congenital Infection. The VDRL or RPR is commonly used to screen newborn infants for possible congenital infection with *T pallidum.* Serum from the infant is preferred to cord blood, since cord blood can produce false-positive results. A nonreactive VDRL in both the infected mother and infant can occur in a neonate with congenital syphilis if the mother acquired the disease late in pregnancy or in the case of a prozone phenomenon. Alternatively, the mother's test can be reactive and the infected infant's test is nonreactive, depending on the timing of maternal infection. A mother who has been treated appropriately for syphilis during pregnancy can still passively transfer both nontreponemal and treponemal antibodies to the fetus, resulting in positive VDRL and FTA-ABS tests in the newborn infant. The neonate's VDRL titer in these circumstances is usually less than or equal to the mother's titer and reverts to negative in 4 to 6 months, whereas a positive FTA-ABS test from passively acquired antibody may not become negative for 1 year or longer. The IgM FTS-ABS test is still experimental and may be unreliable. A reactive FTS-ABS test on the 19S fraction of serum is specific for IgM antibody and, thus, can be useful, but this test is not yet commercially available in the United States. Western blot analysis and ELISA using *T pallidum* surface proteins to detect IgM antibodies in the infants may also be helpful, but these tests are investigational and only available in a few laboratories. Thus, in an asymptomatic infant at birth, distinguishing between early infection and passive transfer of antibody from a previously treated mother remains difficult or impossible.

In a symptomatic infant with clinical and roentgenographic findings (e.g., metaphysitis of the long bones) suggestive of congenital syphilis, a positive VDRL and/or FTA-ABS test in serum strongly supports the diagnosis regardless of the therapy the mother received during the pregnancy.

Cerebrospinal Fluid (CSF) Tests. CFS should be examined in all patients with suspected or proven congenital syphilis, suspected neurosyphilis, or acquired, untreated syphilis of more than 1 year's duration. The CSF abnormalities in patients with neurosyphilis include increased protein and cell count and a reactive VDRL. However, the wide range of normal values for CSF white blood cell counts and protein concentrations in the newborn make interpretation of results difficult. Beyond the neonatal period, normal CSF findings differentiate latent syphilis from asymptomatic neurosyphilis in patients with acquired, untreated syphilis of more than 1 year's duration. The RPR and FTA-ABS tests should not be used for CSF evaluation. Results of CSF VDRL tests should also be interpreted cautiously since a negative VDRL does not exclude neurosyphilis and the CSF VDRL can be positive in an uninfected newborn with a transplacentally acquired high-serum VDRL titer.

In summary, the nontreponemal antibody tests (VDRL, RPR, and ART) are useful for screening; the treponemal specific tests (FTA-ABS, MHA-TP) are used to substantiate the diagnosis. Quantitative nontreponemal antibody tests are used to assess the adequacy of therapy and to detect reinfection and relapse.

Treatment:

Congenital Syphilis (see Table 51 for summary of these recommendations). In infants with proven or highly probable disease, aqueous crystalline penicillin G is preferred. The dosage should be based on chronologic, not gestational age. The recommended dosage is 50,000 U/kg per dose given IV or IM every 12 hours in the first week (100,000 U/kg/d), and every 8 hours up to 28 days of age (150,000 U/kg/d) for 10 to 14 days. Alternatively, some experts recommend aqueous procaine penicillin G (50,000 U/kg, intramuscularly, daily) for a minimum of 10 days.

Because of the difficulty in establishing the diagnosis of neurosyphilis, all infants diagnosed after 4 weeks of age should be treated with aqueous crystalline penicillin, 50,000 U/kg every 6 hours (200,000 U/kg/d) given intravenously for 10 to 14 days. Similarly, children older than 1 year, with late and previously untreated congenital syphilis, should receive intravenous aqueous crystalline penicillin therapy as previously described. Some experts suggest giving such patients three doses of benzathine penicillin G, 50,000 U/kg, intramuscularly, weekly for three weeks if CSF examination has excluded neurosyphilis.

Asymptomatic infants born to mothers who received adequate penicillin treatment for syphilis during pregnancy, although at minimal risk for congenital syphilis, should be examined carefully and at frequent intervals, preferably monthly, until the nontreponemal serologic test results are negative. Recommendations for management are as follows:

1. If maternal treatment was inadequate, unknown, or undocumented, or erythromycin was given, infants should be treated with aqueous crystalline penicillin G (or aqueous procaine penicillin G) for 10 days. Alternatively, for those infants for whom adequate maternal treatment cannot be documented, some experts would give single-dose therapy with benzathine penicillin G, as subsequently described.
2. If adequate treatment was given in the last month of pregnancy and a complete evaluation of the infant, including CSF examination and radiographs, is normal, a single intramuscular dose of 50,000 U/kg of benzathine penicillin G can be given as an alternative to aqueous crystalline penicillin G or aqueous procaine penicillin G.

Table 51. Recommended Treatment of Congenital Syphilis

Clinical Status	Antibiotic Therapy*
Proved or highly probable disease	
Age: ≤ 4 weeks	Aqueous crystalline penicillin G, IV or IM, for 10-14 days†
> 4 weeks	Aqueous crystalline penicillin G, IV or IM, for 10-14 days‡
Asymptomatic infant with normal CSF and radiographic examinations	
Maternal Treatment	
None, inadequate, undocumented, or with erythromycin	Aqueous crystalline penicillin G, IV or IM, for 10 days†,§
Adequate therapy given in last month before delivery	Aqueous crystalline penicillin G, IV or IM, for 10 days† or benzathine penicillin G, IM, single dose
Adequate therapy given > 1 month before delivery	Clinical and serologic follow-up only, OR if follow-up cannot be ensured, benzathine penicillin G, IM, single dose, or aqueous crystalline penicillin G, IV or IM, for 10 days†

*See text for drug dosages and details.

†Some experts recommend aqueous procaine penicillin G, IM, for 10-14 days.

‡For those with late (> 1 year of age) congenital syphilis in whom CSF findings exclude neurosyphilis, some experts recommend benzathine penicillin G IM weekly for 3 weeks.

§Alternatively, for the infant for whom adequate maternal treatment cannot be documented, some experts recommend single-dose therapy with benzathine penicillin G.

3. Asymptomatic infants born to mothers who have received adequate treatment more than 1 month before delivery, with positive nontreponemal tests that are considered secondary to passively transferred antibody can be managed without antibiotic therapy if clinical and serologic follow-up can be ensured. If follow-up cannot be assured but the infant is considered to be at

low risk of having congenital syphilis, treatment should be given with the single-dose regimen of intramuscular benzathine penicillin G (50,000 U/kg). Alternatively, some experts recommend a 10-day course of treatment of aqueous crystalline penicillin G (or aqueous procaine penicillin G) in the previously described regimen, for reasons of possible greater efficacy.

Syphilis in Pregnancy. Regardless of the stage of pregnancy, patients who are not allergic to penicillin should be treated with penicillin according to the dosage schedules appropriate for the stage of syphilis as recommended for nonpregnant patients. For penicillin-allergic patients, penicillin may be given provided (1) their skin test reactions to the major and minor penicillin determinants are negative, or (2) their skin tests are positive, but they are then desensitized to penicillin. Patients can be desensitized and then given standard penicillin doses. Desensitization should be performed in consultation with an expert and only in facilities, such as a hospital, where emergency assistance is available.

Tetracycline is not recommended for pregnant women because of potential adverse effects on the fetus. Erythromycin treatment of syphilis during pregnancy is generally discouraged. It should be considered only for patients who have documented evidence of a penicillin allergy (skin test or history of anaphylaxis) and who are not candidates for penicillin desensitization. Physicians choosing erythromycin treatment assume a major responsibility for close clinical follow-up of both the mother and fetus to assess the possibilities of treatment failure. All infants born to mothers who were diagnosed with syphilis during pregnancy should be evaluated for congenital syphilis, including an examination of the CSF.

Early Acquired Syphilis (primary, secondary, latent syphilis of less than 1 year's duration). Benzathine penicillin G, intramuscularly, in a total dose of 50,000 U/kg, not to exceed 2.4 million units, is the preferred treatment.

For patients allergic to penicillin, tetracycline (adult dose, 500 mg four times a day, orally) or doxycycline (adult dose 100 mg orally twice daily) usually should be given for 2 weeks. Tetracycline or doxycycline should not be given to children younger than 9 years unless the benefits of therapy are clearly greater than the risks of dental staining. Some older patients cannot tolerate this dose of tetracycline. Drugs other than penicillin and tetracycline do not have proven efficacy in the treatment of syphilis. For penicillin-allergic patients, especially children younger than 9 years, consideration must be given to hospitalization and desensitization followed by administration of penicillin. If erythromycin is used, the adult dose recommended is 500 mg four times a day for 2 weeks. If compliance and serologic follow-up cannot be assured, the patient should be hospitalized and managed in consultation with an expert.

Syphilis of More Than 1 Year's Duration (except neurosyphilis). Benzathine penicillin G, at a dose of 50,000 U/kg, intramuscularly, weekly (not to exceed 2.4 million units) for 3 successive weeks, can be used. In patients who are allergic to penicillin, either tetracycline (adult dose, 500 mg four times a day, orally) or doxycycline (adult dose, 100 mg, orally, twice daily) for 4 weeks should be given only if CSF examination has excluded neurosyphilis. Tetracycline or doxycycline should not be given to children younger than 9 years unless the benefits of therapy clearly are greater than the risks of dental staining. Examination of the CSF (VDRL, protein, and cell count) is mandatory for those with suspected or symptomatic neurosyphilis, those who have concurrent HIV infection, those who have failed treatment, and for those receiving antibiotics other than penicillin. CSF examination is recommended for all patients with syphilis for more than 1 year to exclude asymptomatic neurosyphilis.

Neurosyphilis. The recommended regimen for adults is aqueous crystalline penicillin G, 12 to 24 million units daily (2 to 4 million units every 4 hours) intravenously for 10 to 14 days. Many authorities recommend following this regimen with benzathine penicillin G, 2.4 million units, intramuscularly, given weekly for 3 successive weeks. In children, aqueous crystalline penicillin G, 200,000 to 300,000 U/kg/d (50,000 U/kg every 4 to 6 hours) for 10 to 14 days, in doses not to exceed the adult dose, is recommended, possibly followed by benzathine penicillin, 50,000 U/kg per dose (not to exceed 2.4 million units) in three weekly doses.

An alternative regimen, if outpatient compliance can be ensured, is aqueous procaine penicillin G, 2.4 million units, intramuscularly, daily, plus probenecid, 500 mg, orally, four times a day; both should be given for 10 to 14 days, possibly followed by benzathine penicillin G, 2.4 million units, intramuscularly, given weekly for 3 successive weeks.

If the patient has a history of allergy to penicillin, the patient should be managed in consultation with an expert. The allergy should be confirmed and consideration given to desensitization.

Follow-up and Retreatment.

Congenital Syphilis. Infants should have frequent follow-up evaluations, which can be performed at the usual ages of routine infant care (i.e., at 1, 2, 4, 6, and 12 months). Serologic nontreponemal tests should be performed 3, 6, and 12 months after the conclusion of treatment, or until they become nonreactive. Patients with persistent, stable titers, including those with low titers, should be considered for retreatment.

Infants with congenital neurosyphilis and initially positive CSF VDRL tests should undergo repeat clinical evaluation and CSF examination at 6-month intervals for at least 3 years or until their CSF examination is normal. A reactive CSF VDRL at 6 months is an indication for retreatment.

Early Acquired Syphilis. Pregnant women with early acquired syphilis should have quantitative nontreponemal serologic tests performed monthly for the remainder of their pregnancy. Other patients with early acquired syphilis should return for repeat quantitative nontreponemal tests at 3, 6, and 12 months after the conclusion of treatment. Patients with syphilis for more than 1 year should also undergo serologic testing 24 months after treatment. Careful follow-up serologic testing is particularly important in patients treated with antibiotics other than penicillin.

Retreatment is indicated in the following circumstances:

- The clinical signs or symptoms of syphilis persist or recur.
- A sustained, fourfold increase in the titer of a nontreponemal test occurs; in a pregnant woman, a fourfold increase in titer alone is an indication for retreatment.
- An initially high-titer, nontreponemal test fails to decrease fourfold within a year, or in a pregnant woman within a 3-month period.

Retreated patients should be treated with the schedules recommended for patients with syphilis for more than 1 year. In general, only one retreatment course is indicated. The possibility of reinfection or concurrent HIV infection should always be considered when retreating patients with early syphilis.

The CSF should be examined before retreatment unless reinfection and a diagnosis of early syphilis can be established. Patients with neurosyphilis must be followed up with periodic serologic testing and clinical evaluation at 6-month intervals and repeat CSF examinations for at least 3 years or until CSF examination is normal.

Isolation of the Hospitalized Patient: Drainage/secretion precautions in addition to the routinely recommended blood/body fluid precautions (see Isolation Precautions, page 81) are indicated for all infants with suspected or proven congenital syphilis until therapy has been administered for at least 24 hours. Parents, visitors, and medical staff should use gloves when handling the infant. Because moist, open lesions and potentially blood are contagious in all forms of syphilis, these precautions are also required for primary and secondary syphilis with skin and mucous membrane lesions. Precautions are not indicated otherwise, i.e., for those with tertiary syphilis or those who are seropositive but have no lesions.

Control Measures:

- All women should be screened for syphilis during pregnancy (see Diagnostic Tests, page 454).
- Education about sexually transmitted diseases, treatment of sexual contacts, reporting of each case to local public health authorities for contact investigation and appropriate follow-up, and serologic screening of high-risk populations are indicated.
- All recent sexual contacts of a person with acquired syphilis should be identified, examined, serologically tested and treated appropriately. Sexual contacts within the last 3 months who are seronegative are at high risk for early syphilis and should be treated for early acquired syphilis. Every effort, including physical examination and serologic testing, should be made to establish a diagnosis in these patients.
- All individuals, including hospital personnel, who have had close, *unprotected* contact with a patient with early congenital syphilis before identification of the disease or during the first 24 hours of therapy should be examined clinically for the presence of lesions 2 to 3 weeks after contact. Serologic testing should be performed and repeated 3 months after contact, or sooner if symptoms occur.

Tapeworm Diseases

(Taeniasis, Cysticercosis)

Clinical Manifestations: Infection with the adult stage beef or pork tapeworm usually is asymptomatic. Many patients become aware of the infection by noting segments of tapeworm in their stools. Abdominal pain, nausea, diarrhea, excessive appetite, and other symptoms are reported by some patients. Usually only a single tapeworm is present. The larval form of the pork tapeworm also infects humans and causes cysticercosis. This infection results in space-occupying lesions in the muscles, viscera, and brain, frequently manifested by convulsions. In hyperendemic areas, cysticercosis is the most common cause of seizures after the age of 5 years. The eyes can also be involved, resulting in uveitis or retinal masses, which can cause retinal detachment.

Etiology: Intestinal tapeworm infections are caused by *Taenia saginata* (beef tapeworm) and *T solium* (pork tapeworm). Cysticercosis is caused by the larvae of *T solium*.

Epidemiology: *T saginata* is widespread in areas where cattle are raised and disposal of human feces is improper, or where human feces are used as fertilizer. Hence, large areas of Africa and Central and South America, and some parts of Europe and Asia are endemic areas. The infection can be acquired in the United States, but most cases in this country are imported.

T solium has a similar mode of spread, except that it parasitizes pigs instead of cattle. It is prevalent in parts of Southeast Asia, Africa, Micronesia, Mexico, Central and South America, and Eastern Europe. Few cases of the disease are acquired in the United States, but imported cases occur frequently. Consumption of raw or undercooked beef and pork with the encysted parasites results in tapeworm infections. Cysticercosis in humans results from ingestion of eggs from the environment and probably from autoinfection.

Diagnostic Tests: Diagnosis of tapeworm infection is based on demonstration of the proglottids or ova in the feces. In cysticercosis, lesions can be biopsied if they are safely accessible (e.g., subcutaneous), or they may be demonstrated with computed tomography or magnetic resonance imaging if they are not accessible (e.g., intracerebral). Stool examinations are not helpful in evaluating patients for cysticercosis. Serologic tests, available at the Centers for Disease Control, are helpful but require interpretation.

Treatment: Niclosamide,* which is given orally, is a drug of choice for both of these intestinal tapeworm infections. Single-dose praziquantel is also effective but more expensive.

Praziquantel in high doses for 3 to 7 days is the drug of choice in the United States for cerebral cysticercosis. Most experts administer corticosteroids before and during therapy to reduce the intensity of the inflammatory reaction that follows destruction of the worms. However, use of dexamethasone is associated with decreased plasma concentrations of praziquantel. Ocular cysticercosis is usually not treated with praziquantel because severe inflammatory and immune mediated reactions can occur. Albendazole is also effective, but is not yet available in the United States.

Isolation of the Hospitalized Patient: No special precautions are recommended.

Control Measures: Avoidance of ingesting raw or undercooked meat and sanitary disposal procedures for feces are indicated.

---

*Available from Miles Inc., Pharmaceutical Division, West Haven, CT.

Other Tapeworm Infections

Most infections are asymptomatic, but nausea, abdominal pain, and diarrhea have been observed in persons who are heavily infested.

Hymenolepis nana. This tapeworm, also called "dwarf tapeworm," has its entire cycle within humans. Therefore, person-to-person transmission is possible. More problematic is autoinfection, which tends to perpetuate the infection in the host because the eggs can hatch within the intestine and re-initiate the cycle, leading to the development of new worms. This cycle makes eradicating the infection with niclosamide* difficult. If infection persists after treatment with niclosamide, praziquantel should be administered. Repeated treatment may be necessary.

Dipylidium caninum. This tapeworm, with the dog or cat flea as its intermediate host, infects children when they inadvertently swallow a flea while playing with a pet. Diagnosis is made by finding the characteristic eggs or tapeworm segments in the stool. Treatment consists of niclosamide*; praziquantel is an alternative choice, and is given in the same doses as for *Taenia* infections.

Diphyllobothrium latum (and related species). This tapeworm, also called "fish tapeworm," has fish as one of its intermediate hosts. Consumption of infected raw, freshwater fish (including salmon) leads to the infection. The worm sometimes causes megaloblastic anemia. The diagnosis is made by recognition of the characteristic eggs or proglottids passed in the stool. Therapy with niclosamide* is effective; praziquantel is an alternative. Both are given in a single dose. Hydroxocobalamin injections and folic acid supplements may be required.

Echinococcus granulosus* and *E multilocularis. These tapeworms are the causes of hydatid disease. The distribution of *E granulosus* is related to sheep or cattle herding. Countries with the highest prevalence (in alphabetical order) are Argentina, Greece, Italy, Lebanon, Romania, South Africa, Spain, Syria, Turkey, and the Soviet Union. In the United States, small endemic foci exist in Arizona, California, New Mexico, and Utah. Dogs, coyotes, wolves, dingos, and jackals can become infected by swallowing protoscolices of the parasite within hydatid cysts in the organs of sheep or other intermediate hosts. Dogs pass embryonated eggs in their stools, and the sheep become infected by swallowing the eggs. If humans swallow echinococcus eggs, they can become inadvertent intermediate hosts and develop cysts in various organs, such as the liver, lungs, kidney, and spleen. These cysts grow slowly (1 cm in diameter per year) and eventually can contain several liters of fluid. If a cyst ruptures,

*Available from Miles Inc., Pharmaceutical Division, West Haven, CT.

anaphylaxis and multiple secondary cysts from seeding of protoscolices can result. Clinical diagnosis is frequently difficult. A history of contact with dogs in an endemic area is helpful. Space-occupying lesions can be demonstrated by roentgenograms or scanning of various organs. Serologic tests, available at the Centers for Disease Control, are helpful, but they are not always positive. Surgical treatment is indicated in some patients and requires meticulous care to prevent spillage of the cyst contents. Injection of a 0.1% cetrimide solution into the cyst before attempted removal can minimize the risk of dissemination if spillage occurs. Treatment with albendazole (10 mg/kg/d) for several months has been of benefit in many cases. *E multilocularis*, a species whose life cycle involves foxes and rodents, causes the alveolar form of hydatid disease, which is characterized by invasive growth of the larvae in the liver with occasional metastatic spread. The alveolar form of hydatid disease is limited to the Northern hemisphere and is usually diagnosed in persons 50 years or older. The preferred treatment is surgical extirpation of the entire larval mass. In nonresectable cases, continuous treatment with mebendazole has been associated with clinical improvement.

Tetanus (Lockjaw)

Clinical Manifestations: Tetanus (lockjaw) is a neurologic disease with severe muscular spasms caused by the neurotoxin produced by *Clostridium tetani* in a contaminated wound. Onset is gradual, occurring during 1 to 7 days, and progresses to severe generalized muscle spasms, which frequently are aggravated by any external stimulus. Severe spasms persist for 1 week or more and subside in a period of weeks in those who recover. Neonatal tetanus, a common cause of neonatal mortality in developing countries but rare in the United States, arises from contamination of the umbilical stump. Local tetanus is manifested by local muscle spasms in areas contiguous to a wound.

Etiology: *C tetani*, the tetanus bacillus, is a spore-forming, anaerobic, Gram-positive bacillus that produces a potent exotoxin (tetanospasmin), which binds to the central nervous system tissues.

Epidemiology: Tetanus occurs worldwide and is more frequent in warmer climates and months, in part because of the frequency of contaminated wounds. The organism, a normal inhabitant of soil and of animal and human intestines, is ubiquitous in the environment, especially at sites likely to have been contaminated by excreta. Wounds, recognized or unrecognized, are the sites at which the organism multiplies and elaborates toxin. Contaminated wounds, those with devitalized tissue and deep-puncture trauma are at greatest risk. Neonatal tetanus is common in many countries where women do not receive tetanus immunizations. Widespread active immunization against tetanus has vastly modified the epidemiology of the disease in the United States. Tetanus is not transmissible from person to person.

The **incubation period** is 3 days to 3 weeks; the average is 8 days. In neonates it is usually 5 to 14 days. Shorter incubation periods historically have been associated with more heavily contaminated wounds, more severe disease, and a worse prognosis. Recent experience in the United States does not confirm such a relationship.

Diagnostic Tests: The offending wound should be cultured. However, etiologic confirmation is made infrequently by culture. The diagnosis is made clinically by excluding other possibilities.

Treatment:

- Tetanus Immune Globulin (TIG) (Human) is recommended for treatment. A single dose of 3,000 to 6,000 U is recommended; the optimum therapeutic dose has not yet been established. Preparations currently available must be given intramuscularly, with part of the dose infiltrated locally around the wound, although the efficacy of this approach has not been established. The result of studies on the benefit from intrathecal TIG are conflicting. The TIG formulation in use in the United States is not licensed or appropriate for intrathecal or intravenous use.
- Equine tetanus antitoxin (TAT) should be used if TIG is not available. TAT is administered as a single dose of 50,000 to 100,000 U after appropriate testing for sensitivity, and desensitization if necessary (see Sensitivity Tests for Reactions to Animal Sera, page 40, and "Desensitization" for Animal Sera, page 41). Part of this dose (20,000 U) should be given intravenously. Serum sickness occurs in 10 to 20% of recipients of equine serum.
- Immune Globulin Intravenous (IGIV) (Human) contains antibodies to tetanus and can be considered for treatment if TIG is not available. FDA approval has not been given for this use and the dosage has not been determined.
- Parenteral penicillin G (100,000 U/kg/d, given at 4- to 6-hour intervals) or a tetracycline (which should not be given to children younger than 9 years) is effective in reducing the number of vegetative forms of the organism. Therapy for 10 to 14 days is recommended.
- All wounds should be properly cleaned and debrided when indicated, especially if extensive necrosis is present. In neonatal tetanus, wide excision of the umbilical stump is not indicated.
- Supportive care is of major importance.

Isolation of the Hospitalized Patient: No special precautions are recommended.

Control Measures:

Care of Exposed Persons (Table 52). Less than 1% of the recently reported cases of tetanus in the United States have occurred in individuals with adequate, up-to-date immunization. After primary immunization with tetanus toxoid, antitoxin persists at protective levels in most persons for at least 10 years, and for a longer time after a booster immunization. Boosters need to be given as soon as possible after the injury.

- In the management of clean, minor wounds in those who have completed a primary series of tetanus toxoid or received a booster dose within 10 years, a dose of tetanus toxoid is not necessary.
- For other, more serious wounds (such as those contaminated with dirt, feces, soil, and/or saliva, puncture wounds, and those with devitalized tissue, a dose of tetanus toxoid should be given as soon as possible after the injury, according to the guidelines in Table 52. Indications for TIG or antitoxin use in partially immunized persons with more serious wounds are also listed in Table 52. If tetanus immunization is incomplete at the time of wound treatment, a dose should be given, and the series should be completed according to the primary immunization schedule. TIG should be administered for tetanus-prone wounds in AIDS patients, regardless of the history of tetanus immunizations.
- In usual practice, when tetanus toxoid is required for wound prophylaxis in a child 7 years or older, the use of Td instead of tetanus toxoid alone is advisable so that adequate levels of diphtheria immunity can also be maintained. When a booster injection is indicated for wound prophylaxis in a child younger than 7 years, DTP should be used unless pertussis vaccine is contraindicated (see Pertussis, page 366), in which case immunization with DT is recommended.
- Passive protection with TIG or antitoxin is not indicated for patients with clean, minor wounds, regardless of immunization status, or for patients with other wounds who have had three or more previous injections of tetanus toxoid. Patients with more serious wounds who have had less than three previous injections of tetanus vaccine should receive TIG or antitoxin as well as an additional dose of tetanus toxoid within 3 days. TIG is recommended in a dose of 250 to 500 U, intramuscularly. TAT is used if TIG is unavailable; the dose is 3,000 to 5,000 U intramuscularly, after appropriate testing of the patient for sensitivity (see Sensitivity Tests for Reactions to Animal Sera, page 40). If tetanus toxoid and TIG or TAT are given concurrently, separate syringes

Table 52. Guide to Tetanus Prophylaxis in Wound Management

History of Tetanus Immunization (doses)	Clean, Minor Wounds*		All Other Wounds†	
	Td	TIG	Td	TIG
Uncertain or less than 3	Yes	No	Yes	Yes
3 or more‡	No§	No	No‖	No

*Td = adult-type tetanus and diphtheria toxoids. If the patient is younger than 7 years, DT or DTP is given (see text). TIG = tetanus immune globulin.

†Including but not limited to wounds contaminated with dirt, feces, soil, saliva, etc; puncture wounds, avulsions; and wounds resulting from missiles, crushing, burns, and frostbite.

‡If only three doses of fluid toxoid have been received, a fourth dose of toxoid, preferably an adsorbed toxoid, should be given.

§Yes, if more than 10 years since the last dose.

‖Yes, if more than 5 years since the last dose.

and sites should be used. Administration of TIG or TAT does not preclude initiation of tetanus toxoid active immunization. Efforts should be made to both initiate immunization and arrange for its completion.

- Regardless of immunization status, all wounds should be properly cleaned and debrided. Wounds should receive prompt surgical treatment to remove all devitalized tissue and foreign material as an essential part of tetanus prophylaxis.

Immunization. Active immunization with tetanus toxoid is indicated for all persons (see Tables 2 and 3, pages 17 and 18). Adsorbed tetanus toxoid* is preferred to fluid toxoid because of longer lasting immunity.

- Immunization for children from 2 months to the seventh birthday (see Tables 2 and 3, pages 17 and 18) should consist of three initial doses of DTP vaccine given intramuscularly at 2-month intervals; a fourth dose is recommended at 18 months of age; and a fifth dose is given before school entry (kindergarten or elementary school) at 4 to 6 years of age, unless the fourth dose was given after the fourth birthday.† The series should begin at 2 months of age. The fourth dose can be given at 15 months and concurrently with MMR, OPV, and *Haemophilus* conjugate vaccine (HbCV).

*Tetanus toxoid vaccines in use in the United States are adsorbed aluminum salts.

†The Immunization Practices Advisory Committee (ACIP) of the U.S. Public Health Service defines primary immunization as consisting of the first four doses; the fifth dose is considered a booster.

- Children younger than 7 years in whom pertussis immunization is deferred or contraindicated (see Pertussis, page 366) should be immunized with DT instead of DTP. For children younger than 1 year, three doses of DT are given at 2-month intervals; a fourth dose should be given approximately 6 to 12 months after the third dose, usually at 15 to 18 months of age; and the fifth dose is given before school entry at 4 to 6 years of age. Children who have not received prior doses of DT or DTP and who are 1 year or older should receive two doses of DT approximately 2 months apart, followed by a third dose 6 to 12 months after the second dose to complete the initial series. DT can be given concurrently with other vaccines (MMR, OPV, and HbCV). An additional dose is necessary before school entry when the child is 4 to 6 years old, unless the fourth dose was given after the fourth birthday.
- Children who have received one or two doses of DTP (or DT) in the first year of life and for whom further pertussis vaccination is contraindicated should receive additional doses of DT until a total of five doses of diphtheria and tetanus toxoids are received by the time of school entry. The fourth dose is administered 6 to 12 months after the third dose. The preschool (fifth) dose is omitted if the fourth dose was given after the fourth birthday.
- Children 7 years and older and adults not previously immunized should receive Td, i.e., adult-type tetanus and diphtheria toxoids (see Table 3, page 18). The Td preparation contains not more than 2 Lf (flocculating units) of diphtheria toxoid per dose, as compared to 7 to 25 Lf in the DTP and DT preparations for use in infants and younger children. Td is less likely than DTP or DT to produce reactions in older children and adults. Two doses of Td are given 1 to 2 months apart; a third dose should be given 6 to 12 months after the second.
- After the initial immunization series is completed, a booster dose of tetanus toxoid should be given intramuscularly every 10 years. This 10-year period is determined from the last dose administered irrespective of whether it was given earlier in routine childhood immunization or as part of wound management. The immunity conferred by adsorbed preparations of tetanus toxoid has proved to be of long duration; therefore, routine boosters at intervals more frequent than 10 years are not indicated and may be associated with an increased incidence and severity of reactions.
- Prevention of neonatal tetanus can be accomplished by prenatal immunization of the previously unimmunized mother. Two doses should be administered at least 4 weeks apart and the second dose should be given at least 2 weeks before delivery. Booster immunization is not contraindicated during pregnancy.

- Additional measures include community immunization programs for adolescent girls and women of childbearing age and appropriate training of midwives.
- Active immunization against tetanus should always be undertaken during convalescence from tetanus because this exotoxin-mediated disease does not necessarily confer immunity.
- If more than 5 years have elapsed since the last dose, a booster of Td should be considered for persons who are going to summer camps or on wilderness expeditions where tetanus boosters may not be readily available.

Other Control Measures. Sterilization of hospital supplies will prevent the infrequent instances of tetanus which may occur in a hospital from contaminated sutures, instruments, or plaster casts.

Tinea Capitis

(Ringworm of the Scalp)

Clinical Manifestations: Erythema and scaling of the scalp with short broken hairs and localized alopecia are frequent; mild folliculitis or a tender, boggy, suppurative-appearing kerion (a hypersensitivity reaction to the fungal infection) can be seen. The severe inflammatory type of tinea may be associated with fever and regional lymphadenopathy. Tinea capitis can be confused with many other diseases, including seborrheic dermatitis, psoriasis, alopecia areata, trichotillomania, folliculitis, impetigo, and lupus erythematosus.

Etiology: Fungi of the genera *Microsporum* and *Trichophyton* are causes, especially *T tonsurans*, *M canis*, *T mentagrophytes*, and *T verrucosum*. In recent years, *T tonsurans* has been the predominant cause in most areas of the United States.

Epidemiology: Tinea capitis occurs primarily between the ages of 2 and 10 years. It rarely affects infants, and infections beyond puberty are uncommon. Minor trauma can initiate infection. Transmission is by personal contact; combs, brushes and barbers' instruments have also been implicated. Both humans and lower animals are sources of infection. The infection is communicable for as long as fungi can be cultured from the infected area or demonstrated by Wood's light fluorescence.

Diagnostic Tests: Fungal culture or demonstration of fungus by potassium hydroxide wet mount preparation can establish the diagnosis. Dermatophyte test medium (DTM) will turn from yellow to red in the area surrounding a dermatophyte colony and is a useful diagnostic aid. Examination for fluorescence under a Wood's light can aid in diagnosis. Fluorescent fungal species include *M audouini* and *M canis* (brilliant green fluorescence) and *T schoenleini* (pale green fluorescence); infections caused by *T tonsurans* (currently the most common fungus infecting the scalp) and *T violaceum* do not fluoresce. Bluish or purplish fluorescence may be produced by lint, scales, serum exudate, or ointments containing petrolatum. Microscopic examination of a potassium hydroxide preparation of infected hair may reveal tiny arthrospores surrounding the hair shaft in *Microsporum* species infection and chains of arthroconidia within the hair shaft in *T tonsurans* and *T violaceum* infections.

Treatment: Microcrystalline griseofulvin, orally, in a dose of 10 to 20 mg/kg/d (usually 125 to 150 mg/d for children weighing 30 to 50 lb, and 250 to 300 mg/d for those weighing more than 50 lb) is an effective treatment. The dose of ultramicrocrystalline griseofulvin (in polyethylene glycol) is one half the dose of the microcrystalline preparation. The drug is given in two daily doses, and optimally after a meal containing fat (e.g., milk or ice cream). Usually 4 to 8 weeks of treatment are necessary. In rare cases where griseofulvin is not tolerated, ketoconazole in a dose of 3 to 4 mg/kg/d can be given, but side effects are greater. In resistant cases with kerion formation, the combination of oral prednisone and griseofulvin can be helpful.

Concomitant topical therapy with 2.5% selenium sulfide shampoos twice weekly may be beneficial in limiting spread to adjacent areas and to contacts, as it enhances elimination of spores. Topical therapy alone, however, is ineffective.

Isolation of the Hospitalized Patient: No special precautions are recommended.

Control Measures: Detection and treatment of infected persons is indicated. More than a third of adults and children living in the home of an infected child have scalp cultures positive for fungus. Examinations should be performed at regular intervals to detect early cases. Hair cuts, shaving the head, or wearing a cap is not necessary when the patient is treated. Personal contact with hair and the sharing of hair care products should be avoided. Barber tools should be cleaned and sterilized.

Tinea Corporis

(Ringworm of the Body)

Clinical Manifestations: Superficial tinea infections of the nonhairy (glabrous) skin involve the face, trunk, and limbs, but not the scalp, beard, groin, hands, and feet. The lesion is generally circular (hence, the term ringworm) and slightly erythematous; it is well demarcated, and has a scaly, vesicular, or pustular border. Pruritis is common. A frequent source of confusion in diagnosis is an alteration of appearance of lesions resulting from topical corticosteroid application. This atypical presentation has been termed "tinea incognita."

Etiology: The prime causes of the disease are fungi of the genera *Trichophyton*, especially *T rubrum* and *T mentagrophytes*; *Microsporum*, especially *M canis*; and *Epidermophyton floccosum*.

Epidemiology: The fungi occur worldwide and are transmissible by direct contact with infected humans, animals, or fomites. Fungi in the lesions are communicable.

Diagnosis: The organisms can be identified by microscopic examination of the scrapings in a potassium hydroxide mount. They can be isolated by culture on Sabouraud's medium supplemented with cycloheximide and chloramphenicol. Dermatophyte test medium (DTM) will turn from yellow to red in the area surrounding a dermatophyte colony and is a useful diagnostic aid.

Treatment: Topical application of miconazole, clotrimazole, haloprogin, econazole, tolnaftate, naftifine, or ciclopirox preparation twice daily, or ketoconazole, oxiconazole, or sulconazole preparation once daily, is recommended.* Although clinical resolution may be evident within 2 weeks, a minimum duration of 4 weeks is generally indicated. If the lesions are extensive or unresponsive to topical therapy, griseofulvin is administered orally for 4 weeks (see Tinea Capitis, page 471).

Isolation of the Hospitalized Patient: No special precautions are recommended.

Control Measures: Direct contact with known or suspected sources of infection should be avoided. Periodic inspections of contacts for early lesions and prompt therapy are recommended.

---

*See Topical Drugs for Superficial Fungal Infections, page 576.

Tinea Cruris

(Jock Itch)

Clinical Manifestations: Tinea cruris is an extremely common superficial fungal disorder of the groin and upper thighs. The eruption is sharply marginated and usually bilaterally symmetric. Involved skin is erythematous and scaly, and varies in color from red to brown; occasionally it is accompanied by central clearing and a vesiculopapular border. In chronic infections, the active margin can be subtle, and lichenification can be present. Tinea cruris may be extremely pruritic. It should be differentiated from intertrigo, seborrheic dermatitis, psoriasis, primary irritant dermatitis, allergic contact dermatitis (generally caused by the therapeutic agents applied to the area), or erythrasma (a superficial bacterial infection of the skin caused by *Corynebacterium minitussimum*).

Etiology: The fungi *Epidermophyton floccosum*, *Trichophyton rubrum*, and *T mentagrophytes* are the causes. This infection is commonly seen in association with tinea pedis.

Epidemiology: Tinea cruris occurs predominantly in adolescent and adult males. Moisture, close-fitting garments, friction, and obesity are predisposing factors. Direct or indirect person-to-person transmission may occur.

Diagnostic Tests: The fungi responsible for tinea cruris may be detected using potassium hydroxide microscopic examination of scales, and may be identified by fungal cultures. A characteristic, coral-red fluorescence under Wood's light can identify the presence of erythrasma and, thus, exclude tinea cruris.

Treatment: Topical application for 3 to 4 weeks of clotrimazole, haloprogin, econazole, miconazole, tolnaftate, or ciclopirox preparation gently rubbed into the affected areas and surrounding skin twice daily, or topical ketoconazole, naftifine, oxiconazole, or sulconazole preparation once daily is effective.* Topical preparations of antifungal medication mixed with high potency steroids should not be used because the steroids can cause striae and atrophy of the skin. Loose-fitting, washed, cotton underclothes to reduce chafing, as well as the use of a bland, absorbent powder may be helpful adjuvants to therapy. Griseofulvin orally for 2 to 4 weeks may be needed in unresponsive cases (see Tinea Capitis, page 471).

---

*See Topical Drugs for Superficial Infections, page 576.

Isolation of the Hospitalized Patient: No special precautions are recommended.

Control Measures: Infections should be treated promptly. Potentially involved areas should be kept dry, and loose undergarments should be recommended.

Tinea Pedis

(Athlete's Foot, Ringworm of the Feet)

Clinical Manifestations: Tinea pedis consists of fine vesiculopustular or scaly lesions that are frequently pruritic. The lesions can involve all areas of the foot, but usually they are patchy in distribution, with a predisposition to fissures and scaling between the toes. Toenails may be infected and can be dystrophic. Tinea pedis (and many other fungal infections) can be accompanied by a hypersensitivity reaction to the fungi, with resulting vesicular eruptions on the palms and the sides of the fingers, and occasionally by an erythematous vesicular eruption on the extremities and trunk (the dermatophytid or "id" reaction). This condition must be differentiated from foot eczema, juvenile pustular dermatitis, and shoe dermatitis.

Etiology: Fungi of the genera *Microsporum*, *Epidermophyton*, and *Trichophyton*, especially *T rubrum*, *T mentagrophytes*, and *E floccosum*, are the causes.

Epidemiology: Tinea pedis is a common infection in adolescents and adults but is relatively uncommon in young children. It occurs worldwide. The fungi are acquired by contact with skin scales containing fungi or with fungi in damp areas, such as swimming pools, locker rooms, and shower rooms. It is communicable for as long as the infection is present.

Diagnosis: Tinea pedis is usually diagnosed by the clinical manifestations and corroborated by potassium hydroxide examination of the cutaneous scrapings and appropriate fungal cultures.

Treatment: Topical application of miconazole, haloprogin, econazole, clotrimazole, ciclopirox, or tolnaftate preparation twice daily or ketoconazole, naftifine, oxiconazole, or sulconazole preparation once daily may be used for active infections.* Acute vesicular lesions may be treated with intermittent use of open, wet compres-

---

*See Topical Drugs for Superficial Infections, page 576.

ses (e.g., Burrow's solution 1:80). Micronized griseofulvin, similar to that used for tinea capitis (see Tinea Capitis, page 471), administered orally for 6 to 8 weeks, may be necessary for the treatment of severe, chronic, and recalcitrant forms of tinea pedis. "Id" reactions are treated by wet compresses, topical corticosteroids, occasionally systemic corticosteroids, and eradication of the primary source of infection. Recurrence is prevented by proper foot hygiene, which includes keeping the feet dry and cool, gentle cleaning, drying between the toes, the use of absorbent antifungal foot powder, frequent airing of affected areas, and avoidance of occlusive footwear and nylon socks or other fabrics that interfere with dissipation of moisture.

Treatment of most nail infections requires oral antifungal therapy with griseofulvin. Ketaconazole is an alternative. Treatment should be continued for 6 to 24 months or until the entire nail has regrown and is no longer infected.

Isolation of the Hospitalized Patient: No special precautions are recommended.

Control Measures: Treatment of patients with active infections should reduce transmission. Public areas conducive to transmission (e.g., swimming pools) should not be used by those with active infection. Chemical foot baths are of no value and can facilitate spread of infection. Since recurrence after treatment is common, proper foot hygiene is important (see Treatment).

Tinea Versicolor

(Pityriasis Versicolor)

Clinical Manifestations: Tinea (pityriasis) versicolor is a common, superficial disorder of the skin characterized by multiple scaling and oval macular and patchy lesions, usually distributed over the upper portions of the trunk, proximal areas of the arms, and occasionally other areas. The lesions can be hypopigmented or hyperpigmented (fawn-colored or brown); they fail to tan during the summer; they can be somewhat lighter than the surrounding skin; and during the winter they are relatively darker—hence the term "versicolor." Common conditions confused with this disorder include pityriasis alba, postinflammatory hypopigmentation, vitiligo, melasma, seborrheic dermatitis, pityriasis rosea, and secondary syphilis.

Etiology: *Malassezia furfur* is the cause. This lipid-dependent fungus exists on normal skin in the yeast form and causes clinical lesions only when substantial hyphal forms develop.

Epidemiology: Tinea versicolor occurs worldwide. Although primarily a disorder of adolescents and young adults 15 to 30 years of age, it can also be seen in prepubertal children and, at times, infants. The fungus is transmitted by personal contact during periods of scaling.

Diagnosis: Scale scrapings examined microscopically in potassium hydroxide wet mount preparation or stained with methylene blue or May-Grunwald-Giemsa stain reveal the pathognomonic clusters of yeast cells (ranging up to 8 µ in diameter) and short hyphal fragments. Sabouraud's medium overlaid with sterile olive oil is an effective culture medium.

Treatment: Topical treatment with 2.5% selenium sulfide suspension in a shampoo base is recommended. This preparation is applied in a thin layer from face to knees for 1 to 2 hours or overnight, with care to see that the entire body surface is covered, nightly for a period of one to two weeks; followed by monthly applications for three months (in an effort to help prevent recurrences). The preparation is washed off in the morning by bath or shower. Other preparations with therapeutic efficacy include sodium hyposulfite or thiosulfate in 15% to 25% concentrations (e.g., Tinver lotion) applied twice daily for two to four weeks, or topical antifungal agents such as clotrimazole, econazole, haloprogin, ketoconazole, miconazole, or naftifine (see Topical Drugs for Superficial Fungal Infections, page 576). For persistent cases, oral ketoconazole for five days followed by the same dose for three consecutive days once each month for six months can be considered.

Isolation of the Hospitalized Patient: No special precautions are recommended.

Control Measures: Infected individuals should be treated, and their towels and washcloths should be sterilized.

Toxocariasis

(Visceral Larva Migrans; Ocular Larva Migrans)

Clinical Manifestations: The severity of the symptoms of toxocariasis depends on the number of larvae ingested and the degree of allergic response. Most persons who are lightly infected are asymptomatic.

Visceral larva migrans typically occurs in children 1 to 4 years old with history of pica, but it can also occur in older children. Characteristic manifestations include fever, leukocytosis, persistent eosinophilia, hypergammaglobulinemia, and hepatomegaly. Other manifestations include malaise, anemia, cough, and, in rare instances, pneumonia, myocarditis, and encephalitis. When ocular invasion (endophthalmitis or retinal granulomas) occurs, it usually does so without other evidence of the infection, suggesting that the visceral and ocular forms are distinct syndromes. Atypical forms of presentation include hemorrhagic skin rash and convulsions.

Etiology: Toxocariasis is caused by *Toxocara* species, which are common roundworms of dogs and cats (especially puppies or kittens), specifically *T canis* and *T cati* in the United States; most cases are caused by *T canis*. Other nematodes of animals can also cause this syndrome, although they rarely do.

Epidemiology: Humans are infected by the ingestion of eggs in soil containing infective larvae. A history of pica, particularly the eating of soil, is common. Direct contact with dogs is of secondary importance because eggs are not immediately infective when they are shed in the feces. Most reported cases are from North America and Great Britain and involve children. Puppies in the household are the apparent source for most cases, but the eggs are found in many parks and public places, i.e., wherever dogs and cats defecate.

Diagnostic Tests: Hypereosinophilia and hypergammaglobulinemia associated with elevated titers of isohemagglutinins to the A and B blood group antigens are presumptive evidence. Microscopic identification of the larvae in a liver biopsy specimen is diagnostic, but this finding is infrequent. Thus, a negative liver biopsy for larvae does not exclude the diagnosis. An ELISA test, which is available at the Centers for Disease Control, is both specific and sensitive.

Treatment: Thiabendazole or diethylcarbamazine* can be helpful in reducing symptoms, but the effectiveness of either drug has not been demonstrated. Significant toxicity has been observed with diethylcarbamazine. In severe cases such as those with myocarditis or for patients with involvement of the central nervous system, treatment with corticosteroids is indicated. Attention should be given to correcting the underlying causes of pica to prevent reinfection.

Isolation of the Hospitalized Patient: No special precautions are recommended.

---

*Available in the United States from Lederle Laboratories, Pearl River, NY.

Control Measures: Disposal of cat and dog feces is essential. Treatment of puppies and kittens with antihelminthics at 2, 4, 6, and 8 weeks of age prevents excretion of eggs by worms acquired transplacentally or through mother's milk. No specific management of exposed persons is recommended. Covering of sandboxes when not in use is helpful.

Toxoplasma gondii

(Toxoplasmosis)

Clinical Manifestations: In congenital toxoplasmosis, manifestations at birth include all or some of the following: a maculopapular rash, generalized lymphadenopathy, hepatomegaly, splenomegaly, jaundice, and thrombocytopenia. As a consequence of intrauterine meningoencephalitis, the infant can develop hydrocephalus, microcephaly, chorioretinitis, and convulsions. A roentgenogram of the skull or a computed tomogram can show cerebral calcifications. Some severely affected infants die in utero or within a few days of birth. Sequelae of congenital toxoplasmosis include mental retardation, learning disabilities, impaired vision, or blindness. However, congenital infection is usually asymptomatic at birth. In these cases, sequelae can become apparent several years later. Isolated ocular toxoplasmosis most often occurs as a result of congenital infection but can be a result of acquired infection. Ocular disease can become reactivated years after the initial infection, both in healthy and immunocompromised individuals.

In acquired toxoplasmosis, infection is usually asymptomatic. When symptoms do develop, they are nonspecific and include malaise, fever, sore throat, and myalgia. Lymphadenopathy, frequently cervical, is the most common sign. A maculopapular rash and hepatosplenomegaly can also occur. The clinical course is usually benign and self limited. Myocarditis and pneumonitis are also possible complications. Patients with AIDS are at risk for reactivated, severe disease of the central nervous system, which can be fatal.

Etiology: *Toxoplasma gondii* is a protozoan parasite.

Epidemiology: *T gondii* is worldwide in distribution and infects many species of warm-blooded animals. Members of the cat family acquire the organism from mice and are the definitive hosts; the parasite replicates sexually in the feline small intestine. For 2 to 4 weeks after primary infection, cats excrete the oocysts in their stools; oocysts require a maturation phase of 24 to 48 hours in temperate climates after excretion before they are infective by the oral route. Infected animals (including sheep, pigs, and cattle) can have tissue cysts in their brain, myocardium, skeletal muscles, and other organs, which remain viable for the lifetime of the host. Humans become infected either by consumption of poorly cooked meat or by ingestion of sporulated oocysts that have been excreted in cat feces. Transmission by blood product transfusion and from infected organ donors (heart and bone marrow) has been documented. Toxoplasmosis is not otherwise communicable from person to person.

The **incubation period** of the acquired infection, based on a well-studied outbreak, is estimated as approximately 7 days (with a range of 4 to 21 days).

Diagnostic Tests: Serologic tests are the primary means of diagnosis, but results must be carefully interpreted. IgG-specific antibodies are commonly measured by the indirect immunofluorescence assay. IgG-specific antibodies reach peak concentration 1 to 2 months after the infection and remain positive indefinitely. For determination of acute infection, the Centers for Disease Control recommends a capture ELISA for IgM antibodies. Specific IgM antibodies can be detected 2 weeks after the infection, reach their peak concentration in 1 month, decline thereafter, and usually become undetectable within 6 to 9 months; in rare patients IgM-specific antibodies can be detectable for as long as 2 years.

Seroconversion or a fourfold rise in specific IgG antibody titer suggests recently acquired infection, but the results can be misleading if serum specimens are not run in parallel to control for day-to-day laboratory variability. Patients with seroconversion or a fourfold rise in IgG antibody titer should have specific IgM antibody determinations performed by an experienced laboratory.

Congenitally infected infants usually have high concentrations of serum IgG antibodies to *Toxoplasma* organisms and usually show IgM antibodies if tested by a sensitive assay, such as the ELISA. However, absence of IgM-specific antibodies does not exclude congenital *Toxoplasma* infection, especially if the sera are assayed by the IFA test. Parallel testing of an infant's and mother's sera is essential because transplacental passage of IgG results in serum antibodies in both infected and uninfected infants; in uninfected infants, however, IgG antibody concentrations decline with time and become undetectable, and IgM antibodies remain absent.

Patients with AIDS infected with *Toxoplasma* have variable titers of IgG antibody to *Toxoplasma* but rarely have IgM antibody. Seroconversion and fourfold rises in titer frequently do not occur, making serodiagnosis difficult in these individuals. In such patients, typical clinical features of central nervous system disease and any detectable

Toxoplasma antibody in serum are sufficient for a presumptive diagnosis. Demonstration of organisms in tissue, isolation of the organism, or immunologic identification confirms the diagnosis.

Patients with ocular toxoplasmosis may have serologic evidence of either IgM or IgG antibodies.

Treatment: Pyrimethamine and sulfonamides (specifically sulfadiazine and trisulfapyrimidime) act synergistically against *Toxoplasma*. The most widely accepted regimen for children and adults consists of pyrimethamine in a loading dose of 2 mg/kg/d (maximum 100 mg/d), orally, in two doses for 1 to 3 days; followed by 1 mg/kg/d in two doses for 4 weeks, (maximum 25 mg/d); plus sulfadiazine or trisulfapyrimidine, 100 mg/kg/d, orally, in four doses for at least 4 weeks (not to exceed 8 g/d). In infants with congenital infection, the optimal dosage and duration of therapy for pyrimethamine and sulfadiazine are uncertain; consultation with experts should be sought. A national study on treatment of congenital infection is in progress. In patients with AIDS, maintenance therapy is usually given to prevent relapse. Folinic acid (calcium leucovorin) should be administered orally or parenterally (usually 5 to 10 mg/d) to patients receiving pyrimethamine to prevent hematologic toxicity. Clindamycin can be considered as an alternative drug for use in ocular disease. Spiramycin* has been used in Europe and is also an alternative choice. The use of corticosteroids (in conjunction with antimicrobials) in the management of ocular complications is controversial and is usually reserved for acute, progressive chorioretinal lesions in the region of the macula.

Isolation of the Hospitalized Patient: No special precautions are recommended.

Control Measures: Cat litter should be disposed of daily (oocysts are not infective during the first 24 to 48 hours after passage). Domestic cats should be fed commercially prepared cat food, restricted from hunting wild rodents, and should not be allowed to eat raw or partially cooked kitchen scraps. Lamb, beef, and pork should be cooked thoroughly before human consumption. Pregnant women with negative or unknown *Toxoplasma* titers should avoid contact with cat feces, gardening, or yard work in areas to which cats have access, and should not eat undercooked meat.

---

*Available only as an investigational drug in the United States. Contact the Food and Drug Administration (301/295-8012).

Trichinosis (Trichinellosis)

(Trichinella spiralis)

Clinical Manifestations: The clinical manifestations are highly variable, ranging from inapparent infection to fulminating, fatal illness. The severity of the disease is proportional to the infective dose. During the first week after ingesting infected meat, the patient can experience abdominal discomfort, nausea, vomiting, and/or diarrhea. Two to 8 weeks later, as larvae migrate into tissues, fever, myalgia, periorbital edema, urticarial rash, and conjunctival and subungual hemorrhages can develop. In severe infections, myocardial failure, neurologic involvement, and pneumonitis can follow in 1 or 2 months.

Etiology: *Trichinella spiralis*, a nematode capable of infecting only warm-blooded animals, is the cause.

Epidemiology: The infection is enzootic worldwide in many carnivores, especially scavengers. The usual source of human infections is pork; bear meat and other wild carnivorous game can also be sources. Infection occurs as a result of ingestion of raw or insufficiently cooked meat containing encysted larvae of *T spiralis*. Feeding pigs uncooked garbage perpetuates the cycle of infection. In the United States, the incidence of the infection in humans has declined considerably, but infection occurs sporadically, often within a family or among friends who have prepared uncooked sausage from fresh pork. In North America, infection has also resulted from eating undercooked bear or walrus meat. The disease is not transmitted from person to person.

The **incubation period** is usually 1 to 2 weeks.

Diagnostic Tests: Eosinophilia approaching 70%, compatible symptoms, and dietary history suggest the diagnosis. Serologic tests are available through state laboratories and the Centers for Disease Control. Serum antibody titers rarely become positive before the third week of illness. Results of testing paired sera are extremely informative. Beginning 2 weeks after infection, larvae can be seen on muscle biopsy. The tissue is best examined fresh, compressed between two microscope slides. Identification of larvae in leftover, suspect meat can be the most rapid source of diagnostic information.

Treatment: Mebendazole for 10 to 13 days is recommended (see Drugs for Parasitic Infections, page 587). Thiabendazole is an alternative drug. Although thiabendazole kills the adult worms in the small intestine, it appears ineffective against the encysted larvae. Corticosteroids alleviate symptoms of the inflammatory reaction and can be lifesaving when the central nervous system or heart is involved.

Isolation of the Hospitalized Patient: No special precautions are recommended.

Control Measures: Transmission to pigs can be reduced by not feeding them garbage, and by active rat control. People should be educated about the necessity to cook pork thoroughly (until it is no longer pink). Freezing of pork at –23.3°C (–10°F) for 10 days kills the larvae. However, *Trichinella* organisms in Arctic wild animals can survive this procedure. Individuals known to have recently ingested contaminated meat should be treated with mebendazole (or thiabendazole).

Trichomonas vaginalis

(Trichomoniasis)

Clinical Manifestations: Infection with *Trichomonas* is frequently asymptomatic. The usual clinical picture in symptomatic patients consists of a frothy vaginal discharge and mild vulvovaginal itching in postmenarcheal women. Dysuria and lower abdominal pain can occur. Urethritis or prostatitis may be seen in the male. The vaginal discharge is frequently pale yellow to gray-green in color and has a fishy odor. Symptoms are frequently more severe just before or after menstruation. The vaginal mucosa can be edematous and the cervix can be inflamed, with petechiae, and can bleed easily. Recurrence or reinfection is common.

Etiology: *Trichomonas vaginalis* is a flagellated protozoan.

Epidemiology: *Trichomonas* infection is primarily a sexually transmitted disease and frequently coexists with other infections, particularly gonococcal infections. Although trichomoniasis can be acquired without direct sexual contact, its presence in a premenarcheal girl should raise the question of sexual abuse.

The **incubation period** is 4 to 20 days (average, 1 week).

Diagnostic Tests: Diagnosis is usually made by examination of a wet mount preparation of the vaginal discharge. The lashing of the flagella and the motility of the organism are distinctive. Positive preparations are more frequent in symptomatic women and directly related to the number of organisms. Culture of the organism and antibody tests using ELISA or direct or indirect immunofluorescence techniques for demonstration of the organism are possible but not generally indicated.

Treatment: Metronidazole is the treatment of choice. For prepubertal girls, 15 mg/kg/d in three divided doses (maximum dose, 250 mg) is recommended. In adolescents and adults, the dose is 2 g in a single dose. Patients should abstain from alcohol for 48 hours due to the disulfiram-like effects of the drug. Treatment failures should be retreated with metronidazole (500 mg twice daily for adolescents and adults) for 7 days. The sexual partner should be treated concurrently. Metronidazole should not be used in the first trimester of pregnancy. A 100-mg dose of clotrimazole, a vaginal tablet, given at bedtime for 7 nights, may be used during early pregnancy. It improves symptoms but has a low cure rate.

Isolation of the Hospitalized Patient: No special precautions are recommended.

Control Measures: Controls aimed at the prevention of sexually transmitted diseases, particularly the use of condoms, are indicated.

Trichuriasis

(Whipworm infection)

Clinical Manifestations: Whipworm infection is frequently asymptomatic. Symptoms can include abdominal pain, tenesmus, and rectal prolapse. In severe infections, mucous and even bloody diarrhea can occur.

Etiology: The agent is *Trichuris trichiura* (human whipworm).

Epidemiology: Eggs require incubation in the soil for 10 days to 3 weeks to embryonate and become infective. Ingestion of these eggs causes the infection. The disease is not communicable directly from person to person.

Diagnostic Tests: The disease can be diagnosed by microscopic identification of the eggs in the feces.

Treatment: Mebendazole, given orally for 3 days, is the drug of choice.

Isolation of the Hospitalized Patient: No special precautions are recommended.

Control Measures: Sanitary disposal procedures for feces should be followed.

African Trypanosomiasis

(African Sleeping Sickness)

Clinical Manifestations: The rapidity and severity of clinical manifestations vary with the infecting species. With *Trypanosoma gambiense* infection, a nodule or chancre can appear on a person briefly at the site of inoculation within a few days of being bitten by the tsetse fly. Systemic illness occurs months to years later; it is characterized by intermittent fever and posterior cervical lymphadenopathy. Months to years after these signs have developed, the central nervous system can be invaded. This stage is manifested by behavioral changes, cachexia, headache, hallucinations, delusions, and somnolence. With *T rhodesiense* infection, generalized illness develops several weeks after the bite by an infected tsetse fly. The manifestations are much more intense than those in infection by the Gambian variety and can include acute central nervous system and cardiac symptoms, fever, and rapid weight loss. The central nervous system symptoms can develop as early as 3 weeks after the onset of the untreated systemic illness. *T rhodesiense* infection has a high fatality rate; without treatment, the patient usually dies within 1 year.

Etiology: The *Trypanosoma* species, protozoan hemoflagellates, are the cause.

Epidemiology: Approximately 20,000 human cases occur worldwide. Only one or two cases are reported annually in the United States, and they occur in persons who have been traveling in Africa. Infection is confined to an area in Africa between the latitudes of 15° north and 20° south; this area corresponds precisely with the distribution of the tsetse fly (*Glossina* species). Transmission involves the developmental cycle of *Trypanosoma* in tsetse flies, whose bite transmits the infection to humans. Wild game constitutes the major reservoir of *T rhodesiense*, which is found in Central and East Africa, particularly in game reserves. The parasite is present in the blood of infected persons and animals for variable periods up to several years. Humans are postulated to be the only reservoirs of *T gambiense*, which is found in West and Central Africa.

The **incubation period** in *T rhodesiense* is 3 to 21 days, usually 5 to 14 days; in *T gambiense* infection, it is usually longer and extremely variable, ranging from several months to years.

Diagnostic Tests: Diagnosis is made by identification of typical trypanosomes in the blood or in fluid obtained from an involved node or nodule/chancre. Concentration and staining with Giemsa solution of the buffy coat layer of peripheral blood can aid in the diagnosis. *T gambiense* is more likely to be found in lymph node aspirates. With central nervous system involvement, trypanosomes can be found in the cerebrospinal fluid. Increased IgM concentrations in either serum or cerebrospinal fluid can occur, but concentrations of all immunoglobulins can be elevated.

Treatment: The drug of choice for the acute hemolymphatic stage of infection before the involvement of the central nervous system is suramin.* Pentamidine is an alternative drug for early infections due to *T gambiense*. Melarsoprol* is the drug of choice for central nervous system involvement with *T rhodesiense*. Alpha-difluoromethyl ornithine† is available as an investigational drug for the treatment of *T gambiense* infections refractory to melarsoprol.

Isolation of the Hospitalized Patient: Other than the universally recommended blood and body fluid precautions (see Isolation Precautions, page 81), no additional precautions are recommended.

Control Measures: Environmental control measures for tsetse flies should be undertaken, and their contact with infected patients should be prevented. Travelers might consider avoiding highly endemic areas. Infected patients should not breast-feed or donate blood.

American Trypanosomiasis

(Chagas' Disease)

Clinical Manifestations: The early phase of this disease is frequently asymptomatic. However, children are more likely to exhibit symptoms than adults. In some patients, a red nodule known as a chagoma develops at the site of the original inoculation, usually on the face or

*Available in the United States only from the Drug Service, Centers for Disease Control (see Services of the Centers for Disease Control, page 622).
†Available in the United States through Merrell Dow Pharmaceuticals, Cincinnati, OH.

arms. The surrounding skin becomes indurated and later hypopigmented. Unilateral, firm edema of the eyelids, known as Romana's sign, is the earliest indication of the infection, but it is present in fewer than 50% of patients with signs of acute Chagas' disease. The edematous skin is violaceous in color, with conjunctivitis and enlargement of the ipsilateral preauricular lymph node. A few days after the appearance of Romana's sign, fever, generalized lymphadenopathy, and malaise develop. Acute myocarditis, hepatosplenomegaly, edema, and meningoencephalitis can follow. Serious sequelae consisting of cardiomyopathy and heart failure (the major cause of death), megaesophagus, and/or megacolon can develop many years after the initial manifestations. Congenital disease is characterized by low birth weight, hepatomegaly, and meningoencephalitis, with convulsions and tremors.

Etiology: *Trypanosoma cruzi,* a protozoan hemoflagellate, is the cause.

Epidemiology: The parasites are transmitted through the feces of the insects of the triatomid family. These insects defecate while taking a blood meal. The bitten person is inoculated by inadvertently rubbing the insect feces into the site of the bite or mucous membranes of the eye or the mouth. The parasite can also be transmitted congenitally and through blood transfusion. Accidental laboratory infections can result from the handling of infective blood, the vectors, and their excreta, or infected laboratory animals. The disease is limited to the Western hemisphere, predominantly from Mexico to Central and South America; vector-borne transmission is extremely rare in the United States. Infection, however, is common in the United States in immigrants from Central and South America. The disease is a leading cause of death in South America. Between 7 and 15 million people in South America are infected. Small mammals in the southern and southwestern United States harbor *T cruzi.*

The **incubation period** for the acute disease is 1 to 2 weeks. The chronic manifestations do not appear for years.

Diagnostic Tests: During the acute disease, the parasite is demonstrable in blood, either by Giemsa staining or by direct wet-mount preparation. In late infections, which are characterized by low-level parasitemia, parasites in the blood must be cultured on a special medium, inoculated into mice, or identified by xenodiagnosis. Serologic tests include complement fixation, indirect hemagglutination, and indirect immunofluorescence.

Treatment: The acute phase of Chagas' disease is treated with nifurtimox* or benznidazole.† These drugs are not effective against the forms of the parasite usually found in the chronic phase of the disease.

Isolation of the Hospitalized Patient: No special precautions are recommended.

Control Measures: Education about the mode of spread and the methods of prevention should be made available in endemic areas. Homes should be examined for the presence of the vectors. If they are found, thorough disinfection is indicated. Vector control through use of effective insecticides, control of the rodent population on which the vectors feed, and elimination of habitats of the vectors is recommended. Screens on windows and doors exclude the insect vectors. Blood and serologic examinations should be performed on household members with a similar exposure to the vector as that of a known patient.

Blood donors in endemic areas must be screened by serologic tests. Blood recipients can be protected in endemic areas by treatment of the donated blood with gentian violet at a dilution of 1:4,000.

Infected patients should not breast-feed or donate blood because transmission can occur through human milk or blood transfusion.

Tuberculosis

Clinical Manifestations: Most infected children are asymptomatic when the tuberculin reaction is first found to be positive. The primary complex of pulmonary tuberculosis reflecting the initial infection may not be demonstrable on chest roentgenogram, and in most children with primary tuberculosis, the infection is self limited. Early clinical manifestations occurring 1 to 6 months after initial infection can include one or more of the following: lymphadenopathy of hilar, mediastinal, cervical, or other lymph nodes; pulmonary involvement of a segment or lobe, occasionally with consolidation; atelectasis; pleural effusion; miliary tuberculosis; and tuberculous meningitis. Later clinical presentations that can occur at any time after initial infection include tuberculosis of the middle ear and mastoid, bones, joints, and skin. Extrapulmonary disease (e.g., miliary, meningeal, renal, bone, or joint) occurs in approximately 20% of infants and

---

*Available in the United States only from the Drug Service, Centers for Disease Control (see Services for the Centers for Disease Control, page 622).

†Available from Roche Laboratories, Nutley, NJ.

children with tuberculosis. Tuberculosis of the kidney and so-called reactivation or postprimary tuberculosis of the lung usually occur in adolescents or adults.

Etiology: The agent is *Mycobacterium tuberculosis*. Human disease caused by *M bovis*, the agent of bovine tuberculosis, or *M africanum* is rare in the United States. Other mycobacteria rarely cause pulmonary disease in immunocompetent children but usually cause lymphadenopathy (see Disease Due to Nontuberculous Mycobacteria, page 508).

Epidemiology: Although children of all ages are susceptible, infants and postpubertal adolescents are at highest risk of developing tuberculosis in the United States. Case rates for all ages have been highest in urban and nonwhite populations. The highest rates of infection are currently among minority groups (i.e., first-generation immigrants from high-risk countries, Hispanics, Blacks, Asians, American Indians, and Alaskan Natives), the homeless, and institutionalized persons, specifically those in correctional facilities. Many cases occur in geographic areas with a large number of immigrants or minorities. Additional risk factors for progression to active disease among infected persons include recent close contact with an infectious case; recent skin test conversion; immunodeficiency, particularly that associated with HIV infection; Hodgkin's disease; lymphoma; diabetes mellitus; chronic renal failure; malnutrition; and immunosuppression related to accompanying viral infection or induced by drugs (including daily steroid therapy).

Transmission of tuberculosis is usually by inhalation of droplet nuclei produced by an adult with infectious pulmonary tuberculosis. The duration of infectivity of an adult receiving effective treatment depends on the degree of sputum acid-fast smear positivity and cough frequency, and usually lasts only a few weeks. If the sputum is negative on smear and if the cough has disappeared, the person is considered noninfectious. Most authorities consider a patient to be noninfectious within 2 to 4 weeks after starting adequate therapy. The exceptions are children with active primary tuberculosis; they are rarely contagious because the pulmonary lesions are small, discharge of bacilli is small, and cough is minimal or nonexistent. Fomites such as contaminated bronchoscopes, syringes, utensils, and clothing have been rarely implicated in transmission.

The portal of entry is usually the respiratory tract. Skin, gastrointestinal tract, and mucous membranes have been implicated in a few cases. On rare occasions, tuberculosis is transmitted transplacentally from mother to fetus or via infected amniotic fluid.

The **incubation period** from infection to development of a positive reaction to tuberculin skin test is about 2 to 10 weeks. The risk for disease is highest in the first 2 years after infection. However, months to years may elapse between infection and development of disease. In most instances, infection becomes dormant and never progresses to clinical disease.

Diagnostic Tests: Identification of a source case should be intensely sought to support the diagnosis, determine possible drug resistance in the contact (which will influence the choice of drugs in the patient), and find all infected or diseased persons. A chest roentgenogram showing hilar lymph node enlargement suggests the possibility of tuberculous disease. Isolation of tubercle bacilli by culture from gastric washings, sputum, pleural fluid, cerebrospinal fluid, urine, or other body fluids establishes the diagnosis. However, the organism is slow-growing, and recovery of the agent may take as many as 10 weeks by older culture methods and 1 to 2 weeks by the radiometric method. Recovery of *M tuberculosis* in the laboratory can be made even more rapidly if DNA probes, which are available only in a few research laboratories, are combined with radiometric techniques. Attempts should be made to demonstrate acid-fast bacilli (AFB) in body fluids by the Ziehl-Neelsen method or by auramine-rhodamine staining and fluorescent microscopy. Bacteriophage typing, available only through the Centers for Disease Control, can be useful in epidemiologic studies. Histologic examination and demonstration of AFB in specimens from lymph node, pleura, liver, or bone marrow biopsies can be valuable for diagnosis.

Tuberculin Testing. The tuberculin skin test is the only practical tool for diagnosing tuberculous infection. Infection with *M tuberculosis* usually results in development of skin hypersensitivity within 2 to 10 weeks.

Two preparations of tuberculin—Old Tuberculin (OT) and Purified Protein Derivative (PPD)—are available. PPD has largely replaced OT because it is more specific for *M tuberculosis*; OT is currently used only in multiple puncture preparations. The United States Reference Standard is PPD-S. The standard dose of PPD is 5 tuberculin units (5 TU, formerly called "intermediate strength") in 0.1 mL of solution. Tween 80, added to minimize adsorption of the active fraction to glass, plastic bottles, and syringes, is not completely effective. Thus, tuberculin should be administered soon after it is drawn into the syringe. All tuberculins should be kept in a cool, dark location and never transferred from one bottle to another.

PPD is also available in unstandardized dose strengths of 1 TU ("first strength") and 250 TU ("second strength") per 0.1 mL. The 1 TU strength is used rarely and only in patients suspected of having intense tuberculin hypersensitivity (e.g., persons with erythema nodosum). Whether the 250 TU strength skin test should be used to identify persons with tuberculous infection is controversial. A positive reaction to 250 TU (in the absence of a reaction to 5 TU) could indicate tuberculous infection or infection with nontuberculous mycobacteria. The 250 TU test should not be used in any circumstances for the initial skin test.

Techniques of Administration. The current techniques of administration include the Mantoux (intracutaneous) test and several types of multiple-puncture tests. The Mantoux test of 5 TU-PPD (0.1 mL) is the standard tuberculin test. The disadvantage of the multiple-puncture devices with dried or liquid tuberculin is that the exact dose of antigen injected is not controlled. In addition to technical errors in applying the test, a major source of potential error is in reading the reaction. Another concern is the sensitivity and specificity of multiple-puncture tests. With either PPD or OT, approximately 10% to 20% of patients will have false-positive reactions. Of the positive reactions to PPD when the Mantoux method is used, approximately 1% to 10% are false-negative reactions. Conceptually, false-positive reactions are acceptable in a screening test whereas false-negative reactions are not. Positive reactions to a multiple-puncture test should be confirmed by a Mantoux test. Because multiple-puncture tests are also associated with false-negative reactions, they should not be used for tuberculin testing in high-risk populations.

Only the Mantoux test should be used in evaluation of contacts of patients with tuberculosis, in patients suspected of having mycobacterial infection, and in periodic testing of high-risk groups or in areas of high endemic rates of tuberculosis. If current recommendations regarding the frequency and type of tuberculin testing in low-risk groups are implemented, the Mantoux test should completely replace all multiple-puncture tests.

The PPD antigen solution should be aspirated into a disposable plastic syringe with a No. 26 gauge, short-bevel needle no more than 1 hour before use. Antigen solution (0.1 ml) is injected intradermally on the volar aspect of the forearm to produce a 6- to 10-mm wheal. The Mantoux test is read at 48 to 72 hours; however, induration persisting 96 hours or longer is still significant. Measurement of the reaction is easier if the elbow joint is slightly flexed. The margins of induration should be delineated by gentle palpation (not sight) of the injected area, or by using a ball point pen, and measured in millimeters with a ruler held transversely to the long axis of the forearm.

Interpretation of the Mantoux Test. The mean size of positive (significant) tuberculin reactions in adults with clinical tuberculosis is about 15 mm of induration. Among high-risk populations, reactions of 10 mm or more are considered positive; smaller reactions have been attributed to cross-reacting, nontuberculous mycobacterial infection. However, if the patient lives in a geographic area that is not endemic for nontuberculous mycobacterial infection, has clinical or radiographic evidence of tuberculosis, is HIV-seropositive or immunosuppressed from another cause, or is a known contact of an adult with AFB-positive sputum (on smear), a reaction of 5 mm or larger should be considered positive. Some recently infected children, with or without disease, have even smaller reactions; and 5% to 10% of children with clinical, culture-positive tuberculosis have negative Mantoux tuberculin tests. Hence, in some circumstances, if the tuberculin reaction is 5 to 9 mm in induration, or if the child has symptoms suggestive of tuberculosis, the appropriate history should be obtained, a physical examination should be performed, and chest roentgenograms (posteroanterior and lateral) should be taken. Infants younger than 6 months, immunocompromised patients, patients with early disease or infection, and BCG vaccine recipients (see Tuberculin Skin Test Reactivity in BCG Vaccine Recipients) require individual consideration.

Patients who are sensitized to nontuberculous mycobacteria may also react to tuberculin skin tests. Mantoux tuberculin reactions in these individuals are usually smaller than 10-mm induration, but larger reactions can occur, particularly early in the course of the infection. Currently, no skin test preparation is commercially available that will distinguish sensitization by *M tuberculosis* from that caused by nontuberculous mycobacteria.

Skin Test Reactivity in BCG Vaccine Recipients. Vaccination of children with BCG usually induces a positive tuberculin skin test, ranging from 3 mm to 19 mm in diameter. The size of reaction depends on many factors, including age at vaccination, strength of vaccine used, number of doses of vaccine received, and frequency of tuberculin testing. The presence or size of the postvaccination skin tests does not reliably predict the degree of protection afforded by BCG. Skin test reactivity tends to diminish with time, and by 10 years after vaccination, most recipients do not have a significant reaction (10 mm or more of induration). At any time, a reaction greater than 15 mm is not likely to be due to BCG. When evaluating a person for possible tuberculosis who is reported to have received BCG, verification of the history, such as by a vaccination scar or documentation of the history, should be undertaken. Other factors in the evaluation include a history of recent contact with an infectious case of tuberculosis, a family history of tuberculosis, and migration from a country with a high prevalence of tuberculosis.

In interpreting the significance of a positive tuberculin reaction (10 mm or more of induration) in a BCG recipient, no reliable method of distinguishing tuberculin reactions caused by vaccination with BCG from those caused by natural mycobacterial infections exists. Hence, in most cases positive reactions are interpreted as indicative of infection with *M tuberculosis* and should be treated accordingly. However, in select circumstances, treatment may not be indicated, such as in an individual who was recently vaccinated with BCG, who has no history of exposure to tuberculosis, and/or who has emigrated from a country with a low prevalence of tuberculosis. In such cases, consultation with an expert should be obtained.

Recommendations for Tuberculin Testing. In recent years, recommendations regarding the advisability of routine tuberculin testing in infants and children have been conflicting. The Centers for Disease Control, the American Thoracic Society, and the American College of Chest Physicians currently do not recommend routine tuberculin testing of children in low-risk groups in communities with low prevalence of tuberculosis. In these populations, most Mantoux tuberculin reactions of 5 to 9 mm are likely to be false positives, especially if the prevalence of nontuberculous mycobacterial infection is high. Thus, a substantial number of children might be needlessly evaluated and treated with isoniazid because of reactions perceived to be significant. The problem can be circumvented by restricting routine skin testing to high-risk populations. Preventive therapy is reserved for children (not otherwise in high-risk groups) who have reactions of 10 mm or more to the Mantoux test.

The Committee recommends annual tuberculin testing of high-risk children. Those at high risk include Black, Hispanic, Asian, American Indian, and Alaskan Native children, and those who are socioeconomically deprived; children living in neighborhoods where the case rate is higher than the national average; children from, or whose parents have immigrated from high-risk areas of Asia, Africa, the Middle East, Latin America, or the Caribbean; children in households with one or more cases of tuberculosis, and children with medical risk factors for tuberculosis (see Epidemiology, page 488).

Annual testing of low-risk groups (from areas of low prevalence) is not recommended. In low-risk groups, a reasonable alternative to no routine testing is to perform skin tests at three stages of childhood and adolescence which coincide with routine health appraisals or immunizations: (1) at 12 to 15 months of age (before or at the time of administration of MMR), (2) before school entry (4 to 6 years of age), and (3) in adolescence (at 14 to 16 years of age). The tuberculin skin test is always indicated for persons with known contact with a person with tuberculous disease; if the test is negative, it should be repeated 8 to 10 weeks after separation of the patient from the contact.

Pediatricians should consult local and state health departments for assistance in identification, treatment, and follow-up of patients with symptomatic (tuberculosis) and asymptomatic infection and for obtaining periodic summary information concerning prevalence of tuberculous and nontuberculous mycobacterial infection in their locality. Awareness of tuberculosis epidemiology in the community can be a useful guide to frequency of tuberculin testing and intelligent interpretation and investigation of test results.

Tuberculin Testing and Immunizations. Recommendations for tuberculin testing are independent of those for immunization, and tuberculin testing may be done at the same visit at which MMR is given (see Tuberculin Testing, page 21).

Treatment (see Table 53 for summary):

Prevention of Disease. Ample data document that isoniazid (INH) given to persons with a positive tuberculin test but with no evidence of active disease provides substantial protection (54% to 88% efficacy) against the development of active disease for at least 20 years. All infants, children, adolescents, and adults younger than 35 years who have a positive tuberculin test but no other evidence of disease and who have never received antituberculosis therapy should receive INH alone (if INH resistance is not suspected), unless a specific contraindication exists. INH in this circumstance is therapeutic for the infection and preventive against the development of clinical disease. A chest roentgenogram should be obtained at the time preventive therapy is initiated; if the roentgenogram is normal and shows no hilar adenopathy, and the child remains asymptomatic, it need not be repeated.

Children usually do not need pyridoxine supplementation of INH therapy unless they have nutritional deficiencies (see discussion of INH in Specific Drug Therapy, page 499).

Duration of Preventive Chemotherapy. The optimal duration of preventive therapy remains unknown. In the early studies in children, patients received INH for 1 year. Data in adults indicate that after 6 months of continuous medication, a 65% reduction in disease is achieved compared to a 75% reduction with 12 months of treatment. In adults, 6 to 12 months of preventive therapy with INH is now recommended in most cases. **The Committee recommends that in infants and children the duration of INH should be 9 months.** The exceptions are patients with HIV infection, for whom a minimum of 12 months is recommended. INH is given daily, 10 mg/kg (maximum 300 mg), in a single dose. In situations where compliance with daily preventive therapy cannot be assured, twice weekly directly observed administration of INH can be considered, preferably after completion of 1 month of daily therapy. **Direct observation means that a health care worker is present when INH is given to the patient.** Each dose of INH in the twice-weekly regimen is 20 mg/kg, not to exceed a daily maximum of 900 mg.

Table 53. Recommended Treatment Regimens for Tuberculosis in Infants, Children, and Adolescents

Infection or Disease Category	Regimen*	Remarks
Asymptomatic infection (positive skin test, no disease):		At least six consecutive months of therapy should be given, with good compliance by patient.
Isoniazid-susceptible	9 mo of I daily	If daily therapy is not possible, twice weekly therapy may be used for 9 months.
Isoniazid-resistant	9 mo of R daily	
Pulmonary (including hilar adenopathy)	**6-mo regimen (standard):** 2 mo of I,R, and Z daily followed by 4 mo of I and R daily OR 2 mo of I,R, and Z daily followed by 4 mo of I and R twice weekly **9-mo regimen (alternative)**: 9 mo of I and R daily OR 1 mo of I and R daily followed by 8 mo of I and R twice weekly	If possible drug resistance is a concern, another drug (ethambutol or streptomycin) should be added to the initial therapy until drug susceptibility is determined, especially for the 9-month regimen. Drugs can be given two or three times per week under direct observation in the initial phase if noncompliance is likely. For hilar adenopathy, regimens consisting of 6 mo of I and R daily, and 1 mo of I and R daily followed by 5 mo of I and R twice weekly have been successful in areas where drug resistance is rare.

Meningitis, disseminated (miliary), and bone/joint	2 mo of I,R,Z, and S daily followed by 10 mo of I and R daily OR 2 mo of I,R,Z, and S daily followed by 10 mo of I and R twice weekly	Streptomycin is given in initial therapy until drug susceptibility is known. For patients who may have acquired tuberculosis in geographic areas where resistance to streptomycin is common, capreomycin (15-30 mg/kg/d) or kanamycin (15-30 mg/kg/d) may be used instead of streptomycin.
Extrapulmonary other than meningitis, disseminated (miliary), or bone/joint	Same as for pulmonary disease.	See pulmonary.

*I = isoniazid; R = rifampin; Z = pyrazinamide; S = streptomycin.

After completion of preventive therapy, any tuberculin-positive child who undergoes prolonged corticosteroid or other immunosuppressive therapy should also receive INH for the duration of this therapy.

Preventive Therapy for Contacts of Patients With INH-Resistant M *tuberculosis.* Possible INH resistance should always be considered, particularly in children from social, economic, or ethnic groups where drug resistance is high, and especially in foreign-born children from countries of high prevalence of tuberculosis. For contacts who are likely to have been infected by an index case with INH-resistant organisms and in whom the consequences of the infection are likely to be severe (e.g., children younger than 3 years with household exposure), rifampin (10 mg/kg, maximum 600 mg, given daily in a single dose) should be given in addition to INH (10 mg/kg, maximum 300 mg, given daily in a single dose) until susceptibility test results are available. If the index case is proven to be excreting organisms completely resistant to INH, the INH should be discontinued and rifampin given for a total of 9 months; if the organism is only partially resistant, both drugs should be continued for a total of 9 months. INH alone should be given if no proof of exposure to INH-resistant organisms is found. Consultation with an expert in making these decisions is advised.

Treatment of Active (Current) Disease. The goal of treatment is to achieve sterilization of the tuberculous lesion in the shortest possible time. Achievement of this goal maximizes patient compliance, reduces treatment cost, and minimizes the development of resistant organisms. The major problem limiting successful treatment is poor compliance in taking medications. Chemotherapy of tuberculosis is complicated by two characteristics of mycobacteria: (1) spontaneous emergence of drug-resistant mutants and (2) persistence of viable mycobacteria as a result of their slow intermittent growth.

The treatment of children with tuberculosis has always been based on treatment regimens used in adults. The encouraging results of 6-month and 9-month treatment regimens in adults and children with both pulmonary and extrapulmonary tuberculosis have led to the use of these shorter regimens in children in some areas of the world. Published data with the 6-month and 9-month regimens in children in the United States and in developing countries are now available.

The Committee recommends a 6-month regimen consisting of INH, rifampin, and pyrazinamide for the first 2 months and INH and rifampin for the remaining 4 months as standard therapy for treatment of uncomplicated, intrathoracic tuberculosis (pulmonary, pulmonary with hilar adenopathy, or positive tuberculin reaction and hilar adenopathy) in infants, children, and adolescents. When initial drug resistance is suspected, either ethambutol or streptomycin should be added to the initial regimen until drug susceptibilities test results are available (see Chemotherapy for "Drug-Resistant" Tuberculosis). In cases of hilar adenopathy when drug resistance is unlikely, a 6-month regimen of INH and rifampin is usually sufficient. Every effort should be made to perform drug susceptibility studies on the initial isolate or that recovered from the adult contact, especially in cases in which drug resistance is suspected.

In the 6-month regimen with triple drug therapy for the first 2 months, INH in a daily dose of 10 mg/kg (maximum, 300 mg), rifampin in a daily dose of 10 to 15 mg/kg (maximum, 600 mg), and pyrazinamide in a daily dose of 20 to 30 mg/kg (maximum, 2 g) are given. After this 2-month period, a regimen of INH and rifampin given twice weekly is acceptable if directly observed; the doses are 20 to 40 mg/kg (maximum, 900 mg) twice weekly for INH and 10 to 20 mg/kg (maximum, 600 mg) twice weekly for rifampin. **Direct observation means that a health care worker is present when medications are administered to the patient. If the reliability of self-administration of medications is in doubt, directly observed twice weekly therapy administered by a health care professional should be given.**

Chemotherapy for "Drug-Resistant" Tuberculosis. In the United States and Canada, although the incidence of drug resistance in previously untreated patients with tuberculosis has been relatively low, drug resistance is an increasing problem. For example, in certain areas the incidence of resistance to INH can be as high as 15%. Drug resistance is most common in the foreign-born from high-risk areas such as Asia, Africa, and Latin America, in the homeless, in those previously treated for tuberculosis, and in children with tuberculosis whose adult source case is in one of these groups. For all cases of childhood tuberculosis, drug susceptibility information should be sought from the adult source case and/or the child. If the child is at risk for drug resistance, streptomycin or ethambutol should be added to the initial phase of all regimens until the susceptibilities are known. Treatment should always include at least two bactericidal drugs to which the organism is susceptible. Bactericidal drugs include INH, rifampin, streptomycin, and pyrazinamide. In cases of tuberculosis with INH or rifampin resistance, 6-month chemotherapy regimens are not recommended at this time. Consultation with an expert in tuberculosis is strongly advised in cases of drug-resistant disease.

Extrapulmonary Tuberculosis. In general, extrapulmonary tuberculosis, including cervical lymphadenopathy, can be treated with the same regimens as pulmonary tuberculosis. Exceptions may be bone and joint disease, disseminated (miliary) disease, and meningitis, for which the data at present are inadequate to support a 6-month duration of therapy. For these severe forms of extrapulmonary tuberculosis, daily treatment with INH, rifampin, pyrazinamide, and streptomycin for the first 2 months, followed by INH and rifampin administered daily or twice-weekly under direct observation, is recommended for a total of 12 months of therapy. Four drugs are given initially because of the possibility of drug resistance (see Chemotherapy for "Drug-Resistant" Tuberculosis). Based on personal experience and currently unpublished data, some experts recommend a treatment duration of 6 to 9 months.

Pyrazinamide is especially useful in disseminated and meningeal tuberculosis because it achieves better cerebrospinal fluid concentrations than either streptomycin or ethambutol. In cases of severe tuberculosis with vomiting or obtundation, INH or rifampin can be given intramuscularly or intravenously. The dose is the same as the oral dose. (Special investigational new-drug permission must be obtained for intravenous administration of rifampin.)

Tuberculosis and HIV Infection. Adult patients with HIV infection have an increased incidence of tuberculosis. Manifestations in these patients can be unusual and can include multiple disease sites and extrapulmonary involvement. Manifestations of pulmonary tuberculosis in these patients can resemble those of *Pneumocystis carinii* infection, with infiltrates in any area and often without cavitation. Mediastinal or hilar adenopathy is common. A negative tuberculin test due to immunosuppression caused by HIV infection can also occur. Specimens for culture should be obtained in all cases, since infection with atypical mycobacteria is also common and results of mycobacterial drug susceptibility testing is important information for therapeutic decisions. Appropriate specimens include respiratory secretions, blood, urine, stool, bone marrow, liver, lymph node, or other tissue as indicated clinically. Most HIV-infected adult patients with tuberculosis respond well to antituberculosis drugs.

The optimal therapy of tuberculosis in children with HIV infection has not yet been established. Therapy should always include at least three drugs initially, and should be continued for a minimum of 9 months and for at least 6 months beyond documented culture conversion as evidenced by three negative cultures. INH and rifampin plus either ethambutol or pyrazinamide should be given for at least the first 2 months. A fourth drug may be needed for disseminated disease. Consultation with an expert who has experience in managing patients with HIV infection is advised.

HIV testing (with informed consent) is recommended for all children with tuberculosis disease, especially those with risk factors for HIV infection.

Evaluation and Monitoring of Therapy. The duration of antituberculosis therapy is based on the individual patient's clinical and roentgenographic response, smear and culture results, and susceptibility studies of the organism obtained from the patient or the suspect source case. With directly observed intermittent chemotherapy, clinical evaluation is an integral component of each visit for drug administration. Careful monitoring of the clinical and bacteriologic responses to therapy on a monthly basis in sputum-positive patients is important. For bacteriologically sputum-negative pulmonary tuberculosis, chest roentgenograms should be obtained after 2 or 3 months of therapy to evaluate the response to therapy. Follow-up roentgenograms beyond the termination of successful chemotherapy are usually not necessary.

If therapy has been interrupted, the date for completion of therapy will need to be extended. Although guidelines cannot be given for every situation, factors to consider in establishing the date for completion include the following: (1) length of the interruption; (2) the period of therapy (early or late) in which interruption occurred; and (3) the patient's clinical, radiologic, and bacteriologic status before, during, and after interruption. Consultation with an expert is advised.

Untoward effects of INH therapy in children are rare. The incidence of hepatitis during INH therapy is so low in otherwise healthy infants and children that routine determination of serum aminotransferase concentrations is not recommended. However, in cases of severe tuberculosis, especially meningitis and disseminated disease, liver function tests should be monitored during the first several months of treatment. Other indications for liver function tests include concurrent or recent liver disease, high daily dose of INH in combination with rifampin, and clinical evidence of hepatotoxicity (see Specific Drug Therapy). In most circumstances, monthly clinical evaluation for 3 months and every 3 months thereafter directed toward detecting signs or symptoms of hepatitis or other adverse effects of the drug is an appropriate schedule for follow-up. Alternatively, some experts recommend routine evaluation every 4 to 6 weeks throughout the course of therapy.

In all cases, frequent physician-patient contact to assess drug compliance, efficacy and toxicity is an important aspect of management.

Specific Drug Therapy. Administration of antituberculosis drugs kills or inhibits the multiplication of drug-susceptible tubercle bacilli, thereby arresting the progressive tuberculosis and preventing most complications of early, primary tuberculosis. Chemotherapy does not cause rapid disappearance of already caseous or granulomatous lesions (e.g., mediastinal lymphadenitis with endobronchial breakthrough).

Dosage schedules and possible adverse reactions of the antituberculous drugs are as follows (and summarized in Table 54):

Table 54. Commonly Used Drugs for the Treatment of Tuberculosis in Infants, Children, and Adolescents

Drugs	Dosage Forms	Daily Dose (mg/kg/d)	Twice Weekly Dose (mg/kg per dose)	Maximum Dose	Adverse Reactions
Isoniazid*	Scored tablets: 100 mg 300 mg Syrup: 10 mg/mL	10-15†	20-40	Daily: 300 mg Twice weekly: 900 mg	Mild hepatic enzyme elevation, hepatitis, peripheral neuritis, hypersensitivity
Rifampin*	Capsules: 150 mg 300 mg Syrup: formulated in syrup from capsules	10-20	10-20	600 mg	Orange discoloration of secretions/urine, staining contact lenses, vomiting, hepatitis, "flu-like" reaction, and thrombocytopenia; may render birth-control pills ineffective
Pyrazinamide	Scored tablets: 500 mg	20-40	50-70	2 g	Hepatotoxicity, hyperuricemia
Streptomycin (IM administration)	Vials: 1 g 4 g	20-40	20-40	1 g	Ototoxicity, nephrotoxicity, skin rash
Ethambutol	Tablets: 100 mg 400 mg	15-25	50	2.5 g	Optic neuritis (reversible), decreased visual acuity, decreased red-green color discrimination, gastrointestinal disturbance, hypersensitivity

*Rifamate is a capsule containing 150 mg of isoniazid and 300 mg of rifampin. Two capsules provide the usual adult (> 50 kg body weight) daily doses of each drug.

†When isoniazid is used in combination with rifampin, the incidence of hepatotoxicity increases if the isoniazid dose exceeds 10 mg/kg/d.

Isoniazid (10 to 15 mg/kg/d, maximum 300 mg/d; if given twice weekly, 20 to 40 mg/kg per dose, maximum 900 mg per dose). This drug is the keystone of therapy. It is bactericidal, rapidly absorbed, and penetrates well into body fluid, including cerebrospinal fluid. It is metabolized in the liver and excreted primarily through the kidney. The drug is well tolerated by children, who can be given larger doses (on a surface area or kilogram basis) than can adults. In children given therapeutic doses, peripheral neuritis or convulsions caused by inhibition of pyridoxine metabolism have occurred, although rarely.

Children receiving INH usually do not need pyridoxine supplements unless they have nutritional deficiency. Pyridoxine is recommended for children and adolescents on meat- and milk-deficient diets, for those with nutritional deficiencies, and for breast-feeding infants and women during pregnancy (see Tuberculosis in Pregnancy and Lactation, page 503).

Routine liver function tests are not recommended. Liver function studies should be performed, however, if one or more of the following conditions exists: (1) concurrent or recent liver disease; (2) clinical evidence of hepatotoxicity; (3) the higher daily dose of INH is used in combination with rifampin; or (4) the child has disseminated disease or meningitis.

Rifampin (10 to 20 mg/kg/d, maximum 600 mg/d; if given twice weekly, 10 to 20 mg/kg per dose, maximum 600 mg per dose). This drug is a bactericidal antituberculosis agent. Tubercle bacilli initially resistant to rifampin are uncommon. For infants and young children, the contents of the capsules can be suspended in syrup of wild cherry (300 mg capsule in 30 mL provides a 10-mg/mL suspension) or sprinkled on applesauce. Rifampin is excreted in bile and urine and can cause orange urine, sweat, and/or tears. It can also cause discoloration of soft contact lenses and render oral contraceptives ineffective. Hepatotoxicity occurs rarely.

Pyrazinamide (20 to 40 mg/kg/d, maximum 2 g/d). This useful bactericidal drug attains therapeutic concentrations in cerebrospinal fluid and in macrophages. In doses of 30 mg/kg/d or less, it is seldom hepatotoxic and is well tolerated by children.

Streptomycin (20 to 40 mg/kg/d, intramuscularly, maximum 1 g given once daily; if given twice weekly, 20 to 40 mg/kg per dose). This drug to which resistance is relatively common, particularly among immigrants from developing countries such as in Southeast Asia, is bactericidal. Therapeutic concentrations in cerebrospinal fluid are achieved only in meningitis. Streptomycin is usually prescribed for only 4 weeks and for no longer than 12 weeks because the incidence of vestibular and cochlear damage correlates with increasing total dose.

Ethambutol (15 mg/kg/d preferred, maximum 2.5 g/d). This drug is well absorbed, diffuses well, and is excreted in the urine. In this dosage it is bacteriostatic only and its main role is to prevent the emergence of drug-resistant organisms. Because the population of tubercle bacilli is usually smaller in primary tuberculosis than in reinfection tuberculosis, the development of secondary resistance during treatment of primary disease is rare. A dose of 25 mg/kg/d is necessary for bactericidal activity and can be used in older children where appropriate ophthalmologic evaluation is possible. Ethambutol can cause reversible optic neuritis. Hence, patients receiving the drug should be checked monthly for acuity, visual fields, and red-green color discrimination. Because the patient's cooperation is essential for performance of these tests, ethambutol cannot be used safely in small children.

Ethionamide (15 to 20 mg/kg/d, maximum 1 g/d). This bacteriostatic antituberculosis drug is well tolerated by children, achieves therapeutic cerebrospinal fluid concentrations, and is occasionally useful in drug-resistant cases. An expert should be consulted before prescribing.

Other drugs have only limited usefulness because of minimal effectiveness, toxic properties, or both, and should be used only after appropriate consultation has been obtained. Cycloserine, kanamycin, and capreomycin sometimes are helpful in cases of drug resistance or if patients cannot tolerate other drugs.

All of the foregoing therapeutic agents can be responsible for major toxic effects. **The cautions listed in the package insert for each drug should be followed,** and consultation with an expert is advised when the conventional antituberculous regimen is altered.

Of the antituberculosis drugs discussed here and in Table 54, the only two that are approved by the Food and Drug Administration for use in children are INH and streptomycin. Nevertheless, the Committee supports the appropriate use of other drugs as recommended here.

Steroids. Adjuvant treatment with corticosteroids in tuberculous disease is controversial. Corticosteroids have been used for therapy of tuberculous meningitis to reduce vasculitis, inflammation, and, ultimately, intracranial pressure. Recent data indicate that dexamethasone may lower mortality and long-term neurologic impairment, and the administration of dexamethasone should be considered in cases of tuberculous meningitis. Corticosteroids may also be considered in cases of pleural and pericardial effusions (to hasten reabsorption of fluid), in severe miliary disease (to mitigate alveolocapillary block), and in endobronchial disease (to relieve obstruction and atelectasis). Corticosteroids should be given only when accompanied by adequate antituberculosis therapy. Consultation with an expert in the treatment of tuberculosis should be obtained if steroid therapy is being considered.

Immunizations. Patients who are receiving active treatment for tuberculosis can be given measles vaccine or other live virus vaccines as otherwise indicated, unless they are receiving corticosteroids or are otherwise immunocompromised (e.g., due to HIV infection).

Tuberculosis in Pregnancy and Lactation. Tuberculosis in pregnancy should be managed with an expert in the management of tuberculosis. If active disease is diagnosed during pregnancy (positive bacteriology or clinical/radiologic findings compatible with presumptive diagnosis), a 9-month regimen of INH and rifampin, possibly supplemented by an initial phase of ethambutol, is recommended. When INH resistance is a possibility, INH, ethambutol, and rifampin are recommended initially; one of these drugs can be discontinued after 1 or 2 months, depending on the results of susceptibility tests. If rifampin or isoniazid is discontinued, treatment is continued for a total of 18 months; if ethambutol is discontinued, treatment is continued for a total of 9 months. Prompt initiation of chemotherapy is mandatory to protect both the mother and the fetus.

Pregnant women with positive tuberculin skin tests and negative sputum cultures should receive preventive therapy with INH for 9 months if they are HIV-positive, have recently been in contact with an infectious case, or have radiographic evidence of past tuberculosis. If possible, preventive therapy should begin after the first trimester. In other circumstances in which none of these three risk factors is present, although no harmful effects of INH to the fetus have been observed, preventive therapy should be delayed until after delivery.

Pyridoxine should be prescribed for all pregnant women receiving INH. Physicians caring for nursing mothers should be made aware that INH is secreted in human milk; however, adverse effects of INH on nursing infants have not been demonstrated. INH, ethambutol, and rifampin appear to be relatively safe for the fetus. The benefit of ethambutol and rifampin for the therapy of active disease in the mother outweighs the risk to the infant. Streptomycin and pyrazinamide should not be used unless they are essential to control the disease.

Congenital Tuberculosis. This disease is extremely rare. Women who have only pulmonary tuberculosis are not likely to infect their fetus until after delivery. In utero infections with tubercle bacilli, however, can occur after maternal bacillemia at different stages in the course of tuberculosis. Miliary tuberculosis can seed the placenta and thereby gain access to the fetal circulation. In women with tuberculous endometritis, transmission of infection can also result from fetal aspiration of bacilli at the time of delivery. A third mode of transmission is ingestion of infected amniotic fluid in utero.

If an infant is suspected of having congenital tuberculosis, a Mantoux skin test (5 TU PPD) and chest roentgenogram should be performed promptly. Regardless of the skin test results, treatment of the infant should be initiated promptly with INH, pyrazinamide, rifampin, and streptomycin. If the physical examination or chest roentgenogram supports the diagnosis of tuberculosis, the patient should be treated with INH and rifampin for at least 9 to 12 months using the same regimen as that for tuberculous meningitis. The drug susceptibilities of the organism recovered from the mother should be determined.

Management of the Newborn Infant Whose Mother (or Other Household Contact) Has Tuberculosis. Management of a newborn infant whose mother (or other household contact) is suspected of having tuberculosis is based on individual considerations. If possible, separation of the mother (or contact) and infant should be minimized. Differing circumstances and resulting recommendations are as follows:

- *Mother (or Other Household Contact) With a Positive Tuberculin Skin Test Reaction and No Evidence of Current Disease.* Investigation of other members of the household or extended family to whom the infant may later be exposed is indicated. If no evidence of current disease is found in the mother or extended family, the infant should be tested with a Mantoux test (5 TU PPD) at 4 to 6 weeks of age and at 3 to 4 months of age. When the family cannot be promptly tested, consideration should be given to the administration of INH (10 mg/kg/d) to the infant until skin testing of the family has excluded contact with a case of active tuberculosis. The infant does not need to be hospitalized during this time if adequate follow-up can be arranged. The mother should also be considered for INH preventive therapy.
- *Mother With Untreated (Newly Diagnosed) Disease or Disease Which Has Been Treated for 2 or More Weeks* **and** *Who Is Judged to Be Noncontagious at Delivery.* Careful investigation of household members and extended family is mandatory. A chest roentgenogram and Mantoux tuberculin test at 4 to 6 weeks of age should be performed on the infant; if these are negative, the infant should be tested again at 3 to 4 months and at 6 months. Separation of the mother and infant is not necessary if compliance with treatment by the mother is assured. The mother can breast-feed. The infant should receive INH even if the tuberculin skin test and chest roentgenogram do not suggest tuberculous disease, since cell-mediated immunity of a degree sufficient to mount a sig-

nificant reaction to tuberculin skin testing can only develop as late as age 6 months in an infant infected at birth. INH can be discontinued if the Mantoux skin test is negative at 3 to 4 months of age and no active disease exists in family members. The infant should be examined carefully at monthly intervals. If noncompliance is documented, the mother has AFB-positive sputum (or smear), and supervision is impossible, BCG (Bacillus Calmette-Guerin) vaccine may be considered for the infant. However, the response to the vaccine in infants may be inadequate for prevention of tuberculosis.

- *Mother Has Current Disease Suspected of Being Contagious at the Time of Delivery.* The mother and infant should be separated until the mother is judged to be noncontagious. Otherwise, management is the same as when the disease is judged to be noncontagious to the infant at delivery (see preceding paragraph).
- *Mother Has Hematogenous Spread Tuberculosis (e.g., Meningitis, Miliary Disease, or Bone Involvement).* Congenital tuberculosis in the infant is possible. If the infant is suspected of having congenital tuberculosis, a PPD Mantoux skin test and chest roentgenogram should be performed promptly, and treatment of the infant should begin at once (see Congenital Tuberculosis). If clinical or roentgenographic findings do not support the diagnosis of congenital tuberculosis, the infant should be separated from the mother until she is judged to be noninfectious. The infant should be given INH until 6 months of age at which time the skin test should be repeated. If the skin test is positive, INH should be continued for a total of 12 months.

Isolation of the Hospitalized Patient: Children with primary tuberculosis in most cases need not be isolated and can be hospitalized on an open ward if they are receiving chemotherapy. Children and adolescents with infectious pulmonary tuberculosis, i.e., those whose sputum is positive, should be on AFB (tuberculosis) isolation precautions until effective chemotherapy has been initiated, their sputum smears show a diminishing number of organisms, and their cough is abating.

Family members should be managed with AFB (tuberculosis) isolation precautions when visiting until they are demonstrated not to have infectious tuberculosis.

Control Measures:

Day Care and Schools. Children with primary tuberculosis can attend school or day care if they are receiving chemotherapy (see Children in Day Care, page 74). They can return to regular activities as soon as clinical symptoms have disappeared, effective chemotherapy (based on clinical, bacteriologic, and roentgenographic signs) has been instituted, and an acceptable plan for completing the course of therapy has been developed.

Epidemiologic Investigation. Children with positive tuberculin skin tests or with clinically documented tuberculous disease ordinarily should be the starting point for epidemiologic investigation, which is best accomplished with assistance from the local health department. Close associates of the tuberculin-positive child should be skin tested, and persons with a positive result should be investigated for the presence of active tuberculosis. After the presumptive adult source for the child's disease is identified, other contacts of that case should be skin tested to identify those needing antituberculous treatment. Chest roentgenograms of tuberculin-positive contacts should be obtained, and treatment should be started.

Preventive Therapy for Contacts. Persons exposed to a potentially infectious case of tuberculosis, persons with impaired immunity, and all household contacts younger than 6 years who are exposed to any adult with active tuberculosis should undergo tuberculin skin testing, should have a chest roentgenogram, and should be given INH preventive therapy even if the skin test is negative. Infected persons can have a negative skin test because of anergy or because cellular immunity has not yet developed. Persons who are not anergic should be retested 8 to 10 weeks after contact has been broken. If the skin test is still negative, INH can be discontinued. If the skin test becomes positive, INH is continued for a total of 9 months.

Bacillus Calmette-Guerin (BCG).* BCG vaccines are live attenuated strains of *M bovis* that have been developed from multiple substrains cultured for many years in different laboratories. In controlled field trials in humans, efficacy has been shown in some trials and not in others.

The two vaccine strains now licensed in the United States have been derived from the original strain of *M bovis*, but additional culture passages have taken place since efficacy field trials were last conducted in the United States in 1955. Unfortunately, no satisfactory laboratory test for efficacy is available. Therefore, the efficacy of current vaccines is unknown.

The administration of BCG vaccine should be considered only for uninfected children who are at unavoidable risk of exposure and for whom other methods of prevention and control, including INH preventive therapy, have failed or are not feasible. Recommended vaccine recipients include the following: (1) infants and children who are tuberculin skin-test negative and who live in households with

---

*BCG vaccines in the United States are available from the following sources: Quad Pharmaceuticals, Indianapolis, IN (Glaxo strain); Bionetics Research, Inc., Chicago, IL (Tice strain); and Antigen Supply House, Northridge, CA (Tice strain).

repeated exposure to persistently untreated or ineffectively treated patients with sputum-positive tuberculosis or who are continuously exposed to persons with *M tuberculosis* resistant to INH and rifampin; and (2) infants and children in groups in which an excessive rate of new infections (greater than 1% per year) can be demonstrated and the usual surveillance and treatment have failed or are not feasible (e.g., in groups without a source of regular health care). The presently available BCG vaccines are not otherwise indicated for use in countries of low incidence of tuberculosis.

When the vaccine is given, care should be taken to observe the precautions and directions for administration (including dose and route, which is either intradermal or percutaneous, depending on the product) in the package insert. The freeze-dried vaccine should be reconstituted, protected from exposure to light, refrigerated when not in use, and administered within 8 hours of reconstitution.

BCG may be given to infants from birth to 2 months old without tuberculin testing, if the infant is known not to have been exposed; thereafter, BCG is given only to children who have negative Mantoux tests. PPD testing should be repeated 2 to 3 months after vaccination, and vaccination should be repeated if the patient is still skin-test negative. Infants younger than 30 days should receive half the usual dose.

BCG rarely causes serious complications. Side effects occur in 1% to 10% of vaccinated persons and usually include severe or prolonged ulceration at the vaccination site, regional lymphadenitis, and lupus vulgaris. Rare complications have been osteomyelitis with some vaccine strains and disseminated, even fatal BCG infection in persons with impaired immunity.

Contraindications. BCG should not be given to persons who have burns, skin infections, cellular or combined immunodeficiencies, or symptomatic HIV infection, or to persons who are receiving therapy with immunosuppressive agents, including corticosteroids. In the United States where the risk of tuberculosis is low, BCG should not be given to children with known or suspected asymptomatic HIV infection. In populations in which the risk of tuberculosis is high, however, the World Health Organization has recommended that asymptomatic HIV-infected children receive BCG at birth or shortly thereafter.

Although no untoward effects of BCG on the fetus have been observed, vaccination during pregnancy is not prudent. Malnutrition is not considered a contraindication.

Data about whether INH inhibits multiplication (and therefore effectiveness) of BCG are conflicting. INH, which has well-documented efficacy, should not be preempted by BCG which does not.

Reporting of Cases. All cases of active tuberculosis should be reported to the public health authorities, and the physician should assist in a search for a source case and others infected by a source case. Source cases are usually adults or adolescents, such as members of the household (including parents, grandparents, teenage siblings, servants, boarders, baby-sitters, and frequent visitors) or other adults with whom the child has frequent contact.

Disease Due to Nontuberculous Mycobacteria

(Atypical Mycobacteria, Mycobacteria Other Than Tuberculosis)

Clinical Manifestations: Several different syndromes are caused by nontuberculous mycobacteria (NTM). In children, the most common of these syndromes is cervical lymphadenitis. Less commonly, infections are osteomyelitis, cutaneous infection otitis media, and pulmonary disease. More recently, disseminated infections have been described; they are almost always associated with severe congenital or acquired immunodeficiency syndromes characterized by defects in cell-mediated immunity, such as AIDS.

Etiology: Of the many species of NTM that have been identified, only a small number account for most of the infections caused by these organisms. The species most frequently encountered in children are *Mycobacterium avium* complex (includes the Battey bacillus), *M scrofulaceum*, *M kansasii*, and *M marinum* (Table 55). *M fortuitum* and *M chelonei* are frequently referred to as "rapid-growing" mycobacteria because they grow sufficiently in the laboratory to be identified in days whereas other NTM and *M tuberculosis* take weeks. *M fortuitum* and *M chelonei* have occasionally been implicated in wound, soft-tissue, and pulmonary and middle ear infections. Other mycobacterial species, which are usually not considered pathogenic, have caused infections in hosts considered abnormal because of immunologic disorders, immunosuppressive therapy, or the presence of a foreign body.

Epidemiology: Because infections caused by NTM are not reportable in most areas, systematic data concerning their incidence and distribution are fewer than that for infections caused by *M tuberculosis*. In the past, as the incidence of tuberculosis decreased, the relative

Table 55. Nontuberculous Mycobacterial Species Most Commonly Causing Disease in Children

Organism	Syndrome
M avium complex (includes Battey bacillus)	Lymphadenitis, pulmonary infection, disseminated disease in the immunocompromised host
M scrofulaceum	Lymphadenitis
M kansasii	Lymphadenitis, pulmonary infection
M marinum	Cutaneous infection ("swimming pool granuloma")
M fortuitum	Lymphadenitis, cutaneous infection
M chelonei	Cutaneous infection, pulmonary infections, otitis media

proportion of mycobacterial infections caused by NTM increased. Since the advent of HIV infection, however, the incidence of both tuberculosis and NTM infections has increased.

Many NTM species are ubiquitous and are found in soil, food, water, and animals. Most infections appear to be acquired by aspiration or inoculation of the organisms from these natural sources. Skin testing surveys using purified protein derivative (PPD) antigens derived from various NTM indicate that infections occur worldwide. In the United States, a survey in the 1960s suggested that NTM infection is more common in the Southeastern and South Central areas. Although many individuals are exposed to NTM, only a few of these exposures lead either to long-term colonization or overt clinical infection. The usual portals of entry for NTM are believed to be abrasions in the skin (e.g., for the cutaneous lesions caused by *M marinum*), the oropharyngeal mucosa (the presumed portal for cervical lymphadenitis), the gastrointestinal tract for *M avium* complex, and the respiratory tract, including tympanostomy tubes in otitis media and rare cases of mediastinal adenitis and endobronchial disease. Most infections remain localized at the portal of entry or in regional lymph nodes. Severe pulmonary disease and dissemination to distal sites occur primarily in immunocompromised hosts, especially patients with AIDS. No evidence for person-to-person transmission of NTM exists but appropriate studies, especially in the case of HIV-infected and other immunosuppressed patients, have not been performed. Cases of otitis media caused by *M cheloni* has been associated with use of contaminated equipment. A water-borne route of transmission has been incriminated for *M avium* complex in immunodeficient hosts.

Diagnostic Tests: Definitive diagnosis of disease caused by NTM requires isolation and identification of the infecting organism. Caution must be exercised in the interpretation of cultures obtained from sites that are not necessarily sterile, such as from gastric washings, a draining sinus tract, or a single urine specimen. Caution in ascribing illness to the isolated NTM is especially warranted if the species cultured is usually nonpathogenic (e.g., *M gordonae*) and if only a few colonies are recovered from a single specimen. Repeated isolation of numerous colonies of a single species is more likely to be indicative of disease than transient colonization. Most reliable for diagnostic purposes is the recovery of NTM from sites that are otherwise sterile, such as cerebrospinal fluid, pleural fluid, bone marrow, blood, lymph node aspirates, middle ear or mastoid aspirates, or surgically excised tissue. Use of the Du Pont Isolator* system has increased the sensitivity of blood cultures.

Patients with NTM infection can have false positive tuberculin skin tests, since tuberculin preparations (PPD) derived from *M tuberculosis* share a number of antigens with NTM species. These false positive tests occur in otherwise healthy children who have no history of exposure to *M tuberculosis* but may have been sensitized by exposure to NTM in the environment. Those cross-reactions which usually, but not always, result in PPD reactions measuring less than 10 mm of induration may be more common than "true-positive" tuberculin reactions in populations with low prevalence of tuberculosis and a high percentage of NTM infections.

For both clinical and public health reasons, differentiating *M tuberculosis* infection from NTM infections is important. Studies in children had shown that dual Mantoux tests with standard PPD (for *M tuberculosis*) and PPD-Battey sometimes are helpful in distinguishing tuberculous from nontuberculous infections. Skin tests using PPD derived from different NTM species, however, are not commercially available.

A large reaction (15-mm induration) to a standard (5 TU PPD) intradermal tuberculin skin test is more indicative of infection with *M tuberculosis*; a reaction of less than 10 mm suggests NTM infection, especially in the patient with cervical adenitis or other syndromes consistent with NTM disease, a normal chest roentgenogram, and nonreactive PPD tests in other family members. However, exposed children with PPD reactions of 8 to 9 mm could be incubating *M tuberculosis* and should be retested. The identification of family members with positive tuberculin reactions is corroborative

---

*E.I. du Pont de Nemours, Wilmington, DE.

evidence of *M tuberculosis* infection in the index case. Negative results on tuberculin testing, chest roentgenography, and investigation of contacts is consistent with possible NTM infection.

Disseminated NTM disease should prompt a search for an underlying predisposing factor. Tests of immune function and a search for other opportunistic pathogens (e.g., *Pneumocystis carinii*) are indicated. In patients with disseminated NTM disease, history of hemophilia, prior blood transfusion, drug addiction, or a maternal history of drug addiction, prostitution, or sexual intercourse with an intravenous drug user should prompt a diagnostic evaluation for HIV infection.

Treatment: Many NTM are relatively resistant in vitro to antituberculous drugs. In vitro resistance, however, does not necessarily correlate with clinical response. No controlled therapeutic trials have been performed in NTM infections. The approach to therapy should take into account the following factors: (1) the species implicated in the infection, (2) the results of drug susceptibility testing, (3) the site(s) of infection, (4) the nature of the patient's underlying disease (if any), and (5) the occasional need to treat a patient presumptively for tuberculosis while awaiting culture reports that subsequently reveal NTM infection.

For the common problem of NTM lymphadenitis in otherwise healthy children, especially when the disease is caused by *M scrofulaceum* or *M avium* complex, chemotherapy usually offers little benefit, and surgical excision alone is frequently the most effective treatment.

Cutaneous infections with *M marinum* can require a combination of medical and surgical debridement. Minocycline has been successfully used for *M marinum* sporotrichoid skin infections; other tetracyclines can also be given. Tetracyclines, however, should not be given to children younger than 9 years unless the benefits of therapy are clearly greater than the risks of dental staining. The combination of rifampin, ethambutol, and trimethoprim-sulfamethoxazole may also be effective.

Infections caused by *M kansasii* usually respond well to treatment with rifampin, ethambutol, and isoniazid, although the organism may be resistant in vitro to one or more of these agents.

Clinical isolates of *M avium* complex are usually resistant to most of the licensed antituberculous drugs. Nonetheless, empirical therapy with three, four, five, or even six antituberculous agents may be indicated in some patients, such as those with AIDS. Some successes have been reported, although recovery appears to depend on host factors as much as on chemotherapy. Aggressive multidrug therapy is warranted when disease is progressive, severe, or disseminated.

Agents such as clofazamine (an agent used in the treatment of *M leprae* infections) have been used experimentally as part of multidrug regimens, especially in patients with AIDS.

Ciprofloxacin is active in vitro against *M fortuitum* and, to a lesser extent, against *M avium* complex, and may have a role in treating some patients with infections caused by these organisms. Fluroquinolones, however, should not be given to patients younger than 21 years except in circumstances in which no other drug is available and the benefits of therapy are clearly greater than the risks.

Isolates of rapid-growing mycobacteria (*M fortuitum, M chelonei*) should be tested in vitro against antituberculous agents, as well as against other drugs (such as amikacin, imipenem, cefoxitin, ciprofloxacin, erythromycin, and doxycycline) to which they frequently are susceptible and which have been used with some clinical success. Details regarding choice of drugs, dosages, and duration should be reviewed with a consultant experienced in the management of these infections.

Additional information concerning treatment of NTM infections can be obtained from the Division of Tuberculosis Control, Centers for Disease Control (404/639-2530).

Isolation of the Hospitalized Patient: No special precautions are recommended.

Control Measures: No control measures are known, other than use of sterile equipment for middle ear instrumentation including otoscopic equipment for prevention of *M cheloni* otitis media. No specific management of exposed persons is necessary.

Tularemia

Clinical Manifestations: Tularemia is usually characterized by high fever and severe, influenza-like constitutional symptoms of chills, myalgia, and, in older children, headache. However, clinically mild tularemia has been increasingly recognized. Onset frequently is abrupt and conforms to one of the specific tularemic syndromes. The ulceroglandular syndrome, the most common, is characterized by (1) a primary, painful maculopapular lesion at the portal of entry, with subsequent ulceration and slow healing; and (2) painful, acutely inflamed lymph nodes, which may drain spontaneously. Other disease syndromes are the following: oculoglandular (severe conjunctivitis and lymph node involvement), oropharyngeal (severe exudative pharyngitis), glandular (no skin or mucous membrane lesion is present), typhoidal (high fever, hepatomegaly, and splenomegaly), and pneumonia.

Etiology: *Francisella tularensis*, the causative agent, is a small, Gram-negative coccobacillus.

Epidemiology: Sources of the organism include approximately 100 species of wild mammals, including rabbits, hares, muskrats, squirrels, and deer; at least nine species of domestic animals (e.g., sheep, cattle, and cats); blood-sucking insects that bite these animals (e.g., ticks, deerflies, and mosquitoes); and water contaminated by infected animals. In the United States, major reservoirs include rabbits and ticks. Ticks are the most important vectors. Infected animals and insects are infective for prolonged periods: frozen, killed rabbits can remain infective for more than 3 years. Persons at risk are those with direct occupational or indirect recreational exposure to infected animals, such as rabbit hunters and trappers; those with insect bites; and laboratory technicians working with *F tularensis* (which is highly infectious). Transmission is by indirect contact via insect bites; direct contact with infected animals; ingestion of contaminated water or inadequately cooked meat; or inhalation of contaminated particles. Person-to-person transmission has not been documented. Organisms may be found in the blood during the first 2 weeks of the disease and in lesions for up to 1 month if untreated.

The **incubation period** ranges from 1 to 21 days; most cases occur 3 to 5 days after exposure.

Diagnostic Tests: A fourfold or greater rise in the serum *F tularensis* agglutinin titer frequently is evident after the second week of illness and is considered diagnostic. A single convalescent titer of 1:160 or greater is consistent with recent or past infection. Tube titers are more reliable than slide tests; nonspecific cross-agglutination with *Brucella*, *Proteus*, and heterophile antibodies can cause false-positive antibody titers to *F tularensis*. Culture of blood, skin, ulcers, lymph node drainage, gastric washings, and respiratory secretions require special media or guinea pig inoculation. The laboratory should be informed that *F tularensis* is suspected, since the risk of infection in laboratory personnel when cultures are performed is a potential hazard and limits the availability of culture services for establishing the diagnosis. The indirect fluorescent antibody test for ulcer exudate or aspirate can be useful but is not generally available.

Treatment: Streptomycin for 6 to 10 days is the usual therapy. The longer course is given for more severe illness.

Gentamicin also appears effective. The alternative drugs—tetracycline (which should not be given to children younger than 9 years) and chloramphenicol—are more likely to result in clinical relapses.

Isolation of the Hospitalized Patient: Drainage/secretion precautions should be used until the lesions stop draining. Respiratory isolation should be considered for patients with pneumonic tularemia.

Control Measures:

- Persons at risk should minimize opportunities for insect bites by wearing protective clothing and by frequent inspection and removal of ticks from the skin and scalp; insect repellents may be of some value (see Control Measures for Prevention of Tick-Borne Infections, page 112).
- Children should be discouraged from handling sick or dead rabbits and rodents.
- Rubber gloves should be worn when handling wild rabbits and other potentially infected animals.
- Wild rabbit meat should be thoroughly cooked.
- Face masks and rubber gloves should be worn by those working with cultures or infective material in the laboratory.
- Drainage/secretion precautions should be used for handling contaminated articles.
- Interstate or interarea shipment of infected animals should be prohibited.
- A live attenuated vaccine (available from the Centers for Disease Control) is recommended for those repeatedly exposed to the organism, such as laboratory research technicians.

Endemic Typhus

(Murine Typhus)

Clinical Manifestations: Endemic typhus resembles epidemic typhus but is usually milder, with less acute onset and less severe systemic symptoms. In young children, the disease is very mild. Fever can be accompanied by persistent headache and myalgias. The rash is typically macular or maculopapular, appears during days 3 to 5 of illness, lasts 4 to 8 days, and tends to remain discrete, with sparse lesions and no hemorrhage. The disease seldom lasts longer than 2 weeks, and visceral involvement does not usually occur. The disease is rarely fatal.

Etiology: Endemic typhus is caused by *Rickettsia typhi* (formerly *R mooseri*), an organism antigenically similar to *R prowazekii*.

Epidemiology: Rats, in which infection is inapparent, are the natural hosts. The vector for transmission to rats and occasionally and accidentally to humans is the rat flea (usually *Xenopsylla cheopis*). The disease is worldwide in distribution, affects all races, tends to occur more commonly in adults and in males, and is most common from April to October. The disease is infrequent in the United States; most cases occur in focal areas in southern California, the southeastern Gulf Coast and southern border states, and Hawaii. Exposure to rats and their fleas is the major risk factor, although a history of such exposure is frequently absent in infected patients.

The **incubation period** is 6 to 14 days.

Diagnostic Tests: Serum agglutinins against *Proteus* OX-19 peak 2 to 3 weeks after the onset of disease, but these tests lack sensitivity and specificity. Indirect fluorescent antibody, latex agglutination, or complement fixation antibody concentrations peak at a similar or slightly later time. A fourfold titer rise between acute and convalescent serum specimens is diagnostic but can also occur in patients with epidemic typhus. Serologic differentiation between these diseases is possible by cross-absorption of the patient's serum. Isolation of the organism in culture is possible but hazardous, and it requires specialized facilities and experienced personnel.

Treatment: A single dose of tetracycline (5 mg/kg; maximum 200 mg) is the treatment of choice. Although tetracyclines should not be given to children younger than 9 years, the risk of dental staining from a single dose of doxycline is minimal. Chloramphenicol is also an effective drug.

Isolation of the Hospitalized Patient: No special precautions are recommended.

Control Measures: Rat fleas should be controlled by appropriate insecticides, preferably before the use of rodenticides, because the flea will seek alternate hosts when rats are not available. Rat populations should then be controlled by appropriate means. Endemic typhus vaccine is no longer available. No treatment is recommended for exposed persons. This disease is reportable in a few states.

Epidemic Typhus

(Louse-Borne Typhus)

Clinical Manifestations: In epidemic typhus, the onset of high fever, chills, and diffuse aching accompanied by severe headache and malaise is usually abrupt. Influenza-like illness is frequently suspected. The rash appears 4 to 7 days later, beginning on the trunk and spreading to the limbs. A concentrated eruption is present in the axillae. The rash is maculopapular, becomes petechial or hemorrhagic, then develops into brownish, pigmented areas. The face, palms, and soles are usually not affected. Mental changes are common, and delirium or coma may occur. Myocardial and renal failure occur when the disease is severe. Illness varies from moderately severe to fatal (10% to 40% mortality rate); when untreated it typically lasts 2 weeks and ends by lysis of fever and subsidence of symptoms. In untreated cases, mortality is uncommon in children, ranges from 10% to 40% in adults, and increases with increasing age. Brill-Zinsser disease is a relapse of louse-borne typhus that occurs years after the initial episode. Stress or an unknown factor serves to reactivate the rickettsiae. The recrudescent illness is similar to the primary infection, but is generally milder and of shorter duration.

Etiology: *Rickettsia prowazekii* is the cause.

Epidemiology: Humans are the major source of the organism, which is transmitted from person to person by the body louse *Pediculus humanus* subspecies *corporis*. All ages and races and both sexes are affected. Poverty, crowding, poor sanitary conditions, lack of bathing, and poor personal hygiene contribute to the spread of lice, and hence the disease. Currently, cases of typhus are rarely reported but have occurred throughout the world, including Asia, Africa, some parts of Europe, and Central and South America. Typhus was common during winter when conditions favor person-to-person transmission of the vector, the body louse. Rickettsiae are present in the blood and tissues of patients during the early febrile phase but not in secretions. Direct person-to-person spread of the disease does not occur in the absence of the vector.

Serologic evidence of epidemic typhus in flying squirrels in the United States has been reported, and cases in humans have been associated with contact with squirrels, their nests, or their ectoparasites. Squirrel-related epidemic typhus appears to be a milder illness than louse-borne epidemic typhus.

The **incubation period** is 1 to 2 weeks.

Diagnostic Tests: *R prowazekii* can be isolated from the blood by inoculation into guinea pigs and mice or the yolk sac of embryonated hens' eggs, but because isolation is dangerous, it is rarely attempted. Serum agglutinins against *Proteus* OX-19 reach peak titers 2 to 3 weeks after the onset of disease, but an indirect fluorescent antibody or complement fixation antibody test is preferred. A fourfold increase in antibody titer between acute and convalescent serum specimens is diagnostic of either epidemic or endemic typhus (see Endemic Typhus, page 515). An antibody absorption test can often differentiate the two diseases.

Treatment: Tetracycline or chloramphenicol, given intravenously or orally, is the antibiotic of choice. Tetracycline should not be given to children younger than 9 years unless the benefits are clearly greater than the risks of dental staining. Therapy is given until the patient is afebrile for at least 7 days; usual duration is 7 days. Cream and gel pediculocides containing pyrethrins (0.16% to 0.33%) and piperonyl butoxide (2% to 4%), crotamiton (10%), or lindane (1%) can be used for delousing. Convulsions have been reported in children receiving excessive doses of topical lindane.

Isolation of the Hospitalized Patient: No special precautions are recommended.

Control Measures: Thorough delousing in epidemic situations, particularly among exposed contacts of cases, is recommended. Several applications may be needed because the lice eggs are resistant to most insecticides. Washing clothes in hot water kills lice and eggs. During epidemics, insecticides dusted onto the clothes of louse-infested populations are effective in louse control efforts. In some circumstances, preventing flying squirrels from living in human dwellings by sealing their access ports is recommended. Epidemic typhus vaccine is no longer available in the United States. Cases should be reported to public health departments.

Varicella-Zoster Infections

Clinical Manifestations: Primary infection with varicella-zoster virus (VZV) results in chickenpox. Chickenpox is manifest by a generalized, pruritic, vesicular rash, with a mild fever and mild systemic symptoms. A variety of complications occur, including bacterial superinfection, thrombocytopenia, arthritis, hepatitis, encephalitis or meningitis, and glomerulonephritis. Reye syndrome can follow some cases of chickenpox. In immunocompromised children, progressive varicella characterized by continuing eruption of lesions and a high fever into the second week of the illness can occur. Encephalitis, pancreatitis, hepatitis, or pneumonia can develop. Children with AIDS can develop chronic chickenpox with new lesions appearing during a period of months. Chickenpox is often more severe in adults. Pneumonia, although rare in normal children, is the most common complication in older individuals.

The virus persists in a latent form after the primary infection. Reactivation results in zoster or shingles. Grouped vesicular lesions appear in the distribution of one to three sensory dermatomes, sometimes accompanied by pain localized to the area. Systemic symptoms are few. Zoster occasionally can become generalized in immunocompromised children, with lesions appearing outside the dermatomes and with visceral complications.

Fetal infection after maternal varicella in the first or early second trimester of pregnancy may result in varicella embryopathy, which is characterized by limb atrophy and scarring of the skin of the extremity. Central nervous system and eye manifestations can also occur. Children who were exposed to VZV in utero may develop zoster early in life without having had previous varicella. Varicella of the newborn infant can result from maternal varicella shortly before delivery. When maternal varicella occurs between 5 days before delivery and 2 days after delivery, severe disease can result in the newborn with case fatality rates as high as 5%.

Etiology: VZV is a herpesvirus. Only one serotype is recognized.

Epidemiology: Humans are the only source of infection for this highly contagious virus. Person-to-person spread occurs by direct contact with varicella or zoster lesions or by air-borne droplet infection. Patients with zoster, as well as those with varicella, are capable of transmitting infection, but air-borne droplet spread from patients with zoster is rare. Introduction of a VZV infection into a household usually results in infection of nearly all susceptible persons. At present, most reported cases of chickenpox occur in children between 5 and 10 years old, but varicella in adolescents and young adults may be becoming more common. Immunity is generally lifelong. Symptomatic reinfection is rare in normal persons although asymptomatic reinfection may occur. Varicella is most common during the late winter and early spring. Asymptomatic primary infection is rare. Patients are contagious for 1 to 2 days before and shortly after the onset of the rash; contagiousness may be for as long as 5 days after the onset of lesions. Immunocompromised patients with progressive varicella are probably contagious during the entire period of eruption of new lesions.

The **incubation period** is usually 14 to 16 days; some cases occur as early as 11 or as late as 20 days after contact. It may be short in immunocompromised patients. The incubation period may be prolonged to 28 days in Varicella-Zoster Immune Globulin (VZIG) recipients.

Diagnostic Tests: VZV can be isolated from vesicular lesions of normal patients during the first 3 to 4 days of the eruption. Diagnosis can also be accomplished by immunofluorescent staining of vesicular scrapings, and herpesvirus particles can be seen by direct electron microscopic examination. The demonstration of multinucleated giant cells containing intranuclear inclusions in lesions (Tzanck smear) indicates the presence of VZV or another herpesvirus. Infection can be confirmed by staining smears with VZV-specific antibody or by testing acute-phase and convalescent-phase sera for VZ antibody. Serologic ELISA or the fluorescent antibody tests against membrane antigen (FAMA) can be used to determine immune status, but the complement fixation test is not reliable for this purpose.

Treatment: Both intravenous vidarabine and acyclovir are effective in treating varicella or zoster in immunocompromised patients. However, acyclovir is less toxic and is the usual drug of choice. Early therapy is preferable to waiting until progression has occurred. Transfusion of immune plasma or VZIG can prevent or modify the course of disease when given shortly after exposure (see Care of Exposed Persons, page 520) but is not effective in therapy once disease is established.

Oral acyclovir given to children with varicella within 24 hours of the onset of rash results in decrease in the duration and magnitude of fever and in the number and duration of skin lesions. It can be considered for persons at increased risk of severe varicella, such as those older than 14 years and those with chronic respiratory or skin disease.

Children with varicella should not receive salicylates because administration of salicylates in such children increases the risk of subsequent Reye syndrome. Acetaminophen may be used for fever control.

Isolation of the Hospitalized Patient: Strict isolation is indicated for patients with varicella for at least 5 days after the onset of the rash and for the duration of the vesicular eruption, which in immunocompromised patients can be a week or longer. Exposed susceptible inpatients should be in strict isolation from 10 until 21 days after the onset of the rash in the index patient. Those who received VZIG should be kept in isolation until 28 days after exposure.

Neonates born to mothers with active varicella should be placed in isolation at birth and, if still hospitalized, until 21 or 28 days of age, depending on whether they received VZIG. Infants with varicella embryopathy do not require isolation.

Immunocompromised patients who have zoster (localized or disseminated) and normal patients with disseminated zoster should remain in strict isolation for the duration of the illness. For normal patients with localized zoster, drainage/secretion precautions are indicated until all lesions are crusted.

Control Measures:

Day Care and School. Children with uncomplicated chickenpox who have been excluded from school or day care may return on the sixth day after the onset of the rash. In mild cases with only a few lesions and rapid resolution, children may return sooner if all lesions are crusted. Immunocompromised and other children with a prolonged course should be excluded for the duration of the vesicular eruption.

Exclusion of children with zoster whose lesions cannot be covered is based on similar criteria. Those who are excluded may return after the lesions have crusted. Lesions that are covered appear to pose little risk to susceptible individuals. Older children and staff members with zoster should be instructed to wash their hands if they touch potentially infectious lesions.

Care of Exposed Persons. VZIG should be given to susceptible individuals at high risk of developing progressive varicella. VZIG is a licensed product and can be obtained by calling the local office of the American Red Cross Blood Services.

The decision of whether to administer VZIG depends on the following three factors: (1) the likelihood that an individual will develop complications of varicella if infected; (2) the probability that a given exposure to varicella or zoster will result in infection; and (3) the likelihood that the exposed person is susceptible to varicella. Household exposure to varicella poses an almost certain risk of infection; other types of exposure are less likely to result in infection. Exposure more than 5 days after the appearance of the first lesion in normal patients poses a relatively low risk, as does exposure more than 1 to 2 days before the eruption. Persons with history of varicella are usually considered immune. However, persons without such history may still be immune. Careful questioning about history of varicella in other siblings (particularly younger siblings), whether the patient attended an urban school, previous exposure to patients with chickenpox or zoster, or other clues can be helpful in deciding whether a person with a negative history of varicella is susceptible. The use of laboratory tests to determine immune status is useful but should not delay the administration of VZIG beyond 96 hours after exposure. Children with malignancies receiving immunosuppressive therapy who have serum VZV antibody at the time of exposure and a negative history of disease still may be at risk of developing varicella, especially if they recently received blood products. Similarly, children previously immune who receive chemotherapy may become susceptible.

Patients receiving monthly treatments of high dose intravenous immunogobulin (IGIV 100 to 400 mg/kg) should be protected and do not require VZIG if the last dose of IGIV was given within 3 weeks.

Administration and Dose. VZIG is given by intramuscular injection. It contains between 10% and 18% globulin; thimerosal 1:10,000 is included as a preservative. One vial (approximate volume, 1.25 mL) containing 125 units is given for each 10 kg of body weight (and is the minimum dose). The maximum suggested dose is 625 units (i.e., five vials). For maximal effectiveness, VZIG should be given within 48 hours of, and preferably not more than 96 hours after exposure.

Use in patients with a bleeding diathesis should be avoided if possible. VZIG should never be given intravenously. Local discomfort following intramuscular injection is common and is the most frequent adverse effect.

Indications. The following susceptible persons should receive VZIG (also see Tables 56 and 57):

- *High-risk children.* High-risk, immunocompromised, susceptible children younger than 15 years who have had continuing household exposure, shared a hospital room containing four or fewer beds, or played indoors for at least 1 hour with children who are in the contagious state of chickenpox should receive VZIG. Older adolescents and adults who are immunocompromised are likely to be immune, but if susceptible they should also receive VZIG. Hospitalized patients who have been exposed should be discharged before the 10th day after exposure, if possible. If not possible they should be placed in strict isolation (see Isolation of the Hospitalized Patient, page 519).
- *Normal adults.* Administration of VZIG to normal adults who have been in close contact with a person with VZV infection is desirable, particularly if careful questioning indicates that they are likely to be susceptible. However, laboratory testing should be performed whenever possible because most adults with negative or uncertain history of chickenpox have high probability of immunity.
- *Pregnant women.* Varicella-susceptible pregnant women may be at higher risk for serious complications than adults in general. Of major concern is the risk to the fetus when a woman develops varicella-zoster infection during the first half of pregnancy. The composite risk of defects following infection during the first trimester in four studies was 2.3% (3 of 131). The risk for defects after infection at any time during pregnancy was lower. Whether

Table 56. Candidates for VZIG, Provided Significant Exposure* Has Occurred

Immunocompromised, susceptible children.†
Normal, susceptible adolescents (≥ 15 y) and adults, in particular pregnant women. Serologic determination of immune status is advised.
Newborn infant of a mother who had onset of chickenpox within 5 days before delivery or within 48 hours after delivery.
Hospitalized premature infant (≥ 28 wk gestation) whose mother has no history of chickenpox.
Hospitalized premature infants (< 28 wk gestation or ≤ 1,000 g), regardless of maternal history.

*See text and Table 57.

†Immunocompromised adolescents (≥ 15 years) and adults are likely to be immune, but, if susceptible, they should also receive VZIG.

the fetus will be protected against the development of malformations if VZIG is given to a pregnant, susceptible woman after exposure is unknown. VZIG could conceivably modify the maternal infection such that it becomes asymptomatic. Accordingly, protection of the fetus cannot be assumed if a susceptible, exposed woman receives VZIG and does not develop signs of chickenpox.

Antibody administered to a pregnant woman within 5 days before delivery is unlikely to be absorbed and transported across the placenta in sufficient quantities to appreciably protect the infant. Therefore, administration of VZIG to the newborn infant, if otherwise indicated, is preferable.

- *Newborns.* VZIG (125 U) should be given as soon as possible after delivery to infants whose mothers have had onset of varicella within 5 days before or within 2 days after delivery. Approximately half of these infants, if VZIG is not given, can be expected to develop varicella (which can occur as early as 1 day after delivery).

For normal, full-term infants exposed 2 or more days postnatally to varicella, including those whose mothers' rash developed more than 48 hours after delivery, VZIG is not indicated because infants who develop varicella under these conditions are not known to be at any greater risk of complications of chickenpox than older children. However, because of the poor transfer of antibody across the placenta early in pregnancy, all infants born before 28 weeks of gestation (and/or who weigh less than 1,000 g), who still require hospitalization for treatment of prematurity or related conditions, and who are exposed to varicella should receive VZIG (125 U). Premature infants born after 28 weeks'

Table 57. Type of Exposure to Varicella or Zoster for Which VZIG Is Indicated*

One of the following types of exposure to persons with chickenpox or zoster:

- Continuous household contact
- Playmate contact: generally more than 1 hour of play indoors
- Hospital contact: in same 2- to 4-bed room, or adjacent beds in a large ward, or prolonged face-to-face contact with an infectious staff member or patient
- Newborn infant contact: newborn infant whose mother had onset of chickenpox 5 days or less before delivery or within 48 hours after delivery

and

Time elapsed after exposure is such that VZIG can be administered within 96 hours (preferably sooner).

*Patients should meet criteria of both significant exposure and candidacy for receiving VZIG, as given in Table 56.

gestation, who are exposed in the hospital, and whose mothers have negative history of infection should also receive VZIG. Infants in these categories who have been discharged because they have reached mature weight do not need VZIG.

- *Subsequent exposures and follow-up of VZIG recipients.* Since the administration of VZIG can cause the infection to be asymptomatic, testing of recipients 2 months or later after administration of VZIG for infection from chickenpox to ascertain their immune status may be considered. However, whether asymptomatic infection after VZIG administration confers lasting protection is not clear. Thus, the patient in whom asymptomatic infection has been documented, and for whom VZIG is otherwise indicated, probably should still receive VZIG after subsequent recognized varicella exposures.

  The duration for which VZIG recipients are protected against chickenpox is unknown. If a second exposure occurs more than 2 weeks after administration of VZIG in a recipient who did not develop varicella, another dose of VZIG should be given.

Active Immunization. Licensure of live varicella vaccine in the United States is anticipated in the near future. Recommendations from the Committee will be forthcoming at that time.

Vibrio Infections

(Except Cholera)

Clinical Manifestations: Diarrhea is most frequent, characterized by acute onset of watery stools and crampy abdominal pain. About one half of those afflicted will have low-grade fever, headache, and chills; about 30% will have vomiting. Spontaneous recovery follows in 2 to 5 days. Bacteremia is rare.

Infection can develop in contaminated wounds. Immunocompromised patients can develop sepsis from bowel or skin infections, often resulting in shock, bullous or necrotic skin lesions and death. Skin infections in compromised patients can rapidly cause extensive tissue necrosis.

Etiology: Vibrios are aerobic, Gram-negative rods. The most important noncholera *Vibrio* species associated with diarrhea is *V parahaemolyticus*. *V vulnificus* is associated with severe infections in immunocompromised patients. *V alginolyticus* and other species are usually associated with wound infections and otitis externa.

Epidemiology: Noncholera vibrios are commonly found in seawater, increasing in numbers during summer. Most infections occur in summer and fall. Enteritis is usually acquired from seafood eaten raw or undercooked, especially oysters, crabs, and shrimp. Disease is probably not communicable from person to person. Wound infections commonly result from exposure of abrasions to contaminated seawater or from punctures resulting from handling of contaminated shellfish.

The median **incubation period** of enteritis is 23 hours, with a range of 5 to 92 hours.

Diagnostic Tests: These organisms can be isolated from the stool or vomitus of patients with diarrhea, from blood, and from wound exudates. Because identification of the organism requires special techniques, the laboratory should be notified when *Vibrio* infection is suspected.

Treatment: Most episodes of diarrhea are mild and self limited and do not require treatment other than oral rehydration. Antibiotic therapy may benefit those with severe diarrhea or wound infections. Organisms are usually susceptible to cephalexin, tetracycline (which usually should not be used in patients younger than 9 years), chloramphenicol, and gentamicin.

Isolation of the Hospitalized Patient: Enteric precautions are indicated for the duration of diarrheal illness. Contact precautions should be used for draining wounds.

Control Measures: Seafood should be adequately cooked and if not ingested immediately, it should be refrigerated. Uncooked mollusks and crustaceans should be handled with care. Abrasions suffered by ocean bathers should be rinsed well with clean, fresh water. Persons with liver disease or immunodeficiency should be warned to avoid eating raw oysters.

Yersinia enterocolitica and *Yersinia pseudotuberculosis*

(Enteritis and Other Illnesses)

Clinical Manifestations: With *Yersinia enterocolitica*, the most common manifestation is enterocolitis with fever, diarrhea (leukocytes, blood, and mucus frequently in the stool), and abdominal pain lasting 1 to 3 weeks. Other manifestations can include acute mesenteric adenitis, terminal ileitis, pharyngitis, arthritis, erythema nodosum, septicemia, iritis, meningitis, osteomyelitis, hepatic and splenic abscesses, and acute proliferative glomerulonephritis. With *Y pseudotuberculosis*, acute abdominal pain syndromes are most common, resulting from mesenteric adenitis, appendicitis, or terminal ileitis. Other findings can include diarrhea, erythema nodosum, septicemia, sterile pleural and joint effusions, and scarlatiniform rash. Clinical features can mimic those of Kawasaki syndrome.

Etiology: *Y enterocolitica* and *Y pseudotuberculosis* are Gram-negative rods; 34 serotypes of *Y enterocolitica* and 5 serotypes of *Y pseudotuberculosis* are recognized.

Epidemiology: The reservoirs of the organisms are animals, including particularly rodents (*Y pseudotuberculosis*) and swine (*Y enterocolitica*). Infection is believed to be transmitted by the ingestion of contaminated food, especially uncooked pork products and unpasteurized milk, or water; by direct or indirect contact with animals; by transfusion with packed red cells; and possibly by direct fecal-oral, person-to-person transmission. Patients with excessive iron storage syndromes are unusually susceptible to *Yersinia* bacteremia. The period of communicability is unknown; it is probably for the duration of excretion of the specific organisms, which averages 6 weeks after diagnosis.

The **incubation period** is typically 4 to 6 days, and varies from 1 to 14 days.

Diagnostic Tests: *Y enterocolitica* and *Y pseudotuberculosis* can also be recovered from throat swabs, mesenteric lymph nodes, peritoneal fluid, or blood. Stool cultures are generally positive during the first 2 weeks of illness, regardless of the nature of the gastrointestinal manifestations. *Y enterocolitica* has been isolated from synovial fluid, bile, urine, cerebrospinal fluid, sputum, and wounds. Because laboratory identification of organisms from the stool requires special techniques, the laboratory should be notified that *Yersinia* infection is suspected. Pathogenic strains of *Y enterocolitica* are usually pyrazinamidase-negative. Infection can be confirmed by demonstrating serum agglutination antibody titer rises after infection, but these tests are available only in special laboratories. Cross-reactions of these antibodies with *Brucella*, *Vibrio*, *Escherichia coli*, *Salmonella*, and Enterobacteriaceae strains lead to false-positive *Y enterocolitica* and *Y pseudotuberculosis* titers. In patients with thyroid disease, persistently elevated *Y enterocolitica* antibody titers can result from antigenic similarity of the organism with the membrane of the thyroid epithelial cell.

Treatment: Both *Y enterocolitica* and *Y pseudotuberculosis* are susceptible to the aminoglycosides, cefotaxime, and other newer cephalosporins, tetracycline (which usually should not be given to children younger than 9 years), chloramphenicol, and trimethoprim-sulfamethoxazole. Patients with septicemia or sites of infection other than the gastrointestinal tract should receive antibiotic therapy. Benefit from antibiotic therapy in patients with enterocolitis or mesenteric adenitis, other than reduced duration of excretion of the organism in stool, has not been established.

Isolation of the Hospitalized Patient: For patients with enterocolitis, enteric precautions are indicated for the duration of the illness.

Control Measures: Ingestion of uncooked meat, impure water, or unpasteurized milk should be avoided.

PART 4

ANTIMICROBIAL PROPHYLAXIS

Antimicrobial Prophylaxis

Antimicrobial agents are commonly prescribed to prevent infections in infants and children. The efficacy of the prophylactic use of these agents has been documented for some conditions but is unsubstantiated for most. Chemoprophylaxis is directed at different targets: specific pathogens, infection-prone body sites, and vulnerable patients. Effective prophylaxis is more readily achieved with specific pathogens and certain body sites.

Specific Pathogens

Prophylaxis is feasible if the physician can recognize situations associated with an increased risk of serious infection with a specific pathogen and select an antimicrobial agent that will eliminate the pathogen from persons at risk, with minimal adverse effects. For some pathogens that initially colonize the upper respiratory tract, elimination of the carrier state can be difficult and requires the use of an antibiotic, such as rifampin, which achieves effective concentrations in nasopharyngeal secretions. This property is lacking among antibiotics ordinarily used to treat infections caused by such pathogens. Table 58 lists examples of pathogens amenable to antimicrobial prophylaxis in children and provides information about documented efficacy. In cases where prophylaxis is recommended, the regimen is described in the chapter on the specific disease in Part 3.

Infection-Prone Body Sites

Prevention of infection of vulnerable body sites may be possible if (1) the period of risk is defined and brief, (2) the expected pathogens have predictable antibiotic susceptibility, and (3) the site is accessible to antibiotics. Examples of infection-prone body sites amenable to chemo-

Table 58. Examples of Specific Pathogens Amenable to Antimicrobial Prophylaxis

Pathogen	Disease to Be Prevented	Antimicrobial Agent	Efficacy
Bacteria			
Bordetella pertussis	Secondary cases of pertussis in household contacts	Erythromycin	Established
Chlamydia trachomatis	Urogenital infections in exposed persons	Tetracycline,* erythromycin	Proposed
Corynebacterium diphtheriae	Diphtheria in unimmunized contacts	Penicillin, erythromycin	Proposed
Haemophilus influenzae type b	Secondary cases of systemic infection in close contacts < 4 y	Rifampin	Established for household contacts
Mycobacterium tuberculosis	Overt pulmonary or metastatic infection	Isoniazid	Established
Neisseria meningitidis	Meningococcemia in exposed susceptible persons	Rifampin	Established
Neisseria gonorrhoeae	Penicillin-resistant gonococcal infection in exposed persons	Ceftriaxone	Established
Streptococcus pneumoniae	Fulminant pneumococcal infection in those with asplenia	Penicillin	Established for penicillin V in children with sickle-cell anemia
Group A streptococcus	Recurrent rheumatic fever	Penicillin, sulfadiazine	Established
Group B streptococcus	Neonatal infection	Ampicillin (intrapartum)	Established
Vibrio cholerae	Cholera in close contacts of a case	Tetracycline*	Proposed
Treponema pallidum	Syphilis in exposed persons	Penicillin	Established
Yersinia pestis	Plague in household contacts or those exposed to pneumonic disease	Tetracycline* or sulfonamide	Proposed

Table 58. Examples of Specific Pathogens Amenable to Antimicrobial Prophylaxis *(continued)*

Pathogen	Disease to Be Prevented	Antimicrobial Agent	Efficacy
Parasites			
Plasmodium species (Malaria)	Overt infection (chloroquine-sensitive) in endemic areas	Chloroquine	Established
Pneumocystis carinii	Pneumonia in compromised host	Trimethoprim-sulfamethoxazole	Established
Viruses			
Influenza A	Influenza in those at risk of complications	Amantadine	Established

*Tetracycline can cause dental staining in children younger than 9 years.

prophylaxis are listed in Table 59. A more detailed discussion of the prevention of surgical wound infection, bacterial endocarditis, and neonatal ophthalmia is given in related sections in Part 4.

Otitis media recurs less frequently in otitis-prone children treated prophylactically with antibiotics. Studies have demonstrated that either daily amoxicillin or sulfisoxazole is effective.

Protection afforded the urinary tract by chemoprophylaxis is critically dependent on the rate of emergence of antibiotic resistance in the gastrointestinal tract flora, the usual source of bacteria that invade the bladder. The long-term effectiveness of nitrofurantoin and trimethoprim-sulfamethoxazole is explained by the minimal effect of these drugs on the development of resistant flora. Both drugs are concentrated in urine, and adequate inhibitory activity can be obtained with less than the usual therapeutic dose. Use of a single dose at bedtime has been successful.

Chemoprophylaxis of animal bite wounds is usually not necessary, as only about 5% of dog bites become infected. Prophylaxis is recommended for wounds that cannot be adequately debrided or irrigated, for deep wounds of the hand, and for facial wounds where excess scarring from infection would be unacceptable.

Vulnerable Hosts

Most attempts to prevent infection in vulnerable patients have been foiled by the rapid replacement of initial bacteria by others resistant to antibiotics. Table 60 lists circumstances in which antibiotics are frequently given to prevent infection.

Table 59. Examples of Infection-Prone Body Sites Amenable to Antimicrobial Prophylaxis

Body Site	Infection to Be Prevented	Agents Used	Efficacy
Conjunctivae	Neonatal gonococcal ophthalmia	1% silver nitrate,* 0.5% erythromycin,* 1% tetracycline*; penicillin	Established
Abnormal heart valve	Bacterial endocarditis (i.e., following dental extraction)	Penicillin, others	See Prevention of Bacterial Endocarditis (page 536)
Surgical wound	Serious postoperative wound infection	Appropriate for expected contaminants	See Antimicrobial Prophylaxis in Ped. Surg. Pts. (page 531)
Middle ear	Recurrent otitis media	Sulfisoxazole, ampicillin	Established
Urinary tract	Recurrent urinary infection	Trimethoprim-sulfamethoxazole, nitrofurantoin	Established
Animal bite wound	Wound infection, cellulitis	Penicillin, amoxicillin-clavulanate	Proposed

*Topical administration

Table 60. Examples of Chemoprophylaxis for Vulnerable Hosts

Infection to Be Prevented	Agents Used	Efficacy
Pneumocystis carinii pneumonia in immunocompromised host	Trimethoprim-sulfamethoxazole, pentamidine aerosol	Established Data available about adults only.
Fulminant bacteremia in those with asplenia	Penicillin; amoxicillin, trimethoprim-sulfamethoxazole (5 years old only)	Established for penicillin V in children with sickle-cell anemia
Bacterial infection in those with chronic granulomatous disease	Trimethoprim-sulfamethoxazole	Proposed

Antimicrobial Prophylaxis in Pediatric Surgical Patients*

A major use of antimicrobial agents in hospitalized children is prophylaxis of postoperative wound infections. In view of this frequent use and the emerging consensus on recommendations for prevention of surgical wound infections, guidelines for surgical antimicrobial prophylaxis in children have been developed. Prophylaxis is defined as the use of antimicrobial drugs in the absence of suspected or documented infection to prevent the development of infection.

Frequency of Antimicrobial Prophylaxis

In hospitalized patients, approximately one third of antimicrobial courses are initiated for prophylaxis of infection after surgery or an invasive procedure such as cystoscopy or cardiac catheterization. The prevalence and reasons for antimicrobial use have been studied primarily in general or adult hospitals, but the patterns of use in children are similar to those in adults. Two studies have demonstrated that prophylaxis accounts for approximately 75% of the antibiotic use on pediatric surgical services. The efficacy of antimicrobial prophylaxis in lowering the incidence of postoperative infection after certain types of surgery has been demonstrated amply in controlled clinical trials. These and earlier studies in experimental animals have delineated the principles for effective use of antimicrobial agents in surgical prophylaxis, including choice of drugs and when and how long they are to be given.

Inappropriate Antimicrobial Prophylaxis

Prophylaxis has been incriminated as a major cause of inappropriate use of these antimicrobial agents in both adults and children. In a study of children younger than 6 years undergoing surgery in which appropriateness of use was assessed on the basis of commonly accepted guidelines, prophylactic antibiotics were administered inappropriately to 42% of children receiving preoperative prophylaxis, 67% of those receiving intraoperative prophylaxis, and 55% of those receiving postoperative prophylaxis. Similarly, in a large pediatric teaching hospital, 66% of antimicrobial agent use on surgical services was considered inappropriate for reasons of wrong drug, dose, time of initiation, duration,

*Adapted from American Academy of Pediatrics, Committee on Infectious Diseases, Committee on Drugs, and Section on Surgery. Antimicrobial prophylaxis in pediatric surgical patients. *Pediatrics*. 1984;74:437-439.

or lack of indication. These findings indicate that the use of antimicrobial agents in children undergoing surgery and other invasive procedures should be subject to periodic review.

Guidelines for Appropriate Use

Studies documenting the efficacy of systemic prophylaxis in surgical wound infections have been performed primarily in adults. Because the pathogenesis of these infections is the same in children, the principles of surgical prophylaxis in children should be similar. In the absence of studies in children, guidelines recommended by the American College of Surgeons, *The Medical Letter*,* the Veterans Administration Committee on Antimicrobial Drug Use, and the Centers for Disease Control provide the only available standards for use of systemic prophylactic antibiotics in pediatric surgical patients. The following general principles are recommended as guidelines, with the understanding that studies in children may result in changes and that factors unique to children may justify exceptions.

Indications for Prophylaxis

Systemic prophylaxis is indicated when the benefits for prevention of wound infection outweigh the risks of drug reactions and the emergence of resistant bacteria. The latter poses a potential risk not only to the recipient but also to other hospitalized patients, who may develop a nosocomial infection caused by antibiotic-resistant organisms. Procedures in which the benefits justify the risks incurred in antimicrobial prophylaxis are those associated with a significant risk of postoperative infection, and those in which the likelihood of infection may not be great but the consequences of infection can be catastrophic. A determinant of the probability of surgical wound infection is the number of microorganisms in the wound at the completion of the procedure. This concept has led to the classification of surgical procedures (see the Addendum to this section), based on an estimation of bacterial contamination and the risk of subsequent infection, into four broad categories: clean wounds, clean-contaminated wounds, contaminated wounds, and dirty and infected wounds. Within these categories, however, variation in the risk of infection is considerable with resulting effect on the possible need for prophylaxis.

---

*Antimicrobial prophylaxis in surgery. *The Medical Letter*. 1989;31:105-108.

Clean Wounds

In clean wound procedures, the benefit of systemic antimicrobial prophylaxis usually does not justify the potential risk associated with antimicrobial use, except in circumstances in which the consequences of infection are major and life-threatening, such as implantation of a prosthetic foreign body (e.g., insertion of a prosthetic heart valve), open-heart surgery for repair of structural defects, compromised immune status (such as patients receiving high doses of corticosteroids or chemotherapy for a malignancy), and body cavity exploration in neonates. Prophylaxis has been given in these instances, although studies establishing efficacy are lacking. Systemic antimicrobial agents have been empirically recommended for a clean procedure in patients with infection at another site.

Clean-contaminated Wounds

In clean-contaminated wound procedures, the degree of contamination is variable, and prophylaxis is limited to procedures with significant risk of wound contamination and infection. Based on data from adults, recommendations for prophylaxis for pediatric patients include the following: many alimentary tract procedures, selected biliary tract operations (e.g., with obstructive jaundice), and urinary tract surgery or instrumentation in the presence of bacteriuria or obstructive uropathy.

Contaminated, Dirty, and Infected Wounds

In contaminated and in dirty and infected wound procedures, such as those for a perforated abdominal viscus or a compound fracture, or if a major break in sterile technique has occurred, antimicrobial agents are indicated and are considered treatment rather than prophylaxis.

When Should Prophylactic Antibiotics Be Given?

Prophylaxis of infection requires effective drug concentrations in tissues during surgical procedures because maximal bacterial contamination occurs intraoperatively. Except in patients undergoing cesarean sections, the antimicrobial agent should be administered shortly before (within 30 minutes) or at the time of the surgical incision to ensure adequate tissue concentrations at the time of the greatest potential contamination. For patients with cesarean sections, it should be given after the umbilical cord is clamped.

For How Long Should Antibiotics Be Given?

A single antimicrobial dose that provides adequate tissue concentration throughout the procedure usually is sufficient. When surgery is prolonged or massive blood loss occurs, a second dose is advisable during the procedure. Postoperative doses of prophylactic drugs are generally unnecessary. These recommendations are based on studies in adults and may not necessarily apply to all pediatric patients, particularly neonates. However, inasmuch as the pathogenesis of wound infection does not differ with age, the recommendation for brief duration of prophylaxis probably is applicable to patients of all ages.

Which Antibiotics Should Be Given?

The choice of an antimicrobial is based on knowledge of the common bacteria causing infectious complications after the specific procedure, bacterial susceptibility to the drug, proved efficacy of the drug selected, and the safety of the drug. New, costly antimicrobial agents generally should not be used unless prophylactic efficacy has been proved superior to that of drugs of established benefit. The drugs should be active against the most likely pathogens, but they do not have to be active against every potential organism because effective prophylaxis appears to correlate with a decrease in the total number of pathogens rather than eradication of all organisms. Recommended doses and route of administration are based on the need to achieve therapeutic blood and tissue concentrations throughout the procedure, thus necessitating parenteral (usually intravenous) administration.

Conclusion

These principles for surgical antimicrobial prophylaxis in children were originally developed by the Committee in collaboration with the Committee on Drugs and the Section on Surgery of the American Academy of Pediatrics.* They have been slightly revised in accordance with recent recommendations. Because the value of systemic antimicrobial prophylaxis in many pediatric surgical procedures has not been established, additional studies in commonly performed surgical procedures in children (e.g., insertion of neurosurgical shunts and orthopedic procedures) are needed. Pediatricians, pediatric surgeons, and surgical subspecialists should review the prophylactic use of anti-

*Adapted from American Academy of Pediatrics, Committee on Infectious Diseases, Committee on Drugs, and Section on Surgery. Antimicrobial prophylaxis in pediatric surgical patients. *Pediatrics*. 1984;74:437-439.

microbial agents as part of the monitoring review of antibiotic use in their hospitals, and should use the guidelines given here to develop standards for antimicrobial use.

Addendum

Definitions of surgical wounds in the classification scheme are as follows:

Clean Wounds

Clean wounds are uninfected operative wounds in which no inflammation is encountered, and the respiratory, alimentary, or genitourinary tract or the oropharyngeal cavity is not entered. The operative procedures are elective and the wounds are closed primarily, and, if necessary, drained with closed drainage. Operative incisional wounds that follow non-penetrating (blunt) trauma should be included in this category if they meet the criteria.

Clean-contaminated Wounds

In clean-contaminated operative wounds the respiratory, alimentary, or genitourinary tract is entered under controlled conditions and without unusual contamination. Operations involving the biliary tract, appendix, vagina, and oropharynx are included in this category, provided that no evidence of infection is encountered and there is no major break in technique.

Contaminated Wounds

Contaminated wounds include open, fresh, accidental wounds; operative wounds in the setting of major breaks in sterile technique or gross spillage from the gastrointestinal tract; and incisions in which acute, non-purulent inflammation is encountered.

Dirty and Infected Wounds

Dirty and infected wounds include old traumatic wounds with retained devitalized tissue and those that involve existing clinical infection or perforated viscera. This definition suggests that the organisms causing post-operative infection were present in the operative field before surgery.

PREVENTION OF BACTERIAL ENDOCARDITIS

Recommendations by the American Heart Association*

Surgical and dental procedures and instrumentations involving mucosal surfaces or contaminated tissue commonly cause transient bacteremia that rarely persists for more than 15 minutes. Blood-borne bacteria may lodge on damaged or abnormal heart valves or on the endocardium or the endothelium near congenital anatomic defects, resulting in bacterial endocarditis or endarteritis. Although bacteremia is common following many invasive procedures, only a limited number of bacterial species commonly cause endocarditis. It is impossible to predict which patient will develop this infection or which particular procedure will be responsible.

Certain cardiac conditions are more often associated with endocarditis than others (Table 61). Furthermore, certain dental and surgical procedures are much more likely to initiate the bacteremia that results in endocarditis than are other procedures (Table 62). Prophylactic antibiotics are recommended for patients at risk for developing endocarditis who are undergoing those procedures most likely to produce bacteremia with organisms that commonly cause endocarditis.

Prophylaxis is most effective when given perioperatively in doses that are sufficient to assure adequate antibiotic concentrations in the serum during and after the procedure. To reduce the likelihood of microbial resistance, it is important that prophylactic antibiotics be used only during the perioperative period. They should be initiated shortly before a procedure (1 to 2 hours), and should not be continued for an extended period (no more than 6 to 8 hours). In the case of delayed healing, or of a procedure that involves infected tissue, it may be necessary to provide additional doses of antibiotics.

This statement represents recommended guidelines to supplement practitioners in the exercise of their clinical judgment and is not intended as a standard of care for all cases. It is impossible to make recommendations for all clinical situations in which endocarditis may develop. Practitioners must exercise their own clinical judgment in determining the choice of antibiotics and number of doses that are to be administered in individual cases or special circumstances. Furthermore, because endocarditis may occur in spite of appropriate antibiotic prophylaxis,

---

*A statement from the Committee on Rheumatic Fever, Endocarditis, and Kawasaki Disease of the Council on Cardiovascular Disease in the Young of the American Heart Association. Prepared by Dajani AS, Bisno AL, Chung KJ, et al. Reprinted with permission from JAMA (1990;264:2919-2922), Copyright 1990, American Medical Association.

Table 61. Cardiac Conditions*

Endocarditis Prophylaxis Recommended
Prosthetic cardiac valves, including bioprosthetic and homograft valves
Previous bacterial endocarditis, even in the absence of heart disease
Most congenital cardiac malformations
Rheumatic and other acquired valvular dysfunction, even after valvular surgery
Hypertrophic cardiomyopathy
Mitral valve prolapse with valvular regurgitation
Endocarditis Prophylaxis Not Recommended
Isolated secundum atrial septal defect
Surgical repair without residua beyond 6 mo of secundum atrial septal defect, ventricular septal defect, or patent ductus arteriosus
Previous coronary artery bypass graft surgery
Mitral valve prolapse without valvular regurgitation†
Physiologic, functional, or innocent heart murmurs
Previous Kawasaki disease without valvular dysfunction
Previous rheumatic fever without valvular dysfunction
Cardiac pacemakers and implanted defibrillators

*This table lists selected conditions but is not meant to be all-inclusive.
†Individuals who have a mitral valve prolapse associated with thickening and/or redundancy of the valve leaflets may be at increased risk for bacterial endocarditis, particularly men who are 45 years of age or older.

physicians and dentists should maintain a high index of suspicion regarding any unusual clinical events (such as unexplained fever, weakness, lethargy, or malaise) following dental or other surgical procedures in patients who are at risk for developing bacterial endocarditis.

Because no adequate, controlled clinical trials of antibiotic regimens for the prevention of bacterial endocarditis in humans have been done, recommendations are based on in vitro studies, clinical experience, data from experimental animal models, and assessment of both the bacteria most likely to produce bacteremia from a given site and those most likely to result in endocarditis. The substantial morbidity and mortality in patients who have endocarditis and the paucity of controlled clinical studies emphasize the need for continuing research into the epidemiology, pathogenesis, prevention, and therapy of endocarditis.

The current recommendations are an update of those made by the committee in 1984. They incorporate new data and include opinions of national and international experts.

Table 62. Dental or Surgical Procedures*

Endocarditis Prophylaxis Recommended
Dental procedures known to induce gingival or mucosal bleeding, including professional cleaning
Tonsillectomy and/or adenoidectomy
Surgical operations that involve intestinal or respiratory mucosa
Bronchoscopy with a rigid bronchoscope
Sclerotherapy for esophageal varices
Esophageal dilatation
Gallbladder surgery
Cystoscopy
Urethral dilatation
Urethral catheterization if urinary tract infection is present†
Urinary tract surgery if urinary tract infection is present†
Prostatic surgery
Incision and drainage of infected tissue†
Vaginal hysterectomy
Vaginal delivery in the presence of infection†
Endocarditis Prophylaxis Not Recommended‡
Dental procedures not likely to induce gingival bleeding, such as simple adjustment of orthodontic appliances or fillings above the gum line
Injection of local intraoral anesthetic (except intraligamentary injections)
Shedding of primary teeth
Tympanostomy tube insertion
Endotracheal intubation
Bronchoscopy with a flexible bronchoscope, with or without biopsy
Cardiac catheterization
Endoscopy with or without gastrointestinal biopsy
Cesarean section
In the absence of infection for urethral catheterization, dilatation and curettage, uncomplicated vaginal delivery, therapeutic abortion, sterilization procedures, or insertion or removal of intrauterine devices

*This table lists selected procedures but is not meant to be all-inclusive.

†In addition to prophylactic regimen for genitourinary procedures, antibiotic therapy should be directed against the most likely bacterial pathogen.

‡In patients who have prosthetic heart valves, a previous history of endocarditis, or surgically constructed systemic-pulmonary shunts or conduits, physicians may choose to administer prophylactic antibiotics even for low-risk procedures that involve the lower respiratory, genitourinary, or gastrointestinal tracts.

STANDARD PROPHYLACTIC REGIMEN FOR DENTAL, ORAL, AND UPPER RESPIRATORY TRACT PROCEDURES

Poor dental hygiene and periodontal or periapical infections may produce bacteremia even in the absence of dental procedures. Individuals who are at risk for developing bacterial endocarditis should establish and maintain the best possible oral health to reduce potential sources of bacterial seeding. Dentists should make every attempt to reduce gingival inflammation in patients who are at risk by means of brushing, flossing, fluoride rinse, chlorhexidine gluconate mouth rinse, and professional cleaning before proceeding with routine dental procedures. Chlorhexidine that is painted on isolated and dried gingiva 3 to 5 minutes prior to tooth extraction has been shown to reduce postextraction bacteremia. Other agents such as povidone-iodine or iodine and glycerin may also be appropriate. Furthermore, irrigation of the gingival sulcus with chlorhexidine prior to tooth extraction has been shown to reduce postextraction bacteremia in adults. Application of chlorhexidine may be used as an adjunct to antibiotic prophylaxis, particularly in patients who are at high risk and/or have poor dental hygiene.

Antibiotic prophylaxis is recommended with all dental procedures likely to cause gingival bleeding, including routine professional cleaning. If a series of dental procedures is required, it may be prudent to observe an interval of 7 days between procedures to reduce the potential for the emergence of resistant strains of organisms. If possible, a combination of procedures should be planned in the same period of prophylaxis, Edentulous patients may develop bacteremia from ulcers caused by ill-fitting dentures; therefore, denture wearers should be encouraged to have periodic examinations or to return to the practitioner if soreness develops. When new dentures are inserted, it is advisable to have the patient return to the practitioner to correct any overextension that could cause mucosal ulceration. Because the spontaneous shedding of primary teeth or simple adjustment of orthodontic appliances does not present a significant risk of endocarditis, antibiotic prophylaxis is not necessary in these situations. Similarly, endotracheal intubation is not an indication for antibiotic prophylaxis unless it is associated with another procedure for which prophylaxis is recommended.

α-Hemolytic (viridans) streptococci are the most common cause of endocarditis following dental procedures, and prophylaxis should be specifically directed against these organisms. Certain upper respiratory tract procedures, such as tonsillectomy and/or adenoidectomy, bronchoscopy with a rigid bronchoscope, and surgical procedures that involve the respiratory mucosa, may also cause bacteremia with organisms that commonly cause endocarditis and have similar antibiotic susceptibilities to those producing bacteremia following dental procedures. Therefore, the same regimen is recommended for these procedures as is recommended for dental procedures. Endocarditis has not been reported in association with insertion of tympanostomy tubes.

The recommended standard prophylactic regimen for all dental, oral, and upper respiratory tract procedures is amoxicillin (Table 63). The antibiotics amoxicillin, ampicillin, and penicillin V are equally effective in vitro against α-hemolytic streptococci; however, amoxicillin is now recommended because it is better absorbed from the gastrointestinal tract and provides higher and more sustained serum levels. The choice of penicillin V rather than amoxicillin as prophylaxis against α-hemolytic streptococcal bacteremia following dental, oral, and upper respiratory tract procedures is rational and acceptable.

Individuals who are allergic to penicillins (such as amoxicillin, ampicillin, or penicillin) should be treated with the provided alternative oral regimens. Erythromycin ethylsuccinate and erythromycin stearate are recommended because of more rapid and reliable absorption than other erythromycin formulations, resulting in higher and more sustained serum levels. For individuals who cannot tolerate either penicillins or erythromycin, clindamycin hydrochloride is the recommended alternative. Tetracyclines and sulfonamides *are not* recommended for endocarditis prophylaxis.

ALTERNATE PROPHYLACTIC REGIMENS FOR DENTAL, ORAL, AND UPPER RESPIRATORY TRACT PROCEDURES

Table 64 lists alternate prophylactic regimens for individuals who may not be candidates to receive the standard prophylactic regimen. For individuals who are unable to take oral medications, a parenteral agent may be necessary. Ampicillin sodium is recommended because parenteral amoxicillin is not available in the United States. When parenteral administration is needed in an individual who is allergic to penicillin, clindamycin phosphate is recommended.

Individuals who have prosthetic heart valves, a previous history of endocarditis, or surgically constructed systemic-pulmonary shunts or conduits are at high risk for developing endocarditis, and endocardial infection in such individuals is associated with substantial morbidity and mortality. For this reason, previous recommendations of this committee emphasized the use of stringent prophylactic regimens, with a strong preference for the parenteral route of administration. In practice, there are substantial logistic and financial barriers to the use of parenteral regimens. Moreover, oral regimens have now been used in individuals who have prosthetic heart valves in other countries, and failures in prophylaxis have not been a problem. Consequently, this committee recommends the use of the standard prophylactic regimen (Table 63) in

Table 63. Recommended Standard Prophylactic Regimen for Dental, Oral, or Upper Respiratory Tract Procedures in Patients Who Are at Risk*

Drug	Dosing Regimen†
	Standard Regimen
Amoxicillin	3.0 g orally 1 h before procedure; then 1.5 g 6 h after initial dose
	Amoxicillin/Penicillin-Allergic Patients
Erythromycin	Erythromycin ethylsuccinate, 800 mg, or erythromycin stearate, 1.0 g, orally 2 h before procedure; then half the dose 6 h after initial dose
or	
Clindamycin	300 mg orally 1 h before procedure and 150 mg 6 h after initial dose

*Includes those with prosthetic heart valves and other high risk patients.

†Initial pediatric doses are as follows: amoxicillin, 50 mg/kg; erythromycin ethylsuccinate or erythromycin stearate, 20 mg/kg; and clindamycin, 10 mg/kg. Follow-up doses should be one half the initial dose. **Total pediatric dose should not exceed total adult dose.** The following weight ranges may also be used for the initial pediatric dose of amoxicillin: < 15 kg, 750 mg; 15 to 30 kg, 1500 mg; and > 30 kg, 3000 mg (full adult dose).

patients who have prosthetic heart valves and in the other high-risk groups. It is recognized that some practitioners may prefer to use parenteral prophylaxis in these high-risk groups of patients. Accordingly, an alternate regimen is also provided in Table 64.

REGIMENS FOR GENITOURINARY AND GASTROINTESTINAL PROCEDURES

Surgery, instrumentation, or diagnostic procedures that involve the genitourinary or gastrointestinal tracts may cause bacteremia. The rate of bacteremia that is found following urinary tract procedures is high if urinary tract infection is present. Although the risk that any particular patient will develop endocarditis is low, the genitourinary tract is second only to the oral cavity as a portal of entry for organisms that cause endocarditis. The instrumented gastrointestinal tract seems to be less important as a portal of entry for organisms that cause bacterial endocarditis than the oral cavity or genitourinary tract.

Bacterial endocarditis that occurs following genitourinary and gastrointestinal tract surgery or instrumentation is most often caused by *Enterococcus faecalis* (enterococci). Although gram-negative bacil-

Table 64. Alternate Prophylactic Regimens for Dental, Oral, or Upper Respiratory Tract Procedures in Patients Who Are at Risk

Drug	Dosing Regimen*
Patients Unable to Take Oral Medications	
Ampicillin	Intravenous or intramuscular administration of ampicillin, 2.0 g, 30 min before procedure; then intravenous or intramuscular administration of ampicillin, 1.0 g, or oral administration of amoxicillin, 1.5 g, 6 h after initial dose
Ampicillin/Amoxicillin/Penicillin-Allergic Patients Unable to Take Oral Medications	
Clindamycin	Intravenous administration of 300 mg 30 min before procedure and an intravenous or oral administration of 150 mg 6 h after initial dose
Patients Considered High Risk and Not Candidates for Standard Regimen	
Ampicillin, gentamicin, and amoxicillin	Intravenous or intramuscular administration of ampicillin, 2.0 g, plus gentamicin, 1.5 mg/kg (not to exceed 80 mg), 30 min before procedure; followed by amoxicillin, 1.5 g, orally 6 h after initial dose; alternatively, the parenteral regimen may be repeated 8 h after initial dose
Ampicillin/Amoxicillin/Penicillin-Allergic Patients Considered High Risk	
Vancomycin	Intravenous administration of 1.0 g over 1 h, starting 1 h before procedure; no repeated dose necessary

*Initial pediatric doses are as follows: ampicillin, 50 mg/kg; clindamycin, 10 mg/kg; gentamicin, 2.0 mg/kg; and vancomycin, 20 mg/kg. Follow-up doses should be one half the initial dose. **Total pediatric dose should not exceed total adult dose.** No initial dose is recommended in this table for amoxicillin (25 mg/kg is the follow-up dose).

lary bacteremia may follow these procedures, gram-negative bacilli are only rarely responsible for endocarditis. Thus, antibiotic prophylaxis to prevent endocarditis that occurs following genitourinary or gastrointestinal procedures should be directed primarily against enterococci.

Table 65 outlines the recommended regimens for prophylaxis for genitourinary or gastrointestinal tract procedures. The committee continues to recommend parenteral antibiotics, particularly in high-risk patients (eg, those with prosthetic heart valves or a previous history of endocarditis). In low-risk patients, an alternative oral regimen is provided.

Table 65. Regimens for Genitourinary/Gastrointestinal Procedures

Drug	Dosage Regimen*
	Standard Regimen
Ampicillin, gentamicin, and amoxicillin	Intravenous or intramuscular administration of ampicillin, 2.0 g, plus gentamicin, 1.5 mg/kg (not to exceed 80 mg), 30 min before procedure; followed by amoxicillin, 1.5 g orally 6 h after initial dose; alternatively, the parenteral regimen may be repeated once 8 h after initial dose
	Ampicillin/Amoxicillin/Penicillin-Allergic Patient Regimen
Vancomycin and gentamicin	Intravenous administration of vancomycin, 1.0 g, over 1 h plus intravenous or intramuscular administration of gentamicin, 1.5 mg/kg (not to exceed 80 mg), 1 h before procedure; may be repeated once 8 h after initial dose
	Alternate Low-Risk Patient Regimen
Amoxicillin	3.0 g orally 1 h before procedure; then 1.5 g 6 h after initial dose

*Initial pediatric doses are as follows: ampicillin, 50 mg/kg; amoxicillin, 50 mg/kg; gentamicin, 2.0 mg/kg; and vancomycin, 20 mg/kg. Follow-up doses should be half the initial dose. **Total pediatric dose should not exceed total adult dose.**

SPECIFIC SITUATIONS AND CIRCUMSTANCES

Rheumatic Fever

Antibiotic regimens used to prevent the recurrence of acute rheumatic fever are inadequate for the prevention of bacterial endocarditis. Individuals who take an oral penicillin for secondary prevention of rheumatic fever or for other purposes may have viridans streptococci in their oral cavities that are relatively resistant to penicillin, amoxicillin, or ampicillin. In such cases, the physician or dentist should select erythromycin or another of the alternative regimens (listed in Tables 63 and 64), instead of amoxicillin (or another penicillin) for endocarditis prophylaxis.

Patients Who Receive Anticoagulants

Intramuscular injections for endocarditis prophylaxis should be avoided in patients who receive heparin. The use of warfarin sodium is a relative contraindication to intramuscular injections. Intravenous or oral regimens should be used whenever possible.

Patients Who Have Renal Dysfunction

In patients who have a markedly compromised renal function, it may be necessary to modify or omit the second dose of gentamicin sulfate or vancomycin hydrochloride.

Patients Who Undergo Cardiac Surgery

Patients who have cardiac conditions (Table 61) that predispose them to endocarditis are at risk for developing bacterial endocarditis, when undergoing open heart surgery. Similarly, patients who undergo surgery for placement of prosthetic heart valves or prosthetic intravascular or intracardiac materials are also at risk for the development of bacterial endocarditis. Because the morbidity and mortality of endocarditis in such patients are high, perioperative prophylactic antibiotics are recommended.

Endocarditis associated with open heart surgery is most often caused by *Staphylococcus aureus*, coagulase-negative staphylococci, or diphtheroids. Streptococci, gram-negative bacteria, and fungi are less common. No single antibiotic regimen is effective against all these organisms. Furthermore, prolonged use of broad-spectrum antibiotics may predispose to superinfection with unusual or resistant microorganisms.

Prophylaxis at the time of cardiac surgery should be directed primarily against staphylococci and should be of short duration. "First-generation" cephalosporins are most often used, but the choice of an antibiotic should be influenced by the antibiotic's susceptibility patterns at each hospital. For example, high prevalence of infection by methicillin-resistant *S aureus* in a particular institution should prompt consideration of vancomycin for perioperative prophylaxis. Prophylaxis with the chosen antibiotic should be started immediately before the operative procedure, repeated during prolonged procedures to maintain levels intraoperatively, and continued for no more than 24 hours postoperatively to minimize emergence of resistant microorganisms. The effects of cardiopulmonary bypass and compromised postoperative renal function on antibiotic levels in the serum should be considered, and doses timed appropriately before and during the procedure.

A careful preoperative dental evaluation is recommended so that required dental treatment can be completed before cardiac surgery whenever possible. Such measures may decrease the incidence of late postoperative endocarditis.

Status Following Cardiac Surgery

The same precautions should be observed in the years following most heart or valvular surgery that have been outlined for the patient who has not undergone a surgical procedure but is undergoing dental, gastrointestinal, genitourinary, or other procedures. The risk of developing endocarditis appears to continue indefinitely and is particularly significant for patients who have prosthetic heart valves. Furthermore, the morbidity and mortality that result from prosthetic valve endocarditis are high. Patients who have an isolated secundum atrial septal defect that has been surgically repaired, a ventricular septal defect, or patent ductus arteriosus do not seem to be at risk of developing endocarditis following a 6-month healing period after surgery. Data are insufficient to allow recommendations for prophylactic therapy after closure of these lesions by nonsurgical devices. There is no evidence that coronary artery bypass graft surgery introduces a risk for a patient's developing endocarditis.Therefore, antibiotic prophylaxis is not needed for this condition.

Cardiac Transplantation

There are insufficient data to support specific recommendations for patients who have had heart transplants. Some physicians place these patients in the category of people who will need prophylaxis, however.

Selected Readings

Bisno AL, Dismukes WE, Durack DT, et al. Antimicrobial treatment of infective endocarditis due to viridans streptococci, enterococci, and staphylococci. *JAMA*. 1989;261:1471-1477.

Dajani AS, Bisno AL, Chung KJ, et al. Prevention of rheumatic fever. *Circulation*. 1988;78:1082-1086.

Durack DT. Infective and noninfective endocarditis. In: Hurst JW, Schlant RC, Rackley CE, Sonnenblick EH, Wenger NK, eds. *The Heart*. 7th ed. New York, NY: McGraw-Hill Information Services Co; 1990:1230-1255.

Durack DT. Prophylaxis for infective endocarditis. In: Mandell GL, Douglas RG Jr, Bennett JE, eds. *Principles and Practice of Infectious Diseases*. 3rd ed. New York, NY: Churchill Livingstone Inc.; 1990;716-721.

Endocarditis Working Party of the British Society for Antimicrobial Chemotherapy. Antibiotic prophylaxis of infective endocarditis. *Lancet*. 1990;335:88-89.

Horstkotte D, Friedrichs W, Pippert H, Bircks W, Loogen F. Benefit of prophylaxis for infectious endocarditis in patients with prosthetic heart valves [in German with English abstract]. *Z Kardiol*. 1986;75:8-11.

Imperiale TF, Horwitz RI. Does prophylaxis prevent postdental infective endocarditis? *Am J Med*. 1990;88:131-136.

Kaplan EL, Shulman ST. Endocarditis. In: Adams FH, Emmanouilides GC, Riemenschneider TA, eds. *Moss' Heart Disease in Infants, Children, and Adolescents*. 4th ed. Baltimore, MD: Williams & Wilkins; 1989:718-730.

Prevention of Neonatal Ophthalmia

Topical 1% silver nitrate, 0.5% erythromycin, and 1% tetracycline are considered equally effective for prophylaxis of ocular gonorrheal infection in newborn infants. Each is available in single-dose tubes. Silver nitrate causes more chemical conjunctivitis than the others but appears to be the best agent in areas where the incidence of penicillinase-producing *Neisseria gonorrhoeae* (PPNG) is appreciable. Published data on the efficacy of erythromycin prophylaxis against PPNG are not available, and only one study has demonstrated effectiveness of prophylactic tetracycline in an area with a high incidence of PPNG infections.

Neonatal chlamydial ophthalmia, although not as severe as gonococcal conjunctivitis, is common in the United States. In many areas, its frequency equals or surpasses that of gonococcal ophthalmia. The effectiveness of 0.5% erythromycin ophthalmologic ointment in the prevention of chlamydial conjunctivitis has been shown in one study, but it has not been confirmed in subsequent studies. *Chlamydia trachomatis* is also susceptible to tetracyclines, but studies of the clinical efficacy of tetracycline ointment in the prophylaxis of chlamydial conjunctivitis have also given conflicting results. Neither antibiotic prevents *C trachomatis* pneumonia.

Specific recommendations for the prevention of neonatal ophthalmia are as follows:

- *Choice of Drugs.* For prophylaxis of gonococcal ophthalmia neonatorum, a 1% silver nitrate solution in single-dose ampules or single-use tubes of an ophthalmic ointment containing 0.5% erythromycin or 1% tetracycline are each effective and acceptable. The effectiveness of erythromycin or tetracycline in the prevention of ophthalmia caused by PPNG is not established. For gonococcal isolates known to be penicillin-sensitive, intramuscular penicillin G (50,000 units for full-term infants and 20,000 units for low-birth-weight infants) is also effective for prophylaxis. No topical regimen has proven efficacy in the prevention of chlamydial conjunctivitis.
- *Administration.* Prior to administration of local prophylaxis, each eyelid should be wiped gently with sterile cotton. Two drops of a 1% silver nitrate solution or a 1- to 2-cm ribbon of antibiotic ointment are placed in each lower conjunctival sac. The eyelids are then massaged gently to spread the ointment. After 1 minute, excess solution or ointment can be wiped away with sterile cotton. None of the prophylactic agents should be flushed from the eye after instillation. Critical studies have not evaluated the efficacy of silver nitrate prophylaxis with and without flushing, but anecdotal reports suggest that flushing may reduce the efficacy of prophylaxis. In

addition, flushing probably does not reduce the incidence of chemical conjunctivitis.

Prophylaxis should be given shortly after birth. Although some suggest that prophylaxis may be administered more effectively in the nursery than in the delivery room, the efficacy of delaying prophylaxis has not been studied. However, delaying prophylaxis for up to 1 hour after birth is probably not likely to influence efficacy. **Hospitals in which prophylaxis is delayed should establish a check system to ensure that all infants are treated.**

- *Infants born by cesarean section* should receive prophylaxis against neonatal gonococcal ophthalmia. Although gonococcal and chlamydial infections are usually transmitted to the infant during passage through the birth canal, infection by the ascending route also occurs. The risk of these infections occurring in untreated infants born by cesarean section has not been determined.
- *Identification of women who have gonococcal infections by routine cultures and then subsequent treatment is essential.* Gonococcal infections in pregnant women, including those who are asymptomatic, have been associated with septic abortion, early and prolonged rupture of membranes, premature labor, and delivery of low-birth-weight infants. These infections also can result in scalp abscesses in infants receiving intrauterine fetal monitoring and in disseminated neonatal gonococcal infection. Failure to treat an infected woman before or at delivery can result in postnatal transmission of gonococcal infection to infants.
- *Newborn infants whose mothers have gonorrhea at the time of delivery* should receive a single dose of ceftriaxone (125 mg; for low-birth-weight infants, 25 to 50 mg/kg) intravenously or intramuscularly, as occasional cases of gonococcal ophthalmia may occur in infants managed by any of the current modes of prophylaxis.
- *Neonates with clinical evidence of gonococcal ophthalmia or complicated (disseminated) gonococcal infection* should be hospitalized, placed in isolation, and treated appropriately (see Gonococcal Infections, page 213). The emergence of penicillin-resistant strains of *N gonorrhoeae* necessitates culture of specimens from the mother and determination of antibiotic susceptibilities so that appropriate antimicrobial therapy can be given.
- *Treatment of pregnant women who have chlamydial cervicitis* can prevent neonatal chlamydial infection. Oral erythromycin is the only recommended treatment for these women; tetracycline is contraindicated (see *Chlamydia trachomatis*, page 169). Women whose infants develop chlamydial conjunctivitis should be tested and treated if they are positive. Their sexual partners should also receive treatment to prevent reinfection.

- *Chlamydia-positive women can be identified* by screening with one of several rapid antigen detection tests (see *Chlamydia trachomatis*, page 169). Testing is warranted in areas of high prevalence and in women found to have other sexually transmitted diseases.

PART 5

ANTIMICROBIALS AND RELATED THERAPY

Introduction

In some instances, drugs are recommended for specific indications other than those in the package insert approved by the Food and Drug Administration (FDA). An FDA-approved indication means that adequate and well-controlled studies were conducted and reviewed by the FDA. However, accepted medical practice often includes drug use that is not reflected in approved drug labeling. Lack of approval does not necessarily mean lack of efficacy but only that the appropriate studies have not been done; it does not prevent a physician from using an available drug or imply improper use in so doing, provided that reasonable medical evidence, judgment, and prudence are exercised. The decision to prescribe a drug rests with the physician, who must weigh the risks and benefits of the drug in question, whether or not it has full FDA approval.

Some of the antimicrobial agents listed in the tables have not been approved by the FDA for use in pediatric patients. In some cases, application for pediatric use is currently pending FDA decision. However, the broad-spectrum fluroquinolones, such as ciprofloxacin, which are commonly prescribed for adults, are generally contraindicated for children because they cause cartilage damage in immature animals. Although no conclusive data indicate similar toxicity in young children, approval for these drugs for use in subjects younger than 21 years is unlikely in the next several years or more. Nevertheless, special situations arise in which ciprofloxacin or another of the quinolones might be considered for treatment of pediatric patients, such as for infections caused by *Pseudomonas* strains that are resistant to multiple antibiotics or for which an orally administered antibiotic is preferred. In such instances obtaining informed parental consent before use is prudent.

Tables of Drug Dosages

The various antimicrobials for which the following recommended doses are listed are those commonly used for the care of infants and children. The recommendations for antibacterials are separated into two tables—one for older infants and children and the other for newborn infants—because the physiologic immaturity of the newborn infant and resulting different pharmacokinetics necessitate alteration in dosage regimens to achieve maximum efficacy and limit toxicity. The table for older infants and children provides recommendations for both mild and severe infections; that for newborn infants is not divided because infections in this age group, with a few exceptions, are always considered severe. Tables are also given for antiviral agents, drugs for parasitic infections, and antifungal agents.

The recommended doses are not absolute and are intended only as a guide. Clinical judgment about the disease, alterations in renal function, and other factors affecting pharmacokinetics, patient response, and laboratory results may dictate modifications of these recommendations in the individual patient. In some cases, monitoring of serum drug concentrations is recommended to avoid toxicity and to ensure therapeutic efficacy.

Package insert information should be consulted for such details as the diluent for reconstitution of injectable preparations, measures to be taken to avoid incompatibilities, and other precautions.

Antibacterial Drugs for Newborn Infants: Individual Dose (mg/kg or units [U]/kg) and Frequency of Administration

Drug	Route	Infants < 1 week old		Infants ≥ 1 week old	
		BW ≤ 2,000 g	BW > 2,000 g	BW ≤ 2,000 g	BW > 2,000 g
Aminoglycosides*,†					
amikacin	IV, IM	7.5 q 12h	7.5-10 q 12 h	7.5-10 q 8 h	10 q 8 h
gentamicin	IV, IM	2.5 q 12h	2.5 q 12 h	2.5 q 8 h	2.5 q 8 h
kanamycin	IV, IM	7.5 q 12h	7.5-10 q 12 h	7.5-10 q 8 h	10 q 8 h
neomycin sulfate	PO only	25 q 6 h	25 q 6 h	25 q 6 h	25 q 6 h
tobramycin	IV, IM	2 q 12 h	2 q 12 h	2 q 8 h	2 q 8 h
Aztreonam‡	IV, IM	30 q 12 h	30 q 8 h	30 q 8 h	30 q 6 h
Antistaphylococcal penicillins					
methicillin§	IV, IM	25 q 12 h	25 q 8 h	25 q 8 h	25 q 6 h
nafcillin§	IV	25 q 12 h	25 q 8 h	25 q 8 h	25 q 6 h
oxacillin§	IV, IM	25 q 12 h	25 q 8 h	25 q 8 h	25 q 6 h
Cephalosporins					
cefotaxime	IV, IM	50 q 12 h	50 q 8 or 12 h	50 q 8 h	50 q 6 or 8 h

Abbreviations: q = every, BW = body weight, IV = intravenous, IM = intramuscular, PO = oral.

*Optimal dosage should be based on determination of serum concentrations, especially in low-birth-weight (< 1,500 g) infants. In very-low-birth-weight infants (< 1000 g) once daily dosing may be appropriate in the first week of life.

†Dosages for the aminoglycosides may differ from those recommended by the manufacturer in the package insert.

§For meningitis, double the recommended dosage.

‡Approval pending for use in newborn infants (October 1990).

Antibacterial Drugs for Newborn Infants: Individual Dose (mg/kg or units [U]/kg) and Frequency of Administration *(continued)*

		Infants < 1 week old		Infants ≥ 1 week old	
Drug	Route	BW ≤ 2,000 g	BW > 2,000 g	BW ≤ 2,000 g	BW > 2,000 g
ceftazidime	IV, IM	50 q 12 h	30 q 8 h	30 q 8 h	30 q 8 h
ceftriaxone	IV, IM	50 q 24 h	50 q 24 h	50 q 24 h	50-75 q 24 h
Chloramphenicol*	IV, PO	25 q 24 h	25 q 24 h	25 q 24 h	25 q 12 h
Macrolides					
erythromycin	PO	10 q 12 h	10 q 8 h	10-15 q 12 h	10-15 q 8 h
clindamycin	IV, IM, PO	5 q 12 h	5 q 8 h	5 q 8 h	5 q 6 h
Penicillins					
ampicillin§	IV, IM	25 q 12 h	25 q 8 h	25 q 8 h	25 q 6 h
carbenicillin	IV, IM	100 q 12 h	100 q 8 h	100 q 8 h	100 q 6 h
mezlocillin	IV, IM	75 q 12 h	75 q 8 h	75 q 8 or 12 h	75 q 6 h
penicillin G§	IV, IM	25,000 U q 12 h	25,000 U q 8 h	25,000 U q 8 h	25,000 U q 6 h
penicillin G procaine	IM	50,000 U q 24 h	50,000 U q 24 h	50,000 U q 24 h	50,000 U q 24 h
ticarcillin	IV, IM	75 q 12 h	75 q 8 h	75 q 8 h	75 q 6 h
Vancomycin	IV	10 q 12 h	10 q 12 h	10 q 8 h	10 q 8 h

Abbreviations: q = every, BW = body weight, IV = intravenous, IM = intramuscular, PO = oral.

*Optimal dosage should be based on determination of serum concentrations, especially in low-birth-weight (< 1,500 g) infants. In very-low-birth-weight infants (< 1000 g) once daily dosing may be appropriate in the first week of life.

§For meningitis, double the recommended dosage.

Antibacterial Drugs for Pediatric Patients Beyond the Newborn Period

Drug Generic (Trade)	Route	Dosage per kg/d: Mild to Moderate Infections	Dosage per kg/d: Severe Infections	Comments
Penicillin G, crystalline*,† K or NA (numerous)	IV, IM	25,000-50,000 U in 4 doses	100,000-400,000 U in 4-6 doses	1.68 mEq K or Na per 1,000,000 U; use Na salt for large IV doses
Penicillin G, procaine*,† (numerous)	IM	25,000-50,000 U in 1-2 doses	Inappropriate	Contraindicated in procaine allergy
Penicillin G, benzathine*,† (Bicillin, Permapen)	IM	<27.3 kg (60 lb): 600,000 U ≥ 27.3 kg: 1,200,000 U	Inappropriate	Major use is prevention of rheumatic fever by treatment and prophylaxis of streptococcal infections
Penicillin G, potassium*,† oral (numerous)	PO	25,000-50,000 U in 3 or 4 doses	Inappropriate	Absorption variable; optimal to administer unbuffered penicillin G at least 1 h before or 2 h after meals
Penicillin V*,† (numerous)	PO	25,000-50,000 U in 3 or 4 doses	Inappropriate	1,600 U is equivalent to 1 mg; optimal to administer on empty stomach

*Patients with history of allergy to penicillin G or V should be considered for subsequent skin testing. Many such patients can be treated safely with penicillin, since only 10% of children with such history are proven allergic when skin tested.

†In patients with history of allergy to penicillin or one of its many congeners, alternative drugs are recommended. In some circumstances, a cephalosporin may be acceptable. However, these drugs should not be used in patients with an immediate hypersensitivity (anaphylaxis) to penicillin because approximately 5% to 15% of penicillin-allergic patients will also be allergic to the cephalosporins.

Antibacterial Drugs for Pediatric Patients Beyond the Newborn Period *(continued)*

Drug Generic (Trade)	Route	Dosage per kg/d: Mild to Moderate Infections	Dosage per kg/d: Severe Infections	Comments
Penicillinase-resistant penicillins*				
methicillin (Staphcillin)	IV, IM	100-200 mg in 4 doses (daily adult dose, 4-8 g)	150-200 mg in 4-6 doses (daily adult dose, 4-12 g)	Interstitial nephritis (i.e., hematuria) occurs in 0%-4% of patients
oxacillin (Prostaphlin, Bactocill)	IV, IM	100-200 mg in 4 doses (daily adult dose, 2-4 g)	150-200 mg in 4-6 doses (daily adult dose, 4-12 g)	Methicillin-resistant staphylococci are usually resistant to all other semisynthetic antistaphylococcal penicillins and synthetic antistaphylococcal cephalosporins
	PO	50-100 mg in 4 doses (daily adult dose 2-4 g)	Inappropriate	Absorption of oral preparation is variable; administer at least 1 h before or 2 h after meals
nafcillin (Unipen, Nafcil)	IV, IM	50-100 mg in 4 doses (daily adult dose, 2-4 g)	150-200 mg in 4-6 doses (daily adult dose, 4-12 g)	Serum concentrations after oral administration are low compared with those after other orally administered antistaphylococcal drugs
	PO	50-100 mg in 4 doses (daily adult dose 2-4 g)	Inappropriate	

cloxacillin (Tegopen, Cloxapen)	PO	50-100 mg in 4 doses (daily adult dose, 2-4 g)	Inappropriate	
dicloxacillin (Dynapen, Pathocil)	PO	25-50 mg in 4 doses (daily adult dose, 1-2 g)	Inappropriate	Excellent serum concentrations after oral administrations
Broad-spectrum penicillins*				
ampicillin (numerous)	IV, IM	50-100 mg in 4 doses (daily adult dose, 2-4 g)	200-300 mg in 4 doses (daily adult dose, 6-12 g)	Ineffective against beta-lactamase-producing *Haemophilus influenzae*, *Staphylococcus aureus*, and *Moraxella catarrhalis*
	PO	50-100 mg in 4 doses (daily adult dose, 2-4 g)	Inappropriate	
amoxicillin (numerous)	PO	25-50 mg in 3 doses (daily adult dose, 750 mg-1.5 g)	Inappropriate	
amoxicillin-clavulanate (Augmentin)	PO	20-40 mg of amoxicillin in 3 doses (daily adult dose, 750 mg-1.5 g)	Inappropriate	Dosage based on amoxicillin component, should not be exceeded because of potential for diarrhea

*Patients with history of allergy to penicillin G or V should be considered for subsequent skin testing. Many such patients can be treated safely with penicillin, since only 10% of children with such history are proven allergic when skin tested.

Antibacterial Drugs for Pediatric Patients Beyond the Newborn Period *(continued)*

Drug Generic (Trade)	Route	Dosage per kg/d: Mild to Moderate Infections	Dosage per kg/d: Severe Infections	Comments
azlocillin (Azlin)	IV, IM	100-200 mg in 4 doses (daily adult dose, 8-12 g)	200-300 mg in 4-6 doses (daily adult dose, 16-18 g)	Doses as high as 450 mg/kg/d (maximum of 24 g/d) in 6 divided doses have been used in patients with cystic fibrosis; contains 2.17 mEq of Na per gram
bacampicillin (Spectrobid)	PO	25-50 mg in 2 doses (daily adult dose, 1-2 g)	Inappropriate	Prodrug of ampicillin with excellent bioavailability
cyclacillin (Cyclapen)	PO	50-100 mg in 3-4 doses (daily adult dose, 1-2 g)	Inappropriate	Less active in vitro than ampicillin against *H influenzae*
carbenicillin (Geopen, Pyopen)	IV, IM	100-200 mg in 4 doses (daily adult dose, 4-8 g)	400-600 mg in 4-6 doses (daily adult dose, 20-40 g)	Contains 4.7 mEq of Na per gram
(Geocillin)	PO	30-65 mg in 4 doses (daily adult dose, 4-8 tablets)	Inappropriate	Tablets contain 382 mg of indanyl sodium carbenicillin; for treatment of urinary tract infections only
mezlocillin (Mezlin)	IV, IM	50-100 mg in 4 doses (daily adult dose, 6-8 g)	200-300 mg in 4-6 doses (daily adult dose, 12-18 g)	Contains 1.85 mEq of Na per gram

piperacillin (Pipracil)	IV, IM	50-100 mg in 4 doses (daily adult dose, 6-8 g)	200-300 mg in 4-6 doses (daily adult dose, 12-18 g)	Contains 1.85 mEq of Na per gram; experience in infants and children is limited
ticarcillin (Ticar)	IV, IM	50-100 mg in 4 doses (daily adult dose, 2-4 g)	200-300 mg in 4-6 doses (daily adult dose, 12-24 g)	Contains 5.2 mEq of Na per gram
Other beta-lactams				
aztreonam (Azactam)	IV, IM	90 mg in 3 doses (daily adult dose, 3 g)	120 mg in 4 doses (max. daily adult dose, 8 g)	Approval pending (Oct. 1990) for use in children
imipenem-cilastatin (Primaxin)	IV, IM	60 mg in 4 doses (daily adult dose, 1-2 g)	60 mg in 4 doses (daily adult dose, 2-4 g)	Not approved for use in pediatric patients younger than 12 years; not to be used for therapy of meningitis
Cephalosporins				
cefaclor (Ceclor)	PO	20-40 mg in 2 or 3 doses (daily adult dose, 750 mg-1.5 g)	Inappropriate	A twice daily regimen has been shown to be effective for treatment of acute otitis media
cefamandole (Mandol)	IV, IM	50-100 mg in 3-4 doses (daily adult dose, 1.5-3 g)	100-150 mg in 4-6 doses (daily adult dose, 4-12 g)	Inadequate CSF concentrations for treatment of meningitis
cefazolin (Kefzol, Ancef)	IV, IM	25-50 mg in 2-4 doses (daily adult dose, 750 mg-2 g)	50-150 mg in 3 or 4 doses (daily adult dose, 4-6 g)	

Antibacterial Drugs for Pediatric Patients Beyond the Newborn Period *(continued)*

Drug Generic (Trade)	Route	Dosage per kg/d: Mild to Moderate Infections	Dosage per kg/d: Severe Infections	Comments
cefixime (Suprax)	PO	8 mg in 1 or 2 doses (daily adult dose, 400 mg)	Inappropriate	
ceforanide (Precef)	IV, IM	20-40 mg in 2 doses (daily adult dose, 1-2 g)	Not established	Not approved for use in infants younger than 1 year
cefotaxime (Claforan)	IV, IM	75-100 mg in 3 or 4 doses (daily adult dose, 4-6 g)	150-200 mg in 3 or 4 doses (daily adult dose, 8-10 g)	
cefoxitin (Mefoxin)	IV, IM	80-100 mg in 3-4 doses (daily adult dose, 3-4 g)	80-160 mg in 4-6 doses (daily adult dose, 6-12 g)	
ceftazidime (Fortaz, Tazicef, Tazidime)	IV, IM	75-100 mg in 3 doses (daily adult dose, 3 g)	125-150 mg in 3 doses (daily adult dose, 6 g)	Only cephalosporin with anti-*Pseudomonas* activity that has been approved for use in children
ceftizoxime (Cefizox)	IV, IM	100-150 mg in 3 doses (daily adult dose, 3-4 g)	150-200 mg in 3 doses (daily adult dose, 4-6 g)	

ceftriaxone (Rocephin)	IV, IM	50-75 mg in 1 or 2 doses (daily adult dose, 2 g)	80-100 mg in 2 doses (daily adult dose, 4 g)	A single daily dose of 80-100 mg/kg of ceftriaxone can also be used for treatment of serious infections including meningitis
cefuroxime (Zinacef)	IV, IM	75-100 mg in 3 doses (daily adult dose, 2-4 g)	175-240 mg in 3 doses (daily adult dose, 4-6 g)	Activity in CSF is lower than for cefotaxime or ceftriaxone
cefuroxime axetil (Ceftin)	PO	250-500 mg‡ total in 2 doses (daily adult dose is 0.25-1.0 g)	Inappropriate	Available only in tablets
cephalexin (Keflax)	PO	25-50 mg in 4 doses (daily adult dose, 1-4 g)	Inappropriate	
cephalothin (Keflin)	IV, IM	80-100 mg in 4 doses (daily adult dose, 2-4 g)	100-150 mg in 4-6 doses (daily adult dose, 8-12 g)	
cephapirin (Cefadyl)	IV, IM	40 mg in 4 doses (daily adult dose, 2 g)	40-80 mg in 4 doses (daily adult dose, 4-12 g)	
cephradine (Anspor, Velosef)	PO	25-50 mg in 2-4 doses (daily adult dose, 1-4 g)	Inappropriate	

‡Dosage recommendation is daily total (not per kilogram) dose.

Antibacterial Drugs for Pediatric Patients Beyond the Newborn Period *(continued)*

Drug Generic (Trade)	Route	Dosage per kg/d		Comments
		Mild to Moderate Infections	Severe Infections	
(Velosef)	IV, IM	25-50 mg in 4 doses (daily adult dose, 2 g); 50-100 mg in 4 doses (daily adult dose 2-8 g)		
moxalactam (Moxam)	IV, IM	100-150 mg in 4 doses (daily adult dose, 4-6 g)	150-200 mg in 4 doses (daily adult dose, 8-10 g)	Limited pediatric use
Vancomycin (Vancocin, Vancoled, Vancor)	IV	40 mg in 4 doses (daily adult dose, 1-2 g)	40-60 mg in 4 doses (daily adult dose, 2-4 g)	Some experts suggest a dose of 60 mg/kg/d for central nervous system or disseminated infections caused by *Staphylococcus aureus;* dose should be given over a minimum of 60 minutes.
Aminoglycosides§				
amikacin (Amikin)	IV, IM	Inappropriate	15-30 mg in 2 doses (daily adult dose, 15 mg/kg, maximum, 1.5 g)	30 mg in 3 doses is recommended by some consultants

gentamicin (Garamycin)	IV, IM	Inappropriate	3-7.5 mg in 3 doses (daily adult dose is the same)	
kanamycin (Kantrex)	IV, IM	Inappropriate	15-30 mg in 2-3 doses (daily adult dose, 1-1.5 g)	30 mg in 3 doses is recommended by some consultants
neomycin (numerous)	PO only	100 mg in 4 doses	100 mg in 4 doses	For some enteric infections
netilmicin (Netromycin)	IV, IM	Inappropriate	3-7.5 mg in 3 doses (daily adult dose is the same)	
streptomycin (numerous)	IM	Inappropriate	20-40 mg in 2-3 doses (daily adult dose, 1-2 g)	Use limited to treatment of tuberculosis and possibly other conditions
tobramycin (Nebcin)	IV, IM	Inappropriate	3-7.5 mg in 3 doses (daily adult dose, 3-5 mg in 3 doses)	
Chloramphenicol (Chloromycetin)				
palmitate	PO	Inappropriate	50-75 mg in 4 doses (daily adult dose, 1-2 g)	Optimal dosage is determined by measurement of serum concentrations with resulting modifications to achieve therapeutic concentrations

§Dosages for the aminoglycosides may differ from those recommended by the manufacturers (see package insert).

Antibacterial Drugs for Pediatric Patients Beyond the Newborn Period *(continued)*

Drug Generic (Trade)	Route	Dosage per kg/d: Mild to Moderate Infections	Dosage per kg/d: Severe Infections	Comments
succinate	IV	Inappropriate	50-100 mg in 4 doses (daily adult dose, 2-4 g)	Use only for serious infections because of the rare occurrence of aplastic anemia following administration
Clindamycin (Cleocin)	IM, IV	15-25 mg in 3-4 doses (daily adult dose, 600 mg-1.2 g)	25-40 mg in 3-4 doses (daily adult dose, 1.2-2.7 g)	Good activity against anaerobes, especially *Bacteroides* species Should not be used in the treatment of central nervous system infections
	PO	10-20 mg in 4 doses (daily adult dose, 600 mg-1.8 g)	Inappropriate	
Erythromycins (numerous)	PO	20-50 mg in 2-4 doses (daily adult dose, 1-2 g)	Inappropriate	Available in base, stearate, ethyl succinate, and estolate preparations
	IV	Inappropriate	15-50 mg in 4 doses (daily adult dose, 1-4 g)	Administer in a continuous drip or by slow infusion over 60 minutes or longer
Polymyxins colistimethate (Coly-Mycin M)	IM	Inappropriate	2.5-5 mg in 4 doses (daily adult dose, 300 mg)	Limited-purpose drug

colistin sulfate (Coly-Mycin S)	PO	10-15 mg in 3 doses	10-15 mg in 3 doses (daily adult dose, 200-300 mg)	For some enteric infections
polymyxin B (Aerosporin)	IM	Inappropriate	25,000-40,000 U in 4 doses	Limited-purpose drug
	PO	100,000-200,000 U in 3-4 doses	100,000-200,000 U in 3-4 doses	For some enteric infections only
Tetracyclines (numerous)	IV	Inappropriate	10-25 mg in 2-4 doses (daily adult dose, 1-2 g)	Responsible for staining of developing teeth; use only in children 9 years or older except in circumstances in which benefits of therapy exceed risks and alternative drugs are less effective or potentially more toxic
	PO	20-50 mg in 4 doses (daily adult dose, 1-2 g)	Inappropriate	
Sulfonamides				
sulfadiazine	PO, IV	100-150 mg in 4 doses	100-150 mg in 4 doses	The first dose should be doubled; daily adult oral doses, 2-4 g; for IV, same dose as for children
sulfisoxazole (Gantrisin)	PO, IV	100-150 mg in 4 doses	100-150 mg in 4 doses	
triple sulfonamides (numerous)	PO	120-150 mg in 4 doses	120-150 mg in 4 doses	

Antibacterial Drugs for Pediatric Patients Beyond the Newborn Period *(continued)*

Drug Generic (Trade)	Route	Dosage per kg/d		Comments
		Mild to Moderate Infections	Severe Infections	
trimethoprim-sulfamethoxazole (Bactrim, Septra)	PO	8 mg trimethoprim/40 mg sulfamethoxazole in 2 doses (daily adult dose, 320 mg trimethoprim/1.6 g sulfamethoxazole)	20 mg trimethoprim/100 mg sulfamethoxazole in 4 doses (for use only in *Pneumocystis carinii* pneumonia)	For prophylaxis in immunocompromised patients, recommended dose is 5 mg trimethoprim/25 mg sulfamethoxazole per kg/d in 2 doses
trimethoprim-sulfamethoxazole (Bactrim, Septra)	IV	Inappropriate	20 mg trimethoprim/100 mg sulfamethoxazole in 4 doses (for treatment of Pneumocystis infection)	Use intravenous form when oral form cannot be administered
Urinary antiseptic agents				
methenamine mandelate (Mandelamine)	PO	50-75 mg in 3-4 doses (daily adult dose, 2-4 g)	Inappropriate	Should not be used for infants; urine pH must be adjusted to 5-5.5

nitrofurantoin (Furadantin, Macrodantin)	PO	5-7 mg in 4 doses (daily adult dose, 200-400 mg)	Inappropriate	Should not be used for young infants; prophylactic dose is 1-2 mg/kg/d in one dose
Fluoroquinolones				
ciprofloxacin (Cipro)	PO	Inappropriate	30 mg in 2 doses (daily adult dose, 1000-1500 mg)	Not approved for patients younger than 21 years

Dexamethasone Therapy for Bacterial Meningitis in Infants and Children*

Bacterial meningitis affects an estimated 15,000 infants and children in the United States each year. The case-fatality rates for these patients are from 5% to 10%; as many as 20% to 30% of survivors have long-term sequelae, the most common of which is hearing impairment. The reported incidence of hearing loss after meningitis has ranged from 5% to 20% of patients, depending on the selection of patients, techniques used to assess hearing, and etiology. In 1972 to 1977, Dodge and coworkers documented hearing loss in 31% of patients with *Streptococcus pneumoniae* meningitis, 10% with *Neisseria meningitidis* meningitis, and 6% with *Haemophilus influenzae* meningitis. Bilateral sensorineural hearing impairment occurred in 14%, 10%, and 3%, respectively. Newer antimicrobial agents with superior bactericidal activity in cerebrospinal fluid (CSF) have not reduced morbidity and case-fatality rates in comparison to that occurring with conventional antibiotic therapy.

The pathophysiologic events believed to contribute to adverse outcome from bacterial meningitis include alteration of cerebral capillary endothelial cells that comprise the blood-brain barrier, cytotoxic and vasogenic cerebral edema, and increased intracranial pressure. These events can lead to decreased cerebral perfusion pressure with a resultant diminution in cerebral blood flow resulting in regional hypoxia and focal ischemia of brain tissue.

Because of its anti-inflammatory effects, corticosteroid therapy has been evaluated in experimental meningitis and in infants and children with meningitis. Dexamethasone produced significant reductions in intracranial pressure, brain edema, and lactate concentrations in CSF in experimental *H influenzae* and *S pneumoniae* meningitis. Additionally, dexamethasone administration was associated with decreased concentrations of prostaglandin E_2 in CSF, and it lowered mortality and clinically evident neurologic sequelae in rabbits with experimental pneumococcal meningitis. In experimental *H influenzae* meningitis, dexamethasone given concurrently with antimicrobial therapy significantly reduced CSF concentrations of cachectin (tumor necrosis factor), a cytokine that is believed to participate in the host's inflammatory response. By contrast, a study in rats suggested that corticosteroids can potentiate ischemic injury to neurons. Further information on the pathophysiology of bacterial meningitis in children is needed.

---

*Reproduced (with slight modifications) from American Academy of Pediatrics, Committee on Infectious Diseases. Dexamethasone therapy for bacterial meningitis in infants and children. *Pediatrics*. 1990;86:130-133. References have been omitted but are given in the original publication.

The results of two placebo-controlled trials of corticosteroid therapy in children with meningitis were published in 1969. Methylprednisolone was used in one study and dexamethasone in the other. In neither study was hearing specifically evaluated in all patients. The investigators in both studies concluded that no significant beneficial or adverse effects of corticosteroid therapy could be demonstrated. In one study, patients who received dexamethasone, in approximately one third the dose used in the more recent trials, had significantly fewer neurologic complications during hospitalization and at discharge than placebo-treated patients. This effect, however, was discounted because patients in the placebo group were thought to have more serious illness at the time of admission to the hospital. In another study using 40 mg of methylprednisolone, long-term sequelae occurred more frequently in steroid-treated than in placebo-treated children.

The results of two double-blind, placebo-controlled trials of dexamethasone therapy for bacterial meningitis in 200 infants and children 2 months and older have been published (Lebel MH et al. *NEJM.* 1988;319:964-971). Dexamethasone, 0.6 mg/kg/d in four divided doses, or placebo was administered intravenously for the first four days of antibiotic therapy, which consisted of cefuroxime (first study) or ceftriaxone (second study). Dexamethasone-treated patients became afebrile earlier than did placebo-treated patients (1.6 vs 5.0 days; $p<0.001$). The mean increase in glucose concentration (36.0 vs 6.9 mg/dL; $p<0.001$) and decrease in lactate concentration (38.3 vs 19.8 mg/dL; $p<0.005$) in CSF after 24 hours of therapy were significantly greater for dexamethasone-treated than for placebo-treated patients.

Dexamethasone-treated children in those two studies were significantly less likely to have moderate or more severe bilateral sensorineural hearing loss (3 of 92, 3.3% vs 13 of 84, 15.5%; $p<0.01$) and to require hearing aids (1 of 92, 1.1% vs 12 of 84, 14.3%; $p<0.001$) when evaluated 3 to 12 months after illness. The relative risk (95% confidence interval) for developing moderate or greater hearing impairment in placebo-treated patients was 2.54 (95% confidence interval, 1.1 to 5.9) compared to dexamethasone-treated patients using a stratified analysis (Mantel-Haenzel method) of the data from the first and second study considered separately. The relative risk for the combined data was 4.75 (1.6 to 14.1) for the combined data. The relative risks of requiring hearing aids after meningitis were 3.8 (1.4 to 10.3) for the separate data and 13.14 (2.9 to 59.7) when combined. One year after illness, neurologic sequelae other than sensorineural hearing loss were found in 3 of 81 (4%) patients given dexamethasone and 9 of 75 (12%) patients given placebo ($p=0.052$).

These investigators have recently completed a third double-blind placebo-controlled study of dexamethasone therapy in 60 patients who received cefuroxime therapy (McCracken GH and Lebel MH. *Am. J. Dis. Child.* 1989;143:287-289). The data from that study support the findings from the first two trials. For the 260 infants and children enrolled in the three studies, seizures that occurred after admission to the hospital (10 of 133, 7.5% vs 21 of 127, 16.5%; p=0.025) and hemiparesis evident at the time of discharge (3 of 133, 2.3% vs 11 of 127, 8.7%; p=0.022) occurred significantly less frequently in dexamethasone recipients than in placebo recipients. Bilateral moderate or more severe hearing loss occurred in 15 of 113 (13%) placebo-treated patients and 4 of 122 (3%) dexamethasone-treated patients (p<0.005) who had been followed for 3 to 12 months after illness. The relative risk of developing moderate or greater hearing impairment was 4.1 (1.3 to 12.2) for placebo-treated versus dexamethasone-treated children. Because approximately 75% of the study patients had *H influenzae* meningitis, the beneficial effect of dexamethasone on hearing could be determined only in patients with this infection. Too few patients with pneumococcal or meningococcal meningitis were evaluated to determine the effect of steroid therapy on outcome in these other infections.

The effect of dexamethasone in lowering the risk of hearing loss appears to be greater in those with milder illness. To determine whether severity of disease influenced outcome, data from 199 patients with *H influenzae* meningitis were analyzed. When the Herson and Todd prognostic score was ≤ 2.5, indicating a milder illness, the rates of moderate or greater hearing loss in one or both ears (7 of 79 [9%] vs 12 of 56 [21%]; p=0.039) and in both ears only (1 of 79 [1%] vs 9 of 56 [16%]; p=0.001) were significantly smaller in dexamethasone-treated patients than placebo-treated patients. No difference in hearing outcome for the two treatment groups was found in patients whose Herson-Todd score was less than 2.5.

Recently, in a comparative study of ceftriaxone and cefuroxime in the treatment of meningitis, delayed sterilization of CSF and a 17% rate of hearing loss in cefuroxime recipients were reported. In contrast, only 4% of the ceftriaxone group demonstrated hearing loss at follow-up.

A recent meta-analysis of all trials of steroids in *H influenzae* meningitis concluded that dexamethasone probably reduced the risk of hearing loss.

Adverse Effects

Dexamethasone therapy was not associated with delayed sterilization of CSF cultures in these studies. Relapse of meningitis occurred in only one patient, a dexamethasone-treated child who had *H influenzae* meningitis. The rate of relapse of *H influenzae* meningitis (1 of 104 steroid-treated patients, 0.96%) was similar to the 0.8% relapse rate observed in 708 patients with *H influenzae* meningitis treated in Dallas from 1969 to 1980 before initiation of those three dexamethasone studies.

Two patients treated with dexamethasone and ceftriaxone developed gastrointestinal bleeding requiring blood transfusions on the second and third days of steroid treatment. However, whether the bleeding was a result of dexamethasone therapy is uncertain. Secondary, low-grade fever occurred 24 to 48 hours after stopping dexamethasone in approximately two thirds of patients. Fever persisted for 24 to 36 hours. No other adverse effects were observed in the 133 patients who received dexamethasone.

Recommendations

- Dexamethasone therapy probably reduces the likelihood of deafness after *H influenzae* meningitis, although additional placebo-controlled studies are required before the Committee can make unqualified recommendations. Currently, individual consideration of dexamethasone is recommended for bacterial meningitis in infants and children 2 months and older after the physician has weighed the benefits and possible risks. However, the Committee recognizes that some experts have decided not to use dexamethasone therapy until additional data are available.
- The regimen used in the published studies was 0.6 mg/kg/d in four divided doses given intravenously for the first four days of antibiotic treatment. Insufficient data exist to recommend other dosage schedules of dexamethasone or other steroid drugs for therapy of meningitis.
- If dexamethasone is used, it should be administered at the time of the first dose of antibacterial therapy; the effect of dexamethasone therapy when administered more than several hours after the start of parenterally administered antimicrobial therapy has not been determined.
- In the published and current clinical trials of dexamethasone therapy, ceftriaxone, cefotaxime, and cefuroxime have been used for antimicrobial treatment. Because of delayed sterilization of CSF cultures in some infants with *H influenzae* meningitis and of a greater potential for hearing abnormality in cefuroxime-treated patients, the Committee does not recommend cefuroxime for therapy of bacterial meningitis. No a priori reason exists to believe that dexamethasone would not be comparably beneficial when administered with other effective antimicrobial regimens, such as ampicillin and chloramphenicol.
- Dexamethasone therapy should be considered only when the diagnosis of bacterial meningitis has been proven or is strongly suspected on the basis of the CSF examination, Gram-stained smear, or antigen test results.

- The utility of dexamethasone in treating pneumococcal or meningococcal meningitis is not yet known.
- Dexamethasone should not be used for suspected or proved aseptic or nonbacterial meningitis. If the drug had been started before the diagnosis of nonbacterial meningitis, it should be discontinued when a diagnosis of bacterial meningitis becomes unlikely.
- "Partially treated" meningitis with negative cultures is also not an indication for continued dexamethasone therapy.
- The results to date suggest that dexamethasone is effective in those with milder illness; thus, if dexamethasone is used, all patients should be treated, not just those with severe disease.
- No data are currently available on which to recommend the use of dexamethasone for treatment of bacterial meningitis in infants younger than 2 months or of meningitis in those with congenital or acquired abnormalities of the central nervous system, with or without placement of a prosthetic device.
- Measurements of hemoglobin concentrations and examinations of stool for occult blood should be performed regularly during dexamethasone therapy. If melena or gross blood is found, dexamethasone therapy should be stopped and the patient should be observed closely for possible transfusion therapy.

These recommendations and warnings may be modified as the results of additional studies become available.

Drugs of Choice for Invasive and Other Serious Fungal Infections in Children

	Intravenous		Oral Absorbable			Intravenous or Oral
Disease	Miconazole	Amphotericin B	Flucytosine	Ketoconazole	Griseofulvin	Fluconazole*
Aspergillosis		†				
Blastomycosis (North American)		†		‡		
Candidiasis, systemic		‖	‖, ¶			§
Candidiasis: oropharyngeal, gastrointestinal	§	§ (severe cases)	§	†		§
Chronic, mucocutaneous candidiasis	§	§	§	†		
Coccidioidomycosis	§	†		§		
Cryptococcosis		‖	‖			§
Histoplasmosis		†		§		
Mucormycocis (phycomycosis, zygomycosis)		†				
Paracoccidioidomycosis (South American blastomycosis)	§	† (severe cases)		†		

*Efficacy and safety has not been established for children; a small number of children 3-13 years have been treated safely.
†Preferred treatment in most cases.
‡For mild and moderately severe cases.
§Efficacy less well established or alternative drug.
‖Combination recommended.
¶Combination recommended if infection is severe or CNS is involved.

Recommended Doses of Parenteral and Oral Antifungal Drugs

Drug	Route	Dose (per day)	Adverse Reactions
Amphotericin B*	IV	0.25 mg/kg (following test dose†) initially, increase as tolerated to 0.5-1 mg/kg; infuse as single dose during 4-6 h	Fever, chills, phlebitis, renal dysfunction, hypokalemia, anemia, cardiac arrhythmias, anaphylactoid reaction, hematologic abnormalities
	IT	0.025 mg, increase to 0.1-0.5 mg twice weekly	Radiculitis, sensory loss, and foot drop
Clotrimazole troches	PO	10 mg tablet 5 times daily (dissolved slowly in mouth)	Nausea, vomiting, and increase in serum transaminase
Flucytosine	PO	50 to 150 mg/kg in 4 doses at 6-h intervals	Bone marrow suppression; renal dysfunction can lead to drug accumulation; nausea, vomiting, increase in transaminases, BUN, and creatinine
Griseofulvin	PO	Ultramicrosize: 7.3 mg/kg, single dose; maximum dose, 375-750 mg Microsize: 15-20 mg/kg/d divided in 2 doses; maximum dose, 500-1,000 mg	Rash, leukopenia, proteinuria, paresthesias, gastrointestinal symptoms, and mental confusion
Ketoconazole	PO	Children: 3.3-6.6 mg/kg, once daily‡ Adults: 200-400 mg once daily	Rash, anaphylaxis, nausea, vomiting, abdominal pain, fever, gynecomastia, thrombocytopenia, hepatoxicity, and depression of endocrine function (dose-dependent, reversible)

Miconazole	IV	20 to 40 mg/kg, divided into 3 infusions 8 h apart; maximum 15 mg/kg per infusion. Infuse over 30-60 min	Phlebitis, rash, fever, nausea, anemia, hyponatremia, thrombocytopenia, and hyperlipemia
	IT	20 mg per dose for 3 to 7 days	
Nystatin	PO	Infants: 200,000 U 4 times daily Children and adults: 400,000-600,000 U 4 times daily	Nausea, vomiting, and diarrhea
Fluconazole	IV PO	Children§: 3-6 mg/kg daily Adults: 200 mg once followed by 100 mg daily for oropharyngeal, esophageal candidiasis; 400 mg once followed by 200-400 mg daily for cryptococcal meningitis (200 mg daily for maintenance in patients with AIDS).	Rash, nausea, abdominal pain, diarrhea, headache, and possible hepatotoxicity

Abbreviations: IV = intravenous, IT = intrathecal, PO = oral.

*For details, see page 574.

†Test dose is 0.1 mg/kg, with maximum dose of 1 mg/kg (see page 574).

‡For children 2 years and younger, the daily dose has not been established.

§Efficacy has not been established for children. A small number of children aged 3 to 13 years have been treated safely with the dosage given here.

Systemic Treatment With Amphotericin B

Amphotericin B is a key antifungal drug that causes many major and minor adverse reactions, particularly nephrotoxicity. Hence, its parenteral use is primarily restricted to selected, potentially fatal fungal infections. Before using amphotericin B, the physician should consult the manufacturer's package insert for specific precautions, adverse reactions, and infusion information.

Amphotericin B is initially administered intravenously in a single test dose of 0.1 mg/kg (maximum, 1 mg) during a 20-minute to 4-hour period to assess the patient's febrile and hemodynamic responses. The temperature, pulse, respiration, and blood pressure should be carefully monitored during the infusion. The first therapeutic dose is 0.25 mg/kg/d administered during a 2- to 4-hour interval, and is given the same day as the test dose. Patients with severe reactions to the test dose should receive a lower dose. Subsequently, the dose is increased in daily increments of 0.1 to 0.25 mg/kg during a 4-day interval until a total dose of 0.4 to 1 mg/kg is reached. In life-threatening situations, 0.25 mg/kg increments can be given in successive 2- to 4-hour infusions during a 12- to 24-hour period to achieve the maximum total daily dose of 1 mg/kg. Low doses of amphotericin B (e.g., 0.1 to 0.3/kg/d) have been used successfully in infections, such as *Candida* esophagitis, with good results.

The serum concentration is not significantly increased in patients with impaired renal function. Hemodialysis and peritoneal dialysis do not remove significant amounts of the drug.

In some illnesses, doses of 1.25 or 1.5 mg/kg may be necessary. The proper dose for preterm and newborn infants has not been determined, but the doses given here have been used successfully. Amphotericin B must be administered in 5% dextrose in water. The preparation should be discarded if the solution becomes turbid on addition of amphotericin B.

Adequate serum concentrations of the drug can usually be maintained after 1 week of daily therapy by administering double the daily dose (maximum 1.5 mg/kg) on alternate days.

The duration of therapy depends on the type and extent of the specific fungal infection.

Commonly observed adverse reactions include the following: fever (sometimes with shaking chills), nausea and vomiting, generalized body pains, pain at the intravenous administration site (phlebitis), and abnormal renal function (hypokalemia, elevated serum creatinine and BUN levels, decreased creatinine clearance rate, and a diminished ability to concentrate urine). Pretreatment with antipyretics can be helpful in alleviating febrile reactions. Hydrocortisone (25 to 50 mg in adults) can be added to the infusion to reduce febrile and other systemic reactions. Tolerance to the febrile reactions develops with time, allowing tapering and eventual discontinuation of the hydrocortisone. Some experts add heparin to the infusion to decrease phlebitis. Less common severe reactions include anuria, oliguria, anemia and other hematologic abnormalities, hypomagnesemia, cardiovascular toxicity (arrhythmias, hypertension, and hypotension), anaphylactoid reactions, and convulsions and other neurologic symptoms.

For patients with central nervous system fungal infections who do not respond to intravenous therapy, consideration should be given to the concomitant administration of amphotericin B intrathecally, intraventricularly, or intracisternally. Preferably, injections should be into the lateral ventricles through a cisternal Ommaya reservoir. The value of this approach has been clearly established only in coccidioidal meningitis, but it may be justified in the nonresponsive patient with other fungal infections, as cerebrospinal fluid concentrations of the drug are low or undetectable after intravenous administration of the drug. Amphotericin B may be administered twice weekly, or more frequently, in the lumbar, cisternal, or ventricular areas. The usual starting dose in adults is 0.1 mg three times a week; subsequent doses are increased by doubling until a maintenance dose of 0.5 mg is reached. Hydrocortisone (10 to 15 mg in adults) is added as required to relieve headaches. The solution should be freshly prepared and diluted with 2 to 10 mL of sterile 5% dextrose in water (10% dextrose in water for intralumbar injections) without preservatives. Before injection, the solution should be further diluted with spinal fluid so that the final concentration per milliliter is one tenth the dose. Duration of therapy depends on the clinical and mycologic responses. The spinal fluid should be cultured for fungi and bacteria as often as necessary. Nausea, vomiting, urinary retention, leg and back pain, headache, transitory radiculitis, sensory loss, and foot drop have been observed as a result of intrathecal therapy; permanent changes have also occurred.

Topical Drugs for Superficial Fungal Infections

Drug	Strength	Brand Names(s)	Application(s) per Day	Adverse Reactions*/Notes
Amphotericin B	3%	Fungizone	2-4	Drying, local irritation, erythema, pruritus, burning; more effective topical preparations are now available
Ciclopirox	1%	Loprox	2	Irritation, erythema, burning
Clotrimazole	1%	Lotrimin, Mycelex	2	Erythema, stinging, blistering, peeling, edema, itching, hives, burning
Econazole nitrate	1%	Spectazole	2	Burning, itching, stinging, erythema
Haloprogin	1%	Halotex	2	Burning, irritation, erythema, folliculitis, scaling, itching
Ketoconazole	2%	Nizoral	1	Irritation, itching, stinging
Miconazole	2%	Monistat-Derm, Micatin†	2	Irritation, dermatitis
Naftifine	1%	Naftin	2	Burning, stinging, erythema, itching, irritation; fungicidal agent
Nystatin	100,000 U/g	Mycostatin Nystatin Mytrex Mycolog Nystex Nilstat (Others)	2	Rare adverse reactions; effective against yeast only

Oxiconazole	1%	Oxistat	1	Itching, burning, irritation, erythema
Sulconazole	1%	Exelderm	1	Itching, burning, stinging
Tolnaftate	1%	Tinactin†	2	Rare adverse reactions
Undecylenate	10%-20%	Desenex† Caldescene Cruex Quinsano (Others)	2	Irritation
Other Remedies				
Benzoic acid (12%) and salicylic acid (3%)		Whitfield's ointment	2	Irritation, burning; potent keratolytic agent
Castellani's paint	—	—	1-2	Local irritation (contains basic fuchsin, phenol, resorcinol, acetone, alcohol)
Gentian violet	1%-2%	—	2	Staining
Selenium sulfide (shampoo)	2.5%	—	1	For tinea capitis‡
Sodium thiosulfate	25%	Tinver	1-2	For tinea versicolor

*For use in pregnancy, see package insert.
†Nonprescription drug.
‡Primary therapy is oral griseofulvin.

Antiviral Drugs

Drug: Generic (Trade)	Indication	Usually Recommended Dosage
Acyclovir* (Zovirax)	Genital herpes simplex virus (HSV) infection, first episode	Oral - 200 mg, 5 times daily for 10 d Topical - 5% ointment, 4-6 times daily (localized lesions only) for 7 d IV - 15 mg/kg/d in 3 divided doses for 5-7 d
	Genital HSV infection, recurrence	Oral - 200 mg 5 times daily or 800 mg 2 times daily for 5 d
	Recurrent HSV episodes in patients with frequent recurrences:	
	Chronic suppressive therapy	Oral - 200 mg, 2-5 times a day or 400 mg 2 times daily for as long as 12 continuous months
	Intermittent therapy	Oral - 200 mg, 5 times daily for 5 d
	HSV in immunocompromised host (localized, progressive, or disseminated)‡	IV - For children < 1 yr: 15-30 mg/kg/d in 3 divided doses† - For children ≥ 1 yr: 750 mg/m^2/d in 3 divided doses for 7-14 d Oral - 200 mg, 5 times daily for 7-14 days
	HSV encephalitis	IV - For children < 1 yr: 30 mg/kg/d in 3 divided doses† - For children ≥ 1 yr: 750 mg/m^2/d in 3 divided doses for 10-14 d
	Neonatal HSV‡	IV - 30 mg/kg/d in 3 divided doses for 10-21 d. For premature infants, 20 mg/kg/d in 2 divided doses

	Varicella‡ or zoster in immunocompromised host;	IV - For children < 1 yr: 30 mg/kg/d in 3 divided doses. - For children ≥ 1 yr: 1500 mg/m²/d in 3 divided doses for 7-10 d
	Zoster in immunocompetent host‡	IV - Same as for zoster in immunocompromised host Oral - 800 mg, 5 times daily for 5-7 d for patients ≥ 12 y (investigational)
	Varicella in immunocompetent host‡,‖	Oral - 40-80 mg/kg/d according to age§ in 4 divided doses for minimum of 5 d
Vidarabine (Vira-A)	HSV encephalitis¶	IV - 15 mg/kg/d given in 1 dose during 12-24 h for 10 d
	Neonatal HSV¶	IV - 15-30 mg/kg/d given as above for 10-21 d
	Varicella or zoster in immunocompromised host‡,¶	IV - 10 mg/kg/d given as above for 5-10 d
Amantadine* (Symmetrel), Rimantadine*,‡	Influenza A treatment	Oral - For children 1-9 y, 4.4 mg/kg/d in 2 divided doses (maximum, 150 mg/d). For children > 9 y, 200 mg/d in 2 doses; if weight is less than 45 kg, 4.4 mg/kg/d in 2 doses Duration: 2 to 7 d

*Dose should be decreased in patients with impaired renal function.

†Some experts also recommend this dosage for children ≥ 1 year.

‡Drug is not licensed for this indication or is investigational at this time (October 1990).

§5-7 y, 20 mg/kg; 7-12 y, 15 mg/kg; 12-16 y, 10 mg/kg (Balfour et al. Acyclovir treatment of varicella in otherwise healthy children. *J. Ped.* 1990;86:633-639).

‖Selective indications; see Varicella, page 519.

¶Alternative to acyclovir, which is the usual drug of choice.

Antiviral Drugs

Drug: Generic (Trade)	Indication	Usually Recommended Dosage
	Prophylaxis of influenza A	Oral - For children ≤ 20 kg, same dose as for treatment; for children > 20 kg, 100-200 mg in 2 divided doses. Duration is for period of possible exposure; may be used for entire winter season
Ribavirin (Virazole)	Treatment of respiratory syncytial virus (RSV) infection	Aerosol - Given by a small particle generator, in a solution containing 20 mg/mL, for 12-18 h/d for 3-7 days; longer treatment may be necessary in some patients
Ganciclovir* (Cytovene)	Acquired CMV retinitis in immuno-compromised host	IV - 10 mg/kg/d in 2 divided doses or 7.5 mg/kg/d in 3 divided doses, for 14-21 d. For long-term suppression, 25-35 mg/kg/wk given once daily 5 d/wk
Zidovudine (Retrovir, formerly termed azidothymidine [AZT])	Symptomatic HIV infection††	Oral - For children, 720 mg/m²/d in 4 divided doses** For adolescents and adults: starting dose is 200 mg every 4 h

*Dose should be decreased in patients with impaired renal function.

**For infants, dose should be recalculated every 2 months.

††Indications for treatment of children are evolving. Drug is also approved for use in HIV-infected children who are asymptomatic but have laboratory evidence of HIV-related immunosuppression. In adults, zidovudine is indicated for asymptomatic patients with CD4 lymphocyte counts < 500/mm^3.

Ribavirin Therapy of Respiratory Syncytial Virus*

Ribavirin is an antiviral drug approved by the Food and Drug Administration in 1986 for the aerosol treatment of serious respiratory syncytial virus (RSV) infections in hospitalized children who do not require assisted ventilation. Ribavirin is different from other antiviral drugs both in its spectrum of activity and in its mode of administration. The following statement is presented to identify which children should be considered for ribavirin therapy. Questions have also arisen about (1) the benefits of treatment in light of the potential toxicity of the drug, (2) its administration to infants who require assisted ventilation (the package insert has warned against use of the drug by such patients), and (3) the risks to pregnant women or personnel who care for infants receiving ribavirin. Finally, physicians must be aware of the high cost of ribavirin.

Background

RSV Disease

RSV is the most important cause of lower respiratory tract disease in infants and young children. Disease usually appears in yearly winter to spring outbreaks and infects essentially all children during their first 3 years of life. The number of infected infants who require hospitalization has been estimated to range, in different locations, from 1 in 50 to 1 in 1,000. Currently, the mortality in hospitalized infants who were previously healthy is low (less than 1%). In infants with underlying diseases, however, the mortality can be strikingly higher. Conditions that appear to render a child at risk of severe or fatal RSV infection are pulmonary disease, especially bronchopulmonary dysplasia; prematurity; congenital heart disease; and immunodeficiency disease or therapy causing immunosuppression at any age.

Most previously healthy infants infected with RSV improve with only supportive care within a few days and are discharged after an average of 4 to 9 days. Possible long-term sequelae are difficult to assess. Evidence has recently accumulated, however, about abnormalities in pulmonary function that develop in some children. These may be relatively asymptomatic or may manifest as recurrent wheezing or lower respiratory tract disease. Whether treatment of the initial respiratory syncytial virus infection can alter the rate or outcome of such sequelae is unknown.

---

*Revised from American Academy of Pediatrics, Committee on Infectious Diseases. Ribavirin therapy of respiratory syncytial virus. *Pediatrics.* 1987;79:475-478.

Ribavirin

Aerosolized ribavirin is the first specific drug available for the treatment of RSV infections. It is a synthetic nucleoside analogue (1-β-D-ribafuranosyl-1,2,4-triazole-3-carboxamide) resembling guanosine and inosine; it appears to interfere with the expression of messenger RNA and to inhibit viral protein synthesis. It is not significantly incorporated into host cell RNA or DNA.

Safety for Health Care Personnel

Teratogenicity has been observed in rodents administered oral ribavirin, and environmental studies have indicated that absorption in humans, albeit minimal, from aerosol ribavirin exposure can occur. These findings have led to concern among hospital workers about the safety of ribavirin and have led some hospitals to apply very strict precautions in the use of ribavirin to minimize exposure of health care workers. Review of these findings, however, does not support the need for such precautions.

In hamsters after a single dose of 2.5 mg/kg and in rats after a daily oral dose of 10 mg/kg, fetal malformations have been noted. In rabbits, the species most sensitive to the effects of ribavirin, skeletal malformations after daily oral administration of 0.3 mg/kg, and fetal death and resorption after 1.0 mg/kg/d were observed. Blood concentrations associated with fetal damage in these animals are not known. In contrast, the offspring of pregnant baboons treated orally with 60 to 120 mg/kg/d during the time of fetal organogenesis were normal.

Extrapolation from these animal experiments involving oral administration of ribavirin to circumstances of human exposure to ribavirin aerosol is difficult, especially in view of the demonstration of considerable differences in teratogenicity between species. However, blood concentrations in humans given oral ribavirin can be compared with those resulting from aerosol exposure. Whereas plasma concentrations in adults receiving 10 mg/kg/d are 0.4 to 1.2 μg/mL, in infants receiving aerosolized ribavirin by intubation for 20 hours per day, concentrations are less than 1 μg/mg, and much lower than those likely to occur in rodents in whom teratogenicity has been observed.

Incidental exposure of hospital personnel and visitors to ribavirin aerosol while caring for treated infants is likely to occur. In one study 19 nonpregnant nurses were studied who were caring for infants receiving ribavirin by ventilator, in an oxygen tent or in a hood. Nurses were exposed for an average of 8 hours per day during 3 days (a total of 20 to 35 hours). Total air exchanges occurred 5.4 to 24 times per hour in the patient rooms. Bloods for analysis of ribavirin were obtained 1 day before exposure, 1 hour after the final exposure, and 3 to 5 days later;

urine was collected before and 3 to 5 days after exposure. Ribavirin was not detected in any sample of plasma, erythrocytes, or urine. Preexposure and postexposure results did not differ. The lower limit of sensitivity of the drug radioimmunoassay in this study was 0.002 µg/mL. In a similar study of health care personnel caring for infants treated with ribavirin, 90 samples of serum, urine, and erythrocytes were assayed for ribavirin. Ribavirin was detected in a concentration of 0.44 µg/mL in only one erythrocyte sample. Concentrations of the drug in erythrocytes are 100-fold greater than those in serum. The concurrent serum and urine samples on this staff member were negative. No symptoms were reported by any health care workers in this study.

During treatment with aerosolized ribavirin, dissemination of the drug in the environment around the patient is substantial. Some of the escaped ribavirin will be inhaled by those caring for treated children. However, while 60% to 70% of the inhaled drug may be deposited in the lung, absorption from the lung into circulation appears to be minimal and the resulting risk following occupational exposure appears to be negligible. Furthermore, in infants receiving aerosolized ribavirin by endotracheal tube, the peak plasma concentration was less than 0.4 µg/mL at a time when the peak concentrations in endotracheal secretions were greater than 200 µg/mL. Hence, recommendations concerning protection of health care workers based on the assumption that 70% of the inhaled dose is absorbed are not valid.

These findings and the lack of validated reports of adverse efforts in human fetuses after 5 years of clinical use of the drug in the United States indicate that the teratogenicity of ribavirin in humans remains highly questionable.

Clinical Studies

Trials of ribavirin treatment of infants hospitalized with RSV lower respiratory tract diseases have involved both normal infants and those with underlying disease. In the controlled studies involving both healthy infants and those with underlying disease, ribavirin was associated with a greater clinical improvement than placebo treatment. Treatment had a beneficial effect on some signs, such as retraction and rales, but not on others, such as fever and wheezing. However, these latter signs were present in only a minority of patients. The improvement in treated infants' arterial oxygenation has been substantially greater. In one study, the treated group had a mean $Pa0_2$ of 49.4 mm Hg at the start of therapy and 62.4 mm Hg at the end, an increase of 13 mm Hg; the comparable values for the placebo group were 52, 56, and 4 mm Hg. The effect of therapy on persistence of virus in secretions differed in various studies.

Ribavirin has been administered as an aerosol with particles small enough (mass median aerosol diameter, 1 to 2 μm) to reach the lower respiratory tract, and it has been delivered via an oxygen hood or tent for an average of 3 to 5 days for 12 to 20 hours each day. High concentrations of ribavirin were obtained in the respiratory secretions by this method with little systemic absorption. No significant toxicity has been observed in any of these controlled trials. The effect of the ribavirin aerosol on pulmonary function was examined in adult volunteers infected with RSV in a controlled, double-blind study. Serial pulmonary function tests, which included carbachol challenge, showed no alterations in volunteers during the ribavirin therapy or when tested 1 month later.

When ribavirin is administered to mechanically ventilated patients, however, technical difficulties could cause adverse effects if proper precautions are not observed. Deposition of the drug in the delivery system occurs and appears to be dependent on temperature, humidity, and electrostatic forces.

Precipitation of the drug in the respirator tubing and around the expiratory valve of ventilators could, if uncorrected, lead to malfunction or obstruction of the valve, resulting in inadvertently high concentrations of positive end-expiratory pressure. Use of one-way valves on the inspiratory lines and of a breathing circuit filter in the expiratory line, along with careful monitoring, has been effective in preventing these problems.

The long-term effects of ribavirin on pulmonary function and on the sequelae of RSV infection require further investigation. Thus far, when the pulmonary function of the limited number of infants enrolled in the original controlled studies have been examined 4 or more years later, the infants who received ribavirin did at least as well as those who received placebo.

Experience with other antiviral agents has raised the additional concern of the development of resistance to ribavirin by RSV. With limited experience, no change in sensitivity of any viral isolate to ribavirin has been observed, even with prolonged administration.

Cost-Benefit Analysis

Whether the use of this expensive drug (nearly $700, excluding administration, for a 3-day course) will reduce the cost of hospitalization and subsequent pulmonary illness of children with RSV infection is uncertain. Although ribavirin treatment of high-risk patients early in the course of RSV infection will likely yield the greatest benefit, additional studies are needed to quantitate these effects.

Recommendations

Candidates for Ribavirin Treatment

Infants hospitalized with lower respiratory tract disease caused by RSV who are in the following categories should be considered for treatment with ribavirin aerosol:

1. *Infants at high risk for severe or complicated RSV infection*, including infants with congenital heart disease, bronchopulmonary dysplasia, and other chronic lung conditions; those with cystic fibrosis; and certain premature infants. In addition, children with immunodeficiency (especially those with severe combined immunodeficiency disease), recent transplant recipients, and those undergoing chemotherapy for malignancy should also be considered to be at high risk for complicated RSV infection.
2. *Infants hospitalized with RSV lower respiratory tract disease who are severely ill.* Because severity of illness is often difficult to judge clinically in infants with RSV infection, determination of blood gas values is often necessary. Infants with PaO_2 values of less than 65 mm Hg and those with increasing $PaCO_2$ concentrations should be considered candidates for ribavirin therapy. Oximetry may be used as a noninvasive means of determining the arterial oxygen saturation.
3. *Infants who might be considered for treatment* are those hospitalized with lower respiratory tract disease that is not initially severe but who may be at some increased risk of progressing to a more complicated course by virtue of young age (< 6 weeks), or in whom prolonged illness might be particularly detrimental to an underlying condition, such as those with multiple congenital anomalies, or neurologic or metabolic diseases.

Diagnosis of RSV Infection

Institutions planning to use ribavirin should be encouraged to avail themselves of the rapid diagnostic techniques to identify RSV antigen in respiratory secretions (see Respiratory Syncytial Virus, page 400). These tests should be performed when the child is admitted to the hospital. Tissue culture isolation, which requires an average of 3 to 5 days, may not yield results rapidly enough to be useful in making initial decisions about the use of ribavirin. However, the rapid diagnostic tests have variable sensitivity and may miss as many as 45%. If rapid tests are not available, candidates in the three recommended categories for ribavirin therapy who have bronchiolitis or pneumonia clinically compatible with RSV infection and are admitted during the RSV season (generally December to April) might still be considered for ribavirin therapy. If the etiology of the infant's pulmonary disease is subsequently found to be an agent other than RSV, therapy can be discontinued. However, ribavirin may also be effective in influenza virus infections and has in vitro activity against parainfluenza, adenovirus, and measles viruses. If no agent is initially identified as the cause of the lower respiratory tract disease but the most likely clinical diagnosis remains RSV infection and the infant is severely ill, continuation of the treatment while further diagnostic efforts to ascertain the causative agent are undertaken is reasonable. In ventilated infants, confirmation of the diagnosis of RSV infection is particularly important. Although diagnosis by viral isolation can sometimes require more than 7 days, treatment ordinarily should not be continued beyond the usual course of 3 to 7 days without a confirmed diagnosis. Longer durations of therapy may be useful in immunodeficient patients.

Administration of Drug

Ribavirin is nebulized into an oxyhood, tent, or mask from a solution containing 20 mg of ribavirin per milliliter of water by a small-particle aerosol generator supplied with the drug by the manufacturer. The aerosol is administered for 12 to 18 hours per day for 3 to 7 days. In the controlled studies, most children had improved by the third to fifth day of treatment.

Infants Requiring Mechanical Ventilation

Infants who require mechanical ventilation because of severe RSV infection are those who may be most likely to benefit from ribavirin treatment. The technical aspects of delivering ribavirin aerosol via a ventilator require special expertise. Treatment of such infants should be done in facilities whose personnel have specific training and experience in the administration of ribavirin to ventilated infants. The recommended technical precautions must be followed; as with any infant requiring mechanical ventilation, constant monitoring is mandatory.

Isolation of Patients

Implementation of proper isolation procedures for patients with RSV infection is essential. Treatment with ribavirin does not eliminate the need for careful isolation of patients with RSV (see Respiratory Syncytial Virus, page 401).

Precautions for Health Care Personnel and Other Contacts

Until further studies have been performed, pregnant women should be advised not to directly care for patients who are receiving ribavirin via tent or hood. Aerosol administration should be temporarily stopped when the hood is open. Pregnant women should be counseled about not entering the hood and should sit six feet or more from the infant's bed. Other patients are not at increased risk. Use of gloves and gowns by exposed personnel is not necessary since dermal absorption is negligible. The use of a mask designed to block absorption of particulate droplets with ribavirin might provide added protection. Evaluation of a scavenger device to reduce the escape of aerosolized ribavirin into a room is in progress. At present, given the data on absorption of ribavirin from aerosol exposure, more elaborate precautions are not justified.

Future Directions

Additional research is needed to define more accurately the clinical indications, timing of therapy, and safety of ribavirin.

Drugs for Parasitic Infections

The following table is reproduced from the March 23, 1990 issue of *The Medical Letter* (1990;32:23-32) and provides recommendations that are consistent, in most cases, with those of the Committee, given in the chapters on specific diseases in Part 3. However, because of occasional differences, both should be consulted. The Committee thanks the editors of *The Medical Letter* for their courtesy in allowing the table to be reprinted.

In the table, first-choice and alternative drugs with recommended dosages for most parasitic infections are given. In each case, the need for treatment must be weighed against the toxic effects of the drug. A decision to withhold therapy may often be correct, particularly when the drugs can cause severe adverse effects. When the first-choice drug is initially ineffective and the alternative is more hazardous, a second course of treatment with the first drug before giving the alternative may be prudent. Another section of the table lists adverse effects of some antiparasitic drugs.

Several drugs recommended in the table have not been approved by the Food and Drug Administration and are investigational (see footnotes). When a physician prescribes an unapproved drug, the physician should inform the patient of the investigational status and adverse effects of the drug.

DRUGS FOR PARASITIC INFECTIONS[A]

PARTIAL LIST OF ANTIPARASITIC DRUGS

* albendazole — *Zentel* (SKF)
amphotericin B — *Fungizone* (Squibb)
** benznidazole — *Rochagan* (Roche)
† bithionol — *Bitin* (Tanabe, Japan)
chloroquine — *Aralen* (Winthrop-Breon); others
crotamiton — *Eurax* (Westwood)
† dehydroemetine — *Meban* (Hoffmann-LaRoche, Switzerland)
* diethylcarbamazine — *Hetrazan* (Lederle)
† diloxanide furoate — *Furamide* (Boots, England)
* eflornithine (difluoromethylornithine; DFMO) — *Ornidyl* (Merrell Dow)
emetine — (Lilly)
** flubendazole — (Janssen)
furazolidone — *Furoxone* (Norwich Eaton)
hydroxychloroquine — *Plaquenil* (Winthrop-Breon)
iodoquinol (diiodohydroxyquin) — *Yodoxin* (Glenwood); others
* itraconazole — *Sporanox* (Janssen)
† ivermectin — *Mectizan* (Merck)
ketoconazole — *Nizoral* (Janssen)
lindane (gamma benzene hexachloride) — *Kwell* (Reed and Carnrick); others
malathion — *Ovide* (GenDerm)
mebendazole — *Vermox* (Janssen)
mefloquine — *Lariam* (Roche)
† melarsoprol — *Arsobal* (Rhône Poulenc, France)
** metrifonate — *Bilarcil* (Bayer, Germany)
metronidazole — *Flagyl* (Searle); others
niclosamide — *Niclocide* (Miles)
† nifurtimox — *Lampit* (Bayer, Germany)
** ornidazole — *Tiberal* (Hoffman-LaRoche, Switzerland)
oxamniquine — *Vansil* (Pfizer)
paromomycin — *Humatin* (Parke-Davis)
pentamidine isethionate — *Pentam 300* (LyphoMed)
permethrin — *Nix* (Burroughs Wellcome); *Elimite* (Herbert)
piperazine — many manufacturers
praziquantel — *Biltricide* (Miles)
primaquine phosphate — (Winthrop-Breon)
** proguanil — *Paludrine* (Ayerst, Canada; ICI, England)
pyrantel pamoate — *Antiminth* (Pfizer)
pyrethrins and piperonyl butoxide — *RID* (Pfizer); others
pyrimethamine — *Daraprim* (Burroughs Wellcome)
pyrimethamine-sulfadoxine — *Fansidar* (Roche)
quinacrine — *Atabrine* (Winthrop-Breon)
quinidine gluconate — many manufacturers
† quinine dihydrochloride
quinine sulfate — many manufacturers
** spiramycin — *Rovamycine* (Poulenc, Canada)
† stibogluconate sodium (antimony sodium gluconate) — *Pentostam* (Burroughs Wellcome, England)
† suramin — *Germanin* (Bayer, Germany)
thiabendazole — *Mintezol* (Merck)
** tinidazole — *Fasigyn* (Pfizer)
trimethoprim-sulfamethoxazole — *Bactrim* (Roche); *Septra* (Burroughs Wellcome); others
‡ trimetrexate (Parke-Davis)
** tryparsamide

[A] Reprinted with permission from The Medical Letter (1990;32:23-32), Copyright ©1990, The Medical Letter, Inc.
* Available in the USA only from manufacturer
** Not available in the USA
† Available from the CDC Drug Service, Centers for Disease Control, Atlanta, Georgia 30333; 404-639-3670 (evenings, weekends, or holidays: 404-639-2888)
‡ Available from the National Institute of Allergy and Infectious Diseases, 1-800-537-9978

DRUGS FOR TREATMENT OF PARASITIC INFECTIONS

Infection	Drug	Adult Dosage*	Pediatric Dosage*
AMEBIASIS (Entamoeba histolytica)			
asymptomatic			
Drug of choice:	Iodoquinol[1]	650 mg tid x 20d	30-40 mg/kg/d in 3 doses x 20d
Alternatives:	Diloxanide furoate[2]	500 mg tid x 10d	20 mg/kg/d in 3 doses x 10d
	Paromomycin	25-30 mg/kg/d in 3 doses x 7d	25-30 mg/kg/d in 3 doses x 7d
mild to moderate intestinal disease			
Drugs of choice:	Metronidazole[3,4]	750 mg tid x 10d	35-50 mg/kg/d in 3 doses x 10d
	followed by iodoquinol[1]	650 mg tid x 20d	30-40 mg/kg/d in 3 doses x 20d
Alternative:	Paromomycin	25-30 mg/kg/d in 3 doses x 7d	25-30 mg/kg/d in 3 doses x 7d
severe intestinal disease			
Drugs of choice:	Metronidazole[3,4]	750 mg tid x 10d	35-50 mg/kg/d in 3 doses x 10d
	followed by iodoquinol[1]	650 mg tid x 20d	30-40 mg/kg/d in 3 doses x 20d
Alternatives:	Dehydroemetine[2,5]	1 to 1.5 mg/kg/d (max. 90 mg/d) IM for up to 5d	1 to 1.5 mg/kg/d (max. 90 mg/d) IM in 2 doses for up to 5d
	followed by iodoquinol[1]	650 mg tid x 20d	30-40 mg/kg/d in 3 doses x 20d
	OR Emetine[5]	1 mg/kg/d (max. 60 mg/d) IM for up to 5d	1 mg/kg/d in 2 doses (max. 60 mg/d) IM for up to 5d
	followed by iodoquinol[1]	650 mg tid x 20d	30-40 mg/kg/d in 3 doses x 20d

* The letter d indicates day.

1. Dosage and duration of administration should not be exceeded because of possibility of causing optic neuritis; maximum dosage is 2 grams/day.
2. In the USA, this drug is available from the CDC Drug Service, Centers for Disease Control, Atlanta, Georgia 30333; telephone: 404-639-3670 (evenings, weekends, and holidays: 404-639-2888).
3. Metronidazole is carcinogenic in rodents and mutagenic in bacteria; it should generally not be given to pregnant women, particularly in the first trimester.
4. Outside the USA, ornidazole and tinidazole are also used.

Infection	Drug	Adult Dosage*	Pediatric Dosage*
hepatic abscess			
Drugs of choice:	Metronidazole[3,4]	750 mg tid x 10d	35-50 mg/kg/d in 3 doses x 10d
	followed by iodoquinol[1]	650 mg tid x 20d	30-40 mg/kg/d in 3 doses x 20d
Alternatives:	Dehydroemetine[2,5]	1 to 1.5 mg/kg/d (max. 90 mg/d) IM for up to 5d	1 to 1.5 mg/kg/d (max. 90 mg/d) IM in 2 doses for up to 5d
	followed by chloroquine phosphate	600 mg base (1 gram)/d x 2d, then 300 mg base (500 mg)/d x 2-3 wks	10 mg base/kg (max. 300 mg base)/d x 2-3 wks
	plus iodoquinol[1]	650 mg tid x 20d	30-40 mg/kg/d in 3 doses x 20d
	OR Emetine[5]	1 mg/kg/d (max. 60 mg/d) IM for up to 5d	1 mg/kg/d (max. 60 mg/d) IM in 2 doses for up to 5d
	followed by chloroquine phosphate	600 mg base (1 gram)/d x 2d, then 300 mg base (500 mg)/d x 2-3 wks	10 mg base/kg (max. 300 mg base)/d x 2-3 wks
	plus iodoquinol[1]	650 mg tid x 20d	30-40 mg/kg/d in 3 doses x 20d
AMEBIC MENINGOENCEPHALITIS, PRIMARY			
Naegleria			
Drug of choice:	Amphotericin B[6,7]	1 mg/kg/d IV, uncertain duration	1 mg/kg/d IV, uncertain duration
Acanthamoeba			
Drug of choice:	see footnote 8		
Ancylostoma duodenale, see HOOKWORM			
ANGIOSTRONGYLIASIS			
Angiostrongylus cantonensis			
Drug of choice:	Mebendazole[7,9,10]	100 mg bid x 5d	100 mg bid x 5d
Angiostrongylus costaricensis			
Drug of choice:	Thiabendazole[7,9]	75 mg/kg/d in 3 doses x 3 d[11] (max. 3 grams/day)	75 mg/kg/d in 3 doses x 3 d[11] (max.3 grams/d)

Infection	Drug	Adult dosage	Pediatric dosage
ANISAKIASIS (Anisakis)			
Treatment of choice:	Surgical removal		
ASCARIASIS (Ascaris lumbricoides, roundworm)			
Drug of choice:[12]	Mebendazole	100 mg bid x 3d	100 mg bid x 3d
OR	Pyrantel pamoate	11 mg/kg once (max. 1 gram)	11 mg/kg once (max. 1 gram)
BABESIOSIS (Babesia)			
Drugs of choice:[13]	Clindamycin[7]	1.2 grams bid parenteral or 600 mg tid oral x 7d	20-40 mg/kg/d in 3 doses x 7d
	plus quinine	650 mg tid oral x 7d	25 mg/kg/d in 3 doses x 7d
BALANTIDIASIS (Balantidium coli)			
Drug of choice:	Tetracycline[7]	500 mg qid x 10d	40 mg/kg/d in 4 doses x 10d (max. 2 grams/d)[14]
Alternatives:	Iodoquinol[1,7]	650 mg tid x 20d	40 mg/kg/d in 3 doses x 20d
	Metronidazole[3,7]	750 mg tid x 5d	35-50 mg/kg/d in 3 doses x 5d
BAYLISASCARIASIS (Baylisascaris procyonis)			
Drug of choice:	See footnote 15		
BLASTOCYSTIS hominis infection			
Drug of choice:	See footnote 16		

5. Dehydroemetine is probably as effective and probably less toxic than emetine. Because of its toxic effects on the heart, patients receiving emetine should have electrocardiographic monitoring and should remain sedentary during therapy.
6. One patient with a Naegleria infection was successfully treated with amphotericin B, miconazole, and rifampin (JS Seidel et al, N Engl J Med, 306:346, 1982).
7. Considered an investigational drug for this condition by the U.S. Food and Drug Administration.
8. Strains of Acanthamoeba isolated from fatal granulomatous amebic encephalitis are usually sensitive *in vitro* to pentamidine, ketoconazole, paromomycin, 5-fluorocytosine, and (less so) to amphotericin B (RJ Duma et al, Antimicrob Agents Chemother, 10:370, 1976). For treatment of keratitis caused by Acanthamoeba, concurrent topical use of 0.1% propamidine isethionate (*Broline* – Rhône-Poulenc, Canada) plus neosporin, or oral itraconazole plus topical miconazole, has been successful (MB Moore and JP McCulley, Br J Ophthalmol, 73:271, 1989; Y Ishibashi et al, Am J Ophthalmol, 109:121, Feb 1990).
9. Effectiveness documented only in animals
10. Analgesics, corticosteroids, and careful removal of CSF at frequent intervals can relieve symptoms (J Koo et al, Rev Infect Dis, 10:1155, 1988). Albendazole and ivermectin have also been used successfully in animals.
11. This dose is likely to be toxic and may have to be decreased.

Infection	Drug	Adult Dosage*	Pediatric Dosage*
CAPILLARIASIS (Capillaria philippinensis)			
Drug of choice:	Mebendazole[7]	200 mg bid x 20d	200 mg bid x 20d
Alternative:	Albendazole	200 mg bid x 10d	200 mg bid x 10d
	Thiabendazole[7]	25 mg/kg/d in 2 doses x 30d	25 mg/kg/d in 2 doses x 30d
Chagas' disease, see TRYPANOSOMIASIS			
Clonorchis sinensis, see FLUKE infection			
CRYPTOSPORIDIOSIS (Cryptosporidium)			
Drug of choice:	See footnote 17		
CUTANEOUS LARVA MIGRANS (creeping eruption)			
Drug of choice:[18]	Thiabendazole	Topically and/or 50 mg/kg/d in 2 doses (max. 3 grams/d) x 2-5d[11]	Topically and/or 50 mg/kg/d in 2 doses (max. 3 grams/d) x 2-5d[11]
Cysticercosis, see TAPEWORM infection			
DIENTAMOEBA fragilis infection			
Drug of choice:	Iodoquinol[1]	650 mg tid x 20d	40 mg/kg/d in 3 doses x 20d
	OR Paromomycin	25-30 mg/kg/d in 3 doses x 7d	25-30 mg/kg/d in 3 doses x 7d
	OR Tetracycline[7]	500 mg qid x 10d	40 mg/kg/d in 4 doses x 10d (max. 2 grams/d)[14]
Diphyllobothrium latum, see TAPEWORM infection			
DRACUNCULUS medinensis (guinea worm) infection			
Drug of choice:	Metronidazole[3,7,19]	250 mg tid x 10d	25 mg/kg/d (max. 750 mg/d) in 3 doses x 10d
Alternative:	Thiabendazole[7,19]	50-75 mg/kg/d in 2 doses x 3d[11]	50-75 mg/kg/d in 2 doses x 3d[11]
Echinococcus, see TAPEWORM infection			
Entamoeba histolytica, see AMEBIASIS			
ENTAMOEBA polecki infection			
Drug of choice:	Metronidazole[3,7]	750 mg tid x 10d	35-50 mg/kg/d in 3 doses x 10d

ENTEROBIUS vermicularis (pinworm) infection			
Drug of choice:[12]	Pyrantel pamoate	11 mg/kg once (max. 1 gram); repeat after 2 weeks	11 mg/kg once (max. 1 gram); repeat after 2 weeks
	OR Mebendazole	A single dose of 100 mg; repeat after 2 weeks	A single dose of 100 mg; repeat after 2 weeks
Fasciola hepatica, see FLUKE infection			
FILARIASIS			
Wuchereria bancrofti, Brugia (W.) malayi			
Drug of choice:[20]	Diethylcarbamazine[21]	Day 1: 50 mg, oral, p.c. Day 2: 50 mg tid Day 3: 100 mg tid Days 4 through 21: 6 mg/kg/d in 3 doses	Day 1: 25-50 mg, oral, p.c. Day 2: 25-50 mg tid Day 3: 50-100 mg tid Days 4 through 21: 6 mg/kg/d in 3 doses

(continued)

* The letter d indicates day.

12. Albendazole in a single dose of 400 mg has been reported to be highly effective for treatment of intestinal infection (WHO Drug Info, 3:73, 1989).
13. Concurrent use of pentamidine and trimethoprim-sulfamethoxazole has been reported to cure an infection with B. divergens (D Raoult et al, Ann Intern Med, 107:944, 1987).
14. Not recommended for children less than eight years old.
15. Drugs that could be tried include diethylcarbamazine, levamisole, and fenbendazole (KR Kazacos, J Am Vet Med Assoc, 195:894, 1989). Steroid therapy may be helpful, especially in eye or CNS infection. Ocular baylisascariasis has been treated successfully using laser therapy to destroy intraretinal larvae.
16. Clinical significance of these organisms is controversial, but metronidazole 750 mg tid x 10d or iodoquinol 650 mg tid x 20d anecdotally have been reported to be effective (RA Miller and BH Minshew, Rev Infect Dis, 10:930, 1988).
17. Infection is self-limited in immunocompetent patients. In AIDS patients with large-volume intractable diarrhea, octreotide *(Sandostatin)* 300-500 µg tid subcutaneously may control the diarrhea, but not the infection (DJ Cook et al, Ann Intern Med, 108:708, 1988).
18. Albendazole 200 mg bid x 3 days has been reported to be effective (SK Jones et al, Br J Dermatol, 122:99, 1990).
19. Not curative, but decreases inflammation and facilitates removing the worm. Mebendazole 400-800 mg/d for 6d has been reported to kill the worm directly.
20. A single dose of ivermectin, 25-200 µg/kg, has been reported to be effective for treatment of W. bancrofti and M. ozzardi (V Kumaraswami et al, JAMA, 259:3150, 1988; TB Nutman et al, J Infect Dis, 156:662, 1987).

Infection	Drug	Adult Dosage*	Pediatric Dosage*
FILARIASIS (continued)			
Loa loa			
Drug of choice:	Diethylcarbamazine[21]	Day 1: 50 mg, oral, p.c. Day 2: 50 mg tid Day 3: 100 mg tid Days 4 through 21: 9 mg/kg/d in 3 doses	Day 1: 50 mg, oral, p.c. Day 2: 50 mg tid Day 3: 100 mg tid Days 4 through 21: 9 mg/kg/d in 3 doses
Mansonella ozzardi			
Drug of choice:	See footnote 20		
Mansonella perstans			
Drug of choice:[22]	Mebendazole[7]	100 mg bid x 30d	
Tropical eosinophilia			
Drug of choice:	Diethylcarbamazine	6 mg/kg/d in 3 doses x 7-10d	6 mg/kg/d in 3 doses x 7-10d
Onchocerca volvulus			
Drug of choice:	Ivermectin[2,7]	150 µg/kg oral once, repeated every 6 to 12 months	150 µg/kg oral once
FLUKE, hermaphroditic, infection			
Clonorchis sinensis (Chinese liver fluke)			
Drug of choice:	Praziquantel	75 mg/kg/d in 3 doses x 2d	75 mg/kg/d in 3 doses x 2d
Fasciola hepatica (sheep liver fluke)			
Drug of choice:[23]	Bithionol[2]	30-50 mg/kg on alternate days x 10-15 doses	30-50 mg/kg on alternate days x 10-15 doses
Fasciolopsis buski (intestinal fluke)			
Drug of choice:	Praziquantel[7]	75 mg/kg/d in 3 doses x 1d	75 mg/kg/d in 3 doses x 1d
	OR Niclosamide[7]	a single dose of 4 tablets (2 g), chewed thoroughly	11-34 kg: 2 tablets (1 g) >34 kg: 3 tablets (1.5 g)
Heterophyes heterophyes (intestinal fluke)			
Drug of choice:	Praziquantel[7]	75 mg/kg/d in 3 doses x 1d	75 mg/kg/d in 3 doses x 1d
Metagonimus yokogawai (intestinal fluke)			
Drug of choice:	Praziquantel[7]	75 mg/kg/d in 3 doses x 1d	75 mg/kg/d in 3 doses x 1d

Nanophyetus salmincola			
Drug of choice:	Praziquantel	60 mg/kg/d in 3 doses x 1d	60 mg/kg/d in 3 doses x 1d
Opisthorchis viverrini (liver fluke)			
Drug of choice:	Praziquantel	75 mg/kg/d in 3 doses x 1d	75 mg/kg/d in 3 doses x 1d
Paragonimus westermani (lung fluke)			
Drug of choice:	Praziquantel[7]	75 mg/kg/d in 3 doses x 2d	75 mg/kg/d in 3 doses x 2d
Alternative:	Bithionol[2]	30-50 mg/kg on alternate days x 10-15 doses	30-50 mg/kg on alternate days x 10-15 doses
GIARDIASIS (Giardia lamblia)			
Drug of choice:	Quinacrine HCl	100 mg tid p.c. x 5d	6 mg/kg/d in 3 doses p.c. x 5d (max. 300 mg/d)
Alternatives:	Metronidazole[3,4,7]	250 mg tid x 5d	15 mg/kg/d in 3 doses x 5d
	Furazolidone	100 mg qid x 7-10d	6 mg/kg/d in 4 doses x 7-10d
GNATHOSTOMIASIS (Gnathostoma spinigerum)			
Treatment of choice:	Surgical removal		
OR	Mebendazole[7]	200 mg q3h x 6d	
HOOKWORM infection (Ancylostoma duodenale, Necator americanus)			
Drug of choice:[24]	Mebendazole	100 mg bid x 3d	100 mg bid x 3d
OR	Pyrantel pamoate[7]	11 mg/kg (max. 1 gram) x 3d	11 mg/kg (max. 1 gram) x 3d
Hydatid cyst, see TAPEWORM infection			

* The letter d indicates day.

21. Antihistamines or corticosteroids may be required to decrease allergic reactions due to disintegration of microfilariae in treatment of filarial infections, especially those caused by Loa loa. Diethylcarbamazine should be administered with special caution in heavy infections with Loa loa because it can provoke an encephalopathy. Apheresis has been reported to be effective in lowering microfilarial counts in patients heavily infected with loiasis. Diethylcarbamazine, 300 mg once weekly, has been recommended for prevention of loiasis (TB Nutman et al, N Engl J Med, 319:752, 1988).
22. Ivermectin may also be effective.
23. Unlike infections with other flukes, hepatica infections may not respond to praziquantel. Limited data indicate that albendazole may be helpful, and a recent report suggests that triclabendazole *(Fasinex)*, a veterinary fasciolide, may also be effective (L Loutan et al, Lancet, 2:383, Aug 12, 1989).
24. Albendazole is also effective (RNG Pugh, Ann Trop Med Parasitol, 80:565, 1986).
25. In sulfonamide-sensitive patients, such as some patients with AIDS, pyrimethamine 50-75 mg daily has been effective (LM Weiss et al, Ann Intern Med, 109:474, 1988). In immunocompromised patients, it may be necessary to continue therapy indefinitely.

Infection	Drug	Adult Dosage*	Pediatric Dosage*
Hymenolepis nana, see TAPEWORM infection			
ISOSPORIASIS (Isospora belli)			
Drug of choice:	Trimethoprim-sulfamethoxazole[7,25]	160 mg TMP, 800 mg SMX qid x 10d, then bid x 3 wks	
LEISHMANIASIS			
L. braziliensis, L. mexicana (American cutaneous and mucocutaneous leishmaniasis)			
Drug of choice:[26]	Stibogluconate sodium[2]	20 mg/kg/d (max. 800 mg/d) IV or IM x 20d, may be repeated or continued until response	20 mg/kg/d IV or IM (max. 800 mg/d) x 20d
Alternative:	Amphotericin B[7]	0.25 to 1 mg/kg by slow infusion daily or every 2d for up to 8 wks	0.25 to 1 mg/kg by slow infusion daily or every 2d for up to 8 wks
L. donovani (kala azar, visceral leishmaniasis)			
Drug of choice:[27]	Stibogluconate sodium[2,28]	20 mg/kg/d (max. 800 mg/d) IV or IM x 20d (may be repeated)	20 mg/kg/d IV or IM (max. 800 mg/d) x 20d
Alternative:	Pentamidine isethionate	2-4 mg/kg/d IM for up to 15 doses	2-4 mg/kg/d IM for up to 15 doses
L. tropica, L. major (oriental sore, cutaneous leishmaniasis)			
Drug of choice:[29]	Stibogluconate sodium[2]	10 mg/kg/d (max. 600 mg/d) IV or IM x 6-10d (may be repeated)	10 mg/kg/d IV or IM (max. 600 mg/d) x 6-10d
Alternative:	Topical treatment[30]		
LICE infestation (Pediculus humanus, capitis, Phthirus pubis)[31]			
Drug of choice:	1% Permethrin[32]	Topically	Topically
OR	0.5% malathion	Topically	Topically
Alternatives:	Pyrethrins with piperonyl butoxide	Topically[33]	Topically[33]
	Lindane	Topically[33]	Topically[33]
Loa loa, see FILARIASIS			

MALARIA, Treatment of (*Plasmodium falciparum, P. ovale, P. vivax,* and *P. malariae*)

All *Plasmodium* except Chloroquine-Resistant *P. falciparum*

ORAL			
Drug of choice:	Chloroquine phosphate[34,35]	600 mg base (1 gram), then 300 mg base (500 mg) 6 hrs later, then 300 mg base (500 mg) at 24 and 48 hrs	10 mg base/kg (max. 600 mg base), then 5 mg base/kg 6 hrs later, then 5 mg base/kg at 24 and 48 hrs
PARENTERAL			
Drug of choice:	Quinine dihydrochloride[36]	600 mg in 300 ml normal saline IV over 2 to 4 hrs; repeat q8h until oral therapy can be started (max. 1800 mg/d)	25 mg/kg/d; give 1/3 of daily dose over 2 to 4 hrs; repeat q8h until oral therapy can be started (max. 1800 mg/d)
	OR Quinidine gluconate[7,37]	10 mg/kg loading dose (max. 600 mg) in normal saline slowly over 1 hr, followed by continuous infusion of 0.02 mg/kg/min for 3 days maximum	10 mg/kg loading dose (max. 600 mg) in normal saline slowly over 1 hr, followed by continuous infusion of 0.02 mg/kg/min for 3 days maximum
Alternative:	Chloroquine HCl[35]	200 mg base (250 mg) IM q6h if oral therapy cannot be started	0.83 mg base/kg/hr x 30 hrs continuous infusion or 3.5 mg base/kg q6h IM or subcutaneously[38]

(continued)

* The letter d indicates day.

26. Limited data indicate that ketoconazole, 400 to 600 mg daily for 28 days, may be effective for treatment of L. braziliensis panamensis and L. mexicana (cutaneous).
27. Recent studies indicate that stibogluconate (pentavalent antimony)-resistant kala azar may respond to recombinant human gamma interferon in addition to stibogluconate (R Badaro et al, N Engl J Med, 322:16, Jan 4, 1990).
28. For the African form of visceral leishmaniasis, therapy may have to be extended to at least 30 days and may have to be repeated.
29. Ketoconazole, 400 mg daily for four to eight weeks, has also been reported to be effective (J Viallet et al, Am J Trop Med Hyg, 35:491, 1986).
30. Application of heat 39° to 42°C directly to the lesion for 20 to 32 hours over a period of 10 to 12 days has been reported to be effective in L. tropica (FA Neva et al, Am J Trop Med Hyg, 33:800, 1984).
31. For infestation of eyelashes with crab lice, use petrolatum.
32. FDA-approved only for head lice, but see also "Scabies."
33. Some consultants recommend a second application one week later to kill hatching progeny.

Infection	Drug	Adult Dosage*	Pediatric Dosage*
Chloroquine-resistant *P. falciparum*[39]			
ORAL			
Drugs of choice:	Quinine sulfate[40,41]	650 mg tid x 3d	25 mg/kg/d in 3 doses x 3d
	plus pyrimethamine-sulfadoxine[42]	3 tablets at once	<1 yr: 1/4 tablet 1-3 yrs. 1/2 tablet 4-8 yrs: 1 tablet 9-14 yrs: 2 tablets
	OR **plus** tetracycline[7,14]	250 mg qid x 7d	20 mg/kg/d in 4 doses x 7 d[14]
	OR **plus** clindamycin[7]	900 mg tid x 3d	20-40 mg/kg/d in 3 doses x 3d
Alternative:	Mefloquine[43]	1250 mg once	25 mg/kg once
PARENTERAL			
Drug of choice:	Quinine dihydrochloride[36]	same as above	same as above
	OR Quinidine gluconate[7,37]	same as above	same as above
Prevention of relapses: *P. vivax* and *P. ovale* only			
Drug of choice:	Primaquine phosphate[44]	15 mg base (26.3 mg)/d x 14d or 45 mg base (79 mg)/wk x 8 wks	0.3 mg base/kg/d x 14d
MALARIA, Prevention of[45]			
Drug of choice:	Chloroquine phosphate[46]	300 mg base (500 mg salt) orally, once/week beginning 1 wk before and continuing for 4 wks after last exposure	5 mg/kg base (8.3 mg/kg salt) once/week, up to adult dose of 300 mg base
Chloroquine-Resistant Areas[39]			
Drug of choice:	Mefloquine[46,47]	250 mg oral once per week starting one week before travel and continuing for 4 weeks after last exposure.†	15-19 kg: ¼ tablet 20-30 kg: ½ tablet 31-45 kg: ¾ tablet >45 kg: 1 tablet

	OR Chloroquine phosphate[46]	as above	as above
	plus pyrimethamine-sulfadoxine[42] for presumptive treatment[48]	Carry a single dose (3 tablets) for self-treatment of febrile illness when medical care is not immediately available	<1 yr: ¼ tablet 1-3 yrs: ½ tablet 4-8 yrs: 1 tablet 9-14 yrs: 2 tablets
	plus proguanil[49] (in Africa south of the Sahara)	200 mg daily during exposure and for 4 weeks afterwards	<2 yrs: 50 mg daily 2-6 yrs: 100 mg daily 7-10 yrs: 150 mg daily 10 yrs: 200 mg daily
	OR Doxycycline[46,50]	100 mg daily during exposure and for 4 weeks afterwards	>8 years of age: 2 mg/kg/d orally, up to 100 mg/day
Mites, see SCABIES			
MONILIFORMIS moniliformis infection			
Drug of choice:	Pyrantel pamoate[7]	11 mg/kg once, repeat twice 2 wks apart	11 mg/kg once, repeat twice, 2 wks apart

* The letter d indicates day.

† This represents a modified, new recommended therapy, from *MMWR* 1990;39:630.

34. If chloroquine phosphate is not available, hydroxychloroquine sulfate is as effective; 400 mg of hydroxychloroquine sulfate is equivalent to 500 mg of chloroquine phosphate.
35. In *P. falciparum* malaria, if the patient has not shown a response to conventional doses of chloroquine in 48-72 hours, parasitic resistance to this drug should be considered. *P. vivax* with decreased susceptibility to chloroquine has recently been reported from Papua New Guinea (KH Rieckmann et al, Lancet, 2:1183, Nov 18, 1989). Intramuscular injection of chloroquine is painful and can cause abscesses.
36. Available in the USA only from the Centers for Disease Control, telephone 404-488-4046 (nights, weekends, or holidays call 404-639-2888). *P. falciparum* infections with a high parasitemia may require a loading dose of 20 mg/kg (NJ White et al, Am J Trop Med Hyg, 32:1, 1983). IV administration of quinine dihydrochloride can be hazardous; constant monitoring of the pulse and blood pressure is necessary to detect arrhythmia or hypotension. Oral drugs should be substituted as soon as possible.
37. Some experts consider quinidine more effective than quinine (KD Miller et al, N Engl J Med, 321:65, 1989). EKG monitoring is necessary to detect arrhythmias. Oral drugs should be substituted as soon as possible.
38. Intravenous dosage recommendations may change (NJ White et al, N Engl J Med, 319:1493, 1988).
39. Chloroquine-resistant *P. falciparum* infections have been reported in all areas that have malaria except Central America north of Panama, Mexico, Haiti, the Dominican Republic, and the Middle East (including Egypt).

Infection	Drug	Adult Dosage*	Pediatric Dosage*
Naegleria species, see AMEBIC MENINGOENCEPHALITIS, PRIMARY			
Necator americanus, see HOOKWORM infection			
Onchocerca volvulus, see FILARIASIS			
Opisthorchis viverrini, see FLUKE infection			
Paragonimus westermani, see FLUKE infection			
Pediculus capitis, humanus, Phthirus pubis, see LICE			
Pinworm, see ENTEROBIUS			
PNEUMOCYSTIS carinii pneumonia[51]			
Drug of choice:	Trimethoprim-sulfamethoxazole	TMP 20 mg/kg per day, SMX 100 mg/kg/d, oral or IV in 4 doses x 14-21d	TMP 20 mg/kg/d, SMX 100 mg/kg/d, oral or IV in 4 doses x 14d
Alternative:	Pentamidine isethionate	4 mg/kg/d IV x 14-21d	4 mg/kg/d IV x 14d
Roundworm, see ASCARIASIS			
SCABIES (Sarcoptes scabiei)			
Drug of choice:	5% Permethrin	Topically	Topically
Alternatives:	Lindane	Topically	Topically
	10% Crotamiton	Topically	Topically
SCHISTOSOMIASIS			
S. haematobium			
Drug of choice:	Praziquantel	40 mg/kg/d in 2 doses x 1d	40 mg/kg/d in 2 doses x 1d
S. japonicum			
Drug of choice:	Praziquantel	60 mg/kg/d in 3 doses x 1d	60 mg/kg/d in 3 doses x 1d
S. mansoni			
Drug of choice:	Praziquantel	40 mg/kg/d in 2 doses x 1d	40 mg/kg/d in 2 doses x 1d
Alternative:	Oxamniquine	15 mg/kg once[52]	20 mg/kg/d in 2 doses x 1d[52]
S. mekongi			
Drug of choice:	Praziquantel	60 mg/kg/d in 3 doses x 1d	60 mg/kg/d in 3 doses x 1d

Infection	Drug	Adult Dosage*	Pediatric Dosage*
Sleeping sickness, see TRYPANOSOMIASIS			
STRONGYLOIDIASIS (Strongyloides stercoralis)			
Drug of choice:[53]	Thiabendazole	50 mg/kg/d in 2 doses (max. 3 grams /d) x 2d[11,54]	50 mg/kg/d in 2 doses (max. 3 grams/d) x 2d[11,54]
TAPEWORM infection — **Adult (intestinal stage)**			
Diphyllobothrium latum (fish), Taenia saginata (beef), Taenia solium (pork) Dipylidium caninum (dog)			
Drug of choice:	Niclosamide	A single dose of 4 tablets (2 grams), chewed thoroughly	11-34 kg: a single dose of 2 tablets (1 gram); >34 kg: a single dose of 3 tablets (1.5 grams)
	OR Praziquantel[7]	10-20 mg/kg once	10-20 mg/kg once
Hymenolepis nana (dwarf tapeworm)			
Drug of choice:	Praziquantel[7]	25 mg/kg once	25 mg/kg once
Alternative:	Niclosamide	A single daily dose of 4 tablets (2 g), chewed thoroughly, then 2 tablets daily x 6d	11-34 kg: a single dose of 2 tablets (1 gram) x 1d, then 1 tablet (0.5 grams) /d x 6d; >34 kg: a single dose of 3 tablets (1.5 g) x 1d, then 2 tablets (1 gram)/d x 6d

* The letter d indicates day.

40. Quinine alone will usually control an attack of resistant *P. falciparum* but, in a substantial number of infections, particularly with strains from Southeast Asia, it fails to prevent recurrence; addition of pyrimethamine and a sulfonamide lowers the rate of recurrence.
41. For treatment of *P. falciparum* infections acquired in Thailand, quinine should be given for seven days instead of three.
42. *Fansidar* tablets contain 25 mg of pyrimethamine and 500 mg of sulfadoxine.
43. At this dosage, adverse effects including nausea, vomiting, diarrhea, dizziness, disturbed sense of balance, toxic psychosis, and seizures can occur, and information with regard to safety during pregnancy is incomplete. The pediatric dosage has not been approved by the FDA. Mefloquine must not be given together with quinine, and caution is required in using quinine to treat patients with malaria who have taken mefloquine for prophylaxis.
44. Primaquine phosphate can cause hemolytic anemia, especially in patients whose red cells are deficient in glucose-6-phosphate dehydrogenase. This deficiency is most common in Blacks, Orientals, and Mediterranean peoples. Patients should be screened for G-6-PD deficiency before treatment. Primaquine should not be used during pregnancy.
45. Countries with a risk of malaria will be listed in the next issue of The Medical Letter. At present, no drug regimen guarantees protection against malaria. If fever develops within a year (particularly within the first two months) after travel to malarious areas, travelers should be advised to seek medical attention.

Infection	Drug	Adult Dosage*	Pediatric Dosage*
TAPEWORM infection (continued)			
— Larval (tissue stage)			
Echinococcus granulosus (hydatid cysts)			
Drug of choice:	Albendazole[55]	400 mg bid x 28 days, repeated as necessary	10 mg/kg/d x 28 days, repeated as necessary
Echinococcus multilocularis			
Treatment of choice:	See footnote 56		
Cysticercus cellulosae (cysticercosis)			
Drug of choice:[57]	Praziquantel[7]	50 mg/kg/d in 3 doses x 14d	50 mg/kg/d in 3 doses x 14d
	OR Albendazole	15 mg/kg/d in 3 doses x 30d, repeated as necessary	15 mg/kg/d in 3 doses x 30d, repeated as necessary
Alternative:	Surgery		
Toxocariasis, see VISCERAL LARVA MIGRANS			
TOXOPLASMOSIS (Toxoplasma gondii)[58]			
Drugs of choice:	Pyrimethamine[59]	25 mg/d x 3-4 wks	2 mg/kg/d x 3d, then 1 mg/kg/d (max. 25 mg/d) x 4 wks[60]
	plus trisulfapyrimidines	2-6 grams/d x 3-4 wks	100-200 mg/kg/d x 3-4 wks
	OR **plus** sulfadiazine	2-6 grams/d x 3-4 wks	100-200 mg/kg/d x 3-4 wks
Alternative:	Spiramycin	2-4 grams/d x 3-4 wks	50-100 mg/kg/d x 3-4 wks
TRICHINOSIS (Trichinella spiralis)			
Drugs of choice:	Steroids for severe symptoms		
	plus mebendazole[7,61]	200-400 mg tid x 3d, then 400-500 mg tid x 10d	
TRICHOMONIASIS (Trichomonas vaginalis)			
Drug of choice:[62]	Metronidazole[3]	2 grams once or 250 mg tid orally x 7d	15 mg/kg/d orally in 3 doses x 7d

TRICHOSTRONGYLUS infection			
Drug of choice:[12]	Pyrantel pamoate[7]	11 mg/kg once (max. 1 gram)	11 mg/kg once (max. 1 gram)
Alternative:	Thiabendazole[7]	50 mg/kg/d (max. 3 grams/d) in 2 doses[11]	50 mg/kg/d (max. 3 grams/d) in 2 doses[11]
TRICHURIASIS (Trichuris trichiura, whipworm)			
Drug of choice:[12]	Mebendazole	100 mg bid x 3d	100 mg bid x 3d

* The letter d indicates day.

46. For prevention of attack after departure from areas where *P. vivax* and *P. ovale* are endemic, which includes almost all areas where malaria is found (except Haiti), some experts in addition prescribe primaquine phosphate 15 mg base (26.3 mg)/d or, for children, 0.3 mg base/kg/d during the last two weeks of prophylaxis. Others prefer to avoid the toxicity of primaquine and rely on surveillance to detect cases when they occur, particularly when exposure was limited or doubtful. See also footnote 44.
47. Beginning one week before travel and continuing for the duration of stay and for two doses after leaving. For a stay of two weeks or less, Medical Letter consultants recommend four weekly doses followed by one more dose two weeks later. The pediatric dosage has not been approved by the FDA, and the drug has not been approved for use during pregnancy. Women should take contraceptive precautions while taking mefloquine and for two months after the last dose. Mefloquine is not recommended for children weighing less than 15 kg, or for patients taking beta-blockers, calcium-channel blockers, or other drugs that may prolong or otherwise alter cardiac conduction. Patients with a history of seizures or psychiatric disorders and those whose occupation requires fine coordination or spatial discrimination probably should avoid mefloquine (Medical Letter, 31:13, Feb 9, 1990).
48. Resistance to *Fansidar* is widespread in Southeast Asia and the Amazon basin and is frequent in east Africa. Use of *Fansidar* is contraindicated in patients with a history of sulfonamide or pyrimethamine intolerance, in pregnancy at term, and in infants less than two months old.
49. Proguanil (*Paludrine* – Ayerst, Canada; ICI, England), which is not available in the US but is widely available overseas, is recommended mainly for use in Africa south of the Sahara. In addition, concurrent use of proguanil and sulfisoxazole (*Gantrisin*; and others) has been effective prophylactically in areas of mefloquine resistance in Thailand, particularly in young children for whom tetracycline is contraindicated (LW Pang et al, WHO Bull, 67:51, 1989).
50. The FDA considers use of tetracyclines as antimalarials to be investigational. Use of tetracyclines is contraindicated in pregnancy and in children less than eight years old. Physicians who prescribe doxycycline as malaria chemoprophylaxis should advise patients to use an appropriate sunscreen (Medical Letter, 31:59, 1989) to minimize the possibility of a photosensitivity reaction and should warn women that Candida vaginitis is a frequent adverse effect.
51. AIDS patients should be treated for 21 days. For AIDS patients who develop hypersensitivity or resistance to both TMP/SMX and pentamidine, trimetrexate with leucovorin rescue (Medical Letter, 31:5, 1989) or a combination of dapsone and trimethoprim may be effective. Oral TMP/SMX or aerosolized pentamidine is recommended for prophylaxis (Medical Letter, 31:91, 1989; JA Kovacs and H Masur, J Infect Dis, 160:882, Nov 1989).
52. In east Africa, the dose should be increased to 30 mg/kg/d, and in Egypt and South Africa, 30 mg/kg/d x 2d. Neuropsychiatric disturbances and seizures have been reported in some patients (H Stokvis et al, Am J Trop Med Hyg, 35:330, 1986).

Infection	Drug	Adult Dosage*	Pediatric Dosage*
TRYPANOSOMIASIS			
T. cruzi (South American trypanosomiasis, Chagas' disease)			
Drug of choice:	Nifurtimox[2]	8-10 mg/kg/d orally in 4 doses x 120d	1-10 yrs: 15-20 mg/kg/d in 4 doses x 90d; 11-16 yrs: 12.5-15 mg/kg/d in 4 doses x 90d
Alternative:	Benznidazole[63]	5-7 mg/kg/d x 30-120d	
T. brucei gambiense; T. b. rhodesiense (African trypanosomiasis, sleeping sickness) hemolymphatic stage			
Drug of choice:[64]	Suramin[2]	100-200 mg (test dose) IV, then 1 gram IV on days 1,3,7,14, and 21	20 mg/kg on days 1,3,7,14 and 21
Alternative:	Pentamidine isethionate	4 mg/kg/d IM x 10d	4 mg/kg/d IM x 10d
late disease with CNS involvement			
Drug of choice:[64]	Melarsoprol[2,65]	2-3.6 mg/kg/d IV x 3 doses; after 1 wk 3.6 mg/kg per day IV x 3 doses; repeat again after 10-21 days	18-25 mg/kg total over 1 month; initial dose of 0.36 mg/kg IV, increasing gradually to max. 3.6 mg/kg at intervals of 1-5d for total of 9-10 doses
Alternatives:	Tryparsamide	One injection of 30 mg/kg (max. 2g) IV every 5d to total of 12 injections; may be repeated after 1 month	Unknown
	plus suramin[2]	One injection of 10 mg/kg IV every 5d to total of 12 injections; may be repeated after 1 month	
VISCERAL LARVA MIGRANS[66]			
Drug of choice:[67]	Diethylcarbamazine[7]	6 mg/kg/d in 3 doses x 7-10d	6 mg/kg/d in 3 doses x 7-10d
OR	Thiabendazole	50 mg/kg/d in 2 doses x 5d (max. 3 grams/d)[11]	50 mg/kg/d in 2 doses x 5d (max. 3 grams /d)[11]
Alternative:	Mebendazole[7]	100-200 mg bid x 5d[68]	

Whipworm, see TRICHURIASIS

Wuchereria bancrofti, see FILARIASIS

* The letter d indicates day.

53. In immunocompromised patients it may be necessary to continue therapy or use other agents. Albendazole or ivermectin has also been effective.
54. In disseminated strongyloidiasis, thiabendazole therapy should be continued for at least five days.
55. Some patients may benefit from or require surgical resection of cysts. Albendazole may also be useful preoperatively or in case of spill during surgery.
56. Surgical excision is the only reliable means of treatment, although some reports have suggested use of albendazole or mebendazole (JF Wilson et al, Am J Trop Med Hyg, 37:162, 1987; A Davis et al, Bull WHO, 64:383, 1986).
57. Corticosteroids should be given for two to three days before and during drug therapy. Metrifonate, 7.5 mg/kg x 5d, repeated six times at two-week intervals, has been reported to be effective for ocular as well as cerebral and subcutaneous disease. Any cysticercocidal drug, however, may cause irreparable damage when used to treat ocular or spinal cysts, even when corticosteroids are used.
58. In ocular toxoplasmosis, corticosteroids should also be used for anti-inflammatory effect on the eyes.
59. Pyrimethamine is teratogenic in animals. To prevent hematological toxicity from pyrimethamine, it is advisable to give leucovorin (folinic acid), about 10 mg/day, either by injection or orally. Some clinicians have used pyrimethamine 50 to 100 mg daily with a sulfonamide to treat CNS toxoplasmosis in patients with AIDS and, when sulfonamide sensitivity developed, have given clindamycin 1.8 to 2.4 g/d in divided doses instead of the sulfonamide. In AIDS patients, treatment should continue indefinitely.
60. Congenitally infected newborns should be treated with pyrimethamine every two or three days and a sulfonamide daily for about one year.
61. Albendazole or flubendazole may also be effective for this indication.
62. Sexual partners should be treated simultaneously. Outside the USA, ornidazole and tinidazole have been used for this condition. Metronidazole-resistant strains have been reported; higher doses of metronidazole for longer periods are sometimes effective against these strains.
63. Limited data
64. In T. b. gambiense infections, eflornithine (difluoromethylornithine; DFMO – Merrell Dow) has been effective in both the hemolymphatic and CNS stages. Its effectiveness in T. b. rhodesiense infections has been variable. Some clinicians have given 400 mg/kg/d IV in 4 divided doses for 14 days, followed by oral treatment with 300 mg/kg/d for 3-4 wks (F Doua et al, Am J Trop Med Hyg, 37:525, 1987).
65. In frail patients, begin with as little as 18 mg and increase the dose progressively. Pretreatment with suramin has been advocated for debilitated patients.
66. For severe symptoms or eye involvement, corticosteroids can be used in addition.
67. Ivermectin and albendazole may also be effective (D Stürchler et al, Ann Trop Med Parasitol, 83:473, 1989).
68. One report of a cure using 1 gram tid for 21 days has been published (A Bekhti, Ann Intern Med, 100:463, 1984).

ADVERSE EFFECTS OF SOME ANTIPARASITIC DRUGS*

ALBENDAZOLE *(Zentel)*
Occasional: diarrhea; abdominal pain
Rare: leukopenia; alopecia; increased serum transaminase levels

BENZNIDAZOLE *(Rochagan)*
Frequent: allergic rash; dose-dependent polyneuropathy; gastrointestinal disturbance; psychic disturbance

BITHIONOL *(Bitin)*
Frequent: photosensitivity reactions; vomiting; diarrhea; abdominal pain; urticaria
Rare: leukopenia; toxic hepatitis

CHLOROQUINE HCl and CHLOROQUINE PHOSPHATE (*Aralen*; and others)
Occasional: pruritus; vomiting; headache; confusion; depigmentation of hair; skin eruptions; corneal opacity; weight loss; partial alopecia; extraocular muscle palsies; exacerbation of psoriasis, eczema

EFLORNITHINE (Difluoromethylornithine; DFMO; *Ornidyl*)
Frequent: diarrhea; anemia
Occasional: thrombocytopenia
Rare: seizures; hearing loss

EMETINE HCl
Frequent: cardiac arrhythmias; precordial pain; muscle weakness; cellulitis at site of injection
Occasional: diarrhea; vomiting; peripheral neuropathy; heart failure

FLUBENDAZOLE – similar to mebendazole, but frequent inflammation at IM injection site

FURAZOLIDONE *(Furoxone)*
Frequent: nausea; vomiting
Occasional: allergic reactions, including pulmonary infiltration, hypotension, urticaria, fever, vesicular rash; hypoglycemia; headache
Rare: hemolytic anemia in G-6-PD deficiency and neonates; disulfiram-like reaction with alcohol; MAO-inhibitor interactions; polyneuritis

MEFLOQUINE *(Lariam)*
Frequent: vertigo; lightheadedness; nausea; other gastrointestinal disturbances; nightmares; visual disturbances; headache
Occasional: confusion; psychosis
Rare: convulsions; coma

MELARSOPROL *(Mel B; Arsobal)*
Frequent: myocardial damage; albuminuria; hypertension; colic; Herxheimer-type reaction; encephalopathy; vomiting; peripheral neuropathy
Rare: shock

METRIFONATE *(Bilarcil)*
Frequent: reversible plasma cholinesterase inhibition
Occasional: nausea; vomiting; abdominal pain; headache; vertigo

METRONIDAZOLE (*Flagyl*; and others)
Frequent: nausea; headache; dry mouth; metallic taste
Occasional: vomiting; diarrhea; insomnia; weakness; stomatitis; verti-

and other exfoliative dermatoses; myalgias; photophobia
Rare: irreversible retinal injury (especially when total dosage exceeds 100 grams); discoloration of nails and mucous membranes; nerve-type deafness; peripheral neuropathy and myopathy; heart block; blood dyscrasias, hematemesis

CROTAMITON *(Eurax)*
Occasional: skin rash; conjunctivitis

DEHYDROEMETINE – Similar to emetine, but possibly less severe

DIETHYLCARBAMAZINE CITRATE USP *(Hetrazan)*
Frequent: severe allergic or febrile reactions due to the filarial infection; GI disturbances
Rare: encephalopathy; loss of vision in onchocerciasis

DILOXANIDE FUROATE *(Furamide)*
Frequent: flatulence
Occasional: nausea; vomiting; diarrhea
Rare: urticaria; pruritus

IODOQUINOL *(Yodoxin)*
Occasional: rash; acne; slight enlargement of the thyroid gland; nausea; diarrhea; cramps; anal pruritus
Rare: optic atrophy, loss of vision, peripheral neuropathy after prolonged use in high dosage (for months); iodine sensitivity

IVERMECTIN *(Mectizan)*
Occasional: fever; pruritus; tender lymph nodes; headache; joint and bone pain
Rare: hypotension

LINDANE (*Kwell;* and others)
Occasional: eczematous skin rash; conjunctivitis
Rare: convulsions; aplastic anemia

MALATHION *(Ovide)*
Occasional: local irritation

MEBENDAZOLE *(Vermox)*
Occasional: diarrhea; abdominal pain
Rare: leukopenia; agranulocytosis; hypospermia

go; paresthesia; rash; dark urine; urethral burning; disulfiram-like reaction with alcohol
Rare: seizures; encephalopathy; pseudomembranous colitis; ataxia; leukopenia; peripheral neuropathy; pancreatitis

NICLOSAMIDE *(Niclocide)*
Occasional: nausea; abdominal pain

NIFURTIMOX *(Bayer 2502; Lampit)*
Frequent: anorexia; vomiting; weight loss; loss of memory; sleep disorders; tremor; paresthesias; weakness; polyneuritis
Rare: convulsions; fever; pulmonary infiltrates and pleural effusion

ORNIDAZOLE *(Tiberal)*
Occasional: dizziness; headache; gastrointestinal disturbances
Rare: reversible peripheral neuropathy

---

* Drug interactions are generally not included here. See the current edition of *The Medical Letter Handbook of Adverse Drug Interactions.*

OXAMNIQUINE *(Vansil)*
Occasional: headache; fever; dizziness; somnolence; nausea; diarrhea; rash; insomnia; hepatic enzyme changes; ECG changes; EEG changes; orange-red discoloration of urine
Rare: convulsions; neuropsychiatric disturbances

PAROMOMYCIN *(Humatin)*
Frequent: GI disturbance
Rare: eighth-nerve damage (mainly auditory); renal damage

PENTAMIDINE ISETHIONATE *(Pentam 300)*
Frequent: hypotension; hypoglycemia often followed by diabetes mellitus; vomiting; blood dyscrasias; renal damage; pain at injection site; GI disturbances
Occasional: may aggravate diabetes; shock; hypocalcemia; liver damage; cardiotoxicity; delirium; rash
Rare: Herxheimer-type reaction; anaphylaxis; acute pancreatitis; hyperkalemia

PROGUANIL *(Paludrine)*
Occasional: oral ulceration; vomiting; abdominal pain; diarrhea (with large doses); hair loss; scaling of palms and soles
Rare: hematuria (with large doses)

PYRANTEL PAMOATE *(Antiminth)*
Occasional: GI disturbances; headache; dizziness; rash; fever

PYRETHRINS and PIPERONYL BUTOXIDE (*RID*; others)
Occasional: allergic reactions

PYRIMETHAMINE USP *(Daraprim)*
Occasional: blood dyscrasias; folic acid deficiency
Rare: rash; vomiting; convulsions; shock; possibly pulmonary eosinophilia

QUINACRINE HCl USP *(Atabrine)*
Frequent: dizziness; headache; vomiting; diarrhea
Occasional: yellow staining of skin; toxic psychosis; insomnia; bizarre dreams; blood dyscrasias; urticaria;

STIBOGLUCONATE SODIUM *(Pentostam)*
Frequent: muscle pain and joint stiffness; nausea and vomiting
Occasional: colic; diarrhea; rash; pruritus; myocardial damage; liver damage; bradycardia
Rare: hemolytic anemia; renal damage; shock; sudden death

SURAMIN SODIUM *(Germanin)*
Frequent: vomiting; pruritus; urticaria; paresthesias; hyperesthesia of hands and feet; photophobia; peripheral neuropathy
Occasional: kidney damage; blood dyscrasias; shock; optic atrophy

THIABENDAZOLE *(Mintezol)*
Frequent: nausea; vomiting; vertigo
Occasional: leukopenia; crystalluria; rash; hallucinations; olfactory disturbance; erythema multiforme; Stevens-Johnson syndrome
Rare: shock; tinnitus; intrahepatic cholestasis; convulsions; angioneurotic edema

blue and black nail pigmentation; psoriasis-like rash
Rare: acute hepatic necrosis; convulsions; severe exfoliative dermatitis; ocular effects similar to those caused by chloroquine

PERMETHRIN *(Nix; Elimite)*
Occasional: burning; stinging; numbness; increased pruritus; pain; edema; erythema; rash

PIPERAZINE CITRATE USP
Occasional: dizziness; urticaria; GI disturbances
Rare: exacerbation of epilepsy; visual disturbances; ataxia; hypotonia

PRAZIQUANTEL *(Biltricide)*
Frequent: malaise; headache; dizziness
Occasional: sedation; abdominal discomfort; fever; sweating; nausea; eosinophilia; fatigue
Rare: pruritus; rash

PRIMAQUINE PHOSPHATE USP
Frequent: hemolytic anemia in G-6-PD deficiency
Occasional: neutropenia; GI disturbances; methemoglobinemia in G-6-PD deficiency
Rare: CNS symptoms; hypertension; arrhythmias

QUININE DIHYDROCHLORIDE and SULFATE
Frequent: cinchonism (tinnitus, headache, nausea, abdominal pain, visual disturbance)
Occasional: hemolytic anemia; other blood dyscrasias; photosensitivity reactions; hypoglycemia; arrhythmias; hypotension; drug fever
Rare: blindness; sudden death if injected too rapidly

SPIRAMYCIN *(Rovamycine)*
Occasional: GI disturbances
Rare: allergic reactions

TINIDAZOLE *(Fasigyn)*
Occasional: metallic taste; nausea; vomiting; rash

TRIMETREXATE (with "leucovorin rescue")
Occasional: rash; peripheral neuropathy; bone marrow depression; increased serum aminotransferase concentrations

TRYPARSAMIDE
Frequent: nausea; vomiting
Occasional: impaired vision; optic atrophy; fever; exfoliative dermatitis; allergic reactions; tinnitus

APPENDICES

Directory of Telephone Numbers

Organization or Source	Telephone Number
American Academy of Pediatrics	708/228-5005
Centers for Disease Control:	
• Division of Immunization	404/639-1880
• Drug Service	404/639-3670 (weekdays, 8AM-4:30PM) 404/639-2888 (nights, weekends, holidays)
• Disease Information Hotline (includes Travelers Information,* Malaria, Influenza, AIDS, Hepatitis, Rabies, Rickettsial Disease, and Lyme Disease)	404/639-1610
• Division of Vector-Borne Infectious Diseases - Information on Japanese Encephalitis virus activity and vaccine availability	303/221-6400
• Division of Tuberculosis Control	404/639-2530
National Vaccine Compensation Program - For information on filing claims	800/338/2382
Michigan Department of Public Health (for rabies vaccine produced in rhesus diploid cells)	517/335-8050
Food and Drug Administration - Center for Drugs and Experimental Research	301/295-8012
Vaccine Adverse Events Reporting System (VAERS)	800/822-7967
National AIDS Hotline	800/342-AIDS
Pediatric AIDS Drug Trials - Information:	
• Pediatric Branch, National Cancer Institute	301/496-4250
• Pediatric Clinical Trials Group (NIAID-sponsored)	800/TRI-ALSA

*International Health Requirements and Recommendations Hotline

Federal Vaccine Injury Compensation Table

The following excerpt from the National Childhood Vaccine Injury Act of 1986* lists the vaccination-associated events and time period in which the first symptom, manifestation, or significant aggravation occurred for which compensation will be provided.

Sec 2114.(a)
VACCINE INJURY TABLE

I. DTP; P; DTP/Polio Combination; or Any Other Vaccine Containing Whole Cell Pertussis Bacteria, Extracted or Partial Cell Bacteria, or Specific Pertussis Antigen(s).

Illness, disability, injury, or condition covered:	Time period for first symptom or manifestation of onset or of significant aggravation after vaccine administration:
A. Anaphylaxis or anaphylactic shock	24 hours
B. Encephalopathy (or encephalitis)	3 days
C. Shock-collapse or hypotonic-hyporesponsive collapse	3 days
D. Residual seizure disorder in accordance with subsection (b)(2)	3 days
E. Any acute complication or sequela (including death) of an illness, disability, injury, or condition referred to above which illness, disability, injury, or condition arose within the period prescribed	Not applicable

II. Measles, mumps, rubella, or any vaccine containing any of the foregoing as a component; DT; Td; or Tetanus Toxoid.

A. Anaphylaxis or anaphylactic shock	24 hours
B. Encephalopathy (or encephalitis)	15 days (for mumps, rubella, measles, or any vaccine containing any of the foregoing as a component). 3 days (for DT, Td, or tetanus toxoid).

*Public Law 99-660; amended by Public Law 101-239 (1987), effective January 1, 1988.

C. Residual seizure disorder in accordance with subsection (c)(2) . . . . .15 days (for mumps, rubella, measles, or any vaccine containing any of the foregoing as a component). 3 days (for DT, Td, or tetanus toxoid).

D. Any acute complication or sequela (including death) of an illness, disability, injury, or condition referred to above which illness, disability, injury or condition arose within the time period prescribed . . . . .Not applicable

III. Polio Vaccines (other than Inactivated Polio Vaccine).

A. Paralytic polio
– in a nonimmunodeficient recipient . . . . . . .30 days
– in an immunodeficient recipient . . . . .6 months
– in a vaccine-associated community case . . .Not applicable

B. Any acute complication or sequela (including death) of an illness, disability, injury, or condition referred to above which illness, disability, injury, or condition arose within the time period prescribed . . . . .Not applicable

IV. Inactivated Polio Vaccine.

A. Anaphylaxis or anaphylactic shock . . . . .24 hours

B. Any acute complication or sequela (including death) of an illness, disability, injury, or condition referred to above which illness, disability, injury, or condition arose within the time period prescribed . . . . .Not applicable

"(b) Qualifications and Aids to Interpretation.—The following qualifications and aids to interpretation shall apply to the Vaccine Injury Table in subsection (a):

"(1) A shock-collapse or a hypotonic-hyporesponsive collapse may be evidenced by indicia or symptoms such as decrease or loss of muscle tone, paralysis (partial or complete), hemiplegia or hemiparesis, loss of color or turning pale white or blue, unresponsiveness to environmental stimuli, depression of consciousness, loss of consciousness, prolonged sleeping with difficulty arousing, or cardiovascular or respiratory arrest.

"(2) A petitioner may be considered to have suffered a residual seizure disorder if the petitioner did not suffer a seizure or convulsion unaccompanied by fever or accompanied by a fever of less than 102 degrees Fahrenheit before the first seizure or convulsion after the administration of the vaccine involved and if—

"(A) in the case of measles, mumps, or rubella vaccine or any combination of such vaccines, the first seizure or convulsion occurred within 15 days after administration of the vaccine and 2 or more seizures or convulsions occurred within 1 year after the administration of the vaccine which were unaccompanied by fever or accompanied by a fever of less than 102 degrees Fahrenheit, and

"(B) in the case of any other vaccine, the first seizure or convulsion occurred within 3 days after administration of the vaccine and 2 or more seizures or convulsions occurred within 1 year after the administration of the vaccine which were unaccompanied by fever or accompanied by a fever of less than 102 degrees Fahrenheit.

"(3)(A) The term encephalopathy means any significant acquired abnormality of, or injury to, or impairment of function of the brain. Among the frequent manifestations of encephalopathy are focal and diffuse neurologic signs, increased intracranial pressure, or changes lasting at least 6 hours in level of consciousness, with or without convulsions. The neurological signs and symptoms of encephalopathy may be temporary, with complete recovery, or may result in various degrees of permanent impairment. Signs and symptoms such as high pitched and unusual screaming, persistent unconsolable crying, and bulging fontanel are compatible with an encephalopathy, but in and of themselves are not conclusive evidence of encephalopathy. Encephalopathy usually can be documented by slow wave activity on an electroencephalogram.

"(B) If in a proceeding on a petition it is shown by a preponderance of the evidence that an encephalopathy was caused by infection, toxins, trauma, or metabolic disturbances the encephalopathy shall not be considered to be a condition set forth in the table. If at the time a judgment is entered on a petition filed under section 2111(b) for a vaccine-related injury or death it is not possible to determine the cause, by a preponderance of the evidence, or an encephalopathy, the encephalopathy shall be considered to be a condition set forth in the table. In determining whether or not an encephalopathy is a condition set forth in the table, the court shall consider the entire-medical record.

"(4) For purposes of paragraphs (2) and (3), the terms "seizure" and "convulsion" include grand mal, petit mal, absence, myoclonic, tonic-clonic, and focal motor seizures and signs. If a provision of the table to which paragraph (1), (2), (3), or (4) applies is revised under subsection (c) or (d), such paragraph shall not apply to such provision after the effective date of the revision unless the revision specifies that such paragraph is to continue to apply."

Diseases Transmitted by Pets, Rodents, and Other Animals

The transmission of diseases of animals to humans is of special interest in the care of children who may share a household with pets or unwanted rodents, or who are otherwise in contact with animals. Important zoonoses that may be encountered in North America and that are reviewed in the *Red Book* (see chapters on specific diseases in Part 3 for further information) are given in the following table. For a more complete listing of these diseases, see *The Zoonoses* (prepared jointly by the U.S. Department of Health and Human Services, the U.S. Public Health Service, the Centers for Disease Control, the Centers for Infectious Diseases, and the Office of Biosafety, Atlanta, GA 30333; and the University of Texas, School of Public Health, Science Center, Houston, TX 77025). An additional resource is the following: Acha P.M., Szyfres B. *Zoonoses and Communicable Diseases Common to Man and Animals*. Scientific Publication No. 354, 1980. Pan American Health Organization, Pan American Sanitary Bureau, Regional Offices of the World Health Organization, 525 23rd Street, N.W., Washington, DC 20037.

Diseases Transmitted by Pets, Rodents, and Other Animals

Disease or Organism	Common Animal Sources	Vector or Means of Spread
	Bacterial Diseases	
Brucellosis	Pigs, cows, goats, rarely dogs	Direct contact, ingestion of contaminated food, aerosols
Campylobacter jejuni	Dogs, cats, chickens	Ingestion of contaminated food, water
*Capnocytophaga canimorsus**	Dogs, rarely cats	Bites; contact
Cat scratch disease	Cats, infrequently dogs (<10%)	Scratches and bites
Leptospirosis	Dogs, rats, livestock	Contact with water contaminated by urine of infected animal; direct contact with carcasses of infected animals
Lyme disease *(Borrelia burgdorferi)*	Deer, rodents (carriers of ticks)	Bite of tick

*Formerly dysgonic fermenter 2 (DF-2)

Diseases Transmitted by Pets, Rodents, and Other Animals *(continued)*

Disease or Organism	Common Animal Sources	Vector or Means of Spread
Pasteurella multocida	Cats, dogs, rats	Bites and scratches
Plague (*Yersinia pestis*)	Wild and domestic rodents, fleas, cats	Bite of rodent fleas or direct contact with infected animal
Rat-bite fever	Rodents (including mice, rats, guinea pigs, hamsters, and gerbils); rarely dogs and cats	Bites of infected animals, ingestion of contaminated food
Salmonellosis	Poultry, dogs, cats, turtles	Ingestion of contaminated food; direct contact
Tetanus	Any animal, usually indirect via soil	Wound infection, contaminated bites
Tularemia	Rabbits, squirrels, dogs, cats	Direct contact, ingestion of contaminated water, bite of infected insect vector (e.g., tick, deerfly)
Yersinia pseudotuberculosis and *Y enterocolitica*	Rodents; rarely dogs, cats	Direct contact, ingestion of contaminated food, water
Fungal Diseases		
Cryptococcosis	Droppings from pigeons, other birds	Environmental exposure
Histoplasmosis	Droppings from starlings, other birds; bats	Environmental exposure
Ringworm (*Microsporum* and *Trichophyton* species)	Cats, dogs, rodents	Direct contact
Parasitic Diseases		
Babesiosis	Wild rodents (carriers of ticks)	Bite of infected ticks
Cryptosporidiosis	Domestic animals	Ingestion of oocysts shed in feces

Diseases Transmitted by Pets, Rodents, and Other Animals *(continued)*

Disease or Organism	Common Animal Sources	Vector or Means of Spread
Cutaneous larva migrans *(Ancylostoma braziliense)*	Cats, dogs	Contact with larvae which penetrate the skin
Cysticercosis	Hogs (intermediate host for *Taenia solium*)	Ingestion of ova (fecal-oral contact) from contamination with human feces
Dog tapeworm *(Dipylidium caninum)*	Dogs, cats	Ingestion of dog or cat fleas
Giardiasis	Dogs, gerbils, parakeets, beavers	Ingestion of cysts (fecal-oral contact or in contaminated food, water)
Hydatid disease (echinococcosis)	Dogs and other carnivores, livestock	Ingestion of eggs (fecal-oral contact resulting from contamination with dog feces)
Toxoplasmosis	Cats, livestock	Ingestion of oocytes from infected stool, consumption of poorly cooked meat
Toxocariasis (visceral larva migrans)	Dogs, cats	Ingestion of eggs shed in feces
Rickettsial and Chlamydial Diseases		
Psittacosis *(Chlamydia psittaci)*	Birds	Air-borne (aerosol inhalation)
Q fever *(Coxiella burnetii)*	Sheep, other livestock, rabbits	Air-borne (aerosols from infected placentas and birth fluids), ingestion of contaminated milk
Rocky Mountain spotted fever	Dogs (carriers of ticks)	Bites of infected ticks (from any source)
Viral Diseases		
Colorado tick fever	Small rodents, ticks	Bite of tick
Lymphocytic choriomeningitis	Rodents (especially hamsters); rarely dogs	Inhalation or ingestion of dust or contaminated food

Diseases Transmitted by Pets, Rodents, and Other Animals *(continued)*

Disease or Organism	Common Animal Sources	Vector or Means of Spread
Rabies	Dogs, skunks, cats, raccoons, bats, foxes and other wild animals	Bites or scratches of diseased animals
Relapsing fever (some *Borrelia* species)	Small rodents	Bite of tick

Raw Milk*

Serious systemic infections due to *Salmonella* and *Campylobacter* organisms have been attributed to the consumption of raw milk, including certified raw milk. The Committee on Infectious Diseases strongly recommends that parents and public health officials be fully informed of important risks inherent in the consumption of all raw milk, and endorses pasteurized milk for infants and children.

*Interstate sale of raw milk is now banned by the Food and Drug administration in a ruling published in the *Federal Register* of August 10, 1987.

State Immunization Requirements for 1989-1990 School Attendance,* Applicable to Any or All Children From Kindergarten Through Grade 12†

State	Diphtheria	Tetanus	Pertussis	Measles	Mumps	Rubella	Poliomyelitis
Alabama	K-12	K-12	K-6	K-12	K-12	K-12	K-12
Alaska	K-12	K-12	K-6	K-12	not required	K-11	K-12
Arizona	K-12	not required	not required	K-12	not required	K-12	K-12
Arkansas	K-12	K-12	K-6	K-12	not required	K-12	K-12
California	K-12	K-12	K-6	K-12	K-6	K-12	K-12
Colorado	K-12	K-12	K-6	K-12	K	K-6	K-12
Connecticut	K-12	K-12	K-6	K-12	K-12	K-12	K-12
Delaware	K-12	K-12	K-6	K-12	K-10	K-12	K-12
D.C.	K-12	K-12	K-6	K-12	K-12	K-12	K-12
Florida	K-12	K-12	K-6	K-12	K-12	K-12	K-12
Georgia	K-12	K-12	K-6	K-12	K-12	K-12	K-12
Hawaii	K-12	K-12	K-6	K-12	K-12	K-12	K-12
Idaho	K-5	K-5	not required	K-5	K-5	K-5	K-5
Illinois	K-12	K-12	K-5	K-12	K-12	K-12	K-12
Indiana	K-12	K-12	K-6	K-5	K-12	K-12	K-12
Iowa	K-12	K-12	K-6	K-12	not required	K-12	K-12
Kansas	K-12	K-12	K-6	K-12	K-12	K-12	K-12
Kentucky	K-12	K-12	new enterers	K-12	not required	K-12	K-12
Louisiana	new enterers	new enterers	new enterers	new enterers	new enterers	new enterers	new enterers
Maine	K-12	K-12	K-6	K-12	K-10	K-12	K-12
Maryland	K-12	K-12	K-6	K-12	not required	K-12	K-12
Massachusetts	K-12	K-12	K-6	K-12	K-12	K-12	K-12
Michigan	new enterers	new enterers	new enterers	new enterers	new enterers	new enterers	new enterers
Minnesota	K-12	K-12	K-6	K-12	K-12	K-12	K-12
Mississippi	K-12	K-12	K-6	K-12	new enterers	K-12	K-12
Missouri	K-12	not required	not required	K-12	not required	K-12	K-12

*Based on information provided by the U.S. Department of Health and Human Services, Public Health Service, Centers for Disease Control, Center for Prevention Service, Division of Immunization. **Since the requirements for 1990-1991 have been amended (or will be subsequently) in many states to require measles reimmunization, state health departments should be consulted for requirements in local jurisdictions.**

†Denoted as K-12.

State Immunization Requirements for 1989-1990 School Attendance,* Applicable to Any or All Children From Kindergarten Through Grade 12† *(continued)*

State	Diphtheria	Tetanus	Pertussis	Measles	Mumps	Rubella	Poliomyelitis
Montana	K-12	K-12	K-6	K-12	new enterers	K-12	K-12
Nebraska	K-12	K-12	K-6	K-12	K-12	K-12	K-12
Nevada	K-12	K-12	K-6	K-12	new enterers	K-12	K-12
New Hampshire	K-12	K-12	K-6	K-12	K-12	K-12	K-12
New Jersey	K-12	K-12	K-6	K-12	K-15	K-12	K-12
New Mexico	K-12	K-12	K-6	K-12	not required	K-12	K-12
New York	K-12	not required	not required	K-12	K-12	K-12	K-12
North Carolina	K-12	K-12	K-6	K-12	new enterers	K-12	K-12
North Dakota	K-12	K-12	K-6	K-12	K-12	K-12	K-12
Ohio	K-12	K-12	K-6	K-12	K-12	K-12	K-12
Oklahoma	K-12	K-12	K-6	K-12	new enterers	K-12	K-12
Oregon	K-12	K-12	not required	K-12	new enterers	K-12	K-12
Pennsylvania	K-12	K-12	not required	K-12	K-12	K-12	K-12
Puerto Rico	K-12	K-12	K-6	K-12	K-12	K-12	K-12
Rhode Island	K-12	K-12	not required	K-12	K-6	K-12	K-12
South Carolina	K-12	K-12	K-5	K-12	not required	K-12	K-12
South Dakota	K-12	K-12	K-6	K-12	K-12	K-12	K-12
Tennessee	K-12	K-12	K-6	K-12	K-12	K-12	K-12
Texas	K-12	K-12	not required	K-12	K-17	K-11	K-12
Utah	K-12	K-12	K-6	K-12	K-12	K-12	K-12
Vermont	K-12	K-12	K-6	K-12	not required	K-12	K-12
Virginia	K-12	K-12	K-6	K-12	new enterers	K-12	K-12
Washington	K-12	K-12	not required	K-12	K-1	K-12	K-12
West Virginia	new enterers	new enterers	new enterers	new enterers	not required	new enterers	new enterers
Wisconsin	K-12	K-12	K-6	K-12	K-12	K-12	K-12
Wyoming	new enterers	new enterers	K-6	new enterers	new enterers	new enterers	new enterers

*Based on information provided by the U.S. Department of Health and Human Services, Public Health Service, Centers for Disease Control, Center for Prevention Service, Division of Immunization. **Since the requirements for 1990-1991 have been amended (or will be subsequently) in many states to require measles reimmunization, state health departments should be consulted for requirements in local jurisdictions.**

†Denoted as K-12.

Commonly Reportable Infectious Diseases in the United States

Reporting of specific diseases, which are listed below, is required in all states and territories. Additional and specific requirements should be obtained from the responsible health department. A more complete listing of infectious diseases that are reportable to state health departments can be found in the following publication: Chorba TL, Berkelman RL, Safford SK, Gibbs NP, and Hull HT. Mandatory reporting of infectious diseases by clinicians. *JAMA*. 1989;262:3018-3326.*

Acquired immunodeficiency syndrome
Amebiasis
Anthrax
Botulism
Brucellosis
Campylobacteriosis
Chancroid
Chickenpox-herpes zoster
Chlamydia infections
Cholera
Diphtheria
Encephalitis
Giardiasis
Gonorrhea
Granuloma inguinale
Haemophilus influenzae, type b infections (invasive)
Hepatitis A
Hepatitis B
Hepatitis non-A, non-B
Hepatitis, unspecified
Histoplasmosis
HIV infection
Legionellosis
Leprosy
Leptospirosis
Lyme disease
Lymphogranuloma venereum
Malaria
Measles (rubeola)
Meningitis, aseptic
Meningitis, bacterial
Meningococcal disease
Mumps
Pertussis
Plague
Poliomyelitis
Psittacosis
Rabies
Reye syndrome
Rheumatic fever
Rocky Mountain spotted fever
Rubella
Salmonellosis
Shigellosis
Syphilis
Tetanus
Toxic shock syndrome
Trichinosis
Tuberculosis
Tularemia
Typhoid fever
Typhus
Yellow fever

*Reprinted in *MMWR*. 1990;39(No. RR-9):1-17.

In partnership with the Council of State and Territorial Epidemiologists (CSTE), the Centers for Disease Control (CDC) operates the National Notifiable Diseases Surveillance System. The system provides weekly provisional information for reportable diseases. Cases of diseases reported by physicians to state epidemiologists are forwarded to CDC for publication in the *Morbidity and Mortality Weekly Report (MMWR)* and the *Summary of Notifiable Diseases, United States.* Notifiable disease surveillance data are used by public health officials in local, state, and national health departments as part of disease prevention and control activities.

Services of the Centers for Disease Control

The Centers for Disease Control (CDC), U.S. Public Health Service, Department of Health and Human Services, Atlanta, Georgia 30333, is the federal agency charged with protecting the public health of the nation by preventing disease and other disabling conditions. The CDC administers national programs for the prevention and control of infectious diseases, occupational diseases and injury, chronic diseases, and environment-related injury and illness. The CDC also provides consultation to other nations and participates with international agencies in the control of preventable diseases. In addition, the CDC directs and enforces foreign quarantine activities and regulations, and provides consultation and assistance in upgrading the performance of clinical laboratories.

The CDC provides a number of services related to infectious disease management and control. Although the CDC is principally a resource for state and local health departments, it also offers direct and indirect services to hospitals and practicing physicians. The range of services includes reference laboratory diagnosis and epidemiologic consultation, both usually arranged through the state health department. In addition, the CDC Drug Service supplies some specific prophylactic or therapeutic drugs and biologic agents.

Specific immunobiologic products available include botulinal equine (trivalent, ABE) antitoxin, diphtheria equine antitoxin, vaccinia immune globulin (VIG), Japanese encephalitis vaccine (JEV), botulinus pentavalent toxoid, and Western equine encephalitis (WEE) immune globulin.

Additionally, several drugs for the treatment of parasitic disease, which are not currently licensed for use in the United States, are handled under the Investigational New Drug permit. These antiparasitic drugs include suramin, nifurtimox, bithional, dehydroemetine, diloxanide furoate (furamide), ivermectin, melarsoprol, quinine (for parenteral use), and stibogluconate sodium.

Requests for biologic products, antiparasitic drugs, and related information should be directed to the Drug Service, Centers for Disease Control, Atlanta, Georgia 30333. During business hours (8:00 a.m. to 4:30 p.m. EST., Monday through Friday) the telephone number is 404/639-3670; for nights, weekends, or holidays (emergency requests only) the telephone number is 404/639-2888.

INDEX

Page numbers in boldface indicate main discussion.

A

C

D

E

G

H

M

N

Q

R

S

U

V

W

Y

Z